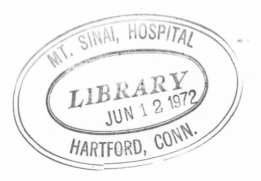

REGIONAL BLOCK

REGIONAL BLOCK

A Handbook for Use in the Clinical

Practice of Medicine and Surgery

(Fourth Edition, Fourth Printing)

By

DANIEL C. MOORE, M.D.

Director, Department of Anesthesiology
The Mason Clinic

Chief of Anesthesia
Virginia Mason Hospital
Seattle, Washington

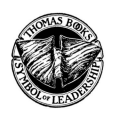

CHARLES C THOMAS • PUBLISHER
Springfield • Illinois • U.S.A.

Published and Distributed Throughout the World by
CHARLES C THOMAS ● PUBLISHER
BANNERSTONE HOUSE
301-327 East Lawrence Avenue, Springfield, Illinois, U.S.A.
NATCHEZ PLANTATION HOUSE
735 North Atlantic Boulevard, Fort Lauderdale, Florida, U.S.A.

First Edition, 1953, 4000 copies
Second Edition, 1957, 3000 copies
Third Edition, First Printing, 1961, 2000 copies
Third Edition, Second Printing, 1962, 2500 copies
Fourth Edition, First Printing, 1965, 3000 copies
Fourth Edition, Second Printing, 1967, 2500 copies
Fourth Edition, Third Printing, 1969, 2500 copies
Fourth Edition, Fourth Printing, 1971, 2500 copies

*With THOMAS BOOKS careful attention is given to all details of
manufacturing and design. It is the Publisher's desire to present books
that are satisfactory as to their physical qualities and artistic possibilities
and appropriate for their particular use. THOMAS BOOKS will be true
to those laws of quality that assure a good name and good will.*

Printed in the United States of America

D-1

To my Mother and Father, who willingly made many sacrifices that I might receive an uninterrupted medical education.

Introduction

THE OBJECTIVE of this book is to present to the general practitioner and to the specialist, particularly the embryonic anesthesiologist, a concise outline of the everyday phases of regional block techniques. Since the book is intended for the beginner, it does not cover all phases and methods of regional anesthesia. But, it does represent the personal and direct experience of the author and his colleagues in the administration of over 55,000 regional block procedures in the past 23 years.

Several reference books on this subject are available; therefore, the purpose here is to provide only a description of those blocks often used in an everyday practice. The procedures included in this text have come to be routine for surgical anesthesia and other block therapy in applicable cases and are now the choice of physicians in the institutions in which the author practices. Block procedures used infrequently, those having a high incidence of serious complications, and certain other blocks in which residual paresthesias occur with a high frequency have been purposely omitted. Included in one or another of these categories are gasserian (semilunar) ganglion block, thoracic sympathetic ganglia block, vagus nerve block, glossopharyngeal nerve block, carotid body block, superficial peroneal nerve block, and anterior and posterior tibial nerve block.

Many of the texts on this subject lack step by step scale illustrations of the procedures, and at times perspectives created by the drawings and photographs are misleading. Also, more than one method is often described for arriving at the same end, i.e., a successful block. It is not uncommon for the neophyte, after he fails in one method, to try the next, and so on until all methods of performing the desired block are exhausted. After a series of failures, he is likely to give up the whole thing and resort to general anesthesia.

If the physician persists in using one method again and again instead of switching from one approach to another, competence is acquired and the percentage of successful blocks approaches 90 to 97 percent. This is true not only for the instructor but also for the pupil. "Practice makes perfect." Therefore, in a book for a beginner, the author feels that for most blocks one technique only should be presented. Once that has been perfected, other methods may be attempted with the confidence that if the new method fails, there is always "an ace in the hole."

The author realizes that with recent advances in anesthetic drugs and techniques, the appearance of an increasing number of well-trained anesthetists who seldom have extensive training in regional block procedures and the need to satisfy the private patient who may be suspicious or afraid of regional procedures, the use of general anesthesia will predominate. Nevertheless, many situations arise in which regional analgesia alone, or in combination with light general anesthesia, is the anesthesia of choice. Therapeutic and diagnostic blocks are being requested more frequently as a means of confirmation, prognostication and palliation. As medicine and surgery progress, these procedures will be in increasing demand. All well-trained anesthetists should have at their finger tips at least the regional procedures of greatest value.

The general practitioners and the specialists in small communities must often furnish their own surgical anesthesia as well as diagnostic and therapeutic blocks. Many of the medical and surgical interns, residents, and fellows are greatly interested in regional anesthesia because the towns in which they plan to practice lack anesthesiologists. Because of the constant interest of such physicians in our everyday techniques, this work was undertaken.

The exclusive use of chemical names of drugs instead of proprietary trade names would have presented impractical difficulties and inconveniences to the reader who wished to order anesthetic agents named. It is not uncommon to find physicians, even specialists in anesthesia, who do not realize that Pentothal is the trade name for thiopental, that Nembutal is the trade name for pentobarbital, that Pontocaine is the trade name for tetracaine, and that Novocain is the trade name for procaine. A similar difficulty arises over the use of centimeters as opposed to inches for the measurements of the lengths of needles and the distances of landmarks and another over the use of the metric system instead of the apothecary system for the dosage of drugs. Therefore, for complete clarity, the author has not hesitated to include in parentheses chemical terms, comparable dosages, comparable measurements, and synonyms wherever one term or system was employed in preference to another.

No claim of originality is made for the methods and procedures described in this book. References at the end of each chapter were not included as this text is designed to serve as a handbook and a quick source of information, not a reference book. The organization is such that a doctor may learn one block technique without reading the entire book, and this organization renders some repetition unavoidable. Some steps which are believed to be new have been added to old methods, as we might expect in the evolution of any science. All drawings and photographs were made from cadavers during dissection or from patients undergoing an anesthetic procedure, except that photographs of the anesthetist's position in relation to the patient used a resident and the author. The one method selected and described for each block has produced successful results in at least 90 percent of the cases in which that technique was used. However, in block procedures where paresthesias are to be elicited, the dictum *no paresthesias*, *no anesthesia,* has been my creed. And, if anesthesia from the first block has proved inadequate, the procedure has been repeated.

Without doubt it is easier to learn regional anesthesia in the operating room under the direction of a competent specialist. It is also admitted that cadaver injection and dissection contribute much to the anesthetist's understanding of nerve distribution and anatomy. Nevertheless, with an adequately illustrated text, practice on corpses prior to the onset of rigor mortis, and perseverance, the techniques of regional anesthesia may be mastered in a reasonable period of time. The author has conscientiously tried to make this book a pictorial review of regional anesthesia so that the verbal description might be adequately supplemented. During the block procedures sterile draping of patients used for illustration was largely omitted so that landmarks and perspective would not be obscured.

It is hoped that this book will be a concise and easily understood text which will allow the beginner to learn the steps necessary for the satisfactory execution of the most useful regional block procedures. But the limits of the book do not permit a full discussion of the complications of regional block. Although the more common complications are concisely outlined, a more complete discussion of these and other complications which may be incurred by any single block procedure will be found in the author's *Complications of Regional Anesthesia,* published by Charles C Thomas, Publisher, in 1955.

The physician attempting to perform regional blocks should remember the following apropos quotations:

"Genius is often perseverance in disguise."

and

"When all else fails, follow directions."

Acknowledgments

For their contributions to this edition, the author wishes to express his deepest appreciation to:

L. Donald Bridenbaugh, M. D., my partner and associate at The Mason Clinic in Anesthesiology, for reading the material presented herein, for his many helpful suggestions, and for his worthy criticisms.

Kay L. Olheiser, medical secretary, for typing the rough and finished manuscript.

Phyllis J. Skoog, medical secretary, for typing the rough and finished manuscript and correcting galley and page proof.

Joy Polis, medical illustrator, for the new and excellent drawings which appear in this edition.

Jack R. Newby, photographer, for the superb reproductions of the new photographs which appear in this edition.

The physicians of The Mason Clinic and the Virginia Mason Hospital.

The private patients whose photographs appear herein.

Charles C Thomas, Publisher, and his staff for their cooperation, attention to details, general counsel, and interest associated with publication of this book.

For their contributions to the first three editions of this book, the author wishes to express his deepest appreciation to:

Donald L. Custis, M. D., surgeon and illustrator.

Robert J. Johnson, M. D., formerly Associate Professor of Anatomy at the University of Washington Medical School, now at the University of Pennsylvania Graduate School.

Clayton P. Wangeman, M. D., anesthesiologist.

Helmut W. Bonheim, Department of English, University of Washington.

Martin Baker, photographer.

Gordon M. Wheeler, M. D., John E. Scheidt, M. D., and LeGrande Anderson, M. D., residents in anesthesiology.

Lucy Jeske, Elizabeth Gustafson, and Phyllis Lindstrom (Phyllis J. Skoog), medical secretaries.

Charles C Thomas, Publisher, and his staff.

D. C. M.

Contents

PART II
Peripheral Nerve Block Anesthesia

SECTION I
Head and Neck

SECTION II
Trunk (Chest, Abdomen, and Perineum)

CONTENTS

SECTION III
Extremities

CONTENTS

REGIONAL BLOCK

PART I

FUNDAMENTAL CONSIDERATIONS

CHAPTER 1

General Information

DEFINITIONS

Regional analgesia (anesthesia) is the abolition of painful impulses from any region or regions of the body by temporarily interrupting the sensory nerve conductivity. Motor function may or may not be involved, but the patient does not lose consciousness.

In this book the terms analgesia and anesthesia are used interchangeably although to the physician anesthetist the term anesthesia usually denotes loss of consciousness while the term analgesia means the patient is conscious.

Local infiltration is the production of regional analgesia by direct infiltration of the incision, wound, or lesion.

Field block is the production of regional analgesia by creating a wall of anesthesia around the operative field.

Nerve block is regional analgesia created by direct injection into or around the nerve or nerves supplying the area involved. Spinal (subarachnoid) block, epidural (peridural) block, and caudal block are nerve blocks by this definition, because the nerves are bathed by the local anesthetic solution in either the subarachnoid or epidural space.

Caudal and Epidural Blocks: When the local anesthetic solution is injected into the epidural space through the sacral hiatus and the caudal canal, the technique is termed *caudal* block.

When the local anesthetic solution is injected into the epidural space through the interspaces of the vertebrae, the technique is termed *epidural* (peridural) block.

Anesthetist: For the purposes of this book, the term refers to the physician administering the anesthesia, regardless of whether he is a general practitioner or specialist.

PREOPERATIVE CONSIDERATIONS

General Information: The patient should enter the hospital the night before surgery in elective major procedures.

All patients should have a complete routine history and physical examination with laboratory work before any anesthesia is given, an emergency being the exception.

Oral Intake: Wherever possible, intake of fluids and solids by mouth should be restricted for at least six hours before the block. This precaution is taken for two reasons. First, in the case of a toxic reaction with accompanying hypoxia, the sequelae of nausea and vomiting with aspiration of undigested food particles may be avoided. Second, if the regional procedure is unsuccessful and general anesthesia must be resorted to, the patient will have little food in the stomach to vomit and cause further complications.

It is important to remember that even if the above precaution is taken, a nervous patient as well as a patient who has pain or has been injured, whether he is in shock or not, may not empty his stomach for 24 hours or longer. A patient in labor (parturient) fits this category.

Preoperative Visit of Anesthetist: It is important in regional analgesia to see the patient before he is under medication and is brought to the operating room. A preoperative visit allows the doctor to evaluate the patient, explain the type of anesthesia, assure him that he will not have pain, and gain his confidence (see Medicolegal Safeguards, page 10).

Premedication: Drugs should be used to blunt consciousness but not abolish it.

Route of Administration.—Intravenous medications, particularly the opiates, usually reach their maximum effect within 15 minutes, while intramuscular medications require 45 minutes and subcutaneous medications 60 to 90 minutes to take effect. Where preoperative oral barbiturate medication cannot be given because of a Levin tube or difficulty in swallowing, intramuscular barbiturates such as phenobarbital (Luminal) in 130 mg. (2 gr.) to 260 mg. (4 gr.) doses may be employed. In these cases the rectal route also may be found useful.

In an emergency where there is not enough time for routine oral, intramuscular, or subcutaneous preoperative medication to become effective, the anesthetist should resort to the intravenous route. Routine drugs such as some barbiturates, opiates, and belladonna derivatives may be given intravenously in the usual dosages if injected *slowly*, *i.e.*, over a period of three to five minutes, and if the patient is observed carefully.

When shock is present prior to the administration of the anesthesia, premedication is usually not needed. If premedication is necessary, the intravenous route should be chosen, since impaired circulation may result in delayed absorption of a subcutaneous or intramuscular injection. Under these circumstances, the anesthetist should always check to be sure the patient has not received previous medication.

Dosage.—There are 65 milligrams (mg.) in 1 grain (gr.). However, this book gives equivalent dosages of drugs as they appear on labels and as they are commonly used. This makes ordering easier; there are fewer insignificant fractions, and the number of milligrams which have been eliminated are of little importance in most medications.

The premedications suggested with each block technique in this book seldom need to be increased; however, often they must be decreased to meet the individual requirements of the debilitated, the aged, the young, and the sick. Morphine, meperedine (Demerol), atropine, scopolamine, pentobarbital (Nembutal), and promethazine (Phenergan) are the author's choice of drugs for premedication. However, comparable doses of other opiates, belladonna derivatives, or barbiturates may be substituted if preferred. In patients over 60 years of age, it is best to omit barbiturates and scopolamine from the premedication as they often cause the elderly patient to become disoriented. If in such a patient a belladonna drug is indicated, atropine is usually satisfactory.

Time of Administration.—Patients in whom it is important to elicit paresthesias are lightly medicated, and additional sedation is given surgical patients when a successful block has been performed. Heavy medication is employed preoperatively in procedures requiring only bony landmarks, such as intercostal nerve block, or no landmarks, as in local infiltration. In these cases if the preoperative sedation is inadequate, small amounts of thiopental (Pentothal), methohexital (Brevital), pentobarbital (Nembutal), or a combination of meperidine (Demerol) and promethazine (Phenergan), are given intravenously in the induction room before the block is undertaken.

The anesthetist doing regional anesthesia should consider *block* time rather than operating time. If the oral medication is not given at least one hour before most intramuscularly or intravenously administered opiates, it will remain in the stomach, since most opiates cause pylorospasm and thus delay the absorption of medication given orally. A satisfactory method for scheduling the preoperative sedation is as follows:

PARESTHESIAS ARE TO BE ELICITED:

If an oral barbiturate is to be used, it is given one and one-half to two hours before the anticipated *block* time. This dosage of the barbiturate often is omitted.

The opiate and belladonna derivative should be administered intramuscularly *on call to surgery* or approximately one-half hour prior to *block* time.

PARESTHESIAS ARE NOT TO BE ELICITED:

The oral barbiturate is given one and one-half to two hours before the anticipated *block* time.

The opiate and belladonna derivative is administered intramuscularly three-quarters to one hour before *block* time.

Wrapping the Legs: Preoperative medicacations cause peripheral vasodilatation and when the normal healthy patient is given these drugs, he often may feel faint or actually faint on rising or on being placed in Fowler's position. This is partially explained by the fact that medication causes the blood to pool in the peripheral vascular system of the lower extremities. Therefore, under many regional blocks where premedication is administered and where an upright type of position, *i.e.,* Fowler's or sitting position, is to be used, the patient's legs should be wrapped from toes to

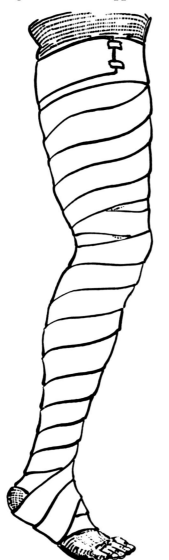

Figure 1. Method of wrapping the legs to prevent pooling of the blood in the superficial venous system.

thigh (Figure 1, page 7). As a substitute elastic stockings may be worn. This is especially true with caudal, epidural, spinal, or celiac plexus blocks, because the vasodilatative effect of these procedures adds to that of the premedicants.

SUPERVISION OF A REGIONAL ANESTHESIA

Placement of the Patient on the Table:

Padding of Table.—The table should be well padded with a sponge rubber mattress. All rests (shoulder braces, etc.), as well as sandbags, should be lined with sponge rubber.

All pressure points should receive special attention, particularly those *involved in the blocked area,* as the patient will not be cognizant of discomfort there. This is mandatory in work on the extremities since residual neurological complications, when they occur, are usually caused by unrelieved compression at pressure points rather than by the nerve block itself.

Restraint of Patient.—The patient should be mildly restrained while on the operating table. The knee strap should be buckled gently but firmly and the arms placed in restraint cuffs. This is advocated for three reasons: (1) the patient may unconsciously contaminate the field; (2) a change of position may cause compression at pressure points with neurological complications; and (3) if the block is unsatisfactory, or if the patient interprets touch and pressure as pain, general anesthesia may have to be instituted—be prepared for this situation.

Additional Sedation: The anesthetist should not hesitate to give additional small doses of barbiturates, opiates, or belladonna drugs intravenously, if: (1) the surgical procedure is prolonged and premedication is dissipated; (2) the patient becomes restless or interprets touch and pressure as pain; (3) the surgeon wishes to discuss the conditions with the referring doctor or pathologist; (4) the patient is annoyed by pounding or sawing as in orthopedic surgery; or (5) a combination of these occur.

When using the intravenous route of administration, the anesthetist should allow three to five minutes for injection of the calculated dose, and if at any time during the injection the desired sedative effect is accomplished, injection should be discontinued. To insure slow administration the intended dose of a drug should be diluted to at least 3 to 5 cc. with normal saline.

When the intravenous route is employed, at least 15 minutes should elapse before giving additional sedation so that the maximal effect of the injection may be realized.

Intravenous Therapy: An intravenous drip using at least an 18-gauge needle is started on all patients except those undergoing minor surgical procedures such as closed manipulations, small tendon repairs, and repairs of superficial lacerations for the following reasons. First, it is best to be prepared for any emergency. Hemorrhage occurs under regional anesthesia as well as general anesthesia. Second, no inconvenience is caused if additional intravenous medication is deemed necessary. And, finally, many patients in a busy surgery may be delayed longer than anticipated, or be too drowsy on return from surgery to eat. Since they may not be fed before major surgical procedures, an effort should be made to maintain fluid balance, if possible.

A plastic needle is preferred—it permits movement (see Figure 2, page 8).

Surgical Considerations: Careful handling of the tissue, minimal packing of the viscera, and careful placing of the retractors are desirable qualities in a surgeon who is operating under regional analgesia. However, most surgeons trained in the United States are accustomed to general anesthesia. Therefore, in good risk patients where the type of anesthesia is elective, it is the anesthetist's responsibility if he chooses a regional procedure, to meet the requirements of the surgeon.

In extremely poor risk patients where it is essential to use regional anesthesia, the surgeon should make every effort to adapt his surgery to the anesthesia.

The surgeon and the anesthetist should confer prior to the operation so that the extent of

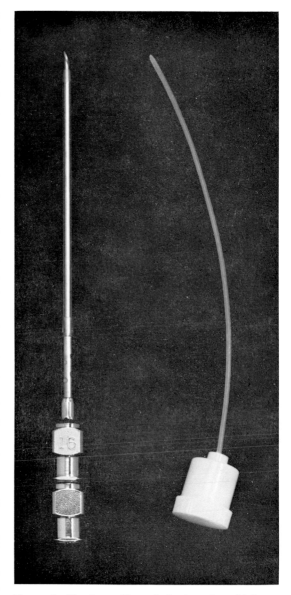

Figure 2. Plastic needle and plastic stylet which are used for intravenous therapy and for intravenous regional analgesia (Chapter 38, page 307).

the surgery may be determined and an adequate regional block assured.

Anesthetist's Responsibility

Preoperative Visit.—A preoperative visit to the patient is a must, except in emergencies.

Monitoring.—Under no circumstance after the block is given, even if the surgeon is his own anesthetist, should the patient be left alone. The anesthetist or a trained technician with a general knowledge of regional block complications should attend the patient during the entire operation. The comfort of the patient and the fluid therapy should be the anesthetist's responsibility during the surgical procedure.

An anesthetic record should be maintained, with blood pressure, pulse, and respirations recorded at frequent intervals. If a tourniquet is used, the surgeon should be informed at hourly intervals until it is released.

Operating Room Personnel Responsibility: The operating personnel should make a minimal amount of noise, and necessary conversation should be carried on in low voices.

POSTOPERATIVE PERIOD

Position of Patient: This will vary with the procedure and condition of the patient, but in general it is no different from general anesthesia. Extreme care should be taken of the anesthetized region in positioning; otherwise neurological complications from pressure may occur during either the operative or postoperative period.

Oral Intake: Patients should be fed according to their tolerance. Solids or liquids should not be forced. It generally is true that patients treated under regional anesthesia will be less of a feeding problem than those who have been treated under general anesthesia.

If a patient does not tolerate liquids or solids following regional block procedures, it usually is the result of the surgery, pain, or of the pre- or postoperative medication. This situation should not be alarming with our present advances in parenteral therapy.

Sedation: Pain is handled in the same method as that following general anesthesia. Generally, patients receiving nerve block require less total sedation than patients receiving general anesthesia—prolonged analgesia from the block obviates the need of opiates for three to six hours following completion of surgery.

REMARKS

Chlorpromazine (Thorazine, Largactil) as Premedication: It has been our observation that when the drug is used for its sedative effect prior to or immediately following a peripheral nerve block, some degree of hypotension may ensue. Such a hypotension is seldom a problem. But if this drug is given before or during a spinal block, epidural (peridural) block, a caudal block, or a celiac plexus block, a severe hypotension may develop. In this case the low blood pressure is of such a nature that it seldom *adequately* responds to the usual dosage of the common vasoconstrictor drugs, *e.g.*, ephedrine sulfate or phenylephrine (Neo-Synephrine). While phenylephrine or levarterenol (Levophed) if run rapidly, may somewhat elevate the pressure, stopping them before either the regional block or the dosage of chlorpromazine has been dissipated may again lower the blood pressure to a precarious level.

Therefore, chlorpromazine has not been used by us with regional block procedures for sedation in: (1) patients who are to receive nerve blocks which in themselves lower blood pressure, such as celiac plexus block, spinal block, epidural block, and caudal block; (2) patients who have hypertension; (3) the elderly; and (4) patients who have had coronary occlusions. An initial dose of 20 mg. of chlorpromazine intravenously is not exceeded in any patient and our usual dose is 10 to 15 mg. Only in the *occasional* patient has it been necessary to add 5 or 10 mg. to this usual dosage to obtain the desired results. At least 15 to 30 minutes should elapse before the initial dose of chlorpromazine is supplemented. By observing these precautions, we have been able to obtain satisfactory sedation with chlorpromazine, yet avoid one of its serious effects —excessive hypotension.

When chlorpromazine is employed for preoperative sedation by us, it is given intravenously by one of the physicians in our department. In those patients receiving regional block procedures *which do not require paresthesias* for a successful block, *e.g.*, local infiltration and certain peripheral nerve blocks (cervical block, etc.), the chlorpromazine is usually administered in the above-noted fashion one-half an hour prior to the block. In those patients receiving blocks *which require that paresthesias be elicited* for a successful block, *e.g.*, brachial plexus block, sciatic nerve block, etc., it is administered immediately upon completion of the block. It is interesting to note that the drug has a retrograde amnesic effect. Often when it has been given following the elicitation of paresthesias, the patient, when seen on postoperative rounds, does not remember the "electric shock-like" sensation caused by stimulating a nerve.

It must be remembered that: (1) there is no effective antidote to chlorpromazine at the present time; (2) the drug is excreted slowly; and (3) the depressing effects on the cardiovascular and respiratory systems may remain for considerable periods after the operation. Therefore, the drug must be administered with care. Furthermore, every patient who is to be operated on under spinal block, epidural block, caudal block or intercostaldeep splanchnic (celiac plexus) block or in whom one of these blocks is to be used in therapy or diagnosis must be asked if he has been on chlorpromazine therapy. The order sheet and nurse's notes must be checked immediately before performing the block. These warnings are emphasized by a death and near fatalities which have occurred because these precautions were not exercised.

Promethazine (Phenergan) with Meperidine (Demerol): Promethazine produces psychic sedation and it is an antiemetic, amnesic, and antihistaminic drug. It does not lower blood pressure and may increase it 10 to 20 millimeters of mercury. Combined with meperidine in the ratio of 10 mg. of meperidine to 2.5 mg. of promethazine per cubic centimeter and administered slowly intravenously in 2 to 5 cc. increments, allowing at least 15 minutes between each increment, excellent sedation may be obtained. Furthermore, the patient will not become restless, uncooperative, hypotensive, or develop an obstructed airway. We rely frequently on this combination of drugs for additional sedation during the execution of the block or during surgery and prefer it to chlorpromazine with or without meperidine.

Medicolegal Safeguards: Regardless of the anesthetic technique selected—regional block or general—precautions to avoid medicolegal suits should be taken and the physician's responsibility to the patient should be understood. The following selected points emphasize the medicolegal aspects of anesthesia. First, the incidences of legal actions against anesthesiologists, as well as other physicians, have risen constantly in the last decade. So precipitous has been the rise that an action in malpractice can be considered as an occupational hazard of every physician. Second, anesthetic mishaps have been singled out as one of the most vulnerable medicolegal hazards. And, third, malpractice actions are not the only suit that may be brought against a physician. Included also are actions for assault and battery (trespass of the person) and abandonment.

Aside from the maintenance of good rapport with the patient, the best way to avoid medicolegal action is to: (1) obtain consent for anesthesia care; (2) review the patient's history and physical examination; (3) keep an accurate anesthetic chart; (4) understand who is responsible for the administration of the anesthesia; (5) use consultation of other physicians; (6) treat complications immediately; and (7) keep the insurance company informed of complications.

Consent for Anesthesia Care.—If circumstances permit, the technique selected and its hazards should be explained to the patient. The patient should sign a consent form for anesthesia. If the patient objects strongly to a specific type of anesthesia, it should be avoided unless the patient's physical status, hospital facilities, or other extenuating circumstances dictate its use. The extenuating circumstances should be documented and confirmed by another physician; if this is not done, the anesthetist may be sued for "assault."

If the patient is considered an adult by the state, he may sign the consent form. The laws of most states differ, but all define who is a minor. If the patient is a minor, his parents, guardian, or responsible person must sign the consent form.

History and Physical Examination.—Regardless of whether a preanesthetic visit is made by the anesthetist, all patients should have a complete routine history and physical examination with laboratory workup before any anesthesia is given—the only exception being a life or death emergency. The findings should be known and understood by the person who is to administer anesthesia. If these findings are not on the chart and are not known to the anesthetist, then they should be ascertained by the anesthetist prior to administration of anesthesia. If a patient dies after being given anesthesia without a preoperative physical, the anesthetist may be charged with murder, not just malpractice.

Anesthetic Record.—A careful, complete anesthetic chart should be kept. This chart should include at least: (1) an evaluation of the patient's physical status prior to anesthesia, during anesthesia, and in the postanesthetic period; (2) a record of the blood pressure and pulse prior to, during, and after anesthesia; (3) vital statistics, *e.g.*, age and weight; (4) type of anesthesia, its conduct, and drugs used; (5) start of anesthesia, start of the surgery, and finish of anesthesia; (6) the surgical procedure; and (7) complications. These details are particularly important with regional block. A note should indicate that the patient was seen both before and after the administration of the regional block.

Responsibility for Administration of Anesthesia.—When a physician other than an anesthetist, *e.g.*, a surgeon, gives the anesthesia and places a nurse in charge of the patient, the physician (surgeon) is responsible for the anesthesia and its complications. When a physician anesthetist gives the anesthesia, he is responsible for its administration.

Consultation.—If a patient has a pre-existing disease that contraindicates regional block or a certain type of regional block but, because of extenuating circumstances or the patient's desire, that regional block is used, consultation should be sought and the method used and the reason for its use confirmed in writing prior to its administration.

If, following anesthesia, complications occur that can be treated better by a specialist, *e.g.*, internist or neurosurgeon, and if their services are available, consultation should be requested immediately. If consultation is not obtained, or if obtaining it is delayed, the patient may charge the responsible physician with "neglect."

Treatment of Complications.—When complications occur, they must be treated effectively and immediately. Good patient rapport and correct treatment will avoid many hours in the courtroom. The physician should notify immediately the insurance company that carries his malpractice insurance. Do not delay; the insurance company often can give valuable assistance in avoiding a lawsuit.

Adequate Insurance Coverage.—Unfortunately, many anesthetists have come to use certain anesthetic procedures on the basis of court decisions and lay opinion rather than on the basis of the type of anesthesia indicated by a particular patient's physical status, operating facilities, and the surgeon's and anesthetist's skill. But, this has not avoided an increase in the number of lawsuits involving anesthetists.

Therefore, regardless of whether regional block or general anesthesia is chosen, the physician anesthetist should have the maximum amount of malpractice insurance that is available. This is his only and ultimate safeguard in a lawsuit.

CHAPTER 2

Local Anesthetic Drugs

GENERAL CONSIDERATIONS

Mixing of Solutions: To avoid inactive solutions and mistakes, all solutions for a regional block should either be freshly mixed by the doctor from crystals of the local anesthetic agent or purchased from a reputable pharmaceutical company. Local anesthetic solutions should be prepared with normal saline or other physiologic solutions, *e.g.*, Ringer's solution. Distilled water makes the procedure more painful.

If an anesthetic solution was mixed by the hospital pharmacist, if it was opened by a nurse, or both, then it should be tasted or meticulously examined by the doctor before injection. This will prevent employing ether, alcohol, or some equally destructive agent by mistake—such mistakes still do occur.

Heat Sterilization: Although refinements in cold sterilization of drugs and equipment have been introduced, autoclaving drugs and equipment to be used in regional block is the accepted technique of sterilization in our institution (see page 50). With the exception of hyaluronidase, all drugs advocated in this text can be sterilized at least once without losing their clinical effectiveness. Most of them can be autoclaved from 3 to 5 times with no alteration in clinical potency. Dextrose (10%) or solutions containing it will not caramelize unless autoclaved more than once—caramelized (yellow) solutions should be discarded.

Dosage and Concentration: While one can state the average and maximum dosage of a drug, dosages should be varied according to age, physical condition, and complicating diseases. Robust young patients usually will tolerate larger doses than the emaciated elderly individual. *The dosage for each patient must be individualized.*

When sensory analgesia without motor involvement is desired, the weakest effective solution of the local agent should be tried. In spite of this precaution motor paralysis often ensues.

Allergy: If a patient is allergic to one anesthetic agent, this is no indication that he will react to a similar drug with a slightly different chemical structure. However, the doctor should not discredit a patient's statement that he is "allergic" to a local anesthetic agent. Such a patient's situation must be evaluated carefully before injection of local anesthetic solutions (see page 32).

AVAILABLE LOCAL ANESTHETIC DRUGS

The available local anesthetic agents are listed in Table I, pages 13 and 14, and they are all hydrochlorides. If a patient is known to have had a true allergic systemic toxic reaction to one specific local anesthetic drug, a local anesthetic drug of another chemical

TABLE I

LOCAL ANESTHETIC DRUGS FOR REGIONAL BLOCK

Chemical and Brand (Trade) Name	Uses and Maximum Dosage			
	Topical for Nose, Pharynx, Trachea	Infiltration or Peripheral Nerve Block	Spinal	Epidural (Caudal or Lumbar Area)
procaine Novocain ethocaine Kerocaine Planocaine Scurocaine Neocaine	Ineffective	200 cc. of 0.5% = 1000 mg. 100 cc. of 1.0% = 1000 mg. 50 cc. of 2.0% = 1000 mg.	4 cc. of 5% = 200 mg.	50 cc. of 2% = 1000 mg.
tetracaine Pontocaine amethocaine Anethaine Decicain Pantocaine Butethanol	5 cc. of 0.5% = 25 mg.	1 mg. per pound body weight—do not exceed 200 mg. or a concentration of 0.25%	2 cc. of 1% = 20 mg.	50 cc. of 0.25% = 125 mg.
lidocaine Xylocaine lignocaine Xylotox	4 cc. of 2% = 80 mg.	100 cc. of 0.5% = 500 mg. 50 cc. of 1.0% = 500 mg. 25 cc. of 2.0% = 500 mg.	4 cc. of 4% = 160 mg.	50 cc. of 1.0% = 500 mg. or 25 cc. of 2% = 500 mg.
mepivacaine Carbocaine	Not established, probably same as lidocaine	100 cc. of 0.5% = 500 mg. 50 cc. of 1.0% = 500 mg. 25 cc. of 2.0% = 500 mg.	4 cc. of 4% = 160 mg.	50 cc. of 1.0% = 500 mg. or 25 cc. of 2% = 500 mg.

Table I is continued on next page.

TABLE I—*Continued*

LOCAL ANESTHETIC DRUGS FOR REGIONAL BLOCK

Chemical and Brand (Trade) Name	Uses and Maximum Dosage			
	Topical for Nose, Pharynx, Trachea	Infiltration or Peripheral Nerve Block	Spinal	Epidural (Caudal or Lumbar Area)
dibucaine Nupercaine Percaine cinchocaine	Not commonly used	200 cc. of 0.02% = 40 mg. 80 cc. of 0.05% = 40 mg. 40 cc. of 0.10% = 40 mg. Not commonly used	20 cc. of 0.0667% = 13.33 mg. or 4 cc. of 0.25% = 10 mg.	Not used
piperocaine Metycaine	Not commonly used	200 cc. of 0.5% = 1000 mg. 100 cc. of 1.0% = 1000 mg. 65 cc. of 1.5% = 1000 mg.	4 cc. of 4% = 160 mg. Not available	65 cc. of 1.5% = 975 mg.
diethoxin Intracaine	Not commonly used	200 cc. of 0.5% = 1000 mg. 100 cc. of 1.0% = 1000 mg. 50 cc. of 2.0% = 1000 mg.	3 cc. of 5% = 150 mg. Seldom used	50 cc. of 2% = 1000 mg.
chloroprocaine Nesacaine	Ineffective	200 cc. of 0.5% = 1000 mg. 100 cc. of 1.0% = 1000 mg. 50 cc. of 2.0% = 1000 mg.	Not established	50 cc. of 2% = 1000 mg.
hexylcaine Cyclaine	5 cc. of 2% = 100 mg.	100 cc. of 0.5% = 500 mg. 50 cc. of 1.0% = 500 mg. 25 cc. of 2.0% = 500 mg.	4 cc. of 1.25% = 50 mg. Seldom used	50 cc. of 1% = 500 mg.
cocaine	3 cc. of 4% = 120 mg.	Not used	Not used	Not used

group may be used in most instances without producing a reaction (see Table II, page 15).

TABLE II

CLASSIFICATION OF LOCAL ANESTHETIC AGENTS ACCORDING TO CHEMICAL STRUCTURE

Chemical Group	Local Anesthetic Drug
para-amino-benzoic acid ester	procaine (Novocain) tetracaine (Pontocaine) chloroprocaine (Nesacaine)
diethylaminoacet-2, 6-xylidide	lidocaine (Xylocaine)
d, 1-N-methylpipecolic acid 2, 6, dimethylanilide	mepivacaine (Carbocaine)
beta-diethyl-amino-ethyl amide	dibucaine (Nupercaine)
benzoic acid ester	cocaine piperocaine (Metycaine)
para-ethoxy-benzoic acid ester	diethoxin (Intracaine)
1-cyclohexylamino-2-propyl benzoate	hexylcaine (Cyclaine)

At the present time, procaine (Novocain), tetracaine (Pontocaine), lidocaine (Xylocaine), mepivacaine (Carbocaine), and dibucaine (Nupercaine) are the local anesthetic agents used most frequently by the author and his colleagues. Cocaine is used by us only to shrink the turbinates of the nose. Piperocaine (Metycaine) and diethoxin (Intracaine) do not have the advantages of lidocaine or mepivacaine and seldom are selected. We do not employ hexylcaine (Cyclaine) because: (1) it has caused prolonged burning sensations, tissue irritation, and swelling, and, in some patients, sloughing and tissue necrosis have resulted following its injection or topical application; and (2) in our series of 100

continuous caudal blocks with a two percent concentration of this agent, three severe systemic toxic reactions have occurred and prolonged numbness of the lateral femoral cutaneous nerve, area around anus, and an area in buttock has ensued. While chloroprocaine (Nesacaine) is a more potent agent than procaine, yet less toxic, and is an excellent agent, we do not use it because: (1) duration of action is short, (2) packaging is inconvenient, and (3) the solutions now available contain preservatives and the manufacturer cautions that they are not be be used for caudal, epidural, or spinal blocks (packaging regulations have presented problems— the drug is easily oxidized).

LOCAL ANESTHETIC DRUGS USED FOR SPINAL (SUBARACHNOID) BLOCK

Procaine (Novocain), tetracaine (Pontocaine), and dibucaine (Nupercaine) are the drugs used by us for spinal block—they are time-tested drugs. Lidocaine (Xylocaine) and mepivacaine (Carbocaine) are effective for spinal block, but are not employed by us because: (1) lack of fixation with cephalad spread, and (2) a gap of four or five dermatomes between sensory and motor paralysis— motor paralysis being at the lower level.

LOCAL ANESTHETIC DRUGS USED FOR CAUDAL AND EPIDURAL (PERIDURAL) BLOCK

Lidocaine (Xylocaine) and mepivacaine (Carbocaine), with or without tetracaine, epinephrine or both, are the agents of choice for these blocks because: (1) onset is more rapid than with the other agents in the volumes and amounts advocated and (2) the establishment of satisfactory analgesia is more predictable.

Tetracaine (Pontocaine), 1 mg. to 2 mg., may be added to lidocaine or mepivacaine solutions to prolong the duration of epidural or caudal block (see page 410 and 441). This ratio for the combination of tetracaine and either lidocaine or mepivacaine has not produced systemic toxic reactions when the recommended dosage with a 1:200,000 concentration of epinephrine (Adrenalin) is used.

LOCAL ANESTHETIC DRUGS USED FOR PERIPHERAL NERVE BLOCK

Procaine (Novocain) has been used for years and is still the drug which many physicians prefer. The author's agent of choice is tetracaine (Pontocaine) for the reasons listed on page 16, or, on occasion, a combination of it and either lidocaine (Xylocaine) or mepivacaine (Carbocaine). Nonetheless, lidocaine and mepivacaine are the two local anesthetic agents which are most frequently employed for these procedures by other anesthetists because: (1) onset is rapid; (2) spreading and penetrating characteristics are excellent —"needle point" accuracy is not necessary; (3) duration of action is moderately prolonged; and (4) convenience of packaging by manufacturers requires minimal preparation prior to block. Using the concentrations of procaine, tetracaine, lidocaine, and mepivacaine with or without the vasoconstrictor drugs advocated in this book for peripheral nerve block, skin slough, severe neuritis, paralysis, or a combination of these has not been observed.

While dibucaine (Nupercaine) provides prolonged anesthesia, it is not used routinely for local infiltration, field block, or peripheral nerve block because the incidence of tissue slough is high when this drug is injected in the superficial tissues.

Procaine (Novocain)

Dosage

Percentage of Procaine	mg./cc.	Average cc. used*	Maximum cc. used*
0.5	5.0	150	200
1.0	10.0	70	100
2.0	20.0	30	50

*It is best never to exceed the average dose, yet in the occasional case it will be necessary. The maximum dosage should never be exceeded.

The use of 2.0 percent procaine should be limited to cases requiring a small volume of anesthetic solution, usually 10 cc. to 25 cc. While amounts as large as 50 cc. may be injected, toxic reactions are more numerous after such dosages.

Onset of Operating Analgesia.—5 to 15 minutes.

Duration of Operating Analgesia.—45 to 90 minutes. Solutions with epinephrine (Adrenalin) produce the longer durations.

Tetracaine (Pontocaine): The use of tetracaine in regional block has been greatly limited by the claim of many that it is too toxic. It is true that mg. for mg. tetracaine is about ten to twelve times as toxic as procaine. However, it is effective for regional block in solutions one-tenth the strength of procaine, so that if it is employed in dilute solutions, it has about the same or slightly more toxicity than procaine. It prolongs operating analgesia, making it the drug of choice for most local infiltrations, field blocks, and peripheral nerve blocks because of the following reasons. First, it allows the patient to have regional analgesia performed with care and minimal trauma, since rapid completion of the block is not necessary to conserve analgesia time. This is especially true when extensive block procedures are required. Second, it allows the anesthesiologist to give valuable instruction to his pupils while performing the block. This is important since it will increase the number of men who can skillfully execute regional procedures. Third, it allows local anesthesia to be used where indicated for the benefit of the patient in spite of the necessity for a slow, careful dissection. This is especially important for the diabetic and the patient with hypertension. Fourth, it allows the operating surgeon to be at ease and less hurried since he knows that the surgical analgesia will be adequate for five to six hours. Fifth, it permits a sudden change in the surgical schedule for an emergency, even if the block has been executed. This is a definite advantage to the patient, since he will not have to be reblocked before operation even if the emergency should require two or three hours of the doctor's time. Sixth, it produces a prolonged postoperative analgesia which reduces the necessity for large amounts of opiates in the immediate postoperative period. This is important because, if free from pain and not under the influence of opiates, the patient will immediately follow the "stir up" regime, i.e., deep breathing, coughing, and moving from side to side. Seventh, it allows the patient to be blocked at the convenience of the anesthetist, a factor of obvious importance in private practice. Eighth, dilute solutions of tetracaine which are effective in producing analgesia cause very little, if any, vasodilatation in the area in which the local anesthetic solution has been injected—adsorption is slowed. Ninth, when tetracaine alone is administered for local infiltration, field block or peripheral nerve block, one seldom sees the minor reactions such as a drop in blood pressure, increased pulse, sweating, and nervousness which often occur when procaine and other agents are employed. Lastly, severe systemic toxic reactions are rare occurrences when the volumes and concentrations listed in this book are administered.

Dosage

Percentage of Tetracaine Solution	Mg. of Agent per cc. of Normal Saline	Average* No. of cc. used	Maximum* No. of cc. used
0.05	0.5	200	400
0.10	1.0	125	200
0.15	1.5	80	130
0.25	2.5	50	80

*It is best never to exceed the average dose; yet in the occasional case it will be necessary. The maximum dosage should never be exceeded.

The maximum dose of tetracaine for an extensive procedure is 1.0 mg. per pound of body weight, not to exceed 200 mg. Solutions stronger than 0.25 percent are dangerous and should not be used even if the volume is small, i.e., 5 cc. or less, for an intravascular injection may occur inadvertently.

Onset of Operating Analgesia.—15 to 45 minutes. Onset may be hastened by adding 1 to 2 mg. of tetracaine to the calculated dose of either 1.0 percent lidocaine or 1.0 percent mepivacaine (see page 18). But, the author seldom does this for peripheral nerve blocks.

Duration of Operating Analgesia.—3½ to 6 hours. Solutions with epinephrine (Adrenalin) may produce the longer durations. When mixed with lidocaine (Xylocaine) or mepivacaine (Carbocaine), duration may be shortened one to two hours depending on the vascularity of the area into which the solution is injected.

Lidocaine (Xylocaine) and Mepivacaine (Carbocaine): These two local anesthetic agents are considered together because: (1) many of their properties (onset, duration, etc.) are similar; (2) both are synthetic base anilids; (3) their toxicity is about the same and is relatively low—a little greater than procaine; (4) they are the most stable of the local anesthetic solutions; and (5) there is little risk of heat sterilization decomposing them.

Dosage.—3 to 5 mg. per pound of body weight and concentrations which do not exceed 1.5 percent. If toxic reactions are to be avoided, 0.5 gm. (500 mg.) should never be exceeded regardless of the patient's weight. Drowsiness from cerebral depressing effects of these drugs is unusual if this dosage schedule is observed.

Onset of Operating Analgesia.—5 to 15 minutes. The rapidity of onset in relatively weak concentrations, i.e., 0.5 to 1.5 percent, is one of the greatest assets of these two drugs.

Duration of Operating Analgesia.—1¼ to 3 hours. The solutions to which epinephrine (Adrenalin) is added produce the longer durations.

Differences Between Lidocaine and Mepivacaine.—Lidocaine solutions can be purchased with or without epinephrine. Because of the acid pH necessary to keep the epinephrine stable, such a lidocaine-epinephrine solution should be injected immediately following its removal from the vial; otherwise, the solution can release metal ions from the syringes, needles, and receptacles and cause neuritis or slough. The author does not use solutions which come with a vasoconstrictor drug. When a vasoconstrictor drug is indicated, he adds a carefully measured amount of epinephrine just before the local anesthetic solution is injected. Carbocaine solutions with epinephrine cannot be purchased.

In continuous techniques (see page 23), mepivacaine has shown a cumulative effect which has resulted in one severe sustained systemic toxic reaction—this has not been observed with lidocaine.

Neuritis, paralysis, and slough as sequelae of local infiltration, field block, and peripheral nerve block have been observed following injection of lidocaine-epinephrine solutions with a concentration of 1.5 percent or greater. This has not been seen with mepivacaine. Because of these sequelae with 1.5 percent lidocaine, seldom do we employ a concentration of this drug in excess of 1.0 percent for local infiltration, field block, or peripheral nerve block.

Mepivacaine seems to have its own "built-in" vasoconstrictor action and, therefore, can be used without the addition of epinephrine. When mepivacaine is used without epinephrine, the duration of action is not altered significantly, i.e., epinephrine may prolong the duration of action by only 15 to 30 minutes. Lidocaine does not have this property.

Lidocaine (Xylocaine) or Mepivacaine (Carbocaine) with Tetracaine (Pontocaine): Lidocaine or mepivacaine may be mixed with tetracaine (Pontocaine) in the ratio of 2 mg. of tetracaine to each 1 cc. of a 1.0 percent solution of either lidocaine or mepivacaine without producing a cloudy or inactive mixture. This combination has the advantages of a rapid onset which is not obtained by weak solutions (0.1 to 0.15 percent) of tetracaine plus the long duration of action of tetracaine. However, it has been noted that when tetracaine is combined in this ratio with either lidocaine or mepivacaine, the duration of anesthesia may not be as great as when stronger solutions (0.25 percent) of tetracaine only are

employed. The ratio listed here for the combination of tetracaine and either lidocaine or mepivacaine has not produced toxic reactions when used in 50 cc. quantities or less provided the solution contains a 1:200,000 concentration of epinephrine (Adrenalin).

Propitocaine (Citanest): Propitocaine is an anilid local anesthetic agent whose potency is comparable to lidocaine (Xylocaine) but whose systemic toxicity is significantly reduced. The drug without epinephrine (Adrenalin) seems to provide a significantly longer duration of operative analgesia than equi-effective doses of lidocaine with epinephrine. The effects of propitocaine on the cardiovascular and respiratory systems appear to be less than with a comparable dose of lidocaine but qualitatively similar to that seen with other local anesthetic agents.

A metabolite of propitocaine is o-toluidine which produces methemoglobin. Methemoglobinemia from 400 mg. of propitocaine does not usually produce clinical signs, but with 600 mg. the mucous membranes and nail beds may appear blue (cyanotic). Methemoglobinemia from such dose levels usually does not need treatment. However, methemoglobinemia may be reversed by 1 to 2 mg. per kilogram of body weight with a 1 percent solution of methylene blue given intravenously over a five-minute period.

Propitocaine may be used in 1 percent solution for local infiltration, 1 to 1.5 per cent for peripheral nerve block, and 1 to 2 percent in epidural and caudal blocks. The manufacturer recommends that no more than 600 mg. be employed. For the present, the use of propitocaine in children under 10 years of age and for continuous techniques probably should be limited to clinical investigation. If in obstetrics a continuous technique is used and if the total dosage of propitocaine approaches 1000 mg., the patient and her infant will be blue (cyanotic).

CHAPTER 3

Systemic Toxic Reactions to High Blood Levels of Local Anesthetic Drugs

ETIOLOGY OF REACTIONS TO LOCAL ANESTHETIC AGENTS

Allergy to the Drug Employed: This comprises a very small fraction, probably less than 1 percent (see Table III, page 19) and is discussed in Chapter 4, page 32. Systemic reactions to local anesthetic drugs applied to the mucous membranes of the nose, mouth, pharynx, and trachea are *not*, in the greater number of instances, an allergic type of systemic reaction, but are due to rapid absorption of highly concentrated solutions and are a high blood level type of reaction.

High Blood Level of the Drug Injected: This causes the majority of reactions, probably 99 percent or better (see Table III, page 19). A high blood level for one individual may be a low blood level for the majority of people, and when a reaction occurs in this one individual, it should not be thought of as a sensitivity to the drug. Usually it is a relative overdose, *i.e.*, hyperergy (see Table III, page 19). That patient may be blocked successfully with smaller amounts of the local anesthetic agent than normal without a reaction. High blood levels of the local anesthetic drug are more likely to occur following those block procedures which require large volumes and high concentrations of the local anesthetic solution, *i.e.*, peripheral nerve block, caudal block, and epidural block; than following those blocks in which small volume and relatively low concentration are employed, *e.g.*, spinal block. A high blood level occurs for one or more of the following reasons.

TABLE III

CLARIFICATION OF TERMS

I. **Allergy** is a condition of unusual or exaggerated specific susceptibility to a substance which is harmless in similar amounts for the majority of members of the same species. This term embraces all types of human hypersensitiveness.

  A. *Anaphylaxis* is an unusual or exaggerated reaction of the organism to foreign protein or other substances. As now used, the term is restricted to a condition of sensitization in laboratory animals produced by the injection of foreign matter such as horse serum.

  B. *Idiosyncrasy* is individual and peculiar susceptibility to some drug, protein or other agent.

  C. *Susceptibility* is the state of being readily affected or acted upon. The condition may be acquired, familial, individual, inherited, racial, specific, etc., the same as immunity.

  D. *Hypersensitivity* is having the specific or general ability to react with characteristic symptoms to application or contact with certain substances (allergens) in amounts innocuous to normal individuals.

II. **High Blood Level**

  A. *True overdosage* is a blood level of a local anesthetic drug which is greater than that which the majority of patients will tolerate.

  B. *Relative overdosage* occurs when a patient who suffers a reaction may be safely blocked with a smaller dosage of the same drug. Such a patient exhibits not *allergy*, but *hyperergy, i.e.*, he reacts in a normal way but overreacts. But if the patient reacts even to an infinitesimal amount of the drug, he exhibits a true allergic reaction (urticaria, wheezing, etc.), *i.e.*, he reacts in an altered manner and is allergic.

Intravascular Injection of the Drug.—An intravascular injection of a large volume, a high concentration, or both of a local anesthetic agent is a frequent cause of a high blood level. Therefore, aspiration for blood is mandatory when performing regional blocks.

Injection Into Highly Vascular Regions With or Without a Vasoconstrictor.—The highly vascular areas which are most frequently injected include the head, neck, epidural space (especially the caudal canal), penis, urethra, trachea, and lung. Absorption from the mucous membrane of the urethra, mouth, pharynx, larynx, trachea, and in particular the alveoli of the lung is almost as rapid as if the solution were injected intravenously. If these structures are inflamed, absorption is even more rapid.

Following an injection into the trachea, the deep breath which precedes a cough sucks the local anesthetic solution into the alveoli—here only a single layer of epithelium is interposed between it and the blood vessels. The addition of epinephrine (Adrenalin) in the solution does not significantly alter absorption from a mucous membrane.

Injection of Averages Doses in Substandard Risks Whose Mechanism of Detoxification is Hindered.—The liver is believed to be the site of detoxification of most local anesthetic agents but some drugs, like cocaine, are excreted by the kidney unchanged. The rapidity with which a local anesthetic drug is detoxified is a determining factor in whether a systemic toxic reaction ensues. And, furthermore, the rate of detoxification governs the duration of a systemic toxic reaction once one has occurred. Of the local anesthetic drugs studied, the rapidity with which they are detoxified is: first, chloroprocaine (Nesacaine); second, procaine (Novocain); third, tetracaine (Pontocaine); and fourth, lidocaine (Xylocaine). Evidence indicated that mepivacaine (Carbocaine) is detoxified more slowly than any of these agents.

Administration of Large or Excessive Concentrations or Amounts of Anesthetic Drugs at One Time.—The toxicity of a local anesthetic drug increases in geometrical, not arithmetical, progression with increase in concentrations or amounts.

Injection of the Wrong Concentrations Due to Error.—If the physician mixes his own solutions from crystals or if he opens the vials of commercially-prepared local anesthetic solutions himself, this complication is less likely to occur.

Injection of Drugs with a Narrow Margin of Safety.—All of the drugs employed by the author and advocated for the block techniques described herein have a wide margin of safety.

Injection of Solutions Containing a Spreading Factor.—Hyaluronidase increases the absorptive area immensely—thus a higher blood level in a shorter period of time.

Injection of Most Local Anesthetic Solutions Without Epinephrine to Slow Absorption.—If local anesthetic solutions are injected into the tissues without epinephrine, the absorption is more rapid.

PRECAUTIONS TO AVOID HIGH BLOOD LEVEL FROM LOCAL ANESTHETIC AGENTS AND ASSURE THEIR IMMEDIATE TREATMENT

While it is difficult to prevent allergic systemic reactions from infinitesimal amounts of local anesthetic agents, those caused by a high blood level of these drugs from overdosage may usually be reduced to a minimum by observing the following prophylactic measures.

Avoid Overmedication with Barbiturates or Other Drugs: For many years barbiturates have been used prophylactically to prevent systemic toxic reactions. However, the following are some practical reasons why barbiturates are not given for this supposedly "protective effect" prior to all regional block analgesia by us. First, they often make the patient uncooperative, and accurate acknowledgment of paresthesias, often necessary for the success of some block procedures, is difficult to elicit. Second, they depress the cortex and thereby often obscure the cortical signs and symptoms of a toxic reaction. This is perfectly all right if the reaction does not progress past the point of cortical stimulation, but if it does, the barbiturates are then actually performing a disservice by hiding the "warning signals" of a reaction. Third, they act synergistically to deepen the depression stage which follows overstimulation of the brain, particularly the vital medullary centers. Thereby they may make the treatment of a reaction more difficult. Lastly, barbiturates do not remove the possibility of toxic reactions and are of little use in preventing those reactions which are a result of rapid absorption.

Barbiturates are used by us only for their sedative effect on the patient and we do not attempt to use doses large enough to prevent the signs of cortical stimulation. As a matter of fact, when paresthesias are to be obtained prior to injecting the drug, we may give no preblock barbiturate. However, after the block has been completed, if the patient wishes to be less aware of his surroundings, a barbiturate, usually 100 mg. (1½ gr.) to 200 mg. (3 gr.) of pentobarbital (Nembutal) or a combination of meperidine (Demerol) and promethazine (Phenergan), is given intravenously (see page 10 for ratio of meperidine to promethazine).

Avoid Overdosage of the Local Anesthetic Agent: This is best accomplished by: (1) using local anesthetic drugs whose toxicities have been well established by clinical and experimental use (see Table I, page 13); (2) not exceeding their recommended doses; (3) using the weakest concentration and the least volume of the drug that will accomplish the desired degree of analgesia; and (4) injecting carefully, that is, aspirating and giving a small test dose so as not to deposit a large amount of the drug intravascularly.

Monitor the Patient: Assure careful observation of the patient throughout the procedure by the doctor or a trained assistant. Keep constant check with the patient so that any change in his sensorium may be immediately detected.

Have Equipment and Drugs Available to Treat Reactions: See pages 25 to 29.

Use Vasoconstrictor Drugs: These drugs constrict the blood vessels, thus slowing absorption. This so-called "physiologic or chemical tourniquet" effect at the site of injection prevents rapid rises in the blood levels of drugs, prolongs the duration of anesthesia, and produces a relatively "bloodless" field at the site of injection. Therefore, when near maximum dosages of local anesthetic agents are to be employed, particularly if the area to be injected is highly vascular, it is usually efficacious to incorporate a vasoconstrictor drug in the anesthetic solution.

Choose the Local Anesthetic Agent Carefully: If the patient is known to have had a systemic toxic reaction to one specific local anesthetic drug, a local anesthetic drug of another chemical group may in most instances be used without producing a reaction (see Table II, page 15).

Avoid Spreading Agents: Spreading agents such as hyaluronidase should not be used unless specifically indicated. When large volumes of a local anesthetic solution are to be injected, and/or they are to be placed in highly vascular areas, hyaluronidase is usually contraindicated.

Stop Injection: Terminate injection of a local anesthetic solution at the slightest indication of an overdose.

Apply a Tourniquet: If regional infiltration of an extremity is being performed and a reaction commences, the application of a tourniquet may prevent further generalized circulation of the drug and prevent or limit a generalized systemic reaction. Once the reaction is controlled, the tourniquet can be intermittently released and reapplied, permitting only small quantities of the local anesthetic agent to gain access to the general circulation at any one time.

Skin Wheals, Lozenge, Patch, and Mucous Membrane Tests: The efficacy of tests to ascertain beforehand whether or not a patient will exhibit a high blood level type of a systemic toxic reaction to that drug is debatable. We have concluded from our own experience that tests to ascertain whether or not a patient will have a high blood level type of systemic toxic reaction or an allergic reaction to a local anesthetic agent prior to infiltration are impractical. First, they are time consuming, and, second, they are not conclusive.

Adequate Personnel: When a severe systemic reaction occurs, the physician who is working alone will find the task of performing all the necessary steps of resuscitation practically impossible. Additional personnel should be immediately available, and he should not hesitate to summon them to start intravenous fluids, prepare necessary drugs, and to hold and pass equipment.

If a reaction occurs with adequate personnel present, the physician must direct the course of treatment. He should give the orders, establish a patent airway, and give oxygen. His assistants should prepare the drugs and other equipment.

SIGNS AND SYMPTOMS OF A HIGH BLOOD LEVEL REACTION TO LOCAL ANESTHETIC DRUGS

Basically, the signs and symptoms of a systemic toxic reaction due to the high blood level of the local anesthetic drug, whether administered parenterally, orally, or topically, are referable to the central nervous system and perhaps the cardiovascular system. They are, first, those of stimulation, *i.e.*, restlessness, tremors, and convulsions, and, secondly, those of depression following overstimulation (see Table IV, page 22). Death is usually attrib-

TABLE IV

SUMMARY OF SIGNS AND SYMPTOMS OF SYSTEMIC TOXIC REACTIONS
FROM LOCAL ANESTHETIC DRUGS

Central Nervous System Effects
  1. Stimulation of
      a. Cerebral cortex ——→ excitement, disorientation, incoherent speech, and convulsions
      b. Medulla
          (1) cardiovascular center ——→ increased blood pressure and pulse
          (2) respiratory center ——→ increased respiratory rate and/or variations in rhythm
          (3) vomiting center ——→ nausea and/or vomiting

  2. Depression of
      a. Cerebral cortex ——→ unconsciousness
      b. Medulla
          (1) vasomotor ——→ fall in blood pressure and rapid or absent pulse (syncope)
          (2) respiratory ——→ variations in respiration and/or apnea

Peripheral Effects
  1. Cardiovascular (syncope)
      a. Heart ——→ bradycardia, *i.e.*, depression from direct action of the local anesthetic
                agent on the myocardium
      b. Blood vessels ——→ vasodilatation from direct action of the local anesthetic agent
                on the blood vessels

Allergic Responses
  1. Skin ——→ urticaria, etc.
  2. Respiration }
  3. Circulation } ——→ depression ("clinical anaphylactic shock")

Miscellaneous Reactions
  1. Psychogenic
  2. To other drugs, *e.g.*, vasoconstrictors, etc.

uted to respiratory depression. However, the direct action of these drugs upon the myocardium cannot be completely ignored as contributing to cardiac depression and collapse.

Onset: Systemic toxic reactions have three types of onset: delayed, immediate, and cumulative. The delayed and immediate type reactions occur following any of the agents listed in Table I, page 13. The cumulative type reaction has been observed by us following only the use of mepivacaine (Carbocaine) in a continuous technique (see page 23).

Delayed Type.—Occurs 5 to 30 minutes after injection. Fortunately, this is the more frequent of the three types of systemic reactions from a high blood level of the anesthetic drug. It is caused by a slow build-up of a toxic blood level, and usually it progresses in stages, *i.e.*, the cortical signs first, then the signs of respiratory collapse, and finally the signs of cardiovascular collapse.

This slow onset permits early recognition and effective treatment usually prevents death.

Immediate Type.—Occurs seconds to minutes after the start of the injection with all the signs and symptoms occurring at once. Such rapid onset is due to an inadvertent intravascular injection of the anesthetic solution or to rapid absorption of a large quantity of the agent in a very short period of time. There is no slow, progressive deterioration of the patient's condition; collapse is rapid and total. Death often results before treatment can be instituted. This type of reaction, where large quantities of the drug are used, should not be confused with the allergic "clinical anaphylactic shock" type occurring from relatively infinitesimal amounts of a drug.

These cases are infrequent, and their treatment is usually unsuccessful, but with rapid institution of resuscitative measures, some cases may be salvaged. Do not overlook the treatment of cardiac arrest in these patients.

Cumulative Type.—The cumulative-type reaction has been observed by us in only three of the more than 40,000 patients who have

received regional blocks (spinal block not included) in the past eighteen years. It has the following characteristics: (1) it has occurred only when mepivacaine (Carbocaine) was used for continuous caudal anesthesia to relieve the pains of labor; (2) the initial signs and symptoms started four to six hours after the initial dose and followed the third reinforcing dose in one patient, the fourth reinforcing dose in the second patient, and the fifth reinforcing dose in the third patient; (3) initially, all three patients exhibited signs of early cortical stimulation, *i.e.*, agitation, disorientation, excitability, and hysteria; and (4) all patients had tonic and clonic convulsions. Each dose of mepivacaine was within the then recommended volume and concentration range for a single injection of mepivacaine. None of the reinforcing doses were given until sensory analgesia from the previous dose was dissipated and labor pains returned. Apparently, a high blood level resulted from either: (1) a slow build up of the mepivacaine or its metabolic by-product; (2) slow hydrolysis, detoxification, etc.; or (3) a combination of these.

One of these patients convulsed for approximately three and one-half hours with evidence of cardiovascular and respiratory depression, *i.e.*, cardiac arrhythmias, pulmonary edema, and hypotension. The other two patients had one convulsion lasting fifteen to twenty seconds with no evidence of cardiovascular or respiratory depression. All three patients lived and had apparently healthy infants—two of the patients had no sequelae from the reaction, but the one who had sustained, persistent convulsions may have had cerebral hypoxia, *i.e.*, she was, and still is, uncooperative, inattentive, etc.

Such reactions following single doses of mepivacaine have not been seen by us. However, two episodes similar to our one case (sustained convulsions) have been reported following single doses of mepivacaine. In one case, 40 cc. of a 2.0 percent solution (800 mg.) was injected to effect a pudendal nerve block. This patient was successfully treated with no subsequent sequelae. In the other instance,

3,000 mg. was used for local infiltration. This patient convulsed and expired.

Nervous System (Cortical) Signs and Symptoms: The early signs and symptoms of cortical stimulation are one or a combination of the following: restlessness, nervousness, apprehension, pugnaciousness, unreasonableness, loquacity, incoherent speech, headache, dizziness, blurred vision, metallic taste, roaring in the ears, nausea and vomiting, choreiform movements, tremors and twitchings. The metallic taste, dizziness, blurred vision, and roaring in the ears have been the most prominent of these early cortical signs and symptoms in the author's experience. If the reaction does not progress past this initial stage, these signs and symptoms are of little clinical importance. However, they do announce the fact that a toxic reaction exists and thereby warn that the reaction may progress to unconsciousness, convulsions, nausea and vomiting, cardiovascular collapse, and respiratory collapse. Convulsions indicate marked stimulation of the cortex with associated increased metabolism, increased oxygen demand, and, since respirations usually cease during a convulsion, hypoxia or anoxia results.

Nausea, vomiting, or both may occur either early or late in the course of a systemic toxic reaction to a local anesthetic drug and may not indicate the severity of the reaction. The vomiting center may be stimulated by hypoxia, by the excessive blood level of the local anesthetic agent, or by a combination of both.

Respiratory System Signs and Symptoms: In the very early stages of a reaction, the patient occasionally may show an increase in the rate and depth of respiration. In almost all cases, irregular respiratory rate and excursion, sighing, dyspnea, periods of apnea, and finally complete respiratory arrest are encountered as a manifestation of depression of the respiratory center in the medulla, presumably from its previous overstimulation. Nevertheless, the part played by tissue hypoxia from the hypotension which invariably accompanies the late stages of this type of reaction cannot be ignored completely. Inasmuch as depressed res-

pirations or apnea usually precede circulatory collapse, the patient becomes cyanotic, *i.e.*, there is 5 gm. or more of reduced hemoglobin present per 100 cc. of blood and since the circulation is reaching the periphery, particularly the dermis, cyanosis is present. While the convulsions which attend this type of reaction are usually attributed to overstimulation of the cortex by the local anesthetic drug, they may be the result of hypoxia, or at least the hypoxia may have had an additive effect.

On rare occasions, the lungs may show signs of hypersecretion, râles, rhonchi, bronchospasm, an asthmatic type of respiration, or a combination of these. Of course, a large dosage of the local anesthetic drug would lead us to suspect that these must be signs of a high blood level systemic reaction, but the use of a large dosage does not *preclude* the possibility that an allergic reaction has taken place. Whether these signs should be classified as an allergic systemic reaction or as a high blood level systemic reaction is debatable.

Cardiovascular System Signs and Symptoms: When a reaction starts, there may be no initial variation in the blood pressure and pulse from that determined prior to the injection. However, as respirations become shallow or cease, the blood pressure rises and a tachycardia ensues. Such a reaction resembles and may easily be confused with a systemic toxic reaction to a vasoconstrictor drug (see Chapter 5, page 40). It reflects either oxygen want or initial stimulation of the cardiovascular center in the medulla by the local anesthetic agent. As the reaction progresses, the following occur: (1) the hypoxia becomes more severe, either from apnea or from the direct depressant effect of the local anesthetic agent on the cardiovascular center or the heart and blood vessels; (2) the blood pressure begins to fall; and (3) a bradycardia appears. If the hypotension is not corrected, the patient usually becomes more cyanotic; he perspires profusely, the skin is clammy, and there ensues syncope and peripheral vascular collapse with a weak and often unobtainable pulse.

Cardiac Failure: Cardiac failure must be diagnosed promptly and treated immediately if good results are to be obtained. Whenever a patient has no pulse, no blood pressure, dilated pupils, a cadaveric appearance, no obtainable heart beat, and absent or gasping respirations, the tentative diagnosis of cardiac failure should be made. Gasping respirations are usually of a reflex nature. A positive diagnosis can be made only by electrocardiography or by direct vision of the heart through a thoracotomy. *Although the incidence is low, cardiac failure does occur under regional analgesia and the possibility must be kept in mind.*

TREATMENT OF A HIGH BLOOD LEVEL REACTION FROM A LOCAL ANESTHETIC DRUG

The signs and symptoms of an overdose of a vasoconstrictor drug may resemble the initial stage, *i.e.*, stimulation stage, of a toxic systemic reaction to a local anesthetic agent (see page 40). However, when the reaction is caused by the vasoconstrictor drug, the blood pressure and pulse rate are increased and remain elevated; but when the reaction is caused by the local anesthetic agent, hypotension may rapidly follow the initial rise in blood pressure and pulse. Therefore, frequent checks of the blood pressure and pulse will usually reveal the cause of the reaction. Haphazard, routine treatment of all reactions is to be condemned and may harm rather than help the patient.

Active treatment of systemic toxic reactions from a high blood level of a local anesthetic drug is aimed at: (1) stopping the signs and symptoms of overstimulation of the central nervous system; (2) supplying oxygen to combat tissue hypoxia, which is a result of the increased cell metabolism caused by overstimulation; (3) correcting the central depression of the cortex and vital medullary centers which follows overstimulation; (4) reversing the peripheral cardiovascular collapse; and (5) re-establishing circulation by closed manual systole in cases of cardiac arrest (standstill) or fibrillation (see Table V, page 26).

When a reaction begins, the physician too commonly gives an intravenous barbiturate and stimulating drugs irrespective of the signs and symptoms. Overtreatment is to be avoided, and analeptic drugs such as caffeine sodium benzoate, picrotoxin, etc., are not to be used, as they merely accentuate the overstimulation and add to the depression of medullary centers. Likewise, the indiscriminate use of barbiturates may be equally disastrous, because they may deepen the depresssion which follows overstimulation.

Treatment of systemic toxic reactions depends on the signs and symptoms exhibited, and these should be treated as they occur. For summary of treatment, see Table V, page 26.

Treatment of Cortical Manifestations: When the signs and symptoms of stimulation of the cortex, *i.e.*, anxiety, disorientation, incoherent speech, etc., appear, *oxygen* by bag and mask should be immediately administered and intravenous fluids started. These should be the first steps in the treatment of any systemic reaction to a local anesthetic agent with or without a vasoconstrictor agent. When the cortex and medulla are stimulated, the metabolic rate of their cells is greatly increased, and therefore the oxygen demand is increased many-fold. If the oxygen requirement of these cells is not met, it follows that hypoxia of the cells with a probable increase in CO_2 concentrations ensues, and this in itself may result in convulsions, cardiovascular collapse and death.

While oxygen is being administered, a careful check of the blood pressure, pulse, and respiration must be maintained, and agents such as muscle relaxants and vasoconstrictor drugs should be readied for immediate injection in case the reaction progresses. Likewise, suction, endotracheal tubes, laryngoscopes, and bronchoscopes should be on hand should the patient vomit and aspirate and/or become apneic. If the patient vomits, the airway must be cleared by tracheal suction; and if aspiration takes place, bronchoscopy may be necessary to clear the trachea and bronchi of food particles (see Table VI, page 27).

TABLE V

SUMMARY OF ACTIVE TREATMENT OF SYSTEMIC TOXIC REACTIONS FROM A HIGH BLOOD LEVEL OF LOCAL ANESTHETIC AGENT

While the following measures apply specifically to a toxic reaction from a high blood level of a local anesthetic agent, they are general principles of resuscitation and are applicable to any reaction which may progress to shock.

I. **Be Sure the Airway is Clear.** If the patient becomes unconscious, establish a clear airway with an *oropharyngeal airway* or preferably a cuffed *endotracheal tube* (Figure 7, page 55).

II. **Clear Vomitus from Pharynx, Larynx, Trachea.** If a cuffed endotracheal tube is in the trachea and the cuff inflated when vomiting occurs, no emergency exists. The vomitus may be cleared from the mouth and pharynx when time permits—the cuffed endotracheal tube prevents the vomitus from entering the tracheobronchial tree. If an endotracheal tube is not in place when the patient vomits, a true emergency may exist—the vomitus must be cleared from the mouth (see page 30).

III. **Administer Oxygen.** Oxygen administration should be performed with a *bag* and *mask* apparatus (Figure 6, page 54) and inadequate respirations supplemented.

IV. **Start Intravenous Fluids.** This is an essential part of the initial treatment of a reaction, and it should be done when the first signs of a reaction occur, because *it assures the physician a means of intravenous administration* of drugs even if the reaction progresses to cardiovascular collapse.

V. **Stop Convulsions.**
    a. Administer oxygen, for oxygen alone may stop the convulsion.
    b. If oxygen alone does not stop the convulsion, use intravenous injections of succinylcholine, 2 cc. (40 mg.) and oxygenate the patient. If convulsions recur after succinylcholine is dissipated (6 to 8 minutes), repeat dose. Then, if convulsions recur, give *d*-tubocurarine 3 to 5 cc. (9 to 15 mg.).
    c. If muscle relaxants are not available or the anesthetist is not familiar with their actions and uses, give small amounts of a short-acting barbiturate, thiopental 50 mg., at one-half to one-minute intervals. In obstetrics a single dose of succinylcholine and oxygenation are preferred. *A barbiturate should not be used unless convulsions are persistent. It merely adds to the depression of both the parturient and the fetus.*

VI. **Raise the Blood Pressure.** When peripheral vascular collapse starts, immediate steps to raise the blood pressure to approximately the preoperative level must be taken—use vasoconstrictor drugs (see page 36).

VII. **Institute Manual Systole.** If cardiac arrest or fibrillation occurs, closed manual systole (cardiac massage) must be rapidly instituted.

Non-sustained Convulsions.—If the minor signs of cerebral stimulation progress to convulsions, which are always accompanied by periods of apnea, or if convulsion is the initial indication of the reaction, oxygen still is the first therapeutic agent to use. This cannot be too strongly emphasized. If the patient is apneic either with or without convulsions, the oxygen must be made available to the pulmonary circulation by artificial respiration. Respirations, per se, are not necessary to life except as a means to supply oxygen to the alveoli of the lungs so that it may be absorbed by the pulmonary circulation. In most instances, respiratory depression precedes circulatory collapse. Cardiovascular collapse will not usually occur if, when respirations become inadequate to supply sufficient oxygen to maintain normal physiological function of the body, oxygen is supplied by artificial means until the local anesthetic agent's action on the respiratory center is dissipated and spontaneous respirations return.

In the greater number of our systemic toxic reactions, oxygen alone has avoided convulsions or corrected them. However, if it does not, then succinylcholine (Anectine, Quellicin) 40 mg. is given intravenously and the

TABLE VI

EQUIPMENT NECESSARY FOR THE IMMEDIATE TREATMENT
OF THE COMPLICATIONS OF REGIONAL BLOCKS

Oxygen Apparatus.—This may consist of nothing more than a bag and mask with a simple reducing needle valve for the oxygen tank, or it may be an anesthetic machine (Figure 6, page 54).

Suction Apparatus.—If vomiting or excessive secretions occur, it is important to clear the airway. Any type of adequate suction is satisfactory (Figure 6, page 54).

Airways.—Oral airways and endotracheal tubes should be available (Figure 7, page 55).

Laryngoscope and Bronchoscope.—Any type of a Jackson or Macintosh laryngoscope will suffice if the doctor can use it effectively. Laryngoscopy or bronchoscopy and intubation are often necessary to clear aspirated material from the tracheobronchial tree and to establish an unobstructed airway (Figure 8, page 56).

Intravenous Apparatus.—Intravenous fluids for supportive therapy should be readily available. Syringes to administer vasoconstrictor drugs, muscle relaxants, and barbiturates should be on hand.

Electrocardiograph.—It is needed to establish diagnosis of cardiac arrest or fibrillation.

Cardiac Defibrillator.—If the heart is fibrillating, it must be brought to arrest before normal rhythm can be re-established.

Drugs.—The following drugs should be readily available: vasoconstrictor drugs, succinylcholine (Anectine), d-tubocurarine; and the barbiturates for treating hypotension and convulsions, respectively; diphenhydramine (Benadryl) for treating allergic reactions; and calcium chloride, potassium chloride, and procainamide (Pronestyl) for treating cardiac failure.

---

patient is oxygenated. With the exception of the one case of a cumulative toxic reaction (page 23), one dose of succinylcholine has been effective. Succinylcholine may be repeated once if necessary—if repeated more than once, bradycardia may ensue. If succinylcholine is not available, then thiopental (Pentothal) in 50 to 100 mg. doses should be used to stop the convulsions and allow oxygenation. An interval of one to three minutes should elapse between doses to permit the barbiturate to be effective. Larger doses of the short-acting barbiturates given rapidly may stop the convulsions sooner, but they also add to the subsequent depression of the medullary centers, resulting in prolonged apnea.

Sustained Convulsions.—Oxygen was given to all three of our patients who had a cumulative-type reaction (see page 23). It was adequate treatment in two of the three patients. The patient who had sustained convulsions was given two 40-mg. doses of succinylcholine, oxygen, and intubated. This treatment controlled the convulsion twice for five

to six-minute periods, *i.e.*, the duration of action of the succinylcholine. On recommendation of the consulting neurologist, 8 cc. of intravenous paraldehyde in divided doses were used to decrease the intensity of the convulsions in this patient. Although the paraldehyde did permit oxygenation, it never completely abolished tonic and clonic contractions, which lasted for approximately three hours. On recovery, this patient was uncooperative, inattentive, and has remained so. The one case of sustained convulsions reported in the literature following a single dose of mepivacaine that lived and had no sequelae on recovery was given general anesthesia immediately, and it was continued until evidence of convulsions subsided three hours later (see page 23).

We have had little experience in treating this type of reaction and the experience of others is no greater if reports in the literature can be considered a criterion. Therefore, an authoritative statement on the treatment of this type of convulsion cannot be given. From experience to date, it can be concluded that regardless of the local anesthetic agent employed, convulsions which do not subside when oxygen, succinylcholine, or both are administered should be treated immediately and rapidly by anesthetizing the patient with 250 mg. of thiopental (Pentothal) intravenously, followed by *d*-tubocurarine 3 to 7 cc. (9 to 20 mg.) intravenously, to permit intubation and oxygenation. If these agents are not readily available or do not control the convulsions, inhalation anesthesia, *i.e.*, halothane (Fluothane), cyclopropane-ether, etc., should be used. Sufficient depth of anesthesia, muscle relaxation, or both must be obtained so that there is no evidence of tonic and clonic convulsions. The patient must be oxygenated and respirations should be assisted. At thirty-minute intervals, anesthesia should be lightened to ascertain if evidence of cortical stimulation (tonic and clonic contractions) is still present. The patient must be kept anesthetized until this evidence of cortical stimulation disappears. Three to four hours of anesthesia may be required.

Treatment of Respiratory Manifestations: The early signs of stimulation of the respiratory center of the medulla by local anesthetic agents is usually only increased respiration—often very transient, seldom noted, and requires no treatment. On the other hand, depression of the respiratory center from overstimulation by these drugs results in respiratory failure. Respiratory failure evidenced by alteration of respiratory rhythm and rate should be treated immediately by administration of oxygen by bag and mask. If the patient should vomit, the airway must be cleared of vomitus prior to giving oxygen by bag and mask (see page 30). If apnea occurs, then artificial respiration must be instituted.

The author has seen respiratory failure occur a number of times as the *only* complication of a high blood level of a local anesthetic drug, namely, tetracaine (Pontocaine), and in these cases, artificial respiration using 100 percent oxygen was the only treatment necessary. Thus, since it is not safe to assume that cardiovascular collapse automatically accompanies, precedes, or follows respiratory failure, the blood pressure and pulse should be checked before aiming treatment at the cardiovascular system, rather than proceeding on the basis of assumption only.

Treatment of Cardiovascular Manifestations: The early signs and symptoms of cardiovascular involvement are hypertension, increase in pulse rate, and occasionally cardiac irregularities. They are usually transient, reflecting a stimulation of the cardiovascular center in the medulla. No special treatment is required other than oxygen therapy and the starting of intravenous fluids.

The signs and symptoms of depression of the cardiovascular center in the medulla, the myocardium, or both may follow those of stimulation; or they may appear as the only signs of a reaction to a local anesthetic drug. The treatment of these signs and symptoms of the depression stage is aimed at the hypotension, the depressed myocardium, and cardiac failure if it occurs. As with cortical and respiratory manifestations of a toxic reaction, the initial treatment is to institute oxygen therapy and start intravenous fluids. Then a vasoconstrictor drug, usually one which will strengthen cardiac action as well as constrict the blood vessels, should be given intravenously to correct the hypotension—we prefer an intravenous infusion of phenylephrine (Neo-Synephrine) (see page 36). If cardiac failure occurs, it must be treated by manual systole. Closed cardiac massage must be instituted immediately. Speed is the essence of successful treatment.

Cardiac arrest rather than ventricular fibrillation is the more frequent type of cardiac failure seen following regional block. Intracardiac epinephrine (Adrenalin) in small doses (¼ cc. of a 1:1000 solution), repeated at one minute intervals, may be beneficial. However, when there is hypoxia of the heart muscle epinephrine tends to produce ventricular fibrillation. Therefore, before injecting epinephrine, manual systole together with oxygen administration should be performed for one minute in an attempt to oxygenate the heart muscle. A 10 percent calcium chloride solution, 3 cc. to 5 cc., injected into the left ventricle may also be of value in cardiac arrest to start the heart beating.

Ventricular fibrillation is the unusual type of cardiac failure seen following a regional block procedure. If it occurs, the first steps in its treatment are to re-establish circulation by closed cardiac massage and assure oxygenation of the tissues by artificial respiration. Once these are done then an effort to defibrillate the heart by electrical stimulation or drug therapy (potassium chloride) or both is indicated. Once the heart is brought to arrest then treatment as outlined, *e.g.*, calcium chloride or epinephrine intracardially, should be instituted in an effort to re-establish a normal heart beat if closed cardiac massage alone does not do so.

If the cardiac arrest is treated successfully and the initial severe period of acute hypoxia corrected, the possibility of chronic edema of the brain with hypoxia of this organ should not be overlooked. Osmotic diuretics, *e.g.*, mannitol, and hypothermia should be considered—they may avoid brain damage.

REMARKS

Psychomotor Responses: This type of reaction is not caused by the local anesthetic agent itself, but the mere mechanics of the procedure of performing the block. It occurs usually in the following group of patients: (1) those who tend to faint at the mere sight of a needle or when the skin is traumatized by the needle; (2) those who do not want a regional procedure and on whom block anesthesia is performed without first convincing the patient that it is the procedure of choice; and (3) those in whom a block procedure is done with the immediate relatives in attendance.

In most instances the reaction is characterized by the patient fainting or pretending to faint. None of the signs and symptoms of a true systemic reaction to a local anesthetic drug appear. The blood pressure, pulse, and respirations remain normal, and the lid reflexes, *i.e.*, movements of the upper eyelid following gentle stroking of its eyelash, are present. On the other hand, a small number of those showing psychomotor responses may become agitated, restless, may sob, and become uncontrollable. Treatment of such a patient consists in watchful waiting. A feigned reaction requires no treatment other than reassurance; but if it is the start of a true toxic systemic reaction, therapy discussed previously must be instituted.

The fact that psychomotor reactions to regional analgesia have been reported to be not infrequent, points to the necessity of correctly preparing the patient for a block procedure. This does not only mean choosing the correct premedication for a block procedure, but explaining the procedure to the patient. On anesthetic preoperative rounds, he should be assured that the anesthetic technique of choice is being used for his particular problem and that he will not be hurt. When he arrives on the surgical floor, he should be reassured that he will not be hurt either during the blocking procedure or during the operation. Gaining the patient's confidence is one of the initial steps in any block procedure. In the past eighteen years we have never had a patient faint. This type of reaction has been averted by: (1) correct premedication, (2) explaining each step in the block technique to the patient prior to and during its execution, and (3) executing the block with the patient in the recumbent position whenever possible. A patient is never permitted to sit in a chair as he is being blocked. If the sitting position facilitates the block, the patient sits on the cart or operating table. This is done so that if the patient feels faint or should faint he may be placed immediately in the recumbent position.

Seldom if ever does loss of consciousness of this nature require treatment for hypotension. Placing the patient in the supine position usually suffices.

Rules To Be Remembered When Performing Regional Blocks:

Carefully Observe the Patient for at Least One-Half Hour Following the Completion of the Injection, Oral Administration, or Topical Application of Local Anesthetic Solutions.—

Some reactions, particularly the mild ones, may be judged by the inexperienced physician to be hysterical in nature and not due to the drug or drugs. Should the reaction progress unobserved, death may occur before treatment can be instituted. When a patient who has been restless and difficult to block suddenly becomes quiet, the physician should not draw a sigh of relief, believing that at last the patient has become cooperative. On the contrary, the physician should immediately become suspicious that a reaction is taking place and make a positive diagnosis without delay.

Objectively Evaluate Any Type of Reaction No Matter How Mild.—Do not treat a reaction without making a definite diagnosis; give only the necessary indicated therapy.

Be Prepared To Treat Any Type of Reaction.—Preparedness to treat all reactions, be they mild and transient in nature or severe, with convulsions, respiratory collapse, cardiovascular collapse, or a combination of these, is essential wherever regional block procedures are performed.

Do Not Overtreat or Undertreat the Reaction.—Some reactions require no treatment; on the other hand, intensive therapy and even closed cardiac massage may be necessary to save the patient's life. Either stimulation or depression of the central nervous system may predominate so that when treatment is instituted it must be "tailored" to the individual signs and symptoms—not administered in "shotgun" doses.

Tell the Patient If He Has a Reaction.—When a reaction to a drug occurs, the patient should be informed of the fact, told the drug or drugs which were employed and the method of administration so that at a later date he may pass this information on to any physician who might choose to give him a regional block.

Do Not Exceed the Recommended Maximum Dosage of the Local Anesthetic Drugs (see Table I, page 13).—Reactions with an immediate onset following the use of a relatively large amount of a local anesthetic drug

are most often seen following the application of local anesthetic agents to the mucous membranes of the nose or mouth, pharynx, larynx, trachea, or urethra. When 5 to 10 cc. of 2.0 percent tetracaine (Pontocaine) is used topically to anesthetize these structures, 100 to 200 mg. of the drug has been administered and if a reaction follows, it must be attributed to too great a dosage—not to an allergy.

When performing topical anesthesia we allow only a measured amount of the local anesthetic solution to be placed at our disposal. The solution is poured into a medicine glass and only this amount is employed. Often the over-zealous resident in an effort to please his chief will exceed the toxic dosage of a local anesthetic agent if more solution is available.

Do Not Rely on Premedications to Prevent Systemic Toxic Reactions.—The protection afforded by heavy doses of barbiturates is unimpressive and, for the reasons previously discussed, the author does not recommend them for this purpose (see page 20).

Vomiting Can Be Catastrophic: The seriousness of this complication will, in most instances, depend on the preoperative preparation and cooperation of the patient.

In the patient who has been prepared for an elective block procedure by restriction of the oral intake and/or by Levin tube suction of the stomach, stimulation of the vomiting center usually presents less of a problem, as the stomach contains little or nothing to expel. When intake has been restricted, the volume regurgitated in most instances is small, and the patient will be able to expel it before he takes an inspiration.

However, the patient whose oral intake has not been restricted and whose stomach has not been emptied presents a greater problem. The volume of stomach contents is usually large and, more likely than not, will contain particles of undigested food. If he vomits he may not be able to expel a large volume of vomitus from the oral cavity before he takes a breath. In that case he aspirates vomitus and the problem is twofold: the hydrochloric acid damages the lungs and the food particles barricade the passage of air or oxygen into the trachea, bronchi, and/or alveoli. If the patient is conscious and will cooperate by opening his mouth, there may be no difficulty in clearing the airway, but if he is uncooperative or unconscious much difficulty may be encountered —a muscle relaxant, succinylcholine (Anectine), may be required to relax the jaw. In the adult 40 mg. (2 cc.) of succinylcholine should be given intravenously; but, if a vein is not accessible, give 40 to 80 mg. (2 to 4 cc.) intramuscularly.

When aspiration occurs, the care during the postoperative period is important and may necessitate: (1) antibiotic and steroid therapy, (2) ventilators, (3) tracheostomy, (4) tracheal suction, and (5) digitalis and vasoconstrictor drugs to support the cardiovascular system.

Common Atypical Systemic Toxic Reactions from a High Blood Level: Lidocaine (Xylocaine) and mepivacaine (Carbocaine) reactions may not be signalled by cerebral stimulation. When doses of over 500 mg. of lidocaine or mepivacaine are employed, central depression without any other signs or symptoms of a toxic reaction may be noted. These patients will not respond to questioning and appear to be in the first plane of surgical anesthesia. Their course during this is usually uneventful; blood pressure, pulse, and respirations remain unchanged and within one-half to three-fourths of an hour they regain consciousness. This type of reaction may also follow the use of large amounts of procaine.

While reactions to tetracaine (Pontocaine) may follow the characteristic pattern, we have found that most of the reactions observed from this drug were atypical, *i.e.*, they were not heralded by restlessness, nervousness, dizziness, sweating, pallor, and tachycardia. As a matter of fact, there was no such warning. They occurred 5 to 10 minutes after the completion of the block and were characterized by drowsiness, shallow respiration, loss of consciousness, and apnea. Blood pressure and pulse did not vary in these patients until apnea occurred, and then they began to increase. When artificial respiration with oxygen by bag and mask was instituted, the blood pressure and pulse returned to normal and remained so. The patients regained consciousness in 30 to 45 minutes and the surgery proceeded as scheduled. Only one of these patients, who was not being carefully observed, started to convulse, and this was corrected by the administration of oxygen alone by bag and mask. In this one case the convulsion was attributed to oxygen want.

RAPID TREATMENT OF SYSTEMIC TOXIC REACTIONS FROM HIGH BLOOD LEVELS OF LOCAL ANESTHETIC AGENTS IS ESSENTIAL TO AVOID DEATHS: BUT CORRECT TREATMENT IS EQUALLY IMPORTANT. INAPPROPRIATE TREATMENT MAY RESULT IN DEATH!

CHAPTER 4

Allergic Reactions to Local Anesthetic Drugs

A REACTION to a drug may be termed allergic with certainty only if small or infinitesimal doses have been administered (see Table III, page 19). The two types of allergic reactions which are of importance in regional nerve block are a generalized systemic allergic reaction and dermatitis. A generalized systemic allergic reaction occurs rarely—less than one percent of systemic toxic reactions from local anesthetic agents are caused by allergy. But, a contact dermatitis is not a rarity.

SIGNS AND SYMPTOMS

Generalized Systemic Allergic Reactions: Such reactions occur within a few minutes after injection of the local anesthetic solution and are characterized by one or more of the following: *generalized angioneurotic edema, urticaria, pruritis, hypotension, joint pains, asthmatic breathing, nausea, and vomiting.* When angioneurotic edema occurs, it may involve the larynx and its associated structures with resultant severe respiratory obstruction. To date, allergic reactions with these signs and symptoms have not been seen by us.

The administration of infinitesimal amounts of local anesthetic solutions, *e.g.*, raising of a skin wheal prior to insertion of large needles, may, on rare occasions, be followed by "clinical anaphylactic shock"—this is a true allergic type reaction. Shock of this type is usually characterized by a sudden cardiovascular and respiratory collapse which, if not adequately treated, may be fatal in 1 to 5 minutes. Only two such cases have been observed by us in over 55,000 regional blocks—both were resuscitated. Equally infrequent is a systemic allergic reaction resulting from the small dosages of local anesthetic drugs required for spinal anesthesia.

Dermatitis: Dermatitis frequently affects those who administer drugs used to produce local analgesia (see Figure 3, page 33). It is an occupational hazard of physicians and dentists. Because of this hazard, gloves should be worn when performing blocks and should the local anesthetic drug come in contact with the physician's or dentist's skin in unprotected areas, the area should be washed as soon as the block is completed even if he is not at the time allergic to the drug. Without this precautionary washing off of the drug, repeated exposure may eventually result in an allergy.

Remember, gloves are not used when injecting local anesthetic solutions only to assure asepsis, which may be obtained by careful scrubbing of the hands, but for the protection of the physician or dentist against the occupational hazard of an acquired allergy to local anesthetic agents used in their daily practice.

PROPHYLAXIS

Prophylaxis of allergy is at best not very satisfactory. It consists of taking an adequate history and performance of a number of time-consuming tests, the results of which are often not significant.

History: If the history is adequately taken, it will prove to be the most valuable source of information, but to be of value the allergic history must be painstakingly obtained. An adequate history does not mean just asking the patient whether he has had a local anesthetic agent injected previously and whether

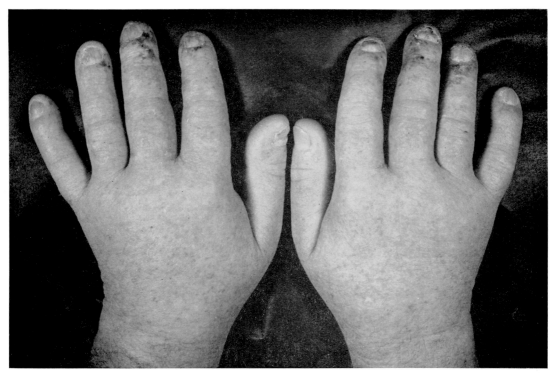

Figure 3. Swelling of the hands following the administration of procaine (Novocain) to a doctor with a known allergy (sensitivity) to cocaine and its derivatives.

or not any untoward effect had followed; the circumstances under which the reaction occurred must be ascertained as well as the drug or drugs used. This is most important, as unpleasant reactions are often caused by high concentrations of vasoconstrictor agents. In addition to a personal history, reactions in other members of the family should be inquired into; such evidence might reveal an important clue, since heredity often plays an important part in allergy.

Skin Wheals, Lozenge, Patch and Mucous Membrane Tests: Intradermal skin wheal tests and tests applied to the mucous membranes may occasionally prove whether or not the patient who is known to be markedly allergic to other substances will have an allergic reaction to the injection or topical application of a local anesthetic agent. But since these tests are time consuming and since serious *allergic* reactions are very infrequent, the practicality of such tests prior to performing local analgesia for an operative procedure or for

diagnostic and therapeutic blocks is questionable.

TREATMENT OF A GENERALIZED ALLERGIC SYSTEMIC REACTION

Treatment consists of the following specific therapy of the signs and symptoms.

Angioneurotic Edema, Wheals (Urticaria), and Pruritis (Itching): These are best treated by an antihistaminic drug such as diphenhydramine (Benadryl) orally and intravenously. The dosage for diphenhydramine is 50 mg. administered either orally or slowly intravenously. This dosage may be repeated at 3 to 4-hour intervals as needed. Larger intravenous doses of diphenhydramine, *i.e.*, 100 mg., should be used with caution, as they are seldom of more therapeutic benefit and may result in nausea and vomiting, convulsions, cardiac irregularities, and even death if given too rapidly.

Epinephrine (Adrenalin) 1:1000 may be given intramuscularly in 0.3 cc. (5 minim) doses and repeated at 15-minute intervals to correct these problems. Ephedrine sulfate 50 mg. may also be effective given intramuscularly.

Intravenous or intramuscular calcium gluconate, 1 to 2 gm. (5 to 10 cc. of a 20 percent solution) may prove valuable to control pruritis. It should be remembered that if calcium chloride is used instead of the gluconate, it must not be given intramuscularly or subcutaneously because of its necrotizing action. Lotions containing calamine and phenols may alleviate the itching, but they are not as effective as the antihistaminic drugs.

Asthmatic Breathing: This may be relieved by the administration of oxygen only or oxygen-helium mixtures. If this treatment does not help within a relatively short period of time, drug therapy should be instituted. A 50 mg. dose of diphenhydramine given intravenously may suffice to stop the attack, but epinephrine or theophylline with ethylenediamine (Aminophylline) is usually more effective. Epinephrine (1:1000) 0.3 cc. (5 minims) may be given intramuscularly and repeated at 15-minute intervals; or if the attack is persistent and seems to be intractable, a dose of 1 cc. of a 1:10,000 concentration may be given *slowly* intravenously. However, theophylline 500 mg. (7.5 gr.) given *slowly* intravenously in the adult is the author's drug of choice. Hydrocortisone may be of value in this type of reaction—200 mg. of hydrocortisone (Solu-cortef) can be given intravenously.

Hypotension: A fall in blood pressure with an associated hypoxia may occur by itself in allergic conditions, or it may accompany "clinical anaphylactic shock." It should be corrected immediately by intravenously administered vasoconstrictor drugs (see page 36).

Laryngeal Edema: Laryngeal edema may arise in the occasional case, and if severe, intubation or tracheotomy may be necessary to obviate respiratory obstruction and prevent oxygen want. However, if angioneurotic edema is treated immediately, laryngeal edema is less likely to occur.

Clinical Anaphylactic Shock: Shock of this type seldom occurs, but when it does, treatment is the same as for a severe systemic reaction from a high blood level of a local anesthetic drug (see pages 25 to 29). In addition, if an allergy to a local anesthetic drug is thought to have caused this reaction, antihistaminic drugs intravenously in the doses noted above may prove valuable. Death is not unusual in this type of reaction, but with the rapid institution of therapy, some fatalities may be avoided. Treatment should include artificial respiration with high concentrations of oxygen, intravenous fluids, vasoconstrictor agents, and closed cardiac massage.

TREATMENT OF DERMATITIS

The treatment of a dermatitis can be handled best by a dermatologist. Treatment includes: (1) relief of itching with antipruritics, sedation, splinting and wrapping the part, avoiding soap, and dehydration; (2) local therapy with wet dressings, lotions, pastes and emulsions; and (3) cortisone therapy.

REMARKS

Acute Delayed Systemic Allergic Reactions: Two cases have been recorded which were labeled as acute systemic allergic reactions because the dose of drug was small. These reactions did not occur for two or more hours after the local anesthetic drug entered the body. This type of an acute systemic allergic reaction, if it is caused by an allergy, is quite unusual because of the delayed onset. These reactions were characterized by coma, cyanosis, soft nonpitting edema, and shallow, slow irregular respirations. One patient died and the other survived. Hydrocortisone was used parenterally in the patient who survived.

Dermatitis from Solutions Used to Aseptically Prepare the Skin: Mercureoles are one of the most potent sensitizing agents. For approximately twelve years, we used thimerosal (Merthiolate) to aseptically prepare the skin prior to a regional block procedure. A number of dermatitises were observed. For the past five years benzalkonium chloride (Zephiran) has been used to prepare the skin with no resulting dermatitis.

Mention of this is made here to emphasize the point that the local anesthetic drug is not always responsible for a dermatitis. Whenever a dermatitis occurs, a patch test to determine the offending drug should be made, and the patient should be told the results so that he can warn another physician who might undertake another block procedure in the future.

Dermatitis from Chlorpromazine: Contact dermatitis following the use of chlorpromazine in personnel administering the drug does occur. The incidence of dermatitis is highest when the drug is given parenterally and lowest when the drug is given orally. This would indicate that repeated spillage of the drug onto the skin of the personnel administering it is responsible for the dermatitis.

Chlorpromazine has been used in regional anesthesia by us and others for sedation following regional nerve blocks (see page 9). Since the drug has been given intravenously in these cases, it is possible that the solution could on occasion come in contact with the skin. This might result in allergy and indicates the necessity of washing the hands when spillage occurs.

CHAPTER 5

Vasoconstrictor Drugs

IN REGIONAL BLOCK techniques, vasoconstrictor drugs are used primarily for two purposes. First, they are injected intramuscularly or intravenously to correct or prevent hypotension. And, second, they are added to the local anesthetic solution to constrict the blood vessels in the area into which the solution is injected.

PREVENTION OR CORRECTION OF HYPOTENSION BY VASOCONSTRICTOR DRUGS

When used "prophylactically" to prevent hypotension, the vasoconstrictor drugs may be given intramuscularly, but when hypotension is present peripheral circulation is slowed and drugs given subcutaneously or intramuscularly are *slowly* absorbed. Therefore, *intravenous administration* is the only rational method of giving a vasoconstrictor drug to correct a severe hypotension rapidly. A vasoconstrictor drug is the "keystone" to the therapy of hypotension which is not a result of blood, plasma, or electrolyte loss, and it behooves the physician to choose one or two of these drugs and become thoroughly familiar with their mechanism of action as well as their usual effect.

All vasoconstrictor drugs do not act in the same way. The vasoconstrictor action may depend on: (1) direct action on the arterioles; (2) myocardial stimulation with increased cardiac output; (3) stimulation of the vasomotor center; (4) constriction of the veins; or (5) a combination of these. The appropriate vasoconstrictor agent must be chosen and the one selected depends to some degree on whether a fast or slow pulse is noted after a regional block procedure. A slow pulse in the presence of hypotension reflects depression of the myocardium as well as peripheral vasodilatation and, therefore, would indicate the use of a drug like ephedrine sulfate, which, in addition to a peripheral vasoconstrictor action, stimulates the heart directly. A fast pulse in the presence of a low blood pressure, on the other hand, would probably indicate increased activity of the heart along with peripheral vasodilatation and suggest the use of a drug which slows the heart rate while producing peripheral constriction of the blood vessels, *e.g.*, phenylephrine (Neo-Synephrine). The more commonly used vasoconstrictors, their dosages, and the fashion in which they act are:

Ephedrine Sulfate

Dosage.—15 to 25 mg. intravenously repeated at 2 to 5-minute intervals until the preblock blood level is approximated; then the dosage is reduced to 10 mg. and given at intervals necessary to maintain the pressure until it is stabilized.

Action.—It constricts the arterioles, stimulates the cerebral cortex, and increases the cardiac output. Ephedrine may produce an actual increase in heart force and does not act on the same basis as phenylephrine or methoxamine (Vasoxyl).

Phenylephrine (Neo-Synephrine, Neophryn)

Dosage.—1 to 2 mg. intravenously when given intermittently. However, it is a powerful drug and in the author's opinion is best given by the drip method. The drip solution is prepared by adding 1 cc. of a 1.0 percent (10 mg./cc.) phenylephrine solution to either 500 cc. or 1000 cc. of intravenous fluid, usually normal saline or 5 percent dextrose in distilled water. Initially this mixture is dripped rapidly (100 to 180 drops per minute) until the blood pressure approaches the preblock level and then it is slowed to a maintenance drip (40 or fewer drops per minute) until the pressure stabilizes. This method of correcting hypotension is the choice of the author because it gives minute-to-minute control and may be continued in the postoperative period with marked safety until the regional block has dissipated itself.

Action.—It raises the blood pressure by peripheral vasoconstriction and cardiac stimulation. In addition, a bradycardia from compensatory reflexes or depression of the sino-auricular node, an increase in the heart size, and increased stroke volume result. Untoward reactions such as apprehension, excitement and headache are negligible.

Methoxamine (Vasoxyl)

Dosage.—2 to 3 mg. intravenously accompanied by 7.5 to 10 mg. intramuscularly to provide for a prolonged action.

Action.—Given intramuscularly, the action of this drug lasts two hours or more. It raises the blood pressure by direct peripheral vascular constriction. Bradycardia ascribed to reflex inhibition arising from pressure receptors of the carotid sinus and aortic arch occurs. Atropine blocks this action, which suggests that it is mediated over the vagus. It is free of central stimulation effects such as nausea, tremor, nervousness, headache, etc. However, it increases the central venous pressure. The small increases in heart force produced by phenylephrine and methoxamine are considered by some to be the results of cardiac dilatation secondary to hypertension and not a result of direct action of these drugs on the myocardium.

Methoxamine in our experience has proven to be a valuable drug for correcting the hypotension following spinal and epidural block.

d-desoxyephedrine, Methamphetamine, (Methedrine, Desoxyn, Pervitin, Norodin)

Dosage.—5 to 10 mg. intravenously followed by 15 to 20 mg. intramuscularly.

Action.—It stimulates the central nervous system, constricts peripheral blood vessels and increases cardiac output. The duration of action following intramuscular injection is about two hours.

Levarterenol (Levophed)

Dosage.—4 to 8 mg. in 1000 cc. of 5 percent dextrose in distilled water administered by the intravenous drip technique.

Action.—It is one of the most powerful of all the peripheral vasoconstrictor drugs and has little or no action on the myocardium. It causes general vasoconstriction of the arterial, capillary, and venous blood vessels with a resultant increase in total peripheral resistance. It should be used in hypotension following regional block only when other vasoconstrictor agents fail, and, if it is administered, an arm vein of the cubital fossa should be used. This is advisable because serious tissue sloughs following the prolonged use of the drug are more frequent when an ankle vein is selected.

Metaraminol (Aramine)

Dosage.—15 to 100 mg. in 500 cc. of isotonic solution of sodium chloride or 5 percent dextrose solution administered by the intravenous technique.

Action.—Metaraminol and levarterenol are the two most powerful vasoconstrictor agents commonly employed. The action of metaraminol is similar to levarterenol (see above) but slough is infrequent. Nevertheless, arm veins are preferred.

Epinephrine (Adrenalin): In general, epinephrine is not commonly employed because it produces tachycardia, anxiety, or cardiac irregularities, and if tissue hypoxia, particularly of the myocardium, is present, ventricular fibrillation may result. If it is used in an emergency when other vasopressor drugs are not available, the intravenous epinephrine drip technique (1:250,000) is the preferable method of administration, *i.e.*, 2.0 cc. of epinephrine 1:1000 in 500 cc. of normal saline.

ADDITION OF VASOCONSTRICTOR DRUGS TO LOCAL ANESTHETIC SOLUTIONS

General Considerations: Vasoconstrictor drugs are incorporated in local anesthetic solutions to constrict the blood vessels, thereby slowing absorption and minimizing toxic reactions: the so-called chemical tourniquet effect. Thus, they accomplish three purposes. First, in local infiltration a vasoconstrictor drug produces a bloodless field. This is not true for field blocking, although capillary oozing is reduced. In nerve blocks a hyperemic condition in the operative field is normal, but this is not detrimental to the surgery. Second, in all types of blocks, rapid absorption of the local anesthetic agent is prevented. This helps to avoid a high blood level of the anesthetic agent and a toxic reaction. And, lastly, in all procedures, it tends to prolong the operating analgesia time. Unless vasoconstrictor drugs are employed for these specific purposes, they should be omitted from the local anesthetic solution.

Drugs of Choice: Epinephrine (Adrenalin) and phenylephrine (Neo-Synephrine) are the author's choice of the presently available vasoconstrictor drugs for incorporation in local anesthetic solutions. Epinephrine is used in solutions for local infiltration, field block, peripheral nerve block, epidural block, caudal block, and spinal block. Phenylephrine is used by us only to prolong the duration of spinal block.

The vasoconstrictor drugs with a prolonged vasoconstrictor action, *e.g.*, methoxamine (Vasoxyl) and levarterenol (Levophed), should not be used to prolong regional blocks until further experimental research assures their safety and establishes the dosage when used in this fashion. One case of cauda equina syndrome (at another hospital) has been seen in consultation which followed the subarachnoid administration of one of these drugs. In this case, 10 mg. (0.5 cc.) of methoxamine had been mixed with the local anesthetic solution to be injected into the subarachnoid space in hopes of prolonging anesthesia time for an appendectomy. This does not necessarily condemn the methoxamine since the paralysis may have been caused by other factors; nevertheless, the action of this drug must be considered as a possible factor.

Measurement: The dose of vasoconstrictor drugs to be used should be measured accurately by the calibrations on the barrel of the syringe. There is a wide difference in dropper shapes and outlets. Also, the drop produced by needles varies according to the gauge of the needle. Therefore, the measuring of these solutions by the drop method is to be condemned unless the dropper is calibrated.

Contamination and Deterioration: To avoid contamination and to prevent deterioration, small ampules of vasoconstrictor drugs should be used rather than large rubber-stoppered bottles, and they should be opened as needed. Epinephrine and phenylephrine are particularly liable to decompose when exposed to air for a period of time. Solutions of epinephrine and phenylephrine are normally clear and colorless; if they are pink, brownish-red, and/or turbid, they are deteriorating and should be discarded.

Maximum Effectiveness: To obtain the maximum effect from a vasoconstrictor drug, it should be added to the anesthetic solution just prior to use. If the anesthetic solution is discolored by the vasoconstrictor drug or if the vasoconstrictor drug itself is discolored, the solution should be discarded. Commercially prepared local anesthetic solutions containing epinephrine are not used by us—they have a high acid pH and the action of epinephrine is not as effective.

Heat Sterilization: Both epinephrine and phenylephrine can be heat sterilized (autoclaved) at least once without deterioration (for method of autoclaving see page 51).

Precautions: Regional procedures performed below the wrist or ankle for operations on the fingers or toes are to be discouraged. However, if they are performed, vasoconstrictor drugs should be omitted from the solution because they increase the chance of gangrene of the part.

In the geriatric patient, the thyrotoxic patient, the outpatient, and the patient with high blood pressure, vasoconstrictor agents usually should be omitted from the local anesthetic solution.

DOSAGE AND CONCENTRATION OF VASOCONSTRICTOR DRUGS USED TO PROLONG DURATION OF LOCAL ANESTHETIC SOLUTIONS

Epinephrine (Adrenalin)

Dosage.—0.1 cc. to 0.25 cc. of 1:1000 solution added to any amount up to 100 cc. or more of local anesthetic solution irrespective of concentration of the latter.

Optimal Concentration.—For the best results in regional block procedures, excluding spinal block, epinephrine should be used in a final concentration of 1:200,000, *i.e.*, 0.1 cc. of 1:1000 epinephrine per 20 cc. of a local anesthetic solution. Exceeding a dose of 0.25 cc. of 1:1000 epinephrine at any one time, raises the incidence of reactions even in those patients who have received adequate premedication. Furthermore, if 0.25 cc. of epinephrine 1:1000 is not exceeded, it is unlikely to cause difficulty even in the patient with heart disease. Therefore, we seldom exceed a dosage of 0.25 cc. of 1:1000 solution of epinephrine even though more than 50 cc. of the local anesthetic solution is employed for a peripheral nerve block. Consequently, the vasoconstrictor concentration of many of our solutions is below the optimal. However, tetracaine (Pontocaine) is our drug of choice for peripheral nerve blocks and, even with concentrations of epinephrine below the optimum level, analgesia lasts from 4 to 6 hours.

For spinal block, 0.2 cc. of epinephrine 1:1000 is added to the local anesthetic solution to be injected into the subarachnoid space regardless of the volume of solution or the milligram dose of the local anesthetic drug. It has been our experience that: (1) this is the optimal dose of epinephrine in the subarachnoid space; (2) increasing the amount of epinephrine will not significantly prolong the duration of analgesia; and (3) this amount of epinephrine prolongs the duration of analgesia, particularly intra-abdominal analgesia, by approximately 50 percent, *i.e.*, tetracaine alone provides approximately 1½ hours of analgesia and tetracaine with 0.2 cc. epinephrine 1:1000 provides 2 to 2¼ hours of analgesia. Analgesia or hypesthesia of the perineum and lower extremities is prolonged for even a longer time, *e.g.*, 2¼ to 5 hours.

Phenylephrine (Neo-Synephrine)

Dosage.—For peripheral nerve block 0.2 to 0.3 cc. of a one percent solution (2 to 3 mg.). For spinal block 0.2 to 0.5 cc. of a one percent solution (2 to 5 mg.).

Optimal Concentration.—Phenylephrine is not employed by us to prolong the duration of local infiltration, field block, peripheral nerve block, caudal block, or epidural block. But, it is used by some physicians and a concentration of 1:20,000 is optimal. However, no more than 2 to 3 mg. of this drug should be added regardless of the volume of solution; otherwise, toxic reactions to this vasoconstrictor drug will occur more frequently.

For spinal block, particularly for a long intra-abdominal procedure (3 to 4 hours), 5 mg. (0.5 cc. of a 1.0 percent solution) of phenylephrine is added to the local anesthetic solution to be injected into the subarachnoid space regardless of the volume of solution or milligram dose of the local anesthetic drug. This amount of phenylephrine has been used by us with procaine (Novocain) and tetracaine (Pontocaine) but not with any other local anesthetic agents, and it prolongs the duration of these two local drugs by 100 percent, *e.g.*, tetracaine alone provides 1½ hours of analgesia and tetracaine with 5 mg. (0.5 cc.) of phenylephrine provides 2¼ to 3½ hours of analgesia. It is our finding in intra-abdominal surgery that, unlike epinephrine, a small amount of phenylephrine 2 mg. (0.2 cc. of a 1 percent solution) does not prolong the duration of analgesia to the same extent as 5 mg. (0.5 cc.). While 5 mg. of phenylephrine injected subcutaneously, intramuscularly, intravenously, or into the epidural space would produce a severe hypertension, it does not do so when injected into the subarachnoid space. This is true probably because the blood supply to the spinal cord is relatively poor and is limited to small blood vessels which are constricted immediately by the vasoconstrictor drug, thereby automatically delaying rapid absorption.

When a solution of tetracaine with 5 mg. of phenylephrine is injected into the subarachnoid space, operating analgesia of the perineum and lower extremities is prolonged 5 to 8 hours. Furthermore, in some cases transient leg hypesthesias may last 8 to 12 hours and this should not cause the anesthetist using this vasoconstrictor drug in the subarachnoid space consternation.

SYSTEMIC TOXIC REACTIONS TO VASOCONSTRICTOR DRUGS

Allergic Reactions: Angioneurotic edema, urticaria, etc., evidence of a true allergy, have not been observed with either epinephrine (Adrenalin) or phenylephrine (Neo-Synephrine).

In the asthmatic patient who has resorted to self-administered epinephrine for relief, skin slough may occur from sensitization when epinephrine is injected into the skin or subcutaneous tissue. This type of local reaction is generally attributed to an Arthus phenomenon. Such a reaction has not been observed by us.

High Blood Level: This type of reaction is not rare and may resemble the initial stage, *i.e.*, stimulation stage, of a toxic systemic reaction to a local anesthetic agent. However, when the reaction is caused by the vasoconstrictor drug, the blood pressure and pulse rate are increased and remain elevated; but when the reaction is caused by the local anesthetic agent, hypotension may rapidly follow the initial rise in blood pressure and pulse. Therefore, frequent checks of the blood pressure and pulse will usually reveal the cause of the reaction.

Signs and Symptoms.—The common signs and symptoms of a high blood level of a vasoconstrictor drug are: pallor, tachycardia, perspiration, palpitation, apprehension, dyspnea and rapid respirations, and hypertension.

Arrhythmias in cardiac rate and rhythm occasionally may occur following the administration of local anesthetic agents, vasoconstrictor drugs or a combination of these. Therefore, when epinephrine or "epinephrine-like" substances are incorporated in local anesthetic solutions and an irregularity develops, it may be due to the vasoconstrictor drug, to the local anesthetic agent, or to both. The type of irregularity usually seen with a vasoconstrictor drug is a coupling of premature auricular contractions with a normal sinus beat. This is not due to any action on the AV node or the conductive system of the heart but is caused by an irritation of the auricle which discharges just after the refractory period of the SA node. With the dosages of local anesthetic and vasoconstrictor drugs advocated in this book, irregularities from either agent are rare.

Treatment.—Oxygen by bag and mask is usually all that is necessary. If apprehension or hypertension is severe, intravenous thiopental (Pentothal) in very small doses, 50 mg., repeated at one minute intervals, is usually sufficient.

Chlorpromazine (Thorazine, Largactil, etc.) reverses the action of epinephrine. Therefore, a small intravenous dosage (12 to 15 mg.) may be administered when the signs and symptoms of a systemic reaction from a high blood level of epinephrine do not subside in response to other therapy. Certainly its use should be considered if a massive dose of epinephrine which may be fatal is injected inadvertently. If the desired effects from the small initial injection are not obtained, additional 5 mg. dosages may be given at intervals of 3 to 5 minutes. It should be warned that a large initial dosage of chlorpromazine (50 mg.) should not be given intravenously as it normally causes a precipitous fall in blood pressure which may respond only to a rapid intravenous drip of levarterenol (Levophed) or phenylephrine (see page 9).

REMARKS

Choice of Agent for Supplementation of Inadequate Regional Analgesia When the Solution Injected Contained Epinephrine: If it is necessary to supplement a regional block procedure other than a spinal block (absorption from the subarachnoid space is slow) with an inhalation agent, the inhalation agent must be chosen carefully. Cyclopropane should not be the agent selected when epinephrine is employed in the blocking solution unless one hour has elapsed from the time the block was completed. Also, a solution containing epinephrine should never be injected when cyclopropane is being administered. Regardless of the amount of epinephrine, the use of cyclopropane in conjunction with it is a perfect combination for bringing on cardiac irregularities, especially ventricular fibrillation.

Whether trichlorethylene (Trilene, Trimar) or halothane (Fluothane) can be administered, is open to debate. The amount of epinephrine used or to be used appears to be the limiting factor. During trichlorethylene or halothane anesthesia, local solutions containing epinephrine may be employed provided: (1) adequate ventilation is assured; (2) epinephrine in a solution of 1:100,000 to 1:200,000 is used; and (3) the dose does not exceed 10 cc. of 1:100,000 epinephrine in any given ten-minute period or 30 cc. within the hour. These criteria would preclude the use of halothane or trichlorethylene to supplement regional analgesia other than a spinal block when the local anesthetic solution contains 0.2 cc. or more of epinephrine 1:1000, unless an interval of one hour has elapsed from the time the block was completed. Whether the other fluorinated hydrocarbons, *e.g.*, methoxyflurane (Penthrane) or fluroxene (Fluoromar), can be used safely in such a situation has not been resolved completely.

Nitrous oxide, barbiturates, muscle relaxants, narcotics, promethazine, or combinations of these are the agents of choice to supplement inadequate regional anesthesia.

Severe Hypertension After the Use of Vasoconstrictor and Oxytocic Drugs: Because of the many advantages for both the mother and the baby, the number of deliveries performed each year with the use of regional block is steadily increasing. When a subarachnoid, caudal, or epidural block is administered, vasoconstrictor drugs may be used intravenously or intramuscularly to prevent or correct a precipitous fall in blood pressure. If local infiltration of the perineum, paracervical block, pudendal nerve block, or a combination of these blocks is used, the local anesthetic solution often contains a vasoconstrictor drug to prolong analgesia and prevent rapid absorption of the local anesthetic agent. During or immediately after the delivery of a baby, it is not unusual for an oxytocic drug to be given.

Too few physicians are aware that a severe, persistent, dangerous hypertension and even rupture of a cerebral blood vessel which may cause brain damage and hemiplegia can result from the combined effect of vasoconstrictor and oxytocic drugs which have been administered to a patient within three to six hours of one another. While such a catastrophe is more likely to result from the combination of these drugs, it may occur from the use of either drug alone.

Because of the adrenolytic action of chlorpromazine (Thorazine), it is the drug of choice to resolve a severe hypertension resulting from the use of a vasoconstrictor, an oxytocic drug, or a combination of these drugs. The dosage of chlorpromazine is 12.5 to 15 mg. This is given immediately intravenously, at a rate of 2.5 mg. every 15 seconds, until there is either a satisfactory reduction in blood pressure or 12.5 to 15 mg. of the drug has been given. To calibrate the administration of the chlorpromazine hydrochloride, 1 cc. (25 mg.) of the drug is diluted to 10 cc. in a 10 cc. syringe by the addition of 9 cc. of isotonic sodium chloride solution or distilled water. Then each cubic centimeter of solution contains 2.5 mg. of chlorpromazine hydrochloride and may easily be injected as stated. If, after injection of 15 mg. of chlorpromazine hydrochloride, the patient's blood pressure has not fallen to normal, at least two minutes should be allowed to pass before more of the drug is given.

Intravenous administration of chlorpromazine hydrochloride must be carefully done, especially if the full effects of a spinal block, an epidural block, or a caudal block are still present. Too large a dose of chlorpromazine or too rapid administration, or both, in the presence of one of these types of analgesia, may result in a precipitous fall in blood pressure. When the full effects of these blocks are present, the initial dose of chlorpromazine should not exceed 6 to 10 mg.

While this problem usually occurs with administration of regional block anesthesia and obstetrical delivery, the hazards of the concomitant use of vasoconstrictor and oxytocic drugs exist regardless of the type of anesthesia induced or whether or not it is given to a pregnant woman or other patient.

Neurologic Sequelae from the Use of Vasoconstrictor Drugs in the Subarachnoid Space: Some neurologists are skeptical about the use of vasoconstrictor drugs in the subarachnoid space and believe that these drugs could produce neurologic sequelae. They base their reasoning on the sparsity and anatomical abnormalities of the blood supply to the spinal cord. During the past twenty-three years, we have performed in excess of 12,000 spinal blocks. In more than 9,000 of these spinal blocks, procaine (Novocain) or tetracaine (Pontocaine) and a vasoconstrictor drug were used without any permanent complications— ephedrine sulfate in 85 patients; epinephrine (Adrenalin) in 7,000 patients; and phenyleph-

rine (Neo-Synephrine) in 2,000 patients. Therefore, it seems reasonable to conclude that when these time-tested vasoconstrictor drugs are used in the subarachnoid space to prolong single-dose spinal block from either procaine or tetracaine, the chances are infinitesimal that these vasoconstrictor drugs will produce spinal cord damage.

Should a Vasoconstrictor Drug Be Used Prophylactically?: The answer is *NO*. It was once believed that vasoconstrictor drugs did no particular harm. Therefore, they have been given by us and others "prophylactically" prior to spinal block, epidural block, caudal block, and celiac plexus block to prevent hypotension. Now, we do not use vasoconstrictor drugs prophylactically because of the following reasons: (1) many patients to whom such blocks are administered do not develop a hypotension; (2) usually, the interval of time between the intramuscular injection of the vasoconstrictor drug and the administration of the regional block is not sufficient to allow the vasoconstrictor drug to exert its full effect; (3) often the dosage of the vasoconstrictor drug is inadequate and does not prevent the hypotension; and (4) the vasoconstrictor drug either alone or in conjunction with another drug, e.g., an oxytocic, may produce a severe complication. However, we carefully monitor all patients and when hypotension occurs, immediately administer intravenously a vasoconstrictor drug, usually a phenylephrine (Neo-Synephrine) drip, until the blood pressure rises to a reasonable level.

CHAPTER 6

Hyaluronidase

GENERAL CONSIDERATIONS

Action: Hyaluronic acid, which is found in the interstitial spaces of the tissues, normally obstructs diffusion of invasive substances. Hyaluronidase is considered to be an enzyme which allows solutions to spread in the tissue by inactivating the hyaluronic acid.

Advantages: *Spreading Effect.*—Hyaluronidase is particularly effective in the subcutaneous and areolar tissues of the body. Hyaluronidase, by allowing rapid spread of the local anesthetic solution, tends to reduce the tumefaction normally caused by local infiltration. This is of particular importance in plastic surgery, especially that of the head and neck.

Nontoxic.—Hyaluronidase is not toxic to the tissues and will not cause them to slough. Allergic reactions to hyaluronidase may occur but they are insignificant.

Speeds Onset of Block.—The interval between the completion of a block and the establishment of operating analgesia seems to be shortened by the hyaluronidase.

Prevention of Hematoma.—When a blood vessel is punctured by the needle and bleeding results, a hematoma will not develop if the local anesthetic solution contains hyaluronidase. Furthermore, the absorption of the blood is facilitated.

Disadvantages: *Anatomic Structures Limit Spread.*—Fasciae, fascial planes, periosteum, and fibrin walls act as barriers to the spread of solutions containing hyaluronidase.

Too Extensive Block.—Therapeutic and diagnostic blocks are not aided by hyaluronidase and its use may result in mistaken diagnosis caused by an extensive spread of anesthetic solution.

May Shorten Duration of Analgesia.—Without a vasoconstrictor drug in the solution in which hyaluronidase is used, the duration of operating analgesia is greatly reduced. When epinephrine (Adrenalin) is added to the local anesthetic solutions, hyaluronidase does not affect the operating analgesia time nor does the epinephrine affect the diffusion caused by the hyaluronidase.

DOSAGE

150 TRU (turbidity reducing units) is adequate for any amount of solution necessary for a regional block. 150 TRU may be used in 10 cc. as well as 200 cc.

REMARKS

No Substitute for Anatomical Knowledge: The use of hyaluronidase is in no way a substitute for anatomical knowledge in regional analgesia. The needles must be placed correctly.

Increases Toxic Reaction: Concentrations and volumes being equal, toxic reactions to local anesthetic agents and vasoconstrictor drugs are more frequent when hyaluronidase is employed. When hyaluronidase is incorporated in the anesthetic solution, smaller volumes of solution may be used. Nevertheless, the large absorptive area caused by the spreading factor, hyaluronidase, may yield a blood concentration of local anesthetic agent equal to or higher than that which occurs when a larger volume of anesthetic agent without hyaluronidase is employed.

Use of Hyaluronidase: In this book, all blocks where hyaluronidase may be used to advantage will have the fact noted under dosage.

CHAPTER 7

Conditions Influencing the Selection of Regional Anesthesia

GENERAL COMMENT

THIS IS a difficult subject to consider since every doctor, not to mention the specialist in anesthesia, has his own method of meeting a particular problem. Field block, local infiltration, and nerve block are probably the safest of all anesthetic procedures. Epidural (peridural), spinal (subarachnoid), and caudal blocks are also classified as regional anesthetic procedures, but are less safe. It is admitted that there are numerous ways of meeting the same anesthetic problem. Nevertheless, the following discussion indicates some situations in which regional anesthesia may or may not be preferred. Obviously, all situations cannot be covered and only the common problems can be considered.

SITUATIONS WHERE REGIONAL ANESTHESIA MAY BE PREFERRED

Availability of Types of Anesthesia: In various localities the equipment and personnel for giving anesthesia differ immensely. Often there is a lack of anesthetic equipment and trained personnel are not available. The general practitioner often finds that providing anesthesia is a responsibility he must assume in addition to his more normal work.

Outpatients: When adult patients are to leave the office following an anesthetic procedure, the use of regional block should be given careful consideration. Inasmuch as general anesthetic agents may leave the patient amnesic for some time, even though he appears normal, they should be used with care. Also, when general anesthesia is employed in an office practice, more anesthetic emergencies arise than with regional methods.

Emergencies: In the face of emergencies where little is known about the patient in regard to his physical status, regional analgesia should always be evaluated. If shock is caused by pain, it may be corrected immediately by relief of the pain by block procedure. This is especially true in the case of a crushed extremity. In cases where shock is caused by blood loss, regional procedures may still be the anesthesia of choice for extremity work, as the hemorrhage may be controlled by a tourniquet. However, spinal, caudal, or epidural blocks should be avoided in most cases of hemorrhage because the vascular dilatation produced by them is usually not limited to a small area.

Food in the Stomach: A patient who comes to an operation, whether for a major or minor procedure, who has recently ingested food, is appraised with great respect by most anesthetists. Vomiting of food with aspiration is a serious complication and should always be thought of in any situation requiring anesthesia. Many doctors have the false impression that if the patient hasn't eaten for six to eight hours before surgery, the stomach has emptied its contents. This is an unjustified assumption. A nervous patient or one who has been injured may not empty his stomach for 24 to 36 hours. This is especially true in an injured patient with pain or shock, and morphine in these patients does not help since it causes a pylorospasm. The stomach pump should be used on these patients, but even then, all the food will probably not be removed. Even if a rapid induction and intubation with a cuffed endotracheal tube avoid the dangers of aspiration during induction, the postoperative period is also to be considered. Vomiting and aspiration may occur at any time. Therefore, regional anesthesia is probably the procedure of choice in these situations as the patient is fully conscious and can maintain his own airway.

Prone Position: When anesthesia is complicated and surgery facilitated by this position, the patient's airway should be established before he is placed on his abdomen. If general anesthesia is employed and this category includes intravenous anesthesia, the patient should be intubated. When personnel or equipment is not available to carry out intubation of the trachea, regional anesthesia is the procedure of choice.

Geriatric Patient: This type of patient is usually ideal for a regional anesthetic procedure if it is not contraindicated by surgery or associated diseases. Many of these patients are stoic and would rather not be put to sleep. Regional analgesia causes minimal disturbances to physiological processes and such patients recover rapidly from the effects of local anesthetic agents.

Climate and Altitude: In extremely hot dry climates administration of general anesthesia may be fraught with complications. CO_2 retention and heat retention, which occur more frequently under general anesthesia, may be difficult to eliminate unless there is adequate personnel and equipment. The ever-present possibility of static electricity with an explosion must be weighed. Where towns are located 8,000 to 9,000 feet above sea level, regional anesthesia is much easier to administer than inhalation techniques because of the laws of partial pressure. In such a situation one should realize that oxygen should be given throughout the procedure, especially if a spinal, caudal, or epidural block has been executed.

Surgery Above the Neck: The main problem in surgery about the head is to establish and keep a patent airway. If general anesthesia is chosen, the patient should be intubated. Situations which require permanent closure of the mouth for a fixed period of time, such as wiring of a fractured jaw, may be done under nasotracheal intubation. Still these patients are a problem postoperatively. They may vomit or aspirate or the mandible may drop posteriorly because of loss of muscular tone, allowing the tongue to obstruct the airway. Should personnel and equipment be inadequate to perform intubation or tracheotomy, then regional analgesia is invaluable as it allows the patient to maintain his own airway.

Cooperation of the Patient: In some operations the assistance of the conscious patient may facilitate surgery. This is true in thyroid surgery, where damage to the laryngeal nerve may be detected immediately by changes in phonation. Also, when repairing tendons, a block may be employed to eliminate sensory sensations while motor function is preserved, for example, a wrist block for repair of lacerated finger tendons.

Diseases

Diabetes.—It is generally agreed that the diabetic who is well controlled will tolerate most anesthetic techniques as long as undue hypoxia is avoided. This is particularly true if the surgery is elective and the patient made to enter the hospital a few days before the operation. However, in the presence of infection or an emergency, the best-controlled diabetic may have difficulty, and in these patients regional anesthesia, especially local infiltration, field block, and nerve block, is the procedure of choice. If spinal block, caudal block, or epidural block is used, oxygen should be administered continuously to avoid hypoxia. It should be remembered that one of the sequelae of diabetes is arteriosclerosis, often with an accompanying hypertension. In these cases, field block, nerve block, or spinal block below the umbilicus (T10) may be used. It is best to avoid high spinal blocks or any regional procedure that may cause a precipitous fall in blood pressure in these cases.

Hypertension and Coronary Heart Disease.— Local infiltration, field block, or nerve block —spinal, caudal, and epidural blocks not included—is ideal for patients whose anesthetic problem is complicated by these diseases. It may be best to omit a vasoconstrictor agent, although the amounts advocated herein have not caused difficulties. Where these blocks cannot be applied, general anesthesia with a high oxygen content is probably the safest. Spinal, caudal, and epidural blocks are best avoided because of the accompanying precipitous and often persistent hypotension which may follow. It is of utmost importance in these patients to prevent a fall of the diastolic pressure, on which the coronary blood flow depends. If spinal, caudal, or epidural block is used, drugs and equipment to correct hypotension must be immediately available.

Decompensated Heart Disease.—These patients should always be evaluated with regional analgesia in mind. There is little question but that local infiltration, field block, and nerve block — spinal, caudal, and epidural blocks not included — are the anesthesia of choice where applicable in these conditions. Many anesthesiologists feel that spinal, caudal, or epidural block is a safe procedure since the load on the heart is reduced. However, these patients tolerate general anesthesia with high oxygen content well, and undue risks should not be undertaken.

Cerebrovascular Accidents.—Patients who fall in this category and come to surgery are problems. If they have any residual paralysis in the region to be operated on, it is best from a medicolegal standpoint to avoid regional anesthesia; otherwise, regional as well as general anesthesia may be given, depending on other complications such as hypertension, arteriosclerosis, etc.

Respiratory Disease.—When a patient with a cold, pneumonia, tuberculosis, or any of the many lung complications comes to surgery, again local infiltration, field block, and nerve block, if applicable, are usually the procedures of choice. Although general anesthesia for intra-abdominal surgery administered by a skilled anesthetist may not be fraught with more postoperative complications than a spinal, caudal, or epidural block,

if a skilled anesthetist is not available, regional analgesia should be carefully considered.

Urinary Diseases.—Any type of anesthesia may be tolerated, but when renal function is poor, it should be remembered that it may be temporarily further embarrassed by general anesthetic agents. Anurias may at times be corrected by regional techniques, *i.e.*, spinal, epidural, caudal, or deep splanchnic (celiac plexus) block.

SITUATIONS WHERE REGIONAL ANESTHESIA MAY NOT BE PREFERRED

Age: In general, the young patient for whom comprehension of the situation and the ability to cooperate is difficult, should be treated under general anesthesia. However, if other situations require a regional block it may be accomplished without difficulty if the patient is correctly sedated. Divided doses of rectal thiopental (Pentothal) or minute doses (50 mg. to 100 mg.) of intravenous thiopental have been very satisfactory in producing just the right level of sedation in young patients. Other barbiturates and opiates may be equally successful. It should be emphasized here that children, if correctly medicated, tolerate all types of regional anesthesia extremely well. However, it is usually best to leave its administration to the specialist in anesthesia who has had experience with pediatric anesthesia.

Hysteria: A patient who is subject to hysterical attacks is usually not a suitable candidate for regional anesthesia, for he may become unmanageable. If regional analgesia in these cases is a necessity, the patient should be heavily medicated or rendered unconscious with intravenous or general anesthesia while the regional procedure is executed.

Malingering: Whenever a patient is known to be a trouble maker, it is best to avoid regional anesthesia. These patients may often feign headaches or backaches following spinal, caudal, and epidural blocks, or weakness and paralysis following other nerve blocks.

Nervous System Diseases: Whenever pre-existing neurological disorders, such as headaches, cerebral accidents, and degenerative conditions of the spinal cord or peripheral nervous system are present, the possibility of a medicolegal suit should be evaluated before administering a spinal, caudal, epidural, or nerve block (see page 10 to 11).

Anemias: Patients with anemias caused by frank hemorrhage usually tolerate spinal, caudal, or epidural block poorly unless the hemorrhage is controlled and adequate replacement therapy is instituted before the anesthesia is given. In pernicious anemia, spinal, epidural, and caudal blocks are avoided since spinal cord degeneration may be accelerated by the procedure. If regional anesthesia is selected in other cases of anemias as the procedure of choice, oxygen should be given and the blood pressure maintained with a vasoconstrictor drug until the anesthetic agent dissipates itself. This will prevent a stagnant hypoxia from being superimposed on the chronic hypoxia which is present from the pre-existing anemia.

Skin Infections: Under no circumstances should one invade an infected area to execute a regional block procedure.

Septicemia: In the presence of septicemia, nerve blocks should be performed only if the anesthetist realizes that he may create an abscess at the site of puncture or any place along the path of the needle.

CHAPTER 8

Regional Anesthesia in an Office Practice

GENERAL COMMENT

One of the routine questions asked by many doctors who are observing the execution of a regional block is: "Can I employ this block in my office?" Most regional procedures can be done in the office, at least those which involve minor surgery and therapeutic and diagnostic blocks. It is assumed that only under unusual circumstances would a doctor give regional anesthesia in the office or home for an intra-abdominal or major procedure.

A patient should never be allowed to leave the doctor's office if regional anesthesia has been employed until he has been observed at least one hour.

EQUIPMENT NECESSARY

Autoclave: Adequate means of sterilizing block equipment and drugs should be available.

Treatment of Complications: Resuscitation facilities as outlined in Chapter 9, page 52, are absolutely necessary.

Recovery Area: It is advisable to have a recovery room where the patient may rest for one to four hours following the block.

Additional Help: The usual amount of help, *i.e.*, a nurse, should be on hand.

INSTRUCTIONS TO THE PATIENT

Oral Intake: Fluids should be withheld for the four hours prior to an elective procedure; solids should be withheld longer. This precaution is emphasized so that the patient will not have a large amount of food or liquid in his stomach should a complication arise.

Premedication: If sedation is indicated which is to be taken before coming to the office, a friend should accompany the patient. It is best to give intravenous sedation when the patient arrives at the office rather than have him take it orally at home. If the patient is treated away from home, whether he is given sedation or not, he should be escorted home. Following the injection of a local anesthetic agent or the administration of sedation, any accident, whether it occurs before the patient enters the office, in the office, or on the way home, may involve the doctor in an embarrassing legal situation.

Recovery Period: Following the injection of a local anesthetic agent, the patient should rest in the doctor's recovery room for a determined period of time and then go directly home to rest.

Position of Anesthetized Part: When an extremity is anesthetized, the patient should be instructed to watch the position in which he places the extremity in order to avoid a neurological complication from pressure. Also, if the extremity has any pressure points from a cast, they should be corrected as soon as noticed.

Inform Patient of Possible Complications: The patient should be warned of complications that may follow block procedures so that he does not become alarmed if they occur; for example, hoarseness following the anterior approach to the stellate ganglion or the tendency to walk toward the anesthetized side following a brachial block. He should be reassured that these are only temporary.

ANESTHETIC DRUG CONSIDERATIONS

Dosage of Local Anesthetic Agent: The weakest concentration and the smallest amount of the anesthetic solution which will produce the desired effect for the contemplated block should be used.

Amount of Vasoconstrictor Drug: Epinephrine (Adrenalin) or other vasoconstrictor agents should be omitted from the solution or a minimal amount used in office procedures. Many reactions seen in outpatients are caused by the vasoconstrictor agent rather than the local anesthetic agent.

CHAPTER 9

Equipment

REGIONAL BLOCK INSTRU-
MENTARIUM

Syringes: Any type of Lok-syringe may be employed in regional anesthesia. A Lok-syringe with finger rings is preferable. Trays should contain more than one size of syringe so that any type of requirement may be met.

Needles: Lok security (bead) type with sharp, short, beveled points are the needles of choice. Most needles break at the junction of the shaft with the hub, and the security (bead) needle prevents insertion to the hub of the needle. The short beveled point assures a more accurate placement of the anesthetic solution and less chance of breakage or bending of the point. A Greene point needle is preferable for spinal anesthesia. Needles should be replaced at least once a year and the old ones discarded. Repeated sterilization tends to make them brittle. When needles are bent below the security bead they should be discarded, not straightened. Bending causes a focal point of weakness and the needles may break at that point under minimal stress.

Measuring Cups: Stainless steel cups are preferred to glass both from the standpoint of durability and because the alkalinity factor does not have to be considered. Many glass receptacles are highly alkaline and may affect the acidity of the local anesthetic solution. Porcelain cups are not recommended because of chipping and consequent rusting of the deporcelainized area.

Trays: A deep-edged instrument tray is preferred to a low-edged one. It protects its contents more efficiently and does not allow needles, etc., to slip over its edges and become contaminated.

Indicators: Each regional tray should contain a sterilizer control or indicator to assure adequate sterilization.

Care of Equipment and Drugs: All the instruments to be used should be carefully and adequately cleaned. Both the instruments and drugs should be heat sterilized.

Cleaning.—A number of detergent products, *e.g.*, Haemo-Sol, Detergex, etc., for cleaning needles and syringes are available, but there is less risk if soap and water or water only are used, for reports show that detergent cleansers have been responsible for cord degeneration. The following steps are meticulously performed by us:

1. The needles and syringes are washed with copious amounts of clear tap water.

2. A rinse with ether follows.

3. The needle hubs are swabbed out with an applicator dipped in ether.

Sterilization.—Every attempt should be made to assure the sterility of the local anesthetic solution. The author never uses hospital-prepared solutions for any regional block procedure. All drugs and solvents are autoclaved in the trays together with the necessary syringes and needles. Autoclaving in this fashion serves a dual purpose: first, it precludes infection should the pharmaceutical manufacturer dispense a contaminated solution; and, second, it resterilizes the crystals should a small, invisible crack in the glass occur during handling of the sealed ampule. Autoclaving also sterilizes a gummed label, although cold sterilization with solutions does not. All the local anesthetic agents in Table I, page 13, and solutions of them can be heat sterilized at least once. It is re-emphasized that epinephrine (Adrenalin) and phenylephrine (Neo-Synephrine) may be heat sterilized. If overheated, dextrose may caramelize; if this happens, it will turn a yellow color and should be discarded. Hyaluronidase cannot be heat sterilized.

Heat sterilization alone is above reproach and consists of the following steps.

1. A sterilizer control (Diack) is placed in each tray as it is wrapped. Sterilizer control tape seals the wrapper.

2. The tray is then autoclaved at 255° to 260° F. under eighteen to twenty-two pounds of pressure for thirty minutes.

3. The pressure is released from the autoclave and the steam evacuated. The tray is dried by creating a vacuum in the sterilizer for ten minutes, following which the sterilizer door is opened and the tray is left in the opened autoclave for an additional ten minutes. With the newest autoclave, steps 2 and 3 are automatically performed and heat temperatures are in the range of 280° F. for three minutes and the entire cycle requires twenty-five minutes.

4. Once the tray is dry, it is stored on a shelf away from all solutions (Figure 5B, page 53). This point is stressed, for if solutions are unsuspectedly spilled on the tray, it may become contaminated even though the sterilizer controls show adequate sterilization when they are checked.

5. When the tray is opened for use, the sterilizer controls are examined to assure adequate sterilization. This precaution serves as a valuable check on the sterilizer and the personnel operating it.

Cold Sterilization: Equipment and drugs should not be sterilized in alcohol, formaldehyde, etc. If in an emergency this is a necessity, the equipment should be rinsed carefully in sterile normal saline before it is used.

Cold sterilization with ethylene oxide freon mixtures will sterilize equipment and the outside of vials and ampules. A period from 24 to 72 hours to permit the ethylene oxide freon mixture to escape should elapse before using the equipment.

Regional Tray (Figure 4, page 52)

Standard Tray.—Trays should be so constructed that they meet the requirements of most regional techniques to be done. One tray to meet most demands can be assembled. Such a tray would include the following items:

1. One 10 cc. Lok-syringe, with finger rings.

2. One 10 cc. Lok-syringe.

3. One 5 cc. Lok-syringe.

4. One 3 cc. Lok-syringe.

5. One tuberculin Lok-syringe to measure epinephrine (Adrenalin).

6. Two ¾-inch (2 cm.), 25-gauge, Huber point security Lok-needles (short bevel).

7. Three 1½-inch (3.8 cm.), 22-guage, security Lok-needles (short bevel).

8. Two 2-inch (5 cm.), 22-gauge, security Lok-needles (short bevel).

9. Three 3-inch (7.5 cm.), 22-gauge, security Lok-needles (short bevel).

10. Three 4-inch (10 cm.), 22-gauge, security Lok-needles (short bevel).

11. One 250 cc. stainless steel graduated measure for mixing solution.

12. Two 60 cc. stainless steel medicine cups.

13. One 1½-inch (3.8 cm.), 18-gauge Lok-needle (for mixing solutions).

14. One Pitkin or thin-walled needle guide.

15. One 3½-inch (9 cm.), 21- or 22-gauge Lok-spinal needle with a Greene point.

16. One 3-inch (7.5 cm.), 19-gauge Lok-spinal needle.

17. One 6-inch (15 cm.) stainless steel ruler.

18. One Allis forceps.

19. One sponge forceps.

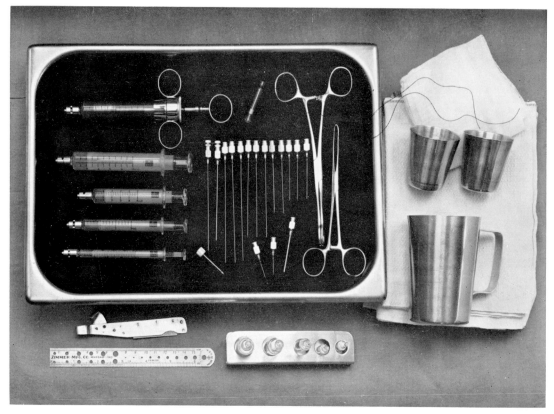

Figure 4. Regional block tray and its contents. The tray is a stainless steel food container for a steam table and may be obtained from any restaurant supply company. Needles, syringes, and needle guides may be obtained from Becton, Dickinson and Company, Rutherford, N. J. The 250 cc. graduated stainless steel measuring cup, the prep cups, the Allis forceps, the sponge forceps, and the sterilizer control (Diack) may be obtained from American Hospital Supply, Evanston, Illinois. The stainless steel can opener and ampule holder are fabricated to our specification in Seattle, Washington. The stainless steel ruler may be obtained from Zimmer Manufacturing Company, Warsaw, Indiana. Sterilizer controls should be encased in glass; otherwise, the chemical(s) used in them may contaminate the equipment in the tray.

20. Four towels.

21. Six 4-inch x 4-inch gauze dressings.

22. One stainless steel can opener with file in handle to open bottles and ampules.

23. One stainless steel ampule holder.

24. One sterilizer control.

25. One stainless steel tray, 14 x 10 x 2½ inches.

Needles Used for Specific Blocks.—For lumbar sympathetic blocks and splanchnic (celiac plexus) blocks the following should be included (Figure 5A, page 53).

1. Three 4-inch (10 cm.), 20-gauge security Lok-needles (short bevel).

2. Three 5-inch (12.5 cm.), 20-gauge security Lok-needles (short bevel).

3. Three 6-inch (15 cm.), 20-gauge security Lok-needles (short bevel).

RESUSCITATION INSTRUMENTARIUM

Every doctor using regional anesthesia should have ready for immediate use the following minimal equipment:

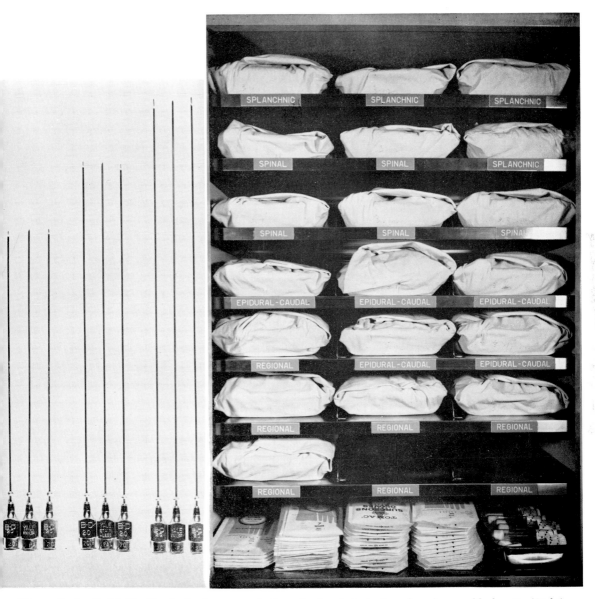

Figure 5. A. *(Left)* Needles for lumbar sympathetic and splanchnic (celiac plexus) nerve blocks. B. *(Right)* Method of storing regional block trays to assure sterility.

Oxygen Apparatus: This need consist of nothing more than a bag and mask with a simple reducing needle valve for the oxygen tank or it may be an anesthetic machine or an Ambu unit (Figure 6A and C, page 54).

Suction Apparatus: If vomiting or excessive secretions occur, it is important to clear the airway. Any type of adequate suction is satisfactory (Figure 6B, page 54).

Airways: Both oral airways and endotracheal tubes should be available (Figure 7, page 55).

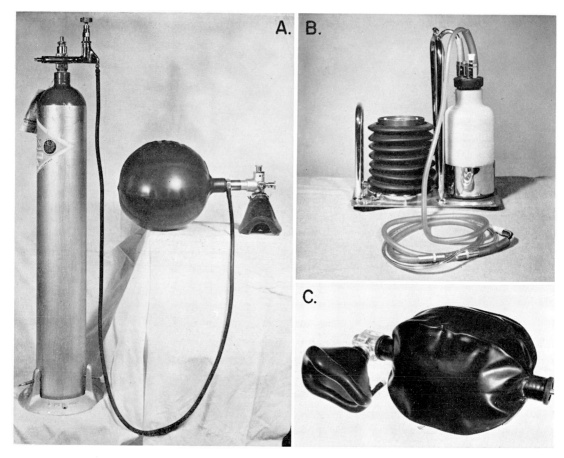

Figure 6. A. Minimal equipment for oxygen therapy, *i.e.*, simple reducing valve, bag, and mask. B. Ambu portable foot suction. This may be used when neither central suction nor an electric suction machine is available. C. Ambu bag. The bag of the Ambu unit automatically expands, eliminating the need of a source of compressed air or oxygen for its inflation. If oxygen is available, a connection on the tail of the bag permits its use. This unit and the unit in illustration B may be obtained from Air Shields, Inc., Hatboro, Pennsylvania.

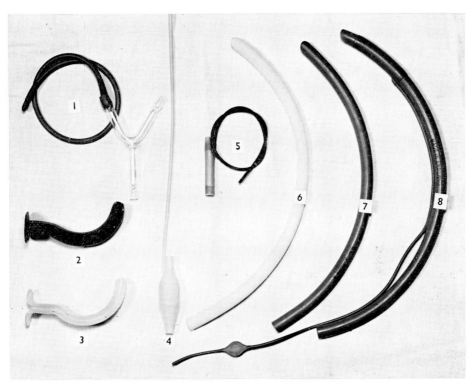

Figure 7. 1. Suction catheter with Y adapter so that intermittent suction may be applied. 2. Guedel oral airway. 3. Berman plastic airway. 4. Sander inflatable cuff for endotracheal tube. 5. Guedel cuff for endotracheal tube. 6. Plastic endotracheal tube. 7. Rubber endotracheal tube. 8. Rubber endotracheal tube with inflatable cuff attached.

Laryngoscope: Laryngoscopy and intubation are often necessary to clear aspirated material from the tracheobronchial tree and to establish an unobstructed airway. Any type of laryngoscope will suffice if the doctor can use it (Figure 8, page 56).

Intravenous Apparatus: Syringes to administer vasoconstrictor drugs, barbiturates, succinylcholine (Anectine) and other drugs should be on hand. Intravenous fluids for supportive therapy should be readily available.

MISCELLANEOUS

"Donuts" (Figure 9, page 56) are not necessary for regional anesthesia, yet they are very convenient when a block of the head is to be performed. They act as a head rest and often stabilize and improve the position.

REMARKS

Lok: The spelling of "lock" in this book as Lok is used since it is the trademark of the lock mechanism which is found on the standard lock syringes and needles used by the author.

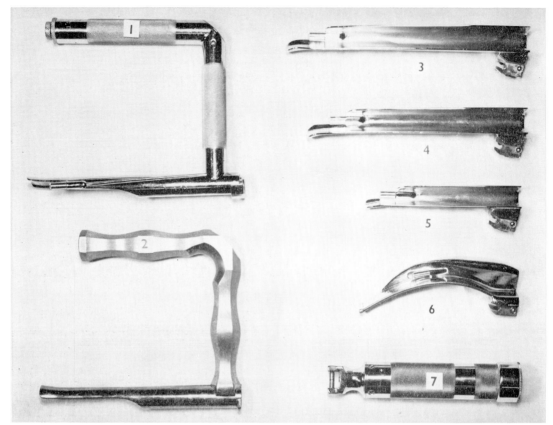

Figure 8. Laryngoscopes. 1. Eversole. 2. Jackson. 3. Large Guedel blade. 4. Medium Guedel blade. 5. Guedel child blade. 6. Macintosh blade. 7. Handle for detachable (hook on) blades.

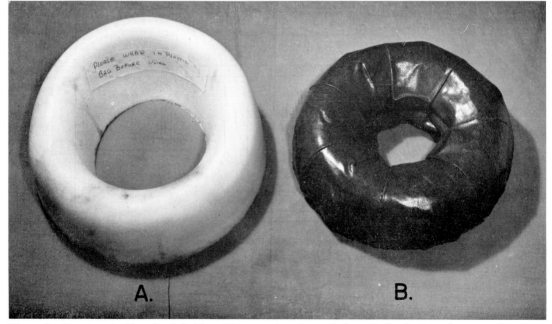

Figure 9. Donuts. A. Shea head holder. This may be obtained from Richards Manufacturing Company, Memphis, Tennessee (Order No. 1248). B. Made by hospital.

CHAPTER 10

Fundamentals of Techniques

PREPARATION FOR REGIONAL BLOCK PROCEDURES

The Patient: The doctor should reassure the patient that he will feel no pain during the surgical procedure and that his cooperation is very important, particularly if the block requires paresthesias.

The patient should be positioned for the block and made as comfortable as possible. The patient should be blocked either on the operating table, operating cart, or examining table. Under no circumstances should the patient sit in a chair. If it is felt that a sitting position facilitates the block, the patient should sit on the operating room cart or table. This precaution is taken in case of a reaction.

Opening of the Tray: Sterile precautions should be used when the block tray is opened, and the mixing graduate and medicine cups should be handled with sterile forceps. The medicine cup should be placed in front of the mixing graduate so that the prep solution will never pass over the anesthetic solution. If any alcoholic solution is dropped in the anesthetic solution and goes unnoticed, a slough of the tissue or a neurological complication may ensue.

The sterilizer control should be examined routinely.

Asepsis: The same sterile precautions should be taken as for an operation.

Use of Gloves and Scrub.—The doctor should wear sterile gloves for at least two reasons: (1) they are no more hindrance to the doctor performing a block than to a surgeon performing a delicate operation, and they do offer an additional safeguard to the aseptic technique; and (2) when a doctor executes a large number of regional procedures it is advisable for his own protection to wear gloves, as occupational allergy to local anesthetic agents is not uncommon (Figure 3, page 33).

Whether a sterile scrub of the hands is a necessity is debatable.

Skin Preparation.—The patient's skin should be prepared with one of the routine surgical preparations (see page 34). If the patient is to leave the office or hospital following the block and cosmetic appearance is a factor, 5 percent iodine solution washed off with alcohol or aqueous merthiolate is satisfactory.

Draping.—The block field should be carefully walled off with sterile towels to assure asepsis. Under no circumstances should this conceal the landmarks or the perspective. Cases used for illustrations in this book were purposely left undraped so that landmarks and positions could be demonstrated.

Types of Landmarks

Superficial.—These may be palpated or visualized and are usually bones, teeth, tendons, or blood vessels.

Deep.—These cannot be seen or palpated and may be felt only with the point of the needle. They are usually bone, periosteum, fascial planes, tendons, or blood vessels. The accuracy of their identification depends for the most part on the educated touch of the anesthetist.

Palpation of Landmarks: The best method of palpation is to feel with one hand and apply pressure with the other (Figure 10, page 58). When the one hand method of palpation is used, the delicate tactile sensitivity of the fingertips is dulled.

Marking of Landmarks: Even the most experienced of regional anesthetists should sketch the landmarks with a skin marking pencil, ball point pen, or a waterproof felt marking pen. The waterproof felt marking pen and the ball point pen are probably the most satisfactory as their marks are the most difficult to erase with aseptic prep solutions.

Once the landmarks are established, the patient should not be allowed to move, since a change of position may alter anatomical relationships.

HANDLING NEEDLES

Check for Patency and Weakness: All needles should be checked for patency before insertion. There is nothing more maddening than to insert a needle, have an excellent placement, and then find that the needle is plugged.

A check for weakness is always a precaution. Most needles break at the junction of the shaft and the hub and if the needle has unconsciously been inserted to the hub, it may require surgery to recover it. This is most embarrassing and may be avoided if security bead needles are employed. If a needle is broken in the tissues, every effort including surgery should be made to recover it.

Use Sharp Needles: The needle point should be checked to be sure it is sharp. A dull point will cause the patient unnecessary pain.

Holding Needles: The open needle should always be held with the thumb and middle (long) finger, grasping the shaft and the index finger resting on the hub (Figure 11, page 59). If the needle is on the end of a syringe as for a brachial plexus or intercostal nerve block, the syringe should be held as shown (Figure 12, page 59). This position

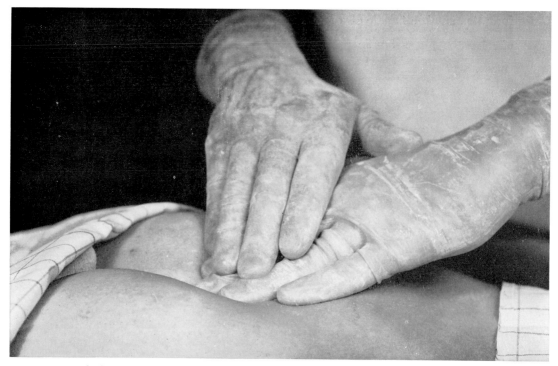

Figure 10. Method of palpating a deep landmark. The anesthetist is right-handed and uses the left hand for feeling while the right hand exerts pressure on the left.

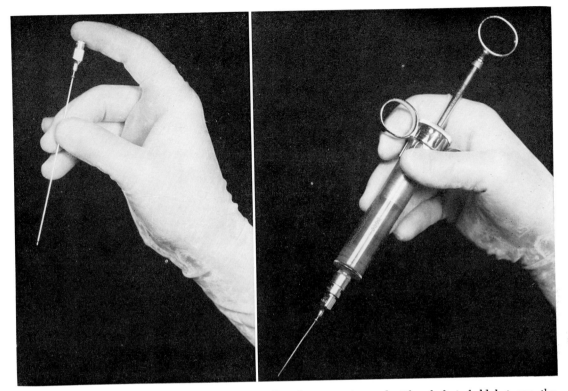

Figure 11. *(Left)* Correct method of holding a needle when it is inserted. The shaft is held between the middle (long) finger and the thumb as the index finger rests on the hub.

Figure 12. *(Right)* Correct method for holding syringe when it contains solution or it is fastened to a needle. The fingers of the anesthetist should not be in the finger controls and the shaft of the plunger should rest against the index finger so that the weight of the plunger does not empty the syringe.

gives good control of the syringe and prevents the plunger from moving.

Insertion of Needle and Changing Its Direction: All needles should be inserted through the hole in the skin made by the needle for the intradermal wheal. There is no reason for having more than one hole per wheal. If it is difficult to insert the needle, the hub should be rotated between the thumb and middle (long) finger, and it will be found to enter easily even the toughest skin.

When changing the direction of a needle, the point should be brought back to the subcutaneous tissues (Figure 13, page 60).

Use of Depth Markers: When care is taken in placing the needles, depth markers are not necessary.

Do Not Bend Point of Needle: Bony landmarks should be approached slowly so as not to damage the point of the needle and tear the tissue on withdrawal (Figure 14, page 60). If a short-beveled point is used as advocated, there is less chance of bending or breaking the point on a bone.

HANDLING THE SYRINGE

Filling the Syringe: The Lok control syringe with finger rings may be filled with ease by inserting the thumb in the piston ring and the index and middle (long) fingers in the barrel rings (Figure 15, page 60). The plunger of the syringe should always be moistened in the anesthetic solution before insertion into the barrel. This will insure a snug-fitting, nonsticking plunger.

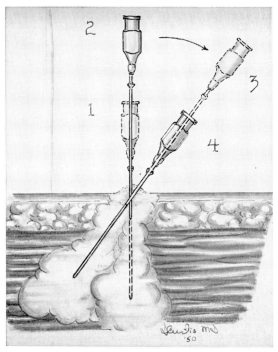

Figure 13. Method of changing direction of the needle. 1. Needle deep in tissue. 2. Needle withdrawn to subcutaneous tissue. 3. Direction of needle changed. 4. Needle reinserted.

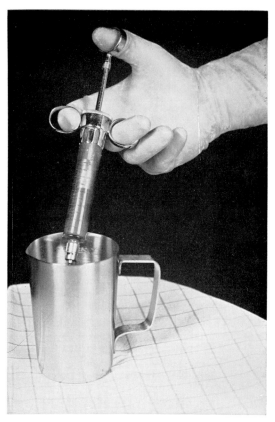

Figure 15. Method of filling the syringe from the stainless steel graduated container.

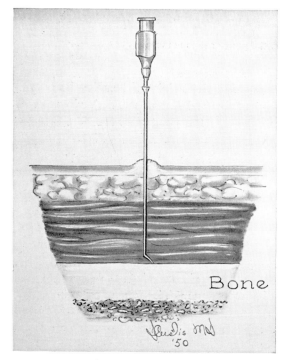

Figure 14. Needle point bent on bone by too rapid insertion of the needle when seeking bony landmarks.

Attaching Needle to the Syringe: When attaching the syringe to the needle, it is best to hold the needle stationary and turn the syringe onto the needle. This will avoid displacement of the needle. In this maneuver the syringe should be held like a pen with the shaft of the plunger resting in the web between the index finger and the thumb (Figure 16, page 61). This prevents the plunger from moving in the syringe. The fingers and thumb should not be kept in the rings since this would make the maneuver clumsy. Occasionally in close quarters it is necessary to spin the needle and hold the syringe stationary to make a tight connection.

METHOD OF MAKING INTRADERMAL WHEALS

The bevel of the needle should be face

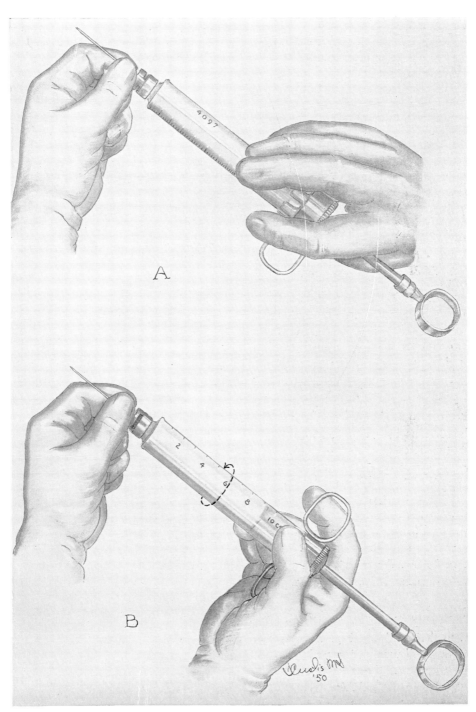

Figure 16. Method of holding syringe and attaching it to needle. A. Syringe placed on needle. B. Syringe rotated 180 degrees to lock the needle to the syringe.

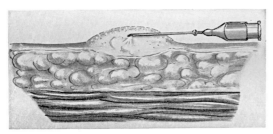

Figure 17. Method of making skin wheal. Note the bevel of the Huber needle points toward the skin surface.

down and parallel to the skin (Figure 17, page 62). A quick thrust of a 25-gauge Huber point needle makes this procedure practically painless.

ASPIRATION TESTS

In any nerve block procedure, whether a large or a small amount of solution is to be placed without movement of the needle, it is imperative to attempt to aspirate blood, spinal fluid, or both in at least two, and preferably four, planes. This is accomplished by rotating the syringe 180 degrees once or 90 degrees three times in a clockwise direction after the first aspiration test, and repeating the aspiration attempt.

After the aspiration test, the open needle should be allowed to remain in position fifteen seconds before injection. It is possible that aspiration may be strong enough to collapse the wall of the vessel or the dura mater against the bevel and not get blood or spinal fluid in the syringe. However, if the above precaution is observed and the needle is in a vessel or subarachnoid space, blood or spinal fluid will usually appear in the allotted fifteen seconds.

Where a field block or local injection is being executed and the needle and syringe are moving backward and forward constantly, aspiration is not important. It is highly unlikely that the needle point will remain in a blood vessel sufficiently long to allow a dangerous amount of anesthetic solution to be injected.

TECHNIQUE OF LOCAL INFILTRATION

This technique requires no explanation as most doctors are already familiar with it. It is merely an infiltrative-as-you-go process. Nevertheless, one cannot expect good anesthesia when the anesthetic solution has been placed haphazardly in the tissues. Injections should be systematic, i.e., first intradermal, then subcutaneous, then intrafascial, then intramuscular, and so on.

The main concern in this type of regional anesthesia is not to exceed the toxic dose of local anesthetic agent.

Hyaluronidase is of value, but not necessary for establishing adequate analgesia with this technique.

TECHNIQUE OF FIELD BLOCK

Field block analgesia is the physiological interruption of the nerve impulses by placing a wall of anesthesia between the operative site and the central nervous system. Here again the anesthesiologist should be careful not to exceed maximum dosage of the local anesthetic agent. No effort is made to anesthetize individual nerves because they are automatically anesthetized in the tissue in which they lie.

Field block may be accomplished in various ways, depending on requirements. First, if the nerves to be anesthetized lie in the subcutaneous tissue, such as the medial brachial cutaneous nerve of the arm, an intracutaneous and subcutaneous infiltration will suffice (Figure 153, page 237). Second, when the nerves supplying a field of operation come from many directions, or where the operation is not extensive, such as small skin grafts (donor or recipient site), papillomas, fibromas, lipomas, and biopsies, the geometrical method is very satisfactory. This consists of outlining the operative site with a geometrical figure, such as a triangle, rhomboid, etc., and projecting the sides to a point in the deep tissues so as to form a pyramid (Figure 18, page 63). Again, it is necessary to be sure all layers are anesthetized, i.e., intradermal, subcutaneous, etc.

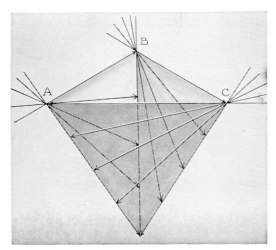

Figure 18. Geometrical method of producing field block analgesia for small operative procedures. Arrows indicate direction of the needle and the placement of the local anesthetic solution.

Lastly, when the nerves supplying the field of operation come from one direction, as in the inguinal region, a wall of anesthesia perpendicular to the surface of the skin involving all the layers (dermal, subcutaneous, fascial, and muscular) in which the nerves lie is adequate (Figure 105, page 170).

Hyaluronidase is of value, but not necessary for establishing adequate analgesia with this technique.

TECHNIQUE OF NERVE BLOCK

This is a reversible chemical section of the nerve supplying a region by injection of the nerve itself. The injection may be either intraneural or extraneural.

Intraneural Injection: Intraneural injection is an injection into the nerve itself. Even though paresthesias occur and one assumes that one is injecting intraneurally, an extraneural injection is usually the result, unless the nerve is large. This is true because by the time the patient reacts to the paresthesia, the needle has passed through the nerve. One can surmise that he is making an intraneural injection if the patient complains of severe paresthesias when the solution is being injected. This pain is caused by distention of the nerve and may be corrected by withdrawing

the needle a millimeter or two. Neurological complications from an intraneural injection are extremely rare. If they occur, the nerve will regenerate. There is no contraindication to obtaining paresthesias where indicated other than the momentary discomfort of the patient.

Intraneural injections may be dangerous, not only on the basis that they may cause nerve damage, but, because solutions injected intraneurally may reach the subarachnoid space or the spinal cord via the perineural spaces of the peripheral nerves. The perineural spaces of the peripheral nerves are actual, not just theoretical, avenues to the spinal cords when solutions are injected intraneurally. Spread centrad of a local anesthetic solution in the perineural spaces is more likely to occur following a paravertebral intraneural injection. When it does, a total spinal block may result.

Extraneural Injection: Extraneural injection is an injection of anesthetic solution in close proximity to the nerve. Onset of operating analgesia is slightly slower than with intraneural injections. Technically speaking, spinal and epidural blocks are in this classification, since the local anesthetic solution is deposited in close proximity to the nerves. This is pointed out since the term "nerve block" is employed by many to mean a block of the nerves peripheral to their emergence from the vertebral column. For the purposes of this book the term also includes spinal and epidural procedures.

TECHNIQUE OF STARTING INTRAVENOUS FLUIDS

The starting of intravenous fluids prior to block procedures is a good prophylactic policy. It is mandatory in those block procedures which are likely to produce hypotension. Often additional help is not available to assist the anesthetist when the patient develops hypotension or a systemic toxic reaction. A plastic needle is best for such a procedure because it has less tendency to be dislodged from the vein during the positioning of the patient for the anesthetic or the surgical procedure.

The author prefers the Rochester (Massa) plastic needle (Figure 2, page 8).

REMARKS

Allow Time for Establishment of Operating Analgesia: *Nerve blocks are like rare old wines: the longer they sit, within reason, the more effective they are.*

Reblock Patient If Analgesia Is Inadequate: In any block procedure, irrespective of the technique employed, *i.e.*, local infiltration, field block, or nerve block, if the block proves unsatisfactory after an adequate time for onset and establishment of anesthesia has passed, do not hesitate to reblock the patient. The following points should be kept in mind when reblocking a patient: (1) the sum of the two doses must not exceed the maximum dose of the local anesthetic drug prescribed for that particular block; and (2) in spinal and epidural blocks, doses smaller than the initial dose should be employed if some anesthesia is present, and only under few circumstances should the initial dose be exceeded.

PART II
PERIPHERAL NERVE BLOCK ANESTHESIA

SECTION I
HEAD AND NECK

CHAPTER 11

Block of Scalp

INDICATIONS

Surgery: Operations of the head, scalp, and brain.

Diagnostic: None.

Therapeutic: None.

ANATOMY

The anterior portion of the scalp is supplied by the supratrochlear, frontal proper, and su-

praorbital branches of the frontal nerve; by the facial and temporal branches of the zygomatic nerve; and by the auriculo-temporal nerve. All the foregoing nerves are branches of the trigeminal. The posterior portion of the scalp is supplied by the greater (major) and lesser (minor) occipital nerves, both of which are branches of the cervical plexus (Figure 19, page 67). The nerves become subfascial approximately at the level of an imaginary circle which passes through the glabella and occiput

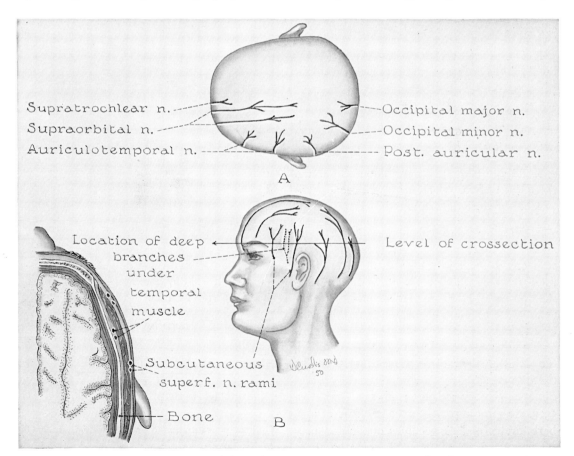

Figure 19. Distribution of the nerves of the scalp. A. Superior view. B. Lateral and cross-sectional view. The more medial portion of the supraorbital nerve as shown above is also called the frontal nerve proper.

(Figure 20, page 69). This circle lies just above the ear.

PREMEDICATION

Premedication depends entirely on the condition of the patient. If the patient is unconscious because of an intracranial lesion or a skull fracture, no premedication before surgery is necessary. If, on the other hand, the patient is conscious and the lesion is superficial, such as a laceration or a scalp tumor, heavy medication is advisable. For intracranial surgery it is best to discuss the premedication with the surgeon.

Heavy Premedication: Where heavy medication is indicated and the patient is average (age 20 to 50, weight 150 pounds or over, approximate height 5 feet, 5 inches or over, and in good physical condition), the patient receives:

1. 200 mg. (3 gr.) of pentobarbital (Nembutal) by mouth at hour of sleep the night previous to surgery.

2. 200 mg. (3 gr.) of pentobarbital by mouth with one ounce of water 1½ to 2 hours before estimated *block* time.

3. 15 mg. (¼ gr.) of morphine and 0.6 mg. (1/100 gr.) of scopolamine intramuscularly ¾ to 1 hour before the estimated *block* time.

Reduction of Premedication: It is seldom necessary to increase this premedication irrespective of the over-all size of the patient until the patient arrives in either the anesthesia or operating room. However, it is very common to reduce this medication under various circumstances; for example, for the geriatric patient, the adolescent patient or child, the debilitated or cachectic patient, and for those whose surgery is complicated by other diseases, e.g., myxedema, diabetes, heart disease, etc. In the patient over 60 years of age, barbiturates and especially scopolamine may often cause disorientation. Therefore, in these patients, atropine is usually substituted for scopolamine and the dosages of barbiturate

omitted or greatly reduced, *i.e.,* to 50 mg. (¾ gr.) or less. *Always err on the light side.*

Inadequate Premedication: If the premedication is inadequate either for the block or the surgical procedure, intravenous pentobarbital 50 mg. (¾ gr.) to 100 mg. (1½ gr.) or intravenous morphine 8 mg. (⅛ gr.) to 15 mg. (¼ gr.) may be given *slowly.* Judicious use of added sedation is extremely important. Often small supplementary doses of morphine or pentobarbital will make a block successful, especially when a patient interprets touch and motion as pain.

DRUGS

Tetracaine (Pontocaine)

Dosage.—10 cc. to 100 cc. of 0.15 percent solution with or without 0.25 cc. of epinephrine (Adrenalin) 1:1000 in 50 cc. of solution.*

Onset.—Operating analgesia is established in 5 to 15 minutes.

Duration.—Operating analgesia lasts 3½ to 6 hours, with solutions containing epinephrine giving the upper limits.

Procaine (Novocain)

Dosage.—10 cc. to 100 cc. of 1.0 percent solution with or without 0.25 cc. of epinephrine (Adrenalin) 1:1000 in 50 cc. of solution.*

Onset.—Operating analgesia is established in 5 to 15 minutes.

Duration.—Operating analgesia lasts 1 to 1½ hours with solutions containing epinephrine giving the upper limits.

Lidocaine (Xylocaine) or Mepivacaine (Carbocaine)

Dosage.—10 cc. to 100 cc. of 0.5 to 1.0 percent solution with or without 0.25 cc. of epinephrine (Adrenalin) 1:1000 in 50 cc.* Do

---

*Optimal concentration of epinephrine is 1:200,000, that is, 0.1 cc. of epinephrine 1:1000 in 20 cc. of the local anesthetic solution. Do not exceed 0.25 cc. of epinephrine 1:1000 even if amount of local anesthetic solution exceeds 50 cc. (see page 39).

not exceed 500 mg. (0.5 gm.) of lidocaine or mepivacaine, *e.g.*, 50 cc. of a 1.0 percent solution.

Onset.—Operating analgesia is established in 5 to 15 minutes.

Duration.—Operating analgesia lasts 1¼ to 3 hours, with stronger concentrations and solutions containing epinephrine giving the upper limits.

MATERIALS

Regional tray (see Chapter 9, page 51) or:

1. One ¾-inch (2 cm.), 25-gauge Huber point security Lok-needle.

2. One 3-inch (7.5 cm.), 22-gauge security Lok-needle.

3. One tuberculin Lok-syringe for adding epinephrine.

4. One 10 cc. Lok-syringe, preferably with finger rings.

5. One graduated measuring cup, preferably stainless steel, for mixing solution.

6. One prep cup, preferably stainless steel.

7. Four sterile towels.

8. Six sterile sponges.

9. One sterilizer control.

TECHNIQUE

Position and Landmarks: The patient may be placed in the desired brain position or may be lying supine with his hands at his sides as in the case of a laceration of the forehead. The glabella and occiput are palpated and marked with X's (Figure 20, page 69).

Precaution: *Aspirate.*—Careful aspiration for blood should be made before injection.

Procedure

1. The sterilizer control must be checked to be sure the equipment has been sterilized.

2. The area is aseptically prepared and draped.

3. An intradermal wheal is raised at the X over the glabella and occiput with a 25-gauge Huber point security Lok-needle.

4. Local infiltration with the 3-inch (7.5 cm.) security Lok-needle is then carried out intradermally, subcutaneously, and intraperiosteally from the two points until a wall of anesthesia from the skull to the skin encircles the head (Figure 20, page 69). The temporal fossa must be carefully infiltrated because there is more muscle in this region and the nerves are a bit more difficult to anesthetize because of their depth (Figure 19, page 67).

EXTENT OF ANALGESIA

A "bowl" or "skull cap" type of analgesia is produced over the head above the line of infiltration (Figure 20, page 69).

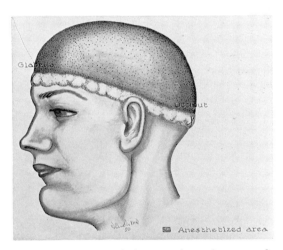

Figure 20. Extent of skin anesthesia from a scalp block.

COMPLICATIONS

Toxic Reactions (intravascular injections, etc.): See Chapter 3, page 19.

REMARKS

Use Epinephrine (Adrenalin): Because of the vascularity of the scalp the addition of epinephrine to the anesthetic solution is advocated because: (1) it reduces the amount of absorption of the local anesthetic agent; and (2) it helps control bleeding.

Do Not Block Entire Scalp If Area To Be Operated Upon Is Small: This block is no more than a local infiltration of the layers of the scalp, and if the operation is confined to a small area it is not necessary to anesthetize the whole scalp. A small section may be easily anesthetized by local infiltration as illustrated in Figure 18, page 63.

Intubate Patient for Intracranial Surgery: Any patient who is to undergo intracranial operation should be intubated before the procedure is started. Once the patient has been put into position, it is very often impossible to pass an endotracheal tube. If the surgeon is opposed to the use of deep inhalation anesthesia for intubation and the patient is conscious or irrational, the endotracheal tube may be inserted while the patient is awake by transtracheal injection (see Chapter 39, page 321) combined with local spray of the mouth and pharynx. It should be noted that after an endotracheal tube lubricated with 2 percent dibucaine (Nupercaine) or 5 percent lidocaine (Xylocaine) ointment has been in place for a short time the patient tolerates it extremely well without coughing unless the position of the head or endotracheal tube is changed. The unconscious patient presents no problem since he usually may be easily tubed. Once the endotracheal tube is situated, light general anesthesia, usually nitrous oxide-oxygen anesthesia or this combined with small amounts of thiopental (Pentothal), will anesthetize the patient adequately. In brain surgery, a scalp block may be a great aid in reducing the amount of inhalation and intravenous anesthesia necessary to control the patient, but is never a substitute for an adequate airway maintained with an endotracheal tube. *In brain surgery, the patient may stop breathing at any time: BE PREPARED.*

Wrap Patient's Legs: The legs of all patients who are to have head surgery should be wrapped from toes to thighs (Figure 1, page 7). It is not uncommon for the surgeon to request Fowler's position in this type of surgery.

Recover Broken Needle(s): All needles should be tested before use. If the needle breaks, every effort to recover it, including surgery, should be made. Unremoved needles have a tendency to migrate and may cause permanent injuries as well as medicolegal complications.

Repeat Block When Analgesia Is Inadequate: If the desired results from the first block attempt are unsatisfactory, do not hesitate to reblock the patient if time permits. Most patients will think nothing about being reblocked if the second attempt is prefaced by a statement such as: "Well, I guess we will have to inject a little more medicine if we are going to freeze this area."

However, do not exceed the maximum safe dosage of the local anesthetic solution for both blocks. If to reblock the patient the maximum safe dose of the local anesthetic solution must be exceeded, 45 minutes should elapse between blocks.

CHAPTER 12

Block of the Supratrochlear and Supraorbital Nerves

INDICATIONS

Surgical: Operations of part of the forehead and scalp as far back as the lamboidal suture.

Diagnostic: Differentiation of trigger areas along the ophthalmic nerve.

Therapeutic: Relief of neuralgias and headaches limited to the distribution of the nerves.

ANATOMY

The supratrochlear, frontal nerve proper, and supraorbital nerves are the terminal branches of the frontal nerve which is the largest branch of the ophthalmic nerve. The supraorbital nerve emerges from the orbit through the supraorbital foramen or notch which lies approximately 1 inch (2.5 cm.) from the midline of the face at the inferior edge of the supraorbital ridge and curves upward onto the forehead. The supratrochlear nerve escapes from the orbit between the pulley (trochlea) of the superior oblique muscle and the supraorbital foramen or notch to course over the lower part of the forehead. (Figure 21A, page 71 and Figure 26, page 78.)

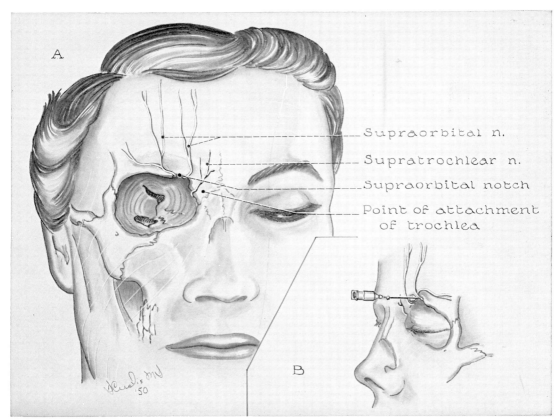

Supraorbital n.

Supratrochlear n.

Supraorbital notch

Point of attachment of trochlea

Figure 21. A. Anatomy of the supraorbital and supratrochlear nerve. B. Needle in place for spot injection of the supraorbital nerve. The more medial portion of the supraorbital nerve as shown above is also called the frontal nerve proper.

PREMEDICATION

Paresthesias are usually sought. Therefore light premedication is advised.

Light Premedication: The average patient (age 20 to 50, weight 150 pounds or over, height 5 feet, 5 inches or over, and good physical status) receives:

1. 200 mg. (3 gr.) pentobarbital (Nembutal) by mouth at hour of sleep the night previous to surgery.

2. 100 mg. (1½ gr.) of pentobarbital by mouth with one ounce of water 1½ to 2 hours before estimated *block* time. This dose of barbiturate is omitted if there is a possibility that the patient will be too heavily sedated to give *an immediate response* when paresthesias are obtained.

3. 10 mg. (⅙ gr.) of morphine and 0.4 mg. (¹⁄₁₅₀ gr.) of scopolamine intramuscularly *on call* to surgery.

Reduction of Premedication: It is seldom necessary to increase this premedication irrespective of the over-all size of the patient until the patient arrives in either the anesthesia or operating room. However, it is very common to reduce this medication under various circumstances; for example, for the geriatric patient, the adolescent patient or child, the debilitated or cachectic patient, and for those whose surgery is complicated by other diseases, *i.e.*, myxedema, diabetes, heart disease, etc. In the patient over 60 years of age, barbiturates and especially scopolamine may often cause disorientation. Therefore, in these patients atropine is usually substituted for scopolamine and the dosages of the barbiturates omitted or greatly reduced, *i.e.*, to 50 mg. (¾ gr.) or less. *Always err on the light side.*

Inadequate Premedication: If the medication is inadequate, either for the block or for the surgical procedure, intravenous pentobarbital 50 mg. (¾ gr.) to 100 mg. (1½ gr.) or intravenous morphine 8 mg. (⅛ gr.) to 15 mg. (¼ gr.) may be given *slowly.* Judicious use of **added sedation is extremely important.** Often

small supplementary doses of morphine or pentobarbital will make a block successful when a patient interprets touch and motion as pain.

DRUGS

Tetracaine (Pontocaine)

Dosage.—1 cc. to 10 cc. of 0.15 to 0.25 percent solution with or without 0.05 cc. of epinephrine (Adrenalin) 1:1000 in each 10 cc. of solution.*

Onset.—Operating analgesia is established in 5 to 15 minutes.

Duration.—Operating analgesia lasts 3½ to 6 hours, with stronger concentrations and solutions containing epinephrine giving the upper limits.

Procaine (Novocain)

Dosage.—1 cc. to 10 cc. of 1.0 to 2.0 percent solution with or without 0.05 cc. of epinephrine (Adrenalin) 1:1000 in each 10 cc. of solution.*

Onset.—Operating analgesia is established in 5 to 15 minutes.

Duration.—Operating analgesia lasts 1 to 1¾ hours, with stronger concentrations and solutions containing epinephrine giving the upper limits.

Lidocaine (Xylocaine) or Mepivacaine (Carbocaine)

Dosage.—1 cc. to 10 cc. of 1.0 to 1.5 percent solution with or without 0.05 cc. of epinephrine (Adrenalin) 1:1000 in each 10 cc. of solution.*

Onset.—Operating analgesia is established in 5 to 15 minutes.

Duration.—Operating analgesia lasts 1¼ to 3 hours, with stronger concentrations and solu-

---

*Optimal concentration of epinephrine is 1:200,000, that is, 0.1 cc. of epinephrine 1:1000 in 20 cc. of the local anesthetic solution (see page 39).

tions containing epinephrine giving the upper limits.

Alcohol

Dosage.—0.25 cc. to 0.5 cc. of absolute alcohol (95 percent) from sterile individual ampules. More than 0.5 cc. should not be injected at any one time for a unilateral block.

Onset.—Analgesia is established in 1 to 5 minutes.

Duration.—Sensory analgesia lasts three weeks to three months. Pain fibers may be analgesic from six months to thirty years. The latter figure is unusual and the average duration is nine to fifteen months.

MATERIALS

Regional tray (see Chapter 9, page 51) or:

1. One ¾-inch (2 cm.), 25-gauge Huber point security Lok-needle.

2. One 1½-inch (3.8 cm.) 22-gauge security Lok-needle, preferably with short bevel.

3. One tuberculin Lok-syringe for measuring epinephrine or alcohol.

4. One 10 cc. Lok-syringe, preferably with finger rings.

5. One graduated measuring cup, preferably stainless steel, for mixing solution.

6. One prep cup, preferably stainless steel.

7. Four sterile towels.

8. Six sterile sponges.

9. One sterilizer control.

TECHNIQUE

Position and Landmarks:

1. The patient lies in the dorsal recumbent position with his arms at his side and a "donut" under his head (Figure 22, page 73).

2. The head should be in a profile position so that a median sagittal section through the nose would be perpendicular to the table.

3. The supraorbital notch (fissure) in the supraorbital ridge of the frontal bone is palpated and the skin overlying it marked with an X. It usually lies 1 inch (2.5 cm.) from the midline.

Precautions: *Aspirate.*—Careful aspiration for blood should be made before injecting the anesthetic solution.

Procedure

1. The sterilizer control must be checked to be sure the equipment has been sterilized.

2. The area is aseptically prepared and draped.

3. The anesthetist stands at the head of the table facing the patient's feet (Figure 22, page 73).

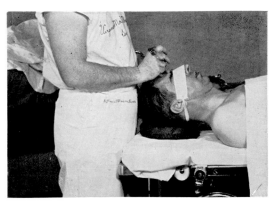

Figure 22. Position of the patient and anesthetist for block of the supraorbital or supratrochlear nerve. Patient rests head on "donut." The anesthetist is not gloved since the illustrations in this book of the anesthetist's position relative to the patient do not depict actual procedures.

4. If accurate spot injection of these nerves is required, as in alcohol blocking, a skin wheal is raised at the X with a 25-gauge, ¾-inch (2 cm.) Huber point security Lok-needle. The needle is then advanced perpendicular to the skin into or medial to the supraorbital notch, depending on which of the nerves is sought, until paresthesias are elicited or bone is struck (Figure 21, page 71). If no paresthesias occur, the maneuver is repeated until they do. Then 1 to 2 cc. of anesthetic so-

lution is injected. *Paresthesias of the supra-orbital, supratrochlear, and frontal nerves are characterized by sharp, spraying, electric shock sensations over the forehead.*

5. If block of these nerves is performed for operating analgesia, no attempt is made to produce paresthesias. A skin wheal is raised at the midline above the level of the bridge of the nose and a wall of anesthetic solution from the skin to the frontal bone lateral to this point for 1½ inches (3.8 cm.) is injected (Figure 23A, page 74). More than 5 to 6 cc. should not be used for each side.

EXTENT OF ANALGESIA

Analgesia extends over part of the forehead and scalp (Figure 23B, page 74).

COMPLICATIONS

Toxic Reactions (intravascular injections, etc.): See Chapter 3, page 19.

Swelling of the Tissue Around the Orbit

Signs and Symptoms.—They are: (1) swelling of the upper lid of the eye and at times the lower lid of the eye; (2) inability of the patient to open the eye; (3) discoloration of the skin if caused by hemorrhage.

Etiology.—This complication occurs from injection of large quantities of local anesthetic solutions, hemorrhage from trauma to the supraorbital vessels, or both.

Course.—If an excessive amount of the local anesthetic solution is the etiology, the swell-

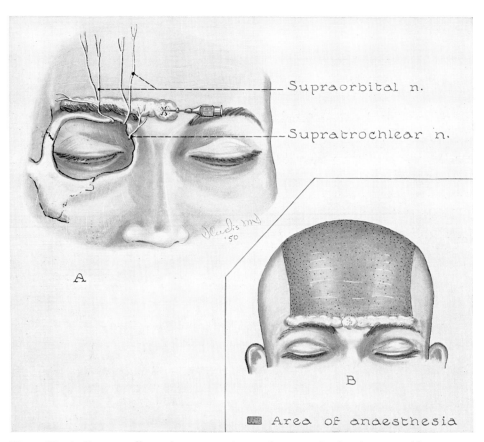

Figure 23. A. Shows needle in place to anesthetize the supraorbital and supratrochlear nerves. B. Area of analgesia produced by a bilateral block of the supraorbital and supratrochlear nerves. The more medial portion of the supraorbital nerve as shown above is also called the frontal nerve proper.

ing will subside in a few hours. When caused by alcohol, the swelling may persist for one to two weeks. And, if it is a result of hemorrhage, the discoloration and the swelling will persist for two days to a week.

Treatment.—None if the local anesthetic solution was the etiology. If caused by hemorrhage or alcohol, warm moist dressing applied constantly will reduce the swelling and discoloration and aid in absorption of the hematoma. If gentle but firm pressure is applied over the supraorbital ridge when hemorrhage is first noted, the swelling will be greatly limited because the loose skin and subcutaneous tissue around the eye will in itself not limit the hemorrhage.

Whatever is the cause, the patient should be reassured that there is nothing to cause concern.

Prophylaxis.—Firm pressure along the supraorbital ridge with fingers of the free hand during the injection and for one or two minutes following the execution of the block will often prevent the swelling (Figure 24, page 75).

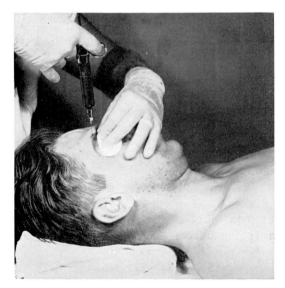

Figure 24.   Method used to prevent swelling of the eyelid from the local anesthetic solution or hemorrhage during a supraorbital or supratrochlear block. Pressure is being exerted along the supraorbital ridge. If hemorrhage occurs or excess solution is used, pressure should be maintained for at least five minutes.

REMARKS

Indication for Bilateral Block: When the lesion is near the midline, bilateral block is necessary because of the crossing of nerve fibers from the opposite side.

Tic Douloureux of Ophthalmic Division Occurs Infrequently: Tic douloureux of the ophthalmic division of the trigeminal nerve is rare. Often pain is referred to the ophthalmic division when the trigger point is in the maxillary nerve. Blocking of the maxillary nerve will usually stop the pain over the eye. If it does not, then injection of the terminal branches of the ophthalmic nerve, *i.e.*, the supratrochlear and supraorbital, is indicated. Block of the ophthalmic nerve at the gasserian ganglion with anesthetic agents of prolonged duration such as alcohol is contraindicated in most cases because of the innumerable sequelae which may be irreparable. The most important of these is corneal ulcer with permanent damage to the cornea (see page 330).

Limit Volume of Solution Injected: One should not inject more than 2 cc. to 6 cc. of the local anesthetic solution depending on whether a spot injection or field block is performed for a unilateral block; otherwise, there is an overflow of solution which causes the lower and upper eyelids to swell. This is of no concern to the anesthetist as the swelling will disappear in ¾ to 1½ hours. When overflow occurs, the patient should be assured that everything is satisfactory, for the lid may swell so much that the patient will not be able to open his eye. This swelling may be limited or avoided by firm pressure along the infraorbital ridge with the fingers of the free hand during injection and for one to two minutes following the execution of the block (Figure 24, page 75).

Use Alcohol with Care: Before using alcohol on either the supraorbital or supratrochlear nerve, consult Chapter 41, page 329.

Supraorbital, Infraorbital, and Mental Foramina Lie On Straight Line: If the supraorbital foramen is difficult to palpate, it should be remembered that the supraorbital foramen, the infraorbital foramen, and the mental fora- men all lie on a straight line approximately 1 inch (2.5 cm.) from the midline of the face. Therefore if one of the last two foramina is palpable and a line is drawn through it par- allel to the midsagittal plane of the body, the supraorbital foramen should be located at a point where this line crosses the supraorbital ridge (Figure 25, page 76 and Figure 29, page 80).

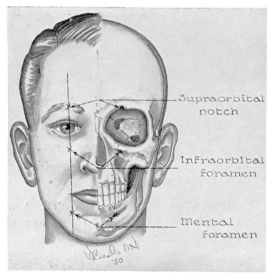

Figure 25. Supraorbital, infraorbital, and mental foramina all lie on a straight line.

Elicit Paresthesias: In this block procedure paresthesias should be elicited for spot injec- tion. Remember the dictum, *"No paresthesias, no anesthesia"* and the failures will be minimal.

Intubate Patient for Long or Tedious Oper- ations: Satisfactory anesthesia for long or te- dious surgical procedures of the face and scalp is perhaps one of the most difficult types of anesthesia to administer in a way that satisfies the requirements of the patient, of the sur-

geon, and of the anesthetist. Regional anal- gesia may be employed satisfactorily for short *superficial* procedures, since the correctly medicated patient will usually tolerate un- comfortable positions, the feeling of suffoca- tion from drapes, and manipulation discom- forts for limited periods. However, during long and/or tedious procedures requiring deep manipulations of the face, nasal pharynx, oral pharynx, pharynx, larynx, or trachea, the con- stant cooperation of the patient must not be relied on. Restlessness and motion at a crucial point by a patient, who was thought to be cooperative, may prove disastrous to the pa- tient or to the operative result being sought. Likewise, the administration of intravenous, rectal, or inhalation anesthesia to a patient who was started under regional block and whose airway has been made inaccessible by the drapes or the surgery may be equally as catastrophic.

Therefore, in long and/or tedious proce- dures of the scalp and face, endotracheal anes- thesia may be a more satisfactory means of establishing anesthesia.

Recover Broken Needle(s): All needles should be tested before use. If a needle breaks, every effort to recover it, including surgery, should be made. Unremoved needles have a tendency to migrate and may cause perma- nent injuries as well as medicolegal complica- tions.

Repeat Block When Analgesia Is Inade- quate: If the desired results from the first block attempt are unsatisfactory, do not hesi- tate to reblock the patient if time permits. Most patients will think nothing about being reblocked if the second attempt is prefaced by a statement such as: "Well, I guess we will have to inject a little more medicine if we are going to freeze this area."

CHAPTER 13

Block of the Infraorbital and Anterior Superior Alveolar Nerves

INDICATIONS

Surgical: Operations and manipulation of the lower eyelid, side of the nose, and septum mobile nasi, upper lip, mucous membrane of the mouth under the lips, and the upper incisor and cuspid teeth.

Diagnostic: Differentiation of trigger areas along the maxillary nerve.

Therapeutic: Relief of neuralgias limited to the infraorbital distribution of the maxillary nerve, relief of intractable root pain following extraction of the incisor and cuspid teeth.

ANATOMY

The infraorbital nerve (terminal part of the maxillary nerve) emerges from the infraorbital foramen and divides into four branches: the inferior palpebral, the external nasal, the internal nasal, and the superior labial (Figure 26A, page 78). They innervate the lower eyelid, lateral inferior portion of the nose and its vestibule, and the upper lip and its mucosa.

The anterior superior alveolar nerve branches from the infraorbital nerve in the anterior part of the infraorbital canal and descends in bony canals to supply the upper incisor and cuspid teeth (Figure 26B, page 78).

The infraorbital canal lies at a 45 degree angle backward and upward at its exit from the maxillary bone. It also lies at a 25 degree angle to the median sagittal plane in an outward direction (Figure 26A, page 78). The anterior portion of the canal in the orbit is usually covered with a thin bone plate.

The infraorbital foramen lies approximately 1 inch (2.5 cm.) from the midline of the face or ¾ inch (2 cm.) lateral to the frontal process of the maxillary bone.

PREMEDICATION

Paresthesias are always sought. Therefore, light medication is advised.

Light Premedication: The average patient (age 20 to 50, weight 150 pounds or over, height 5 feet 5 inches or over, and with good physical status) receives:

1. 200 mg. (3 gr.) of pentobarbital (Nembutal) by mouth at hour of sleep the night previous to surgery.

2. 100 mg. (1½ gr.) of pentobarbital by mouth with one ounce of water 1½ to 2 hours before estimated *block* time. This dose of barbiturate is omitted if there is a possibility that the patient will be too heavily sedated to give *an immediate response* when paresthesias are obtained.

3. 10 mg. (⅙ gr.) of morphine and 0.4 mg. (¹⁄₁₅₀ gr.) of scopolamine intramuscularly *on call* to surgery.

Reduction of Premedication: It is seldom necessary to increase this premedication irrespective of the over-all size of the patient until the patient arrives in either the anesthesia or operating room. However, it is very common to reduce this medication under various circumstances; for example, for the geriatric patient, the adolescent patient or child, the debilitated or cachectic patient, and for those whose surgery is complicated by other disease, *i.e.*, myxedema, diabetes, heart dis-

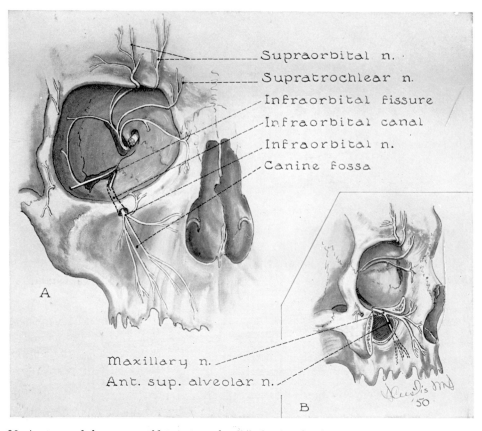

Figure 26. Anatomy of the supratrochlear, supraorbital, and infraorbital nerves. A. Anterior view. B. Lateral view with portion of the maxillary bone removed to show the slope of the infraorbital canal and the anterior superior alveolar nerve. The more medial portion of the supraorbital nerve as shown above is also called the frontal nerve proper.

ease, etc. In the patient over 60 years of age, barbiturates and especially scopolamine may often cause disorientation. Therefore, in these patients atropine is usually substituted for scopolamine and the dosages of the barbiturate omitted or greatly reduced, i.e., to 50 mg. (¾ gr.) or less. *Always err on the light side.*

Inadequate Premedication: If the medication is inadequate, either for the block or for the surgical procedure, intravenous pentobarbital 50 mg. (¾ gr.) to 100 mg. (1½ gr.) or intravenous morphine 8 mg. (⅛ gr.) to 15 mg. (¼ gr.) may be given *slowly.* Judicious use of added sedation is extremely important. Often small supplementary doses of morphine or pentobarbital will make a block successful when a patient interprets touch and motion as pain.

DRUGS

Tetracaine (Pontocaine)

Dosage.—2 cc. to 6 cc. of 0.15 to 0.25 percent with or without 0.05 cc. of epinephrine (Adrenalin) 1:1000 in each 10 cc. of solution.*

Onset.—Operating analgesia is established in 5 to 15 minutes.

Duration.—Operating analgesia lasts 3½ to 6 hours, with stronger concentrations and solutions containing epinephrine giving the upper limits.

---

*Optimal concentration of epinephrine is 1:200,000, that is, 0.1 cc. of epinephrine 1:1000 in 20 cc. of the local anesthetic solution (see page 39).

Procaine (Novocain)

Dosage.—2 cc. to 6 cc. of 1.0 to 2.0 percent solution with or without 0.05 cc. of epinephrine (Adrenalin) 1:1000 in each 10 cc. of solution.*

Onset.—Operating analgesia is established in 5 to 15 minutes.

Duration.—Operating analgesia lasts 1 to 1¾ hours, with stronger concentrations and solutions containing epinephrine giving the upper limits.

Lidocaine (Xylocaine) or Mepivacaine (Carbocaine)

Dosage.—2 cc. to 6 cc. of 1.0 to 1.5 percent solution with or without 0.05 cc. of epinephrine (Adrenalin) in each 10 cc. of solution.*

Onset.—Operating analgesia is established in 5 to 15 minutes.

Duration.—Operating analgesia lasts 1¼ to 3 hours, with stronger concentrations and solutions containing epinephrine giving the upper limits.

Alcohol

Dosage.—0.5 cc. to 1 cc. of absolute alcohol (95 percent) from sterile individual ampules. More than 1.0 cc. should not be injected for a unilateral block since the contents of the orbit and eyelids may become involved.

Onset.—Analgesia is established in 1 to 5 minutes.

Duration.—Sensory analgesia lasts three weeks to three months. Pain fibers may be analgesic from six months to thirty years. The latter figure is unusual and the average duration is nine to fifteen months.

MATERIALS

Regional tray (see Chapter 9, page 51) or:

1. One ¾-inch (2 cm.), 25-gauge Huber point security Lok-needle.

2. One 1½-inch (3.8 cm.), 22-gauge security Lok-needle, preferably with short bevel.

3. One tuberculin Lok-syringe for measuring epinephrine or alcohol.

4. One 10 cc. Lok-syringe, preferably with finger rings.

5. One graduated measuring cup, preferably stainless steel, for mixing solution.

6. One prep cup, preferably stainless steel.

7. Four sterile towels.

8. Six sterile sponges.

9. One sterilizer control.

TECHNIQUE

Position and Landmarks

1. The patient lies in the dorsal recumbent position with his arms at his side and a "donut" under his head (Figure 27, page 79).

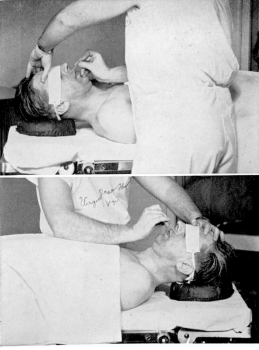

Figure 27.   Position of the patient and right-handed anesthetist for an infraorbital block. A. *(Top)* Right side. B. *(Bottom)* Left side.

---

*Optimal concentration of epinephrine is 1:200,000, that is, 0.1 cc. of epinephrine 1:1000 in 20 cc. of the local anesthetic solution (see page 39).

2. The head should be in a profile position so that a median sagittal section through the middle of the nose would be perpendicular to the table.

3. The infraorbital ridge of the maxillary bone is located and the infraorbital foramen palpated approximately ¾ inch (2 cm.) from the lateral surface of the nose (frontal process of maxillary bone). An X is placed on the skin overlying the foramen (Figure 28, page 80 and Figure 29, page 80). Should it be difficult to feel the foramen, the canine fossa can usually be discerned, above which the infraorbital foramen lies (Figure 26, page 78).

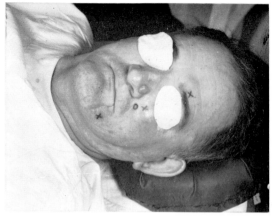

Figure 29. Patient in position for an infraorbital block with the landmarks marked on the skin and the head resting on the donut. The middle X marks the infraorbital foramen, the X on the chin the mental foramen, and the X above the eyebrow the supraorbital notch. These X's lie in a straight line. The O is placed slightly medial to and below the X marking the infraorbital foramen so that the needle may enter and traverse the infraorbital canal. Anesthesia was administered for removal of papilloma on nose. The patient was an outpatient.

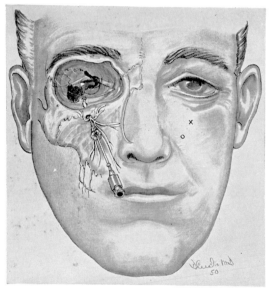

Figure 28. Needle in place in infraorbital canal on right side of face while left side shows the landmarks.

4. An O is marked ¼ inch (0.6 cm.) below and slightly medial to the X (Figure 28, page 80 and Figure 29, page 80). In this manner the anesthetist allows for the slant of the infraorbital canal. If the needle were introduced perpendicularly to the X, the foramen might be felt but it would be difficult to enter and traverse it.

Precautions

Limit Advancement of Needle.—The needle must never advance more than ¼ inch (0.6 cm.) past the infraorbital foramen and more than 3 cc. of anesthetic solution should not be deposited in the infraorbital canal; otherwise, the contents of the orbit can be involved and damaged. The canal in which the anterior superior alveolar nerve lies is usually separated from the orbit by a thin bone plate. However, in some cases this is absent; in any case it is possible to pierce the bone plate with a sharp needle.

Aspirate.—Aspirate carefully for blood before injecting local anesthetic solution.

Procedure

1. The sterilizer control must be checked to be sure the equipment has been sterilized.

2. The area is aseptically prepared and draped.

3. If the anesthetist is right-handed, he stands at the patient's right side irrespective of the side to be blocked, facing the patient's head (Figure 27, page 79). The left side of the face is blocked by reaching across the midline. This is easier than standing at the left

side and working backhanded. A left-handed anesthetist takes the opposite position.

4. A skin wheal is made at the O with a 25-gauge, ¾-inch (2 cm.) Huber point security Lok-needle. Subcutaneous infiltration is carried out along the line XO, using approximately 1 cc. to 2 cc. of the local anesthetic solution.

5. The patient is cautioned to say *"Now"* and not move if he feels paresthesias over the distribution of the infraorbital nerve. *Paresthesias of the infraorbital nerve are characterized by sharp, spraying, electric shock sensations to the upper lip and ala of the nose. As the needle is advanced in the infraorbital canal, paresthesias of the upper front teeth may occur.*

6. If the anesthesiologist is right-handed, the left hand steadies the patient's head, or vice versa (Figure 32, page 82).

7. The 1½-inch (3.8 cm.), 22-gauge, short beveled security Lok-needle with open hub is introduced perpendicular to the skin at O. The hub is then lowered so that the point of the needle will strike the maxillary bone at a point underlying the X. There is usually about a 45-degree angle between the skin and the shaft of the needle (Figure 28, page 80; Figure 30, page 81; and Figure 31, page 81).

8. The needle is advanced outward, up-

ward, and backward until it strikes bone or elicits paresthesias as it slides into the infraorbital foramen. If this does not occur, the anesthetist should redirect the needle point and feel around the portion of the maxilla under the X with the point of the needle until the foramen is located (Figure 28, page 80; Figure 30, page 81; and Figure 31, page 81).

9. The Lok-syringe, with finger rings, is attached to the needle and 1 cc. of anesthetic solution is injected at the opening of the infraorbital foramen. This anesthetizes the infraorbital nerve (Figure 32, page 82).

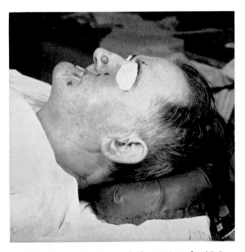

Figure 31. Lateral view of the 1½-inch (3.8 cm.) needle in the infraorbital foramen. Note the 45 degree angle of the shaft of the needle to the skin.

10. Then the needle is slowly advanced down the infraorbital canal, injecting small amounts of the anesthetic solution as the needle moves forward. When it has been introduced ¼ inch (0.6 cm.), 1 cc. of the anesthetic solution is injected (Figure 32, page 82). This anesthetizes the anterior superior alveolar nerve.

11. As the needle is withdrawn, 1 cc. of anesthetic solution is injected.

EXTENT OF ANALGESIA

Analgesia extends over the upper lip and its mucous membrane, part of the upper teeth

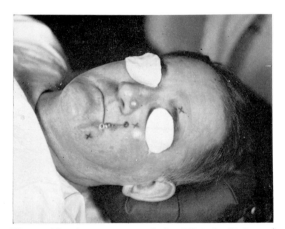

Figure 30. Anterior view of the 1½-inch (3.8 cm.) needle in the infraorbital foramen.

(incisors and cuspids), part of the cheek and nose, and lower eyelid (Figure 33, page 82).

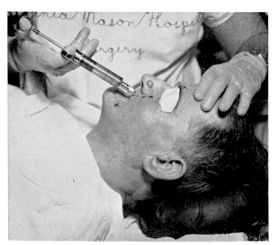

Figure 32. Depositing of the local anesthetic solution in the infraorbital foramen and canal. Note the right-handed anesthetist reaches across the midline to block the left side while the left hand steadies the head. The patient's head rests on a "donut" for stability.

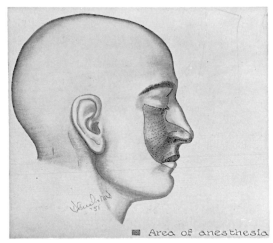

Figure 33. Area of skin anesthesia produced by a unilateral infraorbital nerve block.

COMPLICATIONS

Toxic Reactions (intravascular injections, etc.): See Chapter 3, page 19.

Introduction of Anesthetic Solution or Hemorrhage into the Orbit

Signs and Symptoms.—They are: diplopia, exophthalmus, blurred vision, loss of vision, and pain in the eyeball.

Etiology.—This is a result of advancement of the needle too far up the infraorbital canal, injection of large volumes of anesthetic solutions, and puncture of a blood vessel, or all three.

Course.—The signs and symptoms clear as the anesthetic agent dissipates itself. If alcohol is the anesthetic agent or if hemorrhage is the offender, then the signs and symptoms may be permanent.

Treatment.—None, when a local anesthetic agent was used. If alcohol has been employed and the above signs and symptoms occur, the eye should be treated symptomatically and ophthalmologic consultation obtained immediately.

Swelling of the Tissue Around the Orbit

Signs and Symptoms.—They are: swelling of the lower lid of the eye and at times the upper lid of the eye, inability of the patient to open the eye, discoloration of the skin if caused by hemorrhage, or all three.

Etiology.—It is a result of injection of large quantities of local anesthetic solutions, hemorrhage from trauma to the infraorbital vessels, or both.

Course.—If caused by excessive amounts of the local anesthetic solution, the swelling will subside in a few hours, but, if caused by hemorrhage, the discoloration and the swelling will persist for two days to a week.

Treatment.—None if the local anesthetic solution was the etiology. But, if caused by hemorrhage, warm moist dressings applied constantly will reduce the swelling and discoloration and aid in absorption of the hematoma. Gentle but firm pressure applied over the infraorbital ridge when hemorrhage is first noted will greatly limit the swelling (Figure 34, page 83). This is true because the loose skin and subcutaneous tissue around the eye will not limit the hemorrhage.

Whatever the cause is, the patient should be reassured that there is nothing to cause concern.

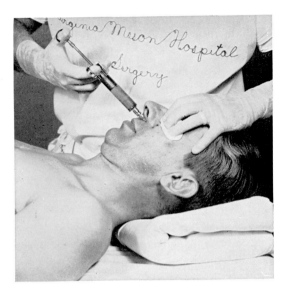

Figure 34. Method used to prevent swelling of the eyelid from the local anesthetic solution or hemorrhage during an infraorbital block. Pressure is being exerted along the infraorbital ridge. If hemorrhage occurs or excess solution is injected, pressure should be maintained for at least five minutes.

Prophylaxis.—Firm pressure along the infraorbital ridge with the fingers of the free hand during injection will often prevent this swelling (Figure 34, page 83).

REMARKS

Complications Minimal: This block is easy to perform, the complications are infrequent, and the analgesia established for facial work is excellent.

Advance Needle into Infraorbital Canal: If the needle is *not* advanced past the opening of the infraorbital canal, the anterior superior alveolar nerve will usually *not* be blocked and analgesia of the gums, teeth, and the inside of the lip will be absent or inadequate.

Indication for Bilateral Block: If the lesion is near the midline, a bilateral block is necessary because of crossing of nerve fibers from the opposite side.

Supraorbital, Infraorbital, and Mental Foramina Lie On Straight Line: When the infraorbital foramen is difficult to palpate, it should be remembered that the supraorbital foramen,

the infraorbital foramen, and the mental foramen all lie on a straight line approximately 1 inch (2.5 cm.) from the midline of the face. Therefore, if either the supraorbital foramen or mental foramen is palpable and a line is drawn through the palpable foramen parallel to the midsagittal plane of the body, the infraorbital foramen should be located at a point where the line crosses the infraorbital ridge (Figure 25, page 76 and Figure 29, page 80).

Limit Volume of Solution Injected: One should not inject more than 6 cc. of anesthetic solution for this entire block; otherwise an overflow of solution will often result which will cause the lower and upper eyelids to swell. This is of no concern to the anesthetist, since such swelling disappears in ¾ to 1½ hours; but overflow should be avoided, if possible, as a matter of technique. The patient should be assured that everything is satisfactory and that he will be able to open his eye in a few hours. This swelling may be limited or avoided by firm pressure along the infraorbital ridge with the fingers of the free hand during injection and for one to five minutes following the execution of the block (Figure 34, page 83).

Use Alcohol with Care: Before injecting alcohol, consult Chapter 41, page 329.

Elicit Paresthesias: In this block procedure, paresthesias should be elicited. Remember the dictum, "*No paresthesias, no anesthesia*" and the failures will be minimal.

Intubate Patient for Long or Tedious Operations: Satisfactory anesthesia for long or tedious surgical procedures of the face is perhaps one of the most difficult types of anesthesia to administer in a way that satisfies the requirements of the patient, of the surgeon, and of the anesthetist. Regional analgesia may be employed satisfactorily for short *superficial* procedures, since the correctly medicated patient will usually tolerate uncomfortable positions, the feeling of suffocation from drapes, and manipulation discomforts for limited periods. However, during long and/or tedious procedures requiring deep manipulations of the face, nasal pharynx, oral pharynx, pharynx, larynx, or trachea, the constant cooperation of the patient must not be relied on. Restlessness and motion at a crucial point by a patient who was thought to be cooperative may prove disastrous to the patient or to the operative result being sought. Likewise, the administration of intravenous, rectal, or inhalation anesthesia to a patient who was started under regional block and whose airway has been made inaccessible by the drapes or the surgery may be equally as catastrophic.

Therefore, in long and/or tedious procedures of the face, endotracheal anesthesia may be a more satisfactory means of establishing anesthesia.

Recover Broken Needle(s): All needles should be tested before use. If a needle breaks, every effort to recover it, including surgery, should be made. Unremoved needles have a tendency to migrate and may cause permanent injuries as well as medicolegal complications.

Repeat Block When Analgesia Is Inadequate: If the desired results from the first block attempt are unsatisfactory, do not hesitate to reblock the patient if time permits. Most patients will think nothing about being reblocked if the second attempt is prefaced by a statement such as: "Well, I guess we will have to inject a little more medicine if we are going to freeze this area."

CHAPTER 14

Block of the Mental and Lower Incisor Nerves

INDICATIONS

Surgical: Operations and manipulations of the lower lip, lower teeth (incisors, cuspids, and bicuspids), and the lower jaw and mandible between the two mental foramina laterally, the lower border of the mental protuberance of the mandibular bone inferiorly, and the lower lip superiorly.

Diagnostic: Differentiation of trigger areas along the mandibular nerve.

Therapeutic: Relief of neuralgias limited to the distribution of the nerve. Relief of intractable root pain following extraction of the lower incisors, the bicuspid, or cuspid teeth. Relief of intractable pain from other pathology.

ANATOMY

The mental and incisor nerves are the terminal branches of the inferior alveolar (dental) nerve, which is a branch of the mandibular nerve. The mental nerve emerges through the mental foramen to supply the skin of the chin, lower lips, and mucous membrane. The incisor nerve continues inside the mandibular bone to the symphysis and supplies the bicuspids and incisor teeth (Figure 35, page 85).

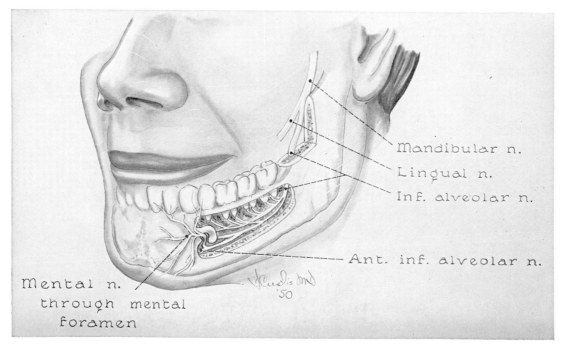

Figure 35. Anatomy of the inferior alveolar and mental nerves. The portion of the inferior alveolar nerve continuing in the above figure beyond the mental foramen within the bony canal is commonly called the incisive branch.

The position of the mental foramen is sometimes difficult to determine since its anatomical position varies with the age of the patient (Figure 36, page 86). In the adult whose jaw has reached maturity and whose teeth have not been pulled, the foramen lies midway between the upper and lower edge of the mandibular bone below the second bicuspid, which is approximately 1 inch (2.5 cm.) from the midline of the face. In the child of seven to eight years of age, the foramen lies closer to the inferior border of the mandible below the first molar posteriorly. In the older patient whose teeth have been pulled, there is atrophy of the mandible, particularly of the alveolar ridge. In these patients the mental foramen lies either on or very near the upper margin of the mandible, approximately 1 inch (2.5 cm.) from the midline of the chin. The distance from the midline of the face varies slightly with the age of the patient.

In its course through the mandibular bone, the mental canal slants posterosuperiorly at a 60-degree angle to the lateral surface of the bone. It makes an angle of 45 degrees with the horizontal plane of the bone (Figure 37, page 87).

PREMEDICATION

Paresthesias are always sought. Therefore, light premedication is advised.

Light Premedication: The average patient (age 20 to 50, weight 150 pounds or over, height 5 feet, 5 inches or over, and in good physical condition) receives:

1. 200 mg. (3 gr.) of pentobarbital (Nembutal) by mouth at hour of sleep the night previous to surgery.

2. 100 mg. (1½ gr.) of pentobarbital by mouth with one ounce of water 1½ to 2 hours before estimated *block* time. This dose of barbiturate is omitted if there is a possibility that the patient will be too heavily sedated to give *an immediate response* when paresthesias are obtained.

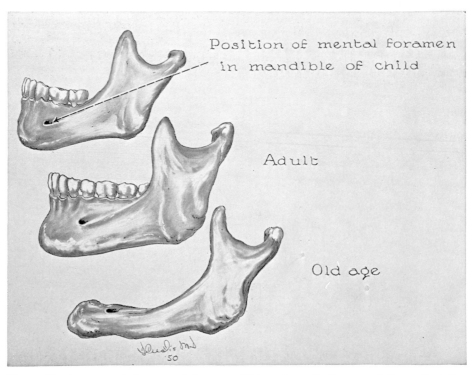

Figure 36. Anatomy of the mental foramen. This varies with the age of the patient, the presence of teeth, and the use of dentures.

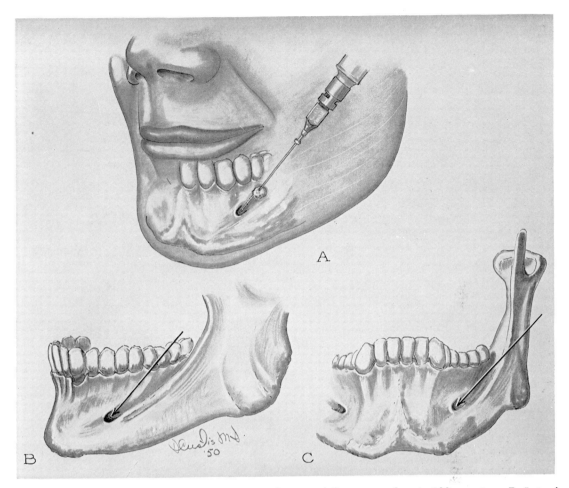

Figure 37. Direction of the needle if it is to enter the mental foramen easily. A. Oblique view. B. Lateral view. C. Front view.

3. 10 mg. (⅙ gr.) of morphine and 0.4 mg. (1/150 gr.) of scopolamine intramuscularly *on call* to surgery.

Reduction of Premedication: It is seldom necessary to increase this premedication irrespective of the over-all size of the patient until the patient arrives in either the anesthesia or operating room. However, it is very common to reduce this medication under various circumstances; for example, for the geriatric patient, the adolescent patient or child, the debilitated or cachectic patient, and for those whose surgery is complicated by other disease, *e.g.*, myxedema, diabetes, heart disease, etc. In the patient over 60 years of age, barbiturates and especially scopolamine often

cause disorientation. Therefore, in these patients atropine is usually substituted for scopolamine and the dosages of the barbiturate omitted or greatly reduced, *i.e.*, to 50 mg. (¾ gr.) or less. *Always err on the light side.*

Inadequate Premedication: If the medication is inadequate, either for the block or for the surgical procedure, intravenous pentobarbital 50 mg. (¾ gr.) to 100 mg. (1½ gr.) or intravenous morphine 8 mg. (⅛ gr.) to 15 mg. (¼ gr.) may be given *slowly.* Judicious use of added sedation is extremely important. Often small supplementary doses of morphine or pentobarbital will make a block successful when a patient interprets touch and motion as pain.

DRUGS

Tetracaine (Pontocaine)

Dosage.—2 cc. to 10 cc. of 0.10 to 0.25 per-cent solution with or without 0.05 cc. of epinephrine (Adrenalin) 1:1000 in each 10 cc. of solution.*

Onset.—Operating analgesia is established in 5 to 15 minutes.

Duration.—Operating analgesia lasts 3½ to 6 hours, with stronger concentrations and solutions containing epinephrine giving the upper limits.

Procaine (Novocain)

Dosage.—2 cc. to 10 cc. of 1.0 to 2.0 per-cent solution with or without 0.05 cc. of epinephrine (Adrenalin) 1:1000 in each 10 cc. of solution.*

Onset.—Operating analgesia is established in 5 to 15 minutes.

Duration.—Operating analgesia lasts 1 to 1¾ hours, with stronger concentrations and solutions containing epinephrine giving the upper limits.

Lidocaine (Xylocaine) or Mepivacaine (Carbocaine)

Dosage.—2 cc. to 10 cc. of 1.0 to 1.5 percent solution with or without 0.05 cc. of epinephrine (Adrenalin) 1:1000 in each 10 cc. of solution.*

Onset.—Operating analgesia is established in 5 to 15 minutes.

Duration.—Operating analgesia lasts 1¼ to 3 hours, with stronger concentrations and solutions containing epinephrine giving the upper limits.

Alcohol

Dosage.—0.5 cc. to 1 cc. of absolute alcohol (95 percent) from sterile individual ampules.

---

*Optimal concentration of epinephrine is 1:200,000, that is, 0.1 cc. of epinephrine 1:1000 in 20 cc. of the local anesthetic solution (see page 39).

More than 1.0 cc. should not be injected at any one time for a unilateral block.

Onset.—Analgesia is established in 1 to 5 minutes.

Duration.—Sensory analgesia lasts three weeks to three months. Pain fibers may be analgesic from six months to thirty years. The latter figure is unusual and the average duration is nine to fifteen months.

MATERIALS

Regional tray (see Chapter 9, page 51) or:

1. One ¾-inch (2 cm.), 25-gauge Huber point security Lok-needle.

2. One 1½-inch (3.8 cm), 22-gauge security Lok-needle, preferably with short bevel.

3. One tuberculin Lok-syringe for measuring epinephrine or alcohol.

4. One 10 cc. Lok-syringe, preferably with finger rings.

5. One graduated measuring cup, preferably stainless steel, for mixing solution.

6. One prep cup, preferably stainless steel.

7. Four sterile towels.

8. Six sterile sponges.

9. One sterilizer control.

TECHNIQUE

Position and Landmarks

1. The patient lies in the dorsal recumbent position with his arms at his sides and his head turned to the side opposite that to be blocked. The head usually rests on a "donut" (Figure 39, page 90).

2. In the adult, the position or the approximate position of the second bicuspid tooth is noted. By direct palpation of the skin overlying the appropriate part of the mandible in this area, the mental foramen is located. An X is made on the skin overlying it. The X is usually located approximately 1 inch (2.5 cm.)

from the midline of the face (Figure 38A and B, page 89).

3. If the mental foramen is not palpable through the skin, an X may be marked on the skin below the second bicuspid at a point midway between the upper and lower margins of the mandible, near the lower margins of the mandible, or near the upper margin of the mandible, depending on the age of the patient.

4. ¼ inch (0.6 cm.) posterior and ¼ inch (0.6 cm.) superior to the X an O is marked on the skin. A straight line is visualized between the X and the O. In this manner the anesthetist takes account of the slant of the mental canal. If the needle were introduced perpendicular to the skin at the X, the foramen might be felt but it would be difficult to enter and traverse it (Figure 38A and B, page 89).

Precautions: *Aspirate.*—Aspirate for blood before injecting anesthetic solution.

Procedure

1. The sterilizer control must be checked to be sure the equipment has been sterilized.

2. The area is aseptically prepared and draped.

3. The anesthetist stands at the head of the table facing the patient's feet. This position is the one of choice as it allows the anesthetist to control the patient's head more easily and obtain the correct angle for the insertion of the needle (Figure 39A and B, page 90).

4. A skin wheal is made at the O with the 25-gauge, ¾-inch (2 cm.) Huber point security Lok-needle. Subcutaneous infiltration is carried along the line XO, using approximately ½ cc. to 1 cc. of the local anesthetic solution.

5. The patient is cautioned to say *"Now"* and not move when he feels paresthesias over the distribution of the mental nerve. *Paresthesias of the mental nerve are characterized by sharp, spraying, electric shock sensations to the lower lip. As the needle is advanced in the mental canal, paresthesias of the lower front teeth may occur.*

6. The 1½-inch (3.8 cm.), 22-gauge short-beveled security Lok-needle with the syringe attached is introduced perpendicularly to the skin. The hub is then lowered so that the

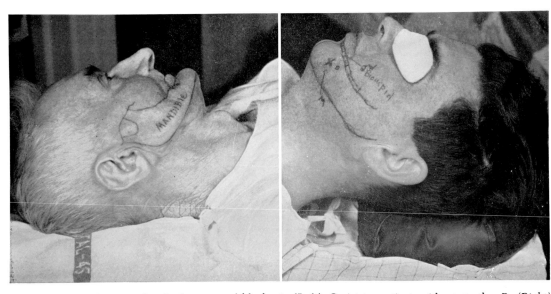

Figure 38. A. and B. Landmarks for a mental block. A. *(Left)* Geriatric patient without teeth. B. *(Right)* Young patient with teeth. The X on the skin overlies the mental foramen.

point of the needle will strike the mandible at a point underlying the X. There is usually a 45-degree angle between the skin and the shaft of the needle (Figure 37A, page 87 and Figure 40A and B, page 90).

7. The needle is advanced inward, downward, and forward until it strikes bone or elicits paresthesias as it slides into the mental foramen. If this does not occur, the anesthetist should redirect the needle point and feel around the portion of the mandible under the X with the needle point until the foramen is located (Figure 37A, page 87 and Figure 40A and B, page 90).

8. 2 cc. of anesthetic solution is injected at the opening of the mental foramen. This anesthetizes the mental nerve.

9. The needle is slowly advanced down the mental canal and small amounts of solution are injected as the needle moves forward. When the needle has been introduced ¼ inch (0.6 cm.), 2 cc. of solution is injected. This anesthetizes the incisor nerve.

10. As the needle is withdrawn, 1 to 3 cc. of anesthetic solution is deposited.

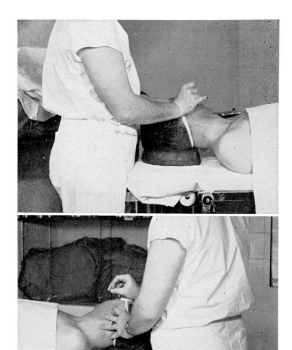

Figure 39. Position of the patient and the right-handed anesthetist for a mental block. A. *(Top)* Right side. B. *(Bottom)* Left side.

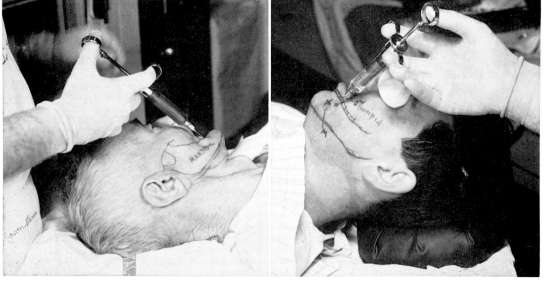

Figure 40. A. and B. Needle rests in the mental foramen and has entered the mental canal. A. *(Left)* The block was performed for biopsy of leukoplakia of the alveolar ridge in a geriatric patient without teeth. Note the position of the anesthetist and the direction and angle of the needle. B. *(Right)* The block was performed for a mucocele of the lower lip on a young patient with teeth.

11. 5 cc. to 10 cc. of solution is usually adequate for a unilateral block.

EXTENT OF ANALGESIA

Analgesia extends over the chin, lower lip, lower teeth (incisors, cuspids, and bicuspids), and the mucous membrane of the lip and inside of the gums (Figure 41, page 91).

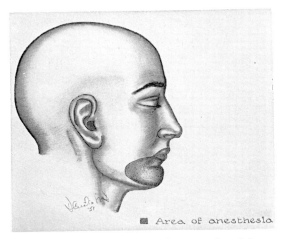

Figure 41. Area of skin anesthesia produced by a unilateral mental nerve block.

COMPLICATIONS

Toxic Reactions (intravascular injections, etc.): See Chapter 3, page 19.

REMARKS

Complications Minimal: This block is simple to perform. Complications are infrequent and the analgesia established is excellent for facial work in the anesthetized area.

Advance Needle into Mental Canal: If the needle is not advanced down the mental canal, the incisor nerve may not be anesthetized.

Indication for Bilateral Block: If the lesion to be operated is near the midline, a bilateral block is necessary because of crossing of nerve fibers from the opposite side.

Indication to Also Block Cervical Nerves: When operative procedures are to extend to or below the lower margin of the mandible, either a line of intradermal and subcutaneous local infiltration along the skin overlying the lower margin of the mandible or a unilateral or bilateral block of the second cervical nerve is necessary to anesthetize overlying filaments of this superficial cervical nerve.

Importance of Alveolar Ridge: The anesthetist should always take into consideration the age of the patient and whether he has teeth. If the patient has no teeth, it is important to know how long he has been without them and how long he has worn a plate. A dental plate tends to prevent atrophy of the alveolar ridge. Such information is a great aid in picturing approximately where the mental foramen is located in relation to the upper and lower margins of the mandible.

Supraorbital, Infraorbital, and Mental Foramina Lie on Straight Line: When the patient is edentulous or the mental foramen is difficult to palpate, it should be remembered that the supraorbital notch, the infraorbital foramen, and the mental foramen all lie on a straight line approximately 1 inch (2.5 cm.) from the midline of the face. Therefore, if either the supraorbital foramen or the infraorbital foramen is palpable and a line is drawn through the palpable foramen parallel to the midsagittal plane of the body, the mental foramen should be located at a point where the line crosses the superior edge or middle of the mandible, depending on whether or not the patient has teeth (Figure 25, page 76 and Figure 29, page 80).

Use Alcohol with Care: Before injecting alcohol, consult Chapter 41, page 329.

Elicit Paresthesias: In this block procedure, paresthesias should be elicited. Remember the dictum, *"No paresthesias, no anesthesia"* and the failures will be minimal.

Intubate Patient for Long or Tedious Operation: Satisfactory anesthesia for long or tedious surgical procedures of the face is perhaps one of the most difficult types of anesthesia to administer in a way that satisfies the requirements of the patient, of the surgeon, and of the anesthetist. Regional analgesia may be employed satisfactorily for short *su-*

perficial procedures, since the correctly medicated patient will usually tolerate uncomfortable positions, the feeling of suffocation from drapes, and manipulation discomforts for limited periods. However, during long and/or tedious procedures requiring deep manipulations of the face, nasal pharynx, oral pharynx, pharynx, larynx, or trachea, the constant cooperation of the patient must not be relied on. Restlessness and motion at a crucial point by a patient who was thought to be cooperative may prove disastrous to the patient or to the operative result being sought. Likewise, the administration of intravenous, rectal, or inhalation anesthesia to a patient who was started under regional block and whose airway has been made inaccessible by the drapes or the surgery may be equally as catastrophic. Therefore, in long and/or tedious procedures of the face, endotracheal anesthesia may be a more satisfactory means of establishing anesthesia.

Recover Broken Needle(s): All needles should be tested before use. If a needle breaks, every effort to recover it, including surgery, should be made. Unremoved needles have a tendency to migrate and may cause permanent injuries as well as medicolegal complications.

Repeat Block When Analgesia Is Inadequate: If the desired results from the first block attempt are unsatisfactory, do not hesitate to reblock the patient if time permits. Most patients will think nothing about being reblocked if the second attempt is prefaced by a statement such as: "Well, I guess we will have to inject a little more medicine if we are going to freeze this area."

CHAPTER 15

Block of the Mandibular Nerve

INDICATIONS

Surgical: Operations or manipulations of the lower jaw including the teeth, gums, mandible and lower lip, and the anterior two-thirds of the tongue.

Diagnostic: Differentiation of neuralgias, especially glossopharyngeal (posterior one-third of the tongue) from trigeminal (anterior two-thirds of the tongue, via mandibular and lingual nerves).

Therapeutic: This block is used for relief of: (1) trigeminal neuralgia (tic douloureux) when limited to mandibular nerve; (2) masseter spasm in cases of trismus, *i.e.*, release of the spasm; (3) neuralgias of alveolar ridge following dental extractions; and (4) intractable pain of the mandible (Figure 42, page 93).

ANATOMY

The mandibular nerve, or third division of the trigeminal nerve, is the largest of three divisions of the trigeminal nerve. It leaves the skull through the foramen ovale and divides into a small motor division and a large sensory division about ½ inch (1.3 cm.) below the foramen ovale. It lies opposite the middle of the mandibular notch between the coronoid and condyloid (head) processes of the mandible (Figure 43, page 94). The internal maxillary artery crosses in front of the mandibular nerve just below the notch in the mandible while the middle meningeal artery lies posterior and in close proximity to it.

The branches of the motor portion of the mandibular nerve are the nerve to the ptery-goideus internus muscle, the masseteric nerve, the nerve to the external pterygoid muscle, the mylohyoid nerve, and the deep temporal nerves. Because of this distribution the motor root is often referred to as the masticator nerve. The branches of the sensory portion of the mandibular nerve are the buccinator nerve, the lingual nerve, the auriculotemporal nerve, and the inferior alveolar nerve.

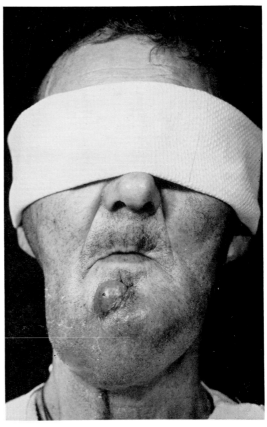

Figure 42. Carcinoma of the mandible with extension, erosion of the tongue, and pain in the mandible and cheek. Bilateral mandibular block with absolute alcohol alleviated the pain.

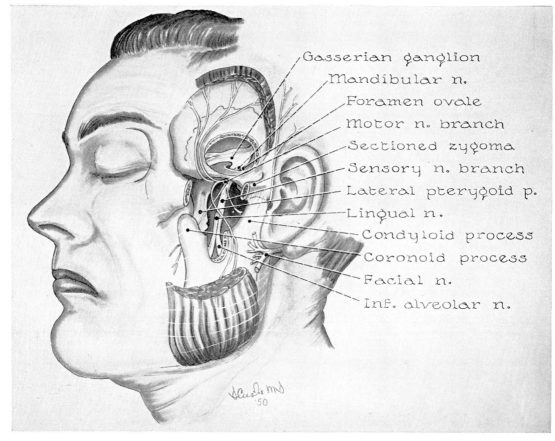

Figure 43. Anatomy of the mandibular nerve.

PREMEDICATION

Paresthesias are always sought. Therefore, light premedication is advised.

Light Premedication: The average patient (age 20 to 50, weight 150 pounds or over, height 5 feet, 5 inches or over, and good physical status) receives:

1. 200 mg. (3 gr.) of pentobarbital (Nembutal) by mouth at hour of sleep the night previous to surgery.

2. 100 mg. (1½ gr.) of pentobarbital by mouth with one ounce of water 1½ to 2 hours before estimated *block* time. This dose of barbiturate is omitted if there is a possibility that the patient will be too heavily sedated to give *an immediate response* when paresthesias are obtained.

3. 10 mg. (⅙ gr.) of morphine and 0.4 mg. (¹⁄₁₅₀ gr.) of scopolamine intramuscularly on call to surgery.

Reduction of Premedication: It is seldom necessary to increase this premedication irrespective of the over-all size of the patient until the patient arrives in either the anesthesia or operating room. However, it is very common to reduce this medication under various circumstances; for example, for the geriatric patient, the adolescent patient or child, the debilitated or cachectic patient, and for those whose surgery is complicated by other disease, *e.g.*, myxedema, diabetes, heart disease, etc. In the patient over 60 years of age, barbiturates and especially scopolamine may often cause disorientation. Therefore, in these patients atropine is usually substituted for scopolamine and the dosages of the barbiturate omitted or greatly reduced, *i.e.*, to 50 mg. (¾ gr.) or less. *Always err on the light side.*

Inadequate Premedication: If the medication is inadequate, either for the block or for the surgical procedure, intravenous pentobarbital 50 mg. (¾ gr.) to 100 mg. (1½ gr.) or intravenous morphine 8 mg. (⅛ gr.) to 15 mg. (¼ gr.) may be given *slowly.* Judicious use of added sedation is extremely important. Often small supplementary doses of morphine or pentobarbital will make a block successful when a patient interprets touch and motion as pain.

DRUGS

Tetracaine (Pontocaine)

Dosage.—10 cc. to 20 cc. of 0.15 to 0.25 percent with or without 0.1 cc. of epinephrine (Adrenalin) 1:1000 in each 20 cc. of solution.*

Onset.—Operating analgesia is established in 10 to 20 minutes.

Duration.—Operating analgesia lasts 3½ to 6 hours, with stronger concentrations and solutions containing epinephrine giving the upper limits.

Procaine (Novocain)

Dosage.—10 cc. to 20 cc. of 1.0 to 2.0 percent solution with or without 0.1 cc. of epinephrine (Adrenalin) 1:1000 in each 20 cc. of solution.*

Onset.—Operating analgesia is established in 5 to 15 minutes.

Duration.—Operating analgesia lasts 1 to 1¾ hours, with stronger concentrations and solutions containing epinephrine giving the upper limits.

Lidocaine (Xylocaine) or Mepivacaine (Carbocaine)

Dosage.—10 cc. to 20 cc. of 1.0 to 1.5 percent with or without 0.1 cc. of epinephrine (Adrenalin) 1:1000 in each 20 cc. of solution.*

Onset.—Operating analgesia is established in 5 to 15 minutes.

Duration.—Operating analgesia lasts 1¼ to 3 hours, with stronger concentrations and solutions containing epinephrine giving the upper limits.

Alcohol

Dosage.—1 cc. to 1.5 cc. of absolute alcohol (95 percent) from sterile individual ampules. More than 1.5 cc. should not be injected at any one time for a unilateral block.

Onset.—Analgesia is established in 1 to 5 minutes.

Duration.—Sensory analgesia lasts three weeks to three months. Pain fibers may be analgesic from six months to thirty years. The latter figure is unusual and the average duration is nine to fifteen months.

MATERIALS

Regional tray (see Chapter 9, page 51) or:

1. One ¾-inch (2 cm.), 25-gauge Huber point security Lok-needle.

2. One 2-inch (5 cm.), 22-gauge security Lok-needle, preferably with short bevel.

3. One tuberculin Lok-syringe for measuring epinephrine or alcohol.

4. One 10 cc. Lok-syringe, preferably with finger rings.

5. One graduated measuring cup, preferably stainless steel, for mixing solution.

6. One prep cup, preferably stainless steel.

7. Four sterile towels.

8. Six sterile sponges.

9. One sterilizer control.

---

*Optimal concentration of epinephrine is 1:200,000, that is, 0.1 cc. of epinephrine 1:1000 in 20 cc. of the local anesthetic solution (see page 39).

TECHNIQUE

Position and Landmarks

1. The patient lies in the dorsal recumbent position with his arms at his sides and a "donut" under his head (Figure 44, page 96).

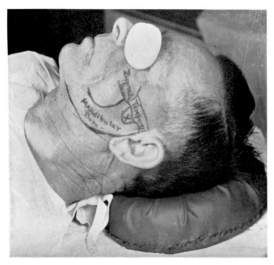

Figure 44. Patient in position for mandibular block with landmarks drawn on the skin. Note position of X slightly below the inferior edge of the zygomatic process of temporal bone. Head rests on 'donut' for stability. This patient was to have a closed reduction of a fractured mandible.

2. The head should be in the profile position so that a sagittal section through the nose would be perpendicular to the table.

3. The zygomatic arch of the zygomatic process of the temporal bone is located.

4. The mandibular notch between the coronoid and condyloid process of the mandibular bone is palpated. This is easily done by exerting gentle pressure with the index finger just anterior to the temporal mandibular articulation and asking the patient to open and close his mouth.

5. An X is made on the skin overlying the middle of the mandibular notch just below the zygomatic arch. This X lies about ½ inch (1.3 cm.) in front of the tragus of the ear and usually at the midpoint between the condyloid and coronoid processes of the mandible (Figure 44, page 96).

Precautions

Aspirate.—Before injection of solutions, very careful aspiration tests must be performed to be sure that the needle point does not rest in the middle meningeal artery, the internal maxillary artery, or inside the dural membrane.

Use of Depth Markers.—Depth markers need not be employed if the anesthetist inserts the 2-inch (5 cm.) needle slowly and is constantly cognizant of its depth.

Avoid Facial Nerve.—Branches of the facial nerve to the eyelids lie in close relationship to the above landmarks, *i.e.*, one fingerbreadth [½ inch (1.3 cm.) to ¾ inch (2 cm.)] anterior and inferior to the tragus of the ear (Figure 43, page 94). For this reason, after the anesthetic solution has been deposited at the mandibular nerve, 2 cc. of air should be injected to expel the remaining solution from the needle before it is withdrawn. This precaution may prevent facial nerve involvement and is mandatory if alcohol is employed for a therapeutic block.

Procedure

1. The sterilizer control must be checked to be sure the equipment has been sterilized.

2. The area is aseptically prepared and draped. Usually one towel placed across the forehead and one across the chin are sufficient.

3. If the anesthetist is right-handed, he stands at the head of the table facing the patient's feet for a right mandibular block and on the left side of the patient facing the head of the table for a left mandibular block (Figure 45, page 97). The opposite is the case for a left-handed operator. This position was selected because it allows the anesthetist to steady the patient's head with his free hand and prevent him from drawing his head away from the advancing needle.

4. A skin wheal is made at the determined

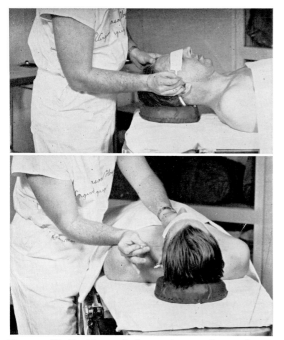

Figure 45. Position of the patient and anesthetist for a maxillary or mandibular block. A. (*Top*) Right side. B. (*Bottom*) Left side.

spot with the 25-gauge, ¾-inch (2 cm.) Huber point security Lok-needle (Figure 46, page 97).

5. The bevel of the needle is checked with the markings on the hub so that the anesthetist knows at all times in which direction the bevel is pointing.

6. The patient is cautioned to say *"Now"* and not move when he feels paresthesias over the distribution of the mandibular nerve. *Paresthesias of the mandibular nerve are characterized by sharp, spraying, electric shock sensations to the lower jaw, the tongue, the lower lip, and occasionally the lower teeth. If the needle is placed too low or too far medially, paresthesias to the tongue from stimulation of the lingual nerve may occur. The needle should be readjusted until paresthesias of the mandibular nerve occur.*

7. The 2-inch (5 cm.), 22-gauge short beveled security Lok-needle without the syringe

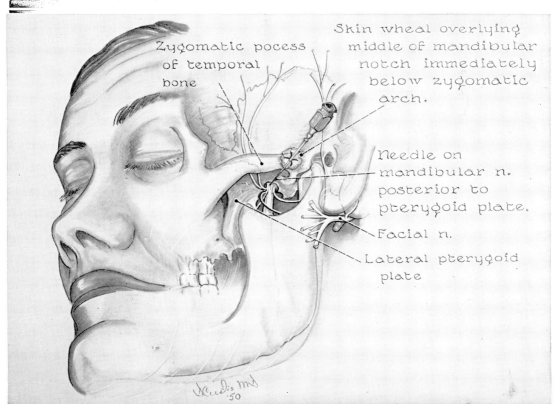

Figure 46. Anatomy of the mandibular nerve at its emergence from the foramen ovale with the needle in place for injection of the local anesthetic solution. The head is slightly tilted in this illustration to demonstrate the anatomy, which would otherwise be hidden by the zygomatic process of the temporal bone.

attached is introduced through the X perpendicular to the skin in all planes and slowly advanced until paresthesias are encountered or the point of the needle impinges on bone (usually the pterygoid plate of the sphenoid bone). This occurs at a depth of 1½ inches (3.8 cm.) to 1¾ inches (4.5 cm.) although in heavy-joweled patients a 2-inch (5 cm.) depth is not uncommon (Figure 46, page 97; Figure 47, page 98; and Figure 48, page 99).

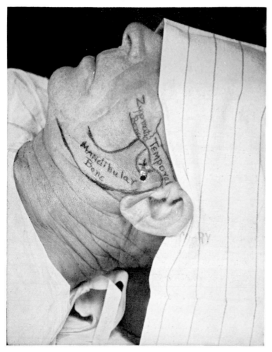

Figure 47. 2-inch (5 cm.) needle in position for mandibular block. Paresthesias were just elicited with a 2-inch (5 cm.) needle. Note that the needle shaft is perpendicular to the skin.

8. If the pterygoid plate is contacted, the needle is too far anterior, since the mandibular nerve passes from the skull through the foramen ovale, which is located posterior to, *i.e.,* ¼ inch (0.6 cm.), and at about the same depth as the pterygoid plate in the base of the sphenoid bone. The distance from the skin to the security bead is carefully noted and the needle withdrawn, redirected posteriorly, and reinserted. This maneuver is repeated until the needle point no longer contacts bone.

When the latter occurs, the needle is slowly and carefully advanced another ⅛ inch (0.3 cm.) to ¼ inch (0.6 cm.). This will usually produce paresthesias of the mandibular nerve or one of its two main branches, the lingual or inferior dental. If paresthesias do not occur, the needle is withdrawn slightly, redirected so that the point is more posterior and superior, and reinserted in an effort to elicit a paresthesia.

If the needle has been inserted 1½ to 1¾ inches (3.8 to 4.5 cm.) into the tissues and if blood appears at its hub, the needle is usually in close proximity to the mandibular nerve—the bevel of the needle lies in either the internal maxillary or middle meningeal arteries (see Anatomy, page 93). The needle is withdrawn from the vessel; the blood is cleared from the needle; the needle is redirected for a slight distance anteriorly, posteriorly, or cephalad and reinserted to approximately the above noted depth in an effort to elicit a paresthesia.

9. When paresthesias of the mandibular nerve occur or when no paresthesias can be elicited after repeated attempts and the needle rests posteriorly and no more than ¼ inch (0.6 cm.) deeper than the pterygoid plate, the bevel of the needle is pointed superiorly and 5 to 10 cc. of local anesthetic solution is deposited (Figure 46, page 97; Figure 47, page 98; and Figure 48, page 99).

Although it is best to have elicited paresthesias, injection of 5 to 10 cc. of the local anesthetic solution in the area through which the mandibular nerve courses often produces an adequate block. If 1.0 to 1.5 cc. of alcohol is to be injected, paresthesias must be elicited.

10. The needle is withdrawn after the anesthetic solution has been cleared from it by the injection of 2 cc. of air.

EXTENT OF ANALGESIA

Analgesia will extend over the temporal region, including the skull and dura mater at the base of the skull, the anterior two-thirds of the tongue, the mucous membrane of the mouth, the lower portion of the face (about

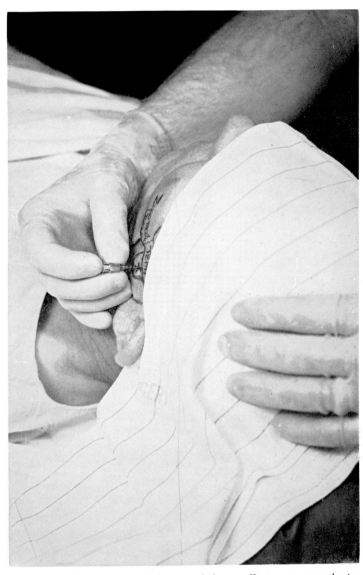

Figure 48. Shows the sagittal view of the needle just as paresthesias of the mandibular nerve were elicited with a 2-inch (5 cm.) needle. Note the perpendicular position of the shaft of the needle in relationship to the skin as well as the method of holding the needle. The anesthetist has changed his position for illustrative purposes.

to the lower edge of the mandibular bone), the lower lip, the auricle of the ear, the external auditory meatus, the mandible, the lower teeth and gums, the temporomandibular joint, the salivary gland, and the lower muscles of the jaw (Figure 49, page 100).

COMPLICATIONS

Toxic Reactions (intravascular injections, etc.): See Chapter 3, page 19. These are infrequent if careful aspiration is practiced and the advised dosage of anesthetic agent is not exceeded.

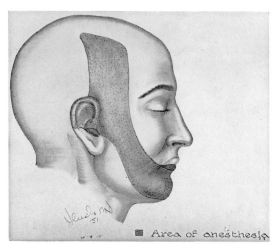

Figure 49. Area of skin anesthesia produced by a unilateral mandibular nerve block.

Subarachnoid Injections: Extremely rare. They are treated as if a high spinal anesthesia had occurred (see Chapter 43, page 353).

Hemorrhage into the Cheek: This is not uncommon since the area is quite vascular and the soft tissues of the cheek do not limit the spread of blood. Therefore, hemorrhage seldom limits itself by its own pressure until a large hematoma has formed.

Signs and Symptoms.—Swelling of the jaw and region around the temporomandibular joint.

Etiology.—Puncture of blood vessel.

Course.—Hematoma is reabsorbed in a few days.

Treatment.—If a blood vessel is known to have been punctured, pressure over the cheek and temporomandibular joint should be applied by means of a folded towel so as to decrease the soft tissue area into which the blood may flow; this avoids a hematoma, or at least decreases its size. When a large hematoma results, then warm moist compresses should be applied to the area.

Tissue Reaction to Alcohol Injection: When alcohol 95 percent is used in a therapeutic block, occasionally a severe tissue reaction will occur.

Signs and Symptoms.—Swelling of the jaw.

Etiology.—Tissue reaction to alcohol.

Course.—Disappears in a few days to a week.

Treatment.—Warm moist compresses and codeine and aspirin for pain.

Facial Nerve Block: Rarely occurs during this procedure and is of no serious consequence unless it occurs in conjunction with an alcohol therapeutic block. However, facial nerve blocks are to be avoided, especially in resection of parotid tumors, for the surgeon often wishes to stimulate the facial nerve in order to identify it and avoid sectioning it. Also, when plastic surgery is to be performed this complication is most disconcerting.

Signs and Symptoms.—Bell's palsy on the affected side, *i.e.,* inability to close eyelid, sagging of face muscles, and expressionless face.

Etiology.—Deposition of too large a volume of the local anesthetic solution in the subcutaneous tissue, incorrect landmark, or both.

Course.—Disappears as the block dissipates itself.

Treatment.—None, if the anesthetic solution is of short duration. When the anesthetic agent is alcohol, the eye should be protected against corneal ulcers and the muscles of the face exercised by electrical stimulation to prevent atrophy until the nerve returns to normal function—obtain consultation of an ophthalmologist.

REMARKS

Indication to Also Block Maxillary or Cervical Nerves: When operations are to be performed under mandibular nerve block, not only must this nerve be anesthetized; but, the second cervical nerve, the maxillary nerve, or both often must be blocked to assure adequate analgesia. Operations for the following conditions, for example, usually require a combination of blocks: (1) to resect a tumor of the parotid gland, a mandibular nerve block, a maxillary nerve block, and a block of the second cervical nerve is needed; (2) to wire a broken jaw—wires must be attached to both upper and lower teeth—blocks of the mandibular and maxillary nerves must be done; and (3) to perform open operation on the lower border of the mandible, a block of the mandibular and second cervical nerves is required.

Indication for Bilateral Block: When operations involving areas near the midline of the chin are to be performed with mandibular nerve block, a bilateral block or local infiltration along the midline is necessary to cover the overlap from the nerves on the opposite side.

Elicit Paresthesias: In this block procedure, paresthesias should be elicited. Remember the dictum, "*No paresthesias, no anesthesia*" and the failures will be minimal.

Accuracy of Paresthesias: Paresthesias of the mandibular nerve may be misleading. Typical paresthesias such as "electric shocks" or "spraying sensations" to the corner of the lip, tongue, lower teeth, or jaw may not occur. The patient may merely complain of pain in the ear, temporomandibular joint, or aching in the cheek when the needle comes in close approximation to the nerve, or the patient may not complain of pain in spite of a correctly placed needle. Periosteal stimulation of the lateral pterygoid plate may be misleading, and the anesthetist ought not to be fooled by it. The patient usually describes the periosteal type of pain as an ache "right where the needle is" and the pain does not radiate. One should always seek typical paresthesias to assure an effective block, but if one cannot produce them after repeated efforts, one should settle for an atypical paresthesia. If the anesthetist cannot produce any paresthesias, he must then rely on the placement of the needle, which to be correct, must be posterior to the lateral pterygoid plate before injection. In this situation, x-ray films of the needle in place may be a great aid.

When alcohol is used, typical paresthesias

must be diligently sought. If they cannot be elicited, it is best not to use alcohol.

Use Donut: The "donut" is employed because: (1) it lends stability to the head and makes the head easier to control, and (2) it allows the operator more working room since the head is raised off the cart 2 inches (5 cm.) to 3 inches (7.5 cm.). The same position cannot be obtained by an ordinary pillow, which allows the head to sink into it, thus decreasing the available working area.

Omit Premedication When Using Alcohol: When performing an alcohol block of the mandibular nerve or its branches in a patient with tic douloureux, premedication should be omitted because: (1) accurate paresthesias are essential and (2) if a complication results and a medicolegal case develops, then the patient cannot claim that he did not want the block but that the sedation made him acquiesce.

Aspirate: During injection of the mandibular nerve the anesthetist should aspirate for air as well as for blood, as the tip of the needle may occasionally be in the pharynx. If this precaution is not observed, the patient may complain of tasting the anesthetic solution. Puncture of the pharyngeal mucosa is of no consequence and is not an indication to discontinue the block procedure. The use of a 2-inch (5 cm.) needle is a safeguard in itself against too deep insertion in most patients.

Method of Entering Mandibular Notch: On occasion it may be difficult to enter the mandibular notch. If this occurs, the patient should be instructed to open his mouth. With this maneuver the anesthetist may determine whether the needle point is resting on the zygomatic process of the temporal bone or on the mandible. If it is on the mandible, the needle will move, and if it is on the zygomatic bone, there will be no change in the position of the needle. On occasion, the opening between the mandibular bone and the zygomatic process may also be extremely small, and by having the patient open his mouth this opening may be enlarged. This maneuver will often facilitate the passage of the needle past the bony landmarks.

Use Alcohol with Care: Before performing alcohol injections of the mandibular nerve, see Chapter 41, page 329.

Intubate Patient for Long or Tedious Operation: Satisfactory anesthesia for long or tedious surgical procedures of the face is perhaps one of the most difficult types of anesthesia to administer in a way that satisfies the requirements of the patient, of the surgeon, and of the anesthetist. Regional analgesia may be employed satisfactorily for short *superficial* procedures, since the correctly medicated patient will usually tolerate uncomfortable positions, the feeling of suffocation from drapes, and manipulation discomforts for limited periods. However, during long and/or tedious procedures requiring deep manipulations of the face, nasal pharynx, oral pharynx, pharynx, larynx, or trachea, the constant cooperation of the patient must not be relied on. Restlessness and motion at a crucial point by a patient who was thought to be cooperative may prove disastrous to the patient or to

the operative result being sought. Likewise, the administration of intravenous, rectal, or inhalation anesthesia to a patient who was started under regional block and whose airway has been made inaccessible by the drapes or the surgery may be equally as catastrophic.

Therefore, in long and/or tedious procedures of the face, endotracheal anesthesia may be a more satisfactory means of establishing anesthesia.

Recover Broken Needle(s): All needles should be tested before use. If a needle breaks, every effort to recover it, including surgery, should be made. Unremoved needles have a tendency to migrate and cause permanent injuries as well as medicolegal complications.

Repeat Block When Analgesia Is Inadequate: If the desired results from the first block attempt are unsatisfactory, do not hesitate to reblock the patient if time permits. Most patients will think nothing about being reblocked if the second attempt is prefaced by a statement such as: "Well, I guess we will have to inject a little more medicine if we are going to freeze this area."

CHAPTER 16

Block of the Maxillary Nerve

INDICATIONS

Surgical: Operations or manipulations of the cheek; upper jaw including the teeth, gums, and maxillary bone; the upper lip; a small portion of the inner angle of the nose; part of the lower eyelid; the antrum; hard and soft palate; and part of the tonsils.

Diagnostic: Differentiation of trigeminal neuralgia (tic douloureux) from psychoneurosis.

Therapeutic: Relief of trigeminal neuralgia (tic douloureux) when limited to the maxillary nerve, relief of neuralgias of the upper alveolar ridge following dental extractions, relief of neuralgias caused by infections or residue of infections in the maxillary sinuses, and relief of intractable pain in areas supplied by the maxillary nerve.

ANATOMY

The maxillary nerve or second division of the trigeminal nerve is a sensory nerve and lies between the ophthalmic and mandibular nerves, in both position and size. It leaves the skull through the foramen rotundum. The foramen rotundum is located in the great wing (base) of the sphenoid bone just superior and slightly posterior to the anterior edge of the pterygoid plate on the posterior wall of the pterygopalatine fissure. The maxillary nerve crosses the pterygopalatine fossa, enters the orbit (under the name of the infraorbital nerve) through the inferior orbital fissure, traverses the infraorbital groove and canal, again leaves the skull through the infraorbital foramen, and then divides into four terminal divisions (Figure 50, page 104). The branches of the maxillary nerve are: the middle meningeal nerve; the sphenopalatine nerve; the zygomatic nerve; the posterior, middle, and anterior superior alveolar nerves; and finally the four terminal divisions which are the inferior palpebral, the external and the internal nasal, and the superior labial nerves.

The internal maxillary artery and its branches furnish the arterial supply to the areas in which the maxillary nerve courses.

PREMEDICATION

Paresthesias are always sought. Therefore, light premedication is advised.

Light Premedication: The average patient (age 20 to 50, weight 150 pounds or over, height 5 feet, 5 inches or over, and good physical status) receives:

1. 200 mg. (3 gr.) of pentobarbital (Nembutal) by mouth at hour of sleep the night previous to surgery.

2. 100 mg. (1½ gr.) of pentobarbital by mouth with one ounce of water 1½ to 2 hours before estimated *block* time. This dose of barbiturate is omitted if there is a possibility that the patient will be too heavily sedated to give *an immediate response* when paresthesias are obtained.

3. 10 mg. (⅙ gr.) of morphine and 0.4 mg. (1⁄150 gr.) of scopolamine intramuscularly *on call* to surgery.

Reduction of Premedication: It is seldom necessary to increase this premedication irrespective of the over-all size of the patient until the patient arrives in either the anesthesia or operating room. However, it is very common to reduce this medication under various circumstances; for example, for the geriatric pa-

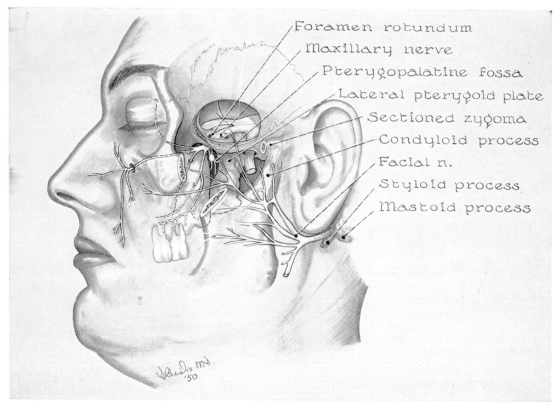

Foramen rotundum
Maxillary nerve
Pterygopalatine fossa
Lateral pterygoid plate
Sectioned zygoma
Condyloid process
Facial n.
Styloid process
Mastoid process

Figure 50. Anatomy of the maxillary nerve. The proximity of the branches of the facial nerve, which innervate the orbicularis oculi muscle, to the mandibular notch should be noted.

tient, the adolescent patient or child, the debilitated or cachectic patient, and for those whose surgery is complicated by other disease, *e.g.*, myxedema, diabetes, heart disease, etc. In the patient over 60 years of age, barbiturates and especially scopolamine may often cause disorientation. Therefore, in these patients atropine is usually substituted for scopolamine and the dosages of the barbiturate omitted or greatly reduced, *i.e.*, to 50 mg. (¾ gr.) or less. *Always err on the light side.*

Inadequate Premedication: If the medication is inadequate, either for the block or for the surgical procedure, intravenous pentobarbital 50 mg. (¾ gr.) to 100 mg. (1½ gr.) or intravenous morphine 8 mg. (⅛ gr.) to 15 mg. (¼ gr.) may be given *slowly*. Judicious use of added sedation is extremely important. Often small supplementary doses of morphine or pentobarbital will make a block successful

when a patient interprets touch and motion as pain.

DRUGS

Tetracaine (Pontocaine)

Dosage.—10 cc. to 20 cc. of 0.15 to 0.25 percent with or without 0.1 cc. of epinephrine (Adrenalin) 1:1000 in each 20 cc. of solution.*

Onset.—Operating analgesia is established in 10 to 20 minutes.

Duration.—Operating analgesia lasts 3½ to 6 hours, with stronger concentrations and solutions containing epinephrine giving the upper limits.

_____

*Optimal concentration of epinephrine is 1:200,000, that is, 0.1 cc. of epinephrine 1:1000 in 20 cc. of the local anesthetic solution (see page 39).

Procaine (Novocain)

Dosage.—10 cc. to 20 cc. of 1.0 to 2.0 per-cent solution with or without 0.1 cc. of epinephrine (Adrenalin) 1:1000 in each 20 cc. of solution.*

Onset.—Operating analgesia is established in 5 to 15 minutes.

Duration.—Operating analgesia lasts 1 to 1¾ hours, with stronger concentrations and solutions containing epinephrine giving the upper limits.

Lidocaine (Xylocaine) or Mepivacaine (Carbocaine)

Dosage.—10 cc. to 20 cc. of 1.0 to 1.5 per-cent solution with or without 0.1 cc. of epinephrine (Adrenalin) 1:1000 in each 20 cc. of solution.*

Onset.—Operating analgesia is established in 5 to 15 minutes.

Duration.—Operating analgesia lasts 1¼ to 3 hours, with stronger concentrations and solutions containing epinephrine giving the upper limits.

Alcohol

Dosage.—1.0 cc. to 1.5 cc. of absolute alcohol (95 percent) from sterile individual ampules. More than 1.5 cc. should not be injected at any one time for a unilateral block.

Onset.—Analgesia is established in 1 to 5 minutes.

Duration.—Sensory analgesia lasts three weeks to three months. Pain fibers may be analgesic from six months to thirty years. The latter figure is unusual and the average duration is nine to fifteen months.

MATERIALS

Regional tray (see Chapter 9, page 51) or:

1. One ¾-inch (2 cm.), 25-gauge Huber point security Lok-needle.

2. One 3-inch (7.5 cm.), 22-gauge security Lok-needle, preferably with a short bevel.

3. One tuberculin syringe for measuring epinephrine or alcohol.

4. One 10 cc. Lok-syringe, preferably with finger rings.

5. One graduated measuring cup, preferably stainless steel, for mixing solution.

6. One prep cup, preferably stainless steel.

7. Four sterile towels.

8. Six sterile sponges.

9. One sterilizer control.

TECHNIQUE

Position and Landmarks

1. The patient lies in the dorsal recumbent position with his arms at his sides and a "donut" under his head (Figure 51, page 105).

2. The head should be in the profile position so that a sagittal section through the nose would be perpendicular to the table (Figure 51, page 105).

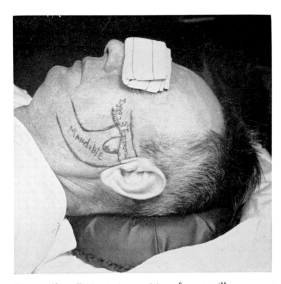

Figure 51. Patient in position for maxillary nerve block with landmarks drawn on the skin. Note the position of X as it lies in posterior inferior portion of the notch of the mandible. Patient received an alcohol injection for trigeminal neuralgia with marked relief. Patient was treated as an outpatient.

*See footnote page 104.

3. The zygomatic arch of the zygomatic process of the temporal bone is located.

4. The mandibular notch between the coronoid and condyloid process of the mandibular bone is palpated (Figure 51, page 105). This is easily done by exerting gentle pressure with the index finger just anterior to the temporal mandibular articulation and asking the patient to open and close his mouth.

5. An X is made on the skin overlying the posterior inferior surface of the mandibular notch (Figure 51, page 105).

Precautions

Aspirate.—Before injection of solutions in this area, careful aspiration tests must be performed to ascertain if the needle point rests in the subarachnoid space, in the maxillary artery, the posterior superior alveolar artery, or the infraorbital artery.

Use of Depth Markers.—Depth markers are not necessary and need not be employed if the anesthetist is constantly cognizant of the depth to which the needle has been inserted. It is seldom necessary to insert the needle deeper than 2¼ inches (5.6 cm.), even in a heavy patient. If the needle is inserted past this depth it may enter the orbit through the inferior orbital fissure.

Avoid Facial Nerve.—The facial nerve lies in close relationship to the above landmarks, i.e., ½ inch (1.3 cm.) anterior and inferior to the tragus of the ear, at a depth of ¼ inch (0.6 cm.) to ½ inch (1.3 cm.) underneath the skin (Figure 50, page 104). Therefore, excessive local infiltration of anesthetic solution in this area is discouraged. For the same reason, after the anesthetic solution has been deposited at the maxillary nerve, 2 cc. of air should be injected to expel the remaining solution from the needle before it is withdrawn. This precaution may prevent facial nerve involvement and is mandatory if alcohol is employed for a therapeutic block.

Avoid Placement of Needle in Orbit.—Should the patient complain of pain in the eye at any time during the procedure, the advancement of the needle should be stopped and the position of the needle carefully checked. If the needle has been advanced too far superiorly in the pterygopalatine fossa, it may enter the inferior orbital fissure and cause pressure in the structures of the orbit.

Procedure

1. The sterilizer control is checked to be sure the equipment has been sterilized.

2. The area is aseptically prepared and draped. Usually one towel placed across the forehead and one across the chin are sufficient.

3. If the anesthetist is right-handed, he stands at the head of the table facing the patient's feet for a right maxillary block. He stands at the left side of the patient facing the head of the table for a left maxillary block (Figure 45, page 97). The opposite position is taken by a left-handed operator. This position was selected because it allows the anesthetist to steady the patient's head with his free hand and prevent the patient from drawing his head away from the advancing needle.

4. A skin wheal is made at the determined spot with a 25-gauge, ¾-inch (2 cm.) Huber point security Lok-needle (Figure 51, page 105 and Figure 52, page 107).

5. The patient is cautioned to say *"Now"* and not move when he feels paresthesias over the distribution of the maxillary nerve. *The paresthesias, characterized by sharp, spraying, electric shock sensations, should radiate to the ala of the nose, the upper lip, and occasionally the upper teeth. Pain or "electrical shocks" occurring in the cheek or lower eyelid may be caused by stimulation of the infraorbital part of the maxillary nerve. However, the anesthetist should be absolutely certain that the pain is not inside the orbit itself, since this may mean that the needle lies within the orbit.*

6. The bevel of the needle is checked with the markings on the hub so that the anesthetist knows at all times in which direction the bevel is pointing.

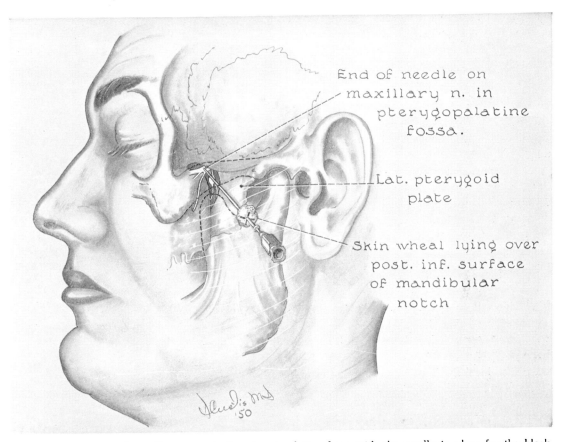

End of needle on
maxillary n. in
pterygopalatine
fossa.

Lat. pterygoid
plate

Skin wheal lying over
post. inf. surface
of mandibular
notch

Figure 52. Anatomy of maxillary nerve in the pterygopalatine fossa with the needle in place for the block.
Note direction of the needle.

7. The 3-inch (7.5 cm.), 22-gauge short beveled security Lok-needle without the syringe attached is introduced through the X at approximately a 45-degree angle to the skin. It is slowly advanced along the direction of an imaginary line between the X and the junction of the optic nerve and sclera. One of the most difficult maneuvers of this block is to get the needle through the mandibular notch and maintain it at a correct angle (Figure 52, page 107 and Figure 53, page 107).

8. At a depth of between 1¾ inches (4.5 cm.) to 2 inches (5 cm.), the needle usually comes in contact with the anterior edge of the lateral pterygoid bone. The distance from the skin to the security bead is carefully noted.

9. After slight withdrawal of the needle and pressure posteriorly and inferiorly on the hub of the needle as the needle is reinserted,

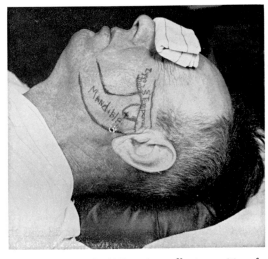

Figure 53. 3-inch (7.5 cm.) needle in position for maxillary block. Paresthesias were just elicited. Note the 45 degree slant of the needle both inferiorly and caudally.

the point will slip anterior to the pterygoid plate and into the pterygopalatine fossa (Figure 52, page 107 and Figure 53, page 107).

10. The needle is now cautiously advanced ¼ inch (0.6 cm.) to ½ inch (1.3 cm.) more deeply than in step 8, until paresthesias are elicited. If no paresthesias occur, the needle should be withdrawn slightly and reintroduced so as to vary the point posteriorly or anteriorly ⅛ inch (0.3 cm.). Paresthesias will in a majority of cases be elicited. Should paresthesias still not occur and if the needle lies at a depth of not more than 2½ inches (6.3 cm.), it is very likely that its point lies in the correct position in the pterygopalatine fissure (Figure 52, page 107 and Figure 53, page 107).

11. The bevel of the needle is pointed superiorly and 5 to 10 cc. of local anesthetic solution is deposited. Although it is best to have elicited paresthesias, injection of 5 to 10 cc. of the local anesthetic solution in the area through which the maxillary nerve courses usually produces an adequate block. If 1.0 to 1.5 cc. of alcohol is to be injected, paresthesias must be elicited.

12. The needle is withdrawn after the anesthetic solution has been cleared from it by the injection of 2 cc. of air.

EXTENT OF ANALGESIA

Analgesia of the upper teeth and gums, upper lip, cheek, lower eyelid, lesser ala of the nose, mucous membrane of the nose and nasopharynx, maxillary sinus, and the soft and hard palate usually ensues (Figure 54, page 108).

COMPLICATIONS

Toxic Reactions (intravascular injections, etc.): See Chapter 3, page 19. These are infrequent if careful aspiration is practiced and the advised dosage of anesthetic agent is not exceeded.

Subarachnoid Injections: Extremely rare. They are treated as if high spinal anesthesia had occurred (see Chapter 43, page 353).

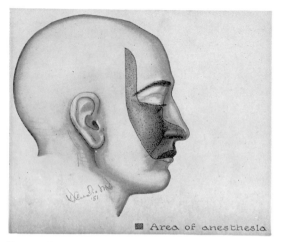

Figure 54. Area of skin anesthesia produced by a unilateral maxillary nerve block.

Hemorrhage into the Cheek: This is not uncommon since the area is extremely vascular and the soft tissues of the cheek do not limit the spread of blood; therefore, it seldom limits itself by its own pressure until a large hematoma has formed.

Signs and Symptoms.—Swelling of the jaw.

Etiology.—Puncture of a blood vessel.

Course.—Hematoma reabsorbs in a few days to a week.

Treatment.—If a blood vessel is known to have been punctured, pressure over the cheek should be applied by means of a folded towel so as to decrease the soft tissue area into which the blood may flow, thereby avoiding or at least decreasing the size of the hematoma. When a large hematoma occurs, warm moist compresses should be applied to the area.

Tissue Reaction to Alcohol Injections: When 95 percent alcohol is used in a therapeutic block, occasionally a severe tissue reaction will occur.

Signs and Symptoms.—Swelling of the jaw.

Etiology.—Tissue reaction to alcohol.

Course.—Disappears in a few days to a week.

Treatment.—Warm moist compresses and codeine and aspirin for pain.

Facial Nerve Palsies: Rarely occur during this procedure and are of no serious consequence unless they occur in conjunction with an alcohol therapeutic block.

Signs and Symptoms.—Bell's palsy on the affected side, *i.e.*, inability to close or tightly close eyelid, sagging of face muscles, and expressionless face.

Etiology.—Block of branches of the facial nerve (Figure 50, page 104).

Course.—Disappears as the block dissipates itself.

Treatment.—None, if the action of the anesthetic solution is of short duration. When the anesthetic agent is alcohol, the eye should be protected against corneal ulcers and the muscles of the face stimulated by electrical stimulation to prevent atrophy until the nerve returns to normal function—obtain consultation of an ophthalmologist.

Orbital Injections or Swelling: These are usually of little consequence provided the solution injected is a short-acting local blocking agent. If alcohol is employed or hemorrhage in the orbit results, the sequelae may be extremely serious with resultant permanent or temporary blindness (Figure 55, page 109 and Figure 56, page 109).

Signs and Symptoms.—They are pain in eye, exophthalmus, diplopia, and loss of vision.

Etiology.—Intraorbital injections of the anesthetic solution, hemorrhage into the orbit caused by trauma to the blood vessels by the needle, or both.

Course.—If local anesthetic drugs are employed, the signs and symptoms will disappear in a matter of hours. When caused by alcohol, the signs and symptoms may be temporary or permanent.

If hemorrhage occurs into the orbit the prognosis is undeterminable.

Treatment.—If signs and symptoms are caused by anesthetic agents no treatment is necessary. Even if alcohol should be deposited on the optic nerve, treatment is of little help.

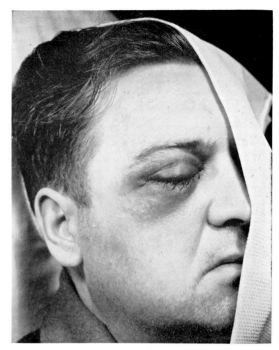

Figure 55. Discoloration and proptosis of an eye following a maxillary nerve block for tic douloureux with alcohol. Acute hemorrhage into the orbit followed the block with slow loss of vision over a period of five minutes. Patient could not open his eyelid.

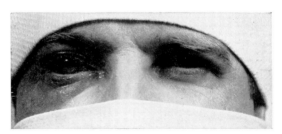

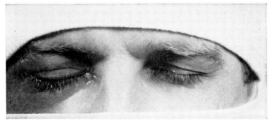

Figure 56. Same patient as in Figure 55 four days later. *(Top)* Shows ability to open eyelid. Motion of the eyeball and action of the pupil is the same as the normal eye. However, the patient did not recover any vision in this eye. *(Bottom)* Shows decrease in swelling of eyelid and discoloration.

When signs and symptoms are caused by hemorrhage, warm moist dressings should be applied to the eye to reduce pressure. Pain should be controlled by sedation as necessary.

An ophthalmologist should be consulted if hemorrhage or alcohol is the causative factor.

Stellate Ganglion Block (see Chapter 18, page 131): Signs and symptoms of this block occasionally accompany a maxillary block. They are of no significance and are corrected when the block dissipates itself. If alcohol has been used, they may persist for a prolonged period of time.

REMARKS

Indication to Also Block Mandibular Nerve: When it is elected to perform operations under maxillary block, it is often necessary to block the mandibular nerve and locally infiltrate around the eye or nose.

Indication for Bilateral Block: When operations involving areas near the midline of the face are to be performed with maxillary nerve block, a bilateral block or local infiltration along the midline of the upper lip and nose is necessary to cover the overlap from the nerves on the opposite side.

Elicit Paresthesias: In this block procedure, paresthesias should be elicited. Remember the dictum, *"No paresthesias, no anesthesia"* and the failures will be minimal.

Accuracy of Paresthesias: Paresthesias of the maxillary nerve may be misleading. Typical paresthesias such as "electric shocks" or "spray sensations" to the upper lip, nose, upper teeth and gums, or upper jaw may not occur. The patient may merely complain of pain at the needle point or of aching in the cheek, or the patient may not complain of pain in spite of a correctly placed needle. Periosteal stimulation of the lateral pterygoid plate may be misleading, and the anesthesiologist should not be fooled by it. The patient usually describes the periosteal type of pain as an ache "right where the needle is" and the pain does not radiate. One should always seek typical paresthesias to assure an effective block, but if one cannot produce them after two or three repeated efforts, one should settle for an atypical paresthesia. If the anesthetist is unable to elicit any paresthesias, he must then rely on the correct placement of the needle at the estimated depth anterior to the pterygoid plate. In this situation, x-ray films of the needle in place may be of great aid. *When alcohol is the anesthetic agent, typical paresthesias must be diligently sought.* If they cannot be elicited, it is best not to use alcohol.

Use Donut: The "donut" is employed because: (1) it lends stability to the head and makes the head easier to control and (2) it allows the operator more working room because the head is raised off the cart 2 inches (5 cm.) to 3 inches (7.5 cm.). The same position cannot be obtained by an ordinary pillow since this allows the head to sink into it, thus decreasing the available working area.

Omit Premedication When Using Alcohol: When performing an alcohol block of the maxillary nerve or its branches in a patient with tic douloureux, premedication should be omitted because: (1) accurate paresthesias are essential and (2) if a complication results and a medicolegal case develops, then the patient cannot claim that he did not want the block but that the sedation made him acquiesce.

Aspirate: During injection of the maxillary nerve, the anesthetist should aspirate for air as well as blood, since the needle tip occasionally may be incorrectly placed posterior to the lateral pterygoid bone and into the pharynx. If this precaution is not observed, the patient may complain of tasting the anesthetic solution. Puncture of the pharyngeal mucosa is of no consequence and is not an indication to discontinue block procedure.

Method of Entering Mandibular Notch: On occasion it may be difficult to enter the mandibular notch. If this occurs, the patient should be instructed to open his mouth. By this maneuver the anesthetist may determine whether the needle is resting on the zygomatic process of the temporal bone or on the mandible. If it is on the mandible, the needle will move, and if it is on the zygomatic bone, there will be no change in the position of the needle. On occasion, the opening between the mandibular bone and the zygomatic process may also be extremely small, and by having the patient open his mouth the opening may be enlarged. This maneuver will often facilitate the passage of the needle past the bony landmarks.

Tic Douloureux of Frontal Nerve Relieved by Maxillary Nerve Block: Often when tic douloureux (trigeminal neuralgia) affects the maxillary nerve, there are referred painful shock-like sensations over the ophthalmic division. If the main trigger area is in the maxillary nerve and if the maxillary nerve is adequately blocked, pain in the ophthalmic division will also disappear. This is probably due to the close association of the fibers of the maxillary and ophthalmic divisions of the trigeminal nerve in the gasserian (semilunar) ganglion.

Use Alcohol with Care: Before performing alcohol injections of the maxillary nerve, see Chapter 41, page 329.

Intubate Patient for Long or Tedious Operation: Satisfactory anesthesia for long or tedious surgical procedures of the face is perhaps one of the most difficult types of anesthesia to administer in a way that satisfies the requirement of the patient, of the surgeon, and of the anesthetist. Regional analgesia may be employed satisfactorily for short *superficial* procedures, since the correctly medicated patient will usually tolerate uncomfortable positions, the feeling of suffocation from drapes, and manipulation discomforts for limited periods. However, during long and/or tedious procedures requiring deep manipulations of the face, nasal pharynx, oral pharynx, pharynx, larynx, or trachea, the constant cooperation of the patient must not be relied on. Restlessness and motion at a crucial point by a patient who was thought to be cooperative may prove disastrous to the patient or to the operative result being sought.

Likewise, the administration of intravenous, rectal, or inhalation anesthesia to a patient who was started under regional block and whose airway has been made inaccessible by the drapes or the surgery, may be equally catastrophic.

Therefore, in long and/or tedious procedures of the face, endotracheal anesthesia is a more satisfactory means of establishing anesthesia.

Recover Broken Needle(s): All needles should be tested before use. If the needle breaks, every effort to recover it, including surgery, should be made. Unremoved needles have a tendency to migrate and may cause permanent injuries as well as medicolegal complications.

Repeat Block When Analgesia Is Inadequate: If the desired results from the first block attempt are unsatisfactory, do not hesitate to reblock the patient if time permits. Most patients will think nothing about being reblocked if the second attempt is prefaced by the statement: "Well, I guess we will have to inject a little more medicine if we are going to freeze this area."

CHAPTER 17

Block of the Cervical Plexus

INDICATIONS

Surgical: Operations on the neck and occipital part of the scalp.

Diagnostic: Differentiation and localization of neuralgias.

Therapeutic: Relief of occipital headaches and neck pain.

ANATOMY

The cervical plexus is formed by the anterior rami of the first four cervical nerves. Each nerve on leaving the intervertebral foramen passes behind the vertebral artery and reaches the tip of the transverse process to lie in the sulcus between the anterior and posterior tubercles of the transverse process (Figure 60, page 116). The tubercle of the transverse processes lie from ½ inch (1.3 cm.) to 1¼ inches (3.2 cm.) below the skin, depending on the size of the patient, with the lower ones more superficially placed. As the nerves leave the sulci, they divide into upper and lower branches, and these in turn unite with each other to form a series of loops known as the cervical plexus. The plexus lies opposite the upper four cervical vertebrae and in front of the levator scapulae muscle and the middle scalene muscle, and is covered by the sternocleidomastoid muscle. Each loop gives rise to a superficial and deep branch. The superficial branches emerge along the posterior margin of the sternocleidomastoid muscle and supply the skin and the superficial structures (Figure 57, page 113). The deep branches innervate the muscles and other deep structures of the neck.

PREMEDICATION

No attempts to elicit paresthesias are made. Therefore, heavy medication is advised for surgical patients.

Heavy Premedication: The average patient (age 20 to 50, weight 150 pounds or over, approximate height 5 feet, 5 inches or over, and good physical condition) receives:

1. 200 mg. (3 gr.) of pentobarbital (Nembutal) by mouth at hour of sleep the night before surgery.

2. 100 mg. (1½ gr.) to 200 mg. (3 gr.) of pentobarbital with one ounce of water by mouth 1½ to 2 hours before estimated *block* time.

3. 15 mg. (¼ gr.) of morphine and 0.6 mg. (¹⁄₁₀₀ gr.) of scopolamine intramuscularly ¾ to 1 hour before estimated *block* time.

Reduction of Premedication: It is seldom necessary to increase this premedication irrespective of the over-all size of the patient until the patient arrives in either the anesthesia or operating room. However, it is very common to reduce this medication under various circumstances; for example, for the geriatric patient, the adolescent patient or child, the debilitated or cachectic patient, and for those whose surgery is complicated by other disease, *i.e.,* myxedema, diabetes, heart disease, etc. In the patient over 60 years of age, barbiturates and especially scopolamine may often cause disorientation. Therefore, in these patients atropine is usually substituted for scopolamine and the dosages of the barbiturate omitted or greatly reduced, *i.e.,* to 50 mg. (¾ gr.) or less. *Always err on the light side.*

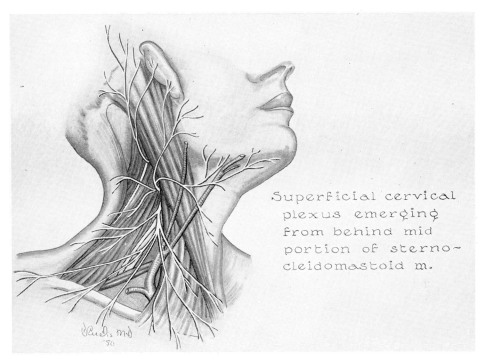

Superficial cervical plexus emerging from behind mid portion of sterno- cleidomastoid m.

Figure 57. Anatomy of the superficial cervical plexus.

Inadequate Premedication: If the medication is inadequate either for the block or for the surgical procedure, pentobarbital 50 mg. (¾ gr.) to 100 mg. (1½ gr.) or morphine 8 mg. (⅛ gr.) to 15 mg. (¼ gr.) may be given slowly intravenously until the desired effect results. Judicious use of added sedation is extremely important. Often small supplementary doses of intravenous morphine or pentobarbital given *slowly* will make a block successful when a patient interprets touch and motion as pain.

DRUGS

Tetracaine (Pontocaine)

Dosage.—80 cc. to 100 cc. of 0.15 percent solution, with or without 0.25 cc. of epinephrine (Adrenalin) 1:1000.*

Onset.—Operating analgesia is established in 15 to 45 minutes with an average of 20 minutes.

Duration.—Operating analgesia lasts 3 to 4 hours, with solutions containing epinephrine giving the upper limits.

Procaine (Novocain)

Dosage.—80 cc. to 100 cc. of 1.0 percent solution with or without 0.25 cc. of epinephrine (Adrenalin) 1:1000.*

Onset.—Operating analgesia is established in 5 to 15 minutes with an average of 10 minutes.

Duration.—Operating analgesia lasts ¾ to 1¼ hours, with solutions containing epinephrine giving the upper limits.

Lidocaine (Xylocaine) or Mepivacaine (Carbocaine)

Dosage.—80 cc. to 100 cc. of 0.5 percent solution with or without 0.25 cc. of epinephrine (Adrenalin) 1:1000.*

---

*Optimal concentration of epinephrine is 1:200,000, that is, 0.1 cc. of epinephrine 1:1000 in 20 cc. of the local anesthetic solution. Do not exceed 0.25 cc. of epinephrine 1:1000 even if amount of local anesthetic solution exceeds 50 cc. (see page 39).

Onset.—Operating analgesia is established in 5 to 15 minutes.

Duration.—Operating analgesia lasts 1¼ to 2 hours, with stronger concentrations and solutions containing epinephrine giving the upper limits.

MATERIALS

Regional tray (see Chapter 9, page 51) or:

1. One ¾-inch (2 cm.), 25-gauge Huber point security Lok-needle.

2. Three 1½-inch (3.8 cm.), 22-gauge security Lok-needles, preferably with short bevel.

3. One 2-inch (5 cm.), 22-gauge security Lok-needle, preferably with short bevel.

4. One 3-inch (7.5 cm.), 22-gauge security Lok-needle, preferably with short bevel.

5. One tuberculin Lok-syringe for measuring epinephrine.

6. One 10 cc. Lok-syringe, preferably with finger rings.

7. One graduated measuring cup, preferably stainless steel, for mixing solution.

8. One prep cup, preferably stainless steel.

9. Four sterile towels.

10. Six sterile sponges.

11. One sterilizer control.

TECHNIQUE

Position and Landmarks

1. The patient lies in the dorsal recumbent position without a pillow, his arms at his sides, and his head turned to the side opposite the one being blocked (Figure 61, page 116).

2. The tip of the mastoid process of the temporal bone is located and the overlying skin is marked with an X (Figure 58, page 114 and Figure 59, page 115).

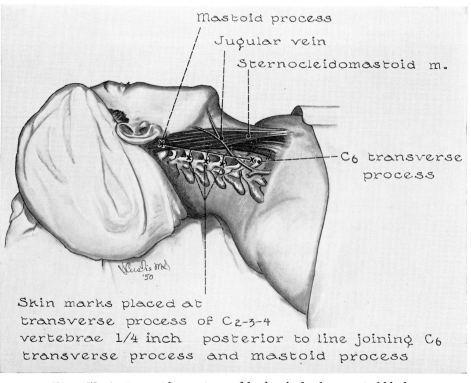

Figure 58. Anatomy with superimposed landmarks for deep cervical block.

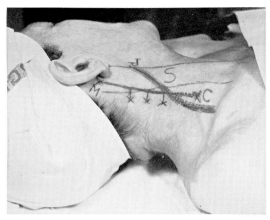

Figure 59. Patient in position for a deep cervical block. M, mastoid process. J, external jugular vein. S, sternocleidomastoid muscle. C, Chassaignac's tubercle (tubercle on the transverse process of the sixth cervical vertebra). Anesthesia administered for a thyroidectomy.

3. Chassaignac's tubercle, the anterior tubercle on the transverse process of the sixth cervical vertebra, is palpated and an X marked on the overlying skin. This tubercle is easily felt since it makes the sixth transverse process the most prominent of the cervical transverse processes (Figure 58, page 114 and Figure 59, page 115).

4. A straight line is drawn between the two X's. This gives the approximate plane in which the cervical transverse processes lie (Figure 58, page 114 and Figure 59, page 115).

5. Approximately ⅝ inch (1.5 cm.) below the tip of the mastoid process and usually ¼ inch (0.6 cm.) posterior to the line drawn between the X's, the second cervical transverse process usually may be palpated. The skin overlying it is marked with an X (Figure 58, page 114 and Figure 59, page 115).

6. In a like fashion the third and fourth transverse processes are marked *after palpation*. They are ½ inch (1.3 cm.) to ⅝ inch (1.5 cm.) apart (Figure 58, page 114 and Figure 59, page 115). These transverse processes should always be felt, since they usually can be palpated even in a thick necked patient.

7. The landmarks are checked by again locating the sixth transverse process and counting the transverse processes in a cephalad direction.

Precautions

Maintain Position of Patient's Head.—Once the landmarks have been located, caution should be taken so that the patient does not move his head; otherwise the landmarks may be misleading.

Aspirate.—The neck is a highly vascular area of the body and great care should be taken to avoid intravascular injections. Also, if the needle is placed too deeply and incorrectly, spinal fluid may be aspirated.

Avoid Subarachnoid Injection.—When each needle is inserted, the point should be inclined slightly caudad. This will avoid subarachnoid injections. In the cervical region the slant of the parts of the vertebrae are such that the needle must be pointed cephalad to go easily between them and puncture the dura.

Place Needle on Anterior Surface of Transverse Process.—Great care to place the needle on the anterior surface of the transverse process in the region of the sulcus should be exerted (Figure 60, page 116). If the needle lies on the posterior side of the transverse process, analgesia will be poor. If it lies too far anteriorly on the transverse process, puncture of the vertebral artery or carotid sheath is likely. Should it become necessary to insert the 1½-inch (3.8 cm.) needle so that its security bead rests on or almost on the skin, the position of the needle should be questioned.

Variations in Depth of Transverse Processes.—The depth of the tip of the transverse process from the skin varies from ½ inch (1.3 cm.) to 1¼ inch (3.2 cm.) depending on the pressure of the palpating finger, the build of the patient, and the region, *e.g.*, the transverse processes become more superficial as they descend in the neck.

Observe Needle for Pulsations, Blood, or Spinal Fluid.—While placing the point of the needle on the tip of the transverse process the syringe should not be attached to the needle.

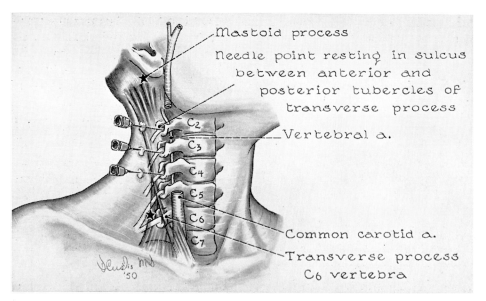

Figure 60. Correct position for the needles for a deep cervical block. Note their positions in the sulci between the anterior and posterior tubercles of the transverse processes.

Before injecting or aspirating, the needle should be observed for pulsations as well as for the appearance of blood or spinal fluid at the open hub. Pulsations or blood usually indicate that the needle is placed too anteriorly and too medially. Spinal fluid indicates too deep placement of the needle.

Procedure

1. The sterilizer control is checked to be sure the equipment has been sterilized.

2. The area is aseptically prepared and draped.

3. The anesthetist stands at the head of the table or cart facing the feet of the patient. This position allows him to control the patient's head as well as to palpate the transverse process (Figure 61, page 116).

4. Intradermal skin wheals are raised over the second, third, and fourth transverse processes with the ¾-inch (2 cm.) Huber point security Lok-needle. Subcutaneous infiltration is carried out with the ¾-inch needle to make the procedure less painful. If a transverse process is encountered at this time, the needle is fixed and 3 cc. of anesthetic solution injected.

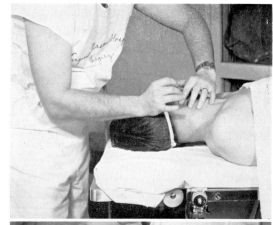

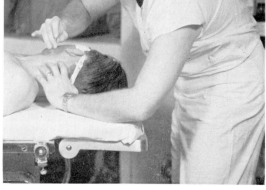

Figure 61. Position of the patient and the right-handed anesthetist for a cervical plexus block. A. (*Top*) Right side. B. (*Bottom*) Left side.

5. If the anesthetist is right-handed, the index finger of the left hand palpates the second transverse process, the middle (long) finger the third, and the ring finger the fourth (Figure 61, page 116 and Figure 62, page 117).

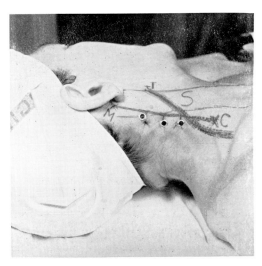

Figure 63. Lateral view of the 1½-inch (3.8 cm.) needles resting on the transverse processes just previous to injection. Note the perpendicular relationship of the shaft of the needle to the skin. M, mastoid process. J, external jugular vein. S, sternocleidomastoid muscle. C, Chassaignac's tubercle (tubercle of the transverse process of the sixth cervical vertebra).

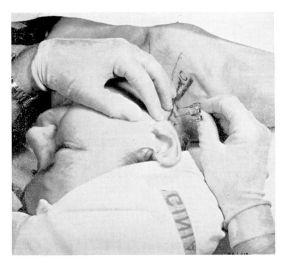

Figure 62. Placing of the needles at the sulci of the second, third, and fourth cervical transverse processes. Note that the anesthetist is right-handed and the index finger of the left hand palpates the second cervical transverse process, the middle (long) finger the third cervical transverse process, and the ring finger the fourth cervical transverse process. The points of the 1½-inch (3.8 cm.) needles lie on the transverse processes. This view is that seen by the anesthetist.

6. The 1½-inch (3.8 cm.), 22-gauge Lokneedles are inserted perpendicular to the skin wheal, then slightly tilted caudad and pushed downward until they rest on the transverse process of the second, third, and fourth cervical vertebrae under the palpating fingers (Figure 62, page 117 and Figure 63, page 117). Should paresthesias occur during the placement of a needle, that needle should be fixed and 2 cc. to 3 cc. of the local anesthetic solution injected before proceeding with the placement of the needle point on the transverse process. Paresthesias to the back of the head indicate stimulation of the second or third cervical nerves while those to the arm and lower neck indicate stimulation of the fourth cervical nerve. If the second cervical transverse process is difficult to palpate, nee-

dles should be placed on the third and fourth cervical transverse processes since this will help the anesthetist to visualize the position and depth of the second cervical transverse process.

7. The position of the needles should be checked to be sure they rest on the transverse processes (Figure 60, page 116). This is easily accomplished by first slightly withdrawing the needle and reinserting it cephalad, and then repeating the maneuver caudad. If the needle is felt to slide off bone or fails to contact bone at all, the anesthetist may confidently assume the needle's position was correct.

8. Each needle in turn is held gently against the transverse process with the left hand. The full 10 cc. Lok-syringe is connected and after careful aspiration, 7 cc. of the anesthetic solution is injected. As the needle is withdrawn, the remaining 3 cc. is injected.

9. This step and step 10. are now performed to facilitate and hasten analgesia. A 2-inch (5 cm.) needle is now introduced through the skin wheal over the third cervi-

cal transverse process and a total of 10 cc. of anesthetic solution is injected for 1½ inches (3.8 cm.) both cephalad and caudad along the posterior inferior border of the sternocleidomastoid muscle. By this simple infiltration the superficial cervical plexus may be anesthetized (Figure 57, page 113 and Figure 64, page 118). Do not inject deeper than the posterior inferior border of the sternocleidomastoid muscle or more than 1½ inches (3.8 cm.) caudad to the skin wheal over the third cervical transverse process. Otherwise it is possible to anesthetize the recurrent laryngeal nerve.

10. The line of incision should be infiltrated intradermally and subcutaneously with the anesthetic solution (Figure 65, page 119). This allows the surgeon to make the incision earlier and insure a local block of the cervical branch of the facial nerve which innervates the platysma muscle.

DISTRIBUTION OF ANALGESIA

Skin analgesia is established which includes the area from the inferior surface of the man-

dible, the posterior one-third of the ear, and occipital region of the skull over the neck and shoulders to the level of the second rib. The deep and superficial muscles of the neck are profoundly relaxed (Figure 66, page 119).

COMPLICATIONS

Toxic Reactions (intravascular injections, etc.): See Chapter 3, page 19. The neck is highly vascular and this type of complication is the most frequent offender. Although the diagnosis of other complications is made, in all probability the reaction is a variation of this type.

Subarachnoid Injection: See Chapter 43, page 353. This should seldom occur if the anesthetist keeps the needle pointing slightly caudad and is cognizant at all times of its depth.

Block of the Phrenic Nerve: This occurs frequently.

Signs and Symptoms.—Absent or decreased

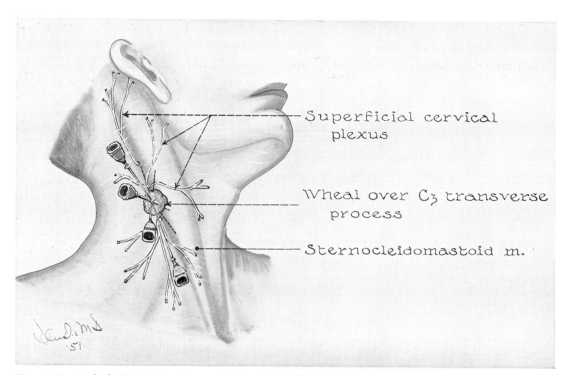

Figure 64. Method of injecting the superficial cervical plexus as it emerges along the posterior lateral border of the sternocleidomastoid muscle.

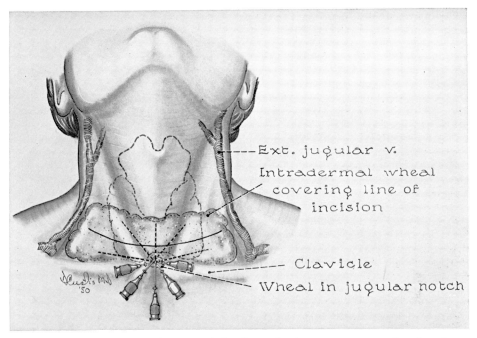

Figure 65. Method of local infiltration of the skin and subcutaneous tissue of neck to insure block of the nerves innervating the platysma muscle.

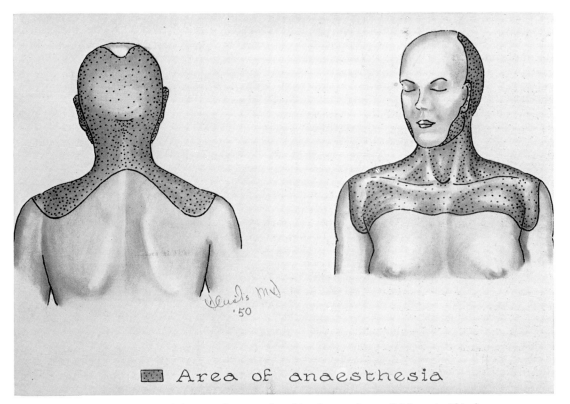

Figure 66. Area of skin anesthesia produced by deep and superficial cervical block.

diaphragmatic motion and slight cyanosis may be present.

Etiology.—The phrenic nerve arises chiefly from the fourth cervical nerve and receives small branches from the third and fifth cervical nerves. Therefore, block of the third and fourth cervical nerves usually decreases the activity of the phrenic nerve. The branch from the fifth cervical nerve will usually sustain partial diaphragmatic action.

Course.—Clears as the block dissipates itself.

Treatment.—Usually none is necessary since the intercostals will supply adequate oxygenation. If there is hypoxia, oxygen should be administered.

Compression of the Carotid Sheath: This seldom occurs. Diagnosis of this complication is difficult. That unilateral compression will cause no symptoms has been proven experimentally by unilateral ligation of the carotid artery. Also, it is questionable, considering the volume of solution used and the usual amount of diffusion and absorption of the local anesthetic solution, whether bilateral compression could occur other than very rarely.

Block of the Recurrent Laryngeal Nerve: This occurs in 2 to 3 percent of the cases and is usually unilateral. When this complication occurs, it is most annoying to the anesthetist and surgeon because the cervical block is usually performed so that any change in phonation during thyroidectomy may be noted immediately. What is called block of the recurrent laryngeal nerve is more probably in reality a block of the vagus nerve, since the main trunk of the vagus nerve is much closer to the deposited fluid than is the recurrent nerve. The latter enters the larynx at the level of the sixth cervical vertebra.

Signs and Symptoms.—They are hoarseness, aphonia, and difficult breathing.

Etiology.—Block of the recurrent laryngeal nerve usually is caused by too deep infiltration along the posterior border of the sternocleido-

mastoid muscle. The vagus nerve itself should be affected first unless the needle point has really strayed far and is much too medial and too low.

Course.—Clears as the block dissipates itself.

Block of the Vagus Nerve: Very infrequent and difficult to diagnose as it is most often unilateral. The signs and symptoms are usually an increase in pulse rate and the loss of phonation. These may easily occur from one of the above complications or from the drugs injected.

Horner's Syndrome: See Chapter 18, Effects, page 131.

REMARKS

Supplementation of Cervical Block with Nitrous Oxide-Oxygen Mixture: When strenuous manipulation or traction is exerted on the thyroid gland, trachea, or deep muscles of the neck, or if there is extreme extension of the head and neck, most patients will complain of being uncomfortable, even under the most complete cervical block. If these annoyances are present, it is best to supplement the block before the patient becomes restless. Nitrous oxide-oxygen combinations are very satisfactory, since the patient rapidly regains consciousness and can answer questions within a few minutes after its withdrawal. This is an important point, for many surgeons feel that local anesthesia is the procedure of choice because it permits the detection of any change in the patient's voice immediately and enables the surgeon to avoid a paralyzed vocal cord. This is not true of other anesthetic agents, such as thiopental (Pentothal) and cyclopropane, from which a patient usually requires at least ten minutes to recover and respond.

First Cervical Nerve Not Injected: The first cervical nerve is not injected since it has no sensory branch.

Palpation of Second Cervical Transverse Process Is Difficult: The second cervical transverse process is the most difficult to palpate as it is often deeply located.

Locate Cervical Transverse Processes by Palpation: *It should be stressed that the most effective means of accurately locating the transverse processes is by direct palpation, not relative projection of lines.* If spasm or contraction of the sternocleidomastoid muscle prevents palpation of the transverse processes of the cervical vertebrae, a superficial cervical block as described under procedure, step 9, page 117, may be used to relax the sternocleidomastoid muscle before proceeding with the blocking of the deep cervical plexus.

Intubate Patient Who Has Compression of Trachea: Where tracheal compression or the possibility of tracheal collapse is imminent, the anesthesia should be conducted with an endotracheal tube in place. A block may be done in these patients to reduce the amount of intravenous or inhalation anesthetic agents, but an endotracheal tube should be placed.

Problems Encountered When Cervical Block Is Used for Thyroidectomy: 95 percent of cervical plexus blocks are performed for thyroidectomies. Therefore, the following pertinent points should be emphasized.

First, the superficial tissues around the superior poles of the thyroid gland are innervated by branches of the superior laryngeal nerve and branches from the cervical plexus. The superior laryngeal nerve is not anesthetized by a cervical block. Blind blocking of the superior laryngeal nerve might alter the quality of phonation. Therefore, the surgeon should be informed of this possibility and asked to inject the superior pole under direct vision.

Second, a patient with a toxic thyroid has a high basal metabolic rate and a very labile blood pressure. Such a patient requires heavy medication and a high oxygen intake. Oxygen should be administered during surgery and postoperatively for 12 to 24 hours. Remember that paralysis of the phrenic nerve usually occurs and this also adds to the necessity of a high oxygen intake. Even if the thyrotoxic patient is well controlled, drugs increasing the pulse rate should be avoided. Therefore, it is best to employ scopolamine routinely instead of atropine.

Third, the fact that a rapid pulse and a thyroid crisis may occur, even if the patient is well controlled preoperatively, should not be overlooked. In general, correct medical preparation has greatly lowered the mortality rate of patients undergoing toxic thyroid surgery; nevertheless, under regional block or inhalation anesthesia, the patient may "break through" the preoperative therapy.

Finally, vasoconstrictor agents should be omitted from the solution in cervical plexus blocks for thyroidectomies in toxic patients, because the combination of the vasoconstrictor drug, the rapid absorption from the neck, and the existing thyrotoxicosis forms an ideal situation for a systemic reaction to the vasoconstrictor drug.

Duration of Action of Local Anesthetic Solutions Shorter When Injected into Neck: It will be noted that the duration of operating analgesia is somewhat less in this block than in others. This may be due to two factors. First, the high vascularity of the neck may cause rapid absorption and dissipation of the local anesthetic agent. Second, the vasoconstrictor drug often is omitted from the local anesthetic solution.

Importance of Vascularity of the Neck: The neck is extremely vascular for its size in comparison to other areas of the body. Therefore, the following statements are important: (1) greater absorption of the anesthetic solution with a higher blood level of the local anesthetic agent as well as the vasoconstrictor agent often results in more toxic reactions in this procedure than in other blocks; and (2) hyaluronidase *should not* be incorporated in the anesthetic solution since it will increase this normally rapid rate of absorption.

Wrap Legs: Wrapping of the legs is essential in thyroidectomy, because the heavily medicated patient is often placed in Fowler's position, which tends to cause pooling of the blood in the lower extremities (see Chapter 1, page 7).

Tetracaine (Pontocaine) Is Local Anesthetic Agent of Choice: Tetracaine solutions are the local anesthetic solutions of choice in cervical plexus block for the thyrotoxic patient, the geriatric patient, and the patient with high blood pressure because prolonged anesthesia, *i.e.*, at least three hours, is assured without the use of a vasoconstrictor agent. Furthermore, *weak, effective* tetracaine solutions do not cause vasodilatation, which is a characteristic physiological response when solutions of most other local anesthetic agents are injected. Therefore, a tetracaine solution, even without a vasoconstrictor drug, usually does not increase its own rate of absorption as do most other local anesthetic solutions.

Headache Following Cervical Block: Occasionally following cervical block for a thyroidectomy the patient may complain of an occipital headache which may persist for one to two days. In such cases, the headache should not be blamed on the block procedure. The identical type of headache may follow the use of general anesthesia for this surgical procedure. The headache and neck pain are caused by hyperextension of the neck muscles due to a position used by many surgeons for thyroidectomy. These headaches may last two days to a week, and then spontaneously disappear.

Recover Broken Needle(s): All needles should be tested before use. If a needle breaks, every effort to recover it, including surgery, should be made. Unremoved needles have a tendency to migrate and may cause permanent injuries as well as medicolegal complications.

Repeat Block When Analgesia Is Inadequate: If the desired results from the first block attempt are unsatisfactory, do not hesitate to reblock the patient if time permits. Most patients will think nothing about being reblocked if the second attempt is prefaced by the statement: "Well, I guess we will have to inject a little more medicine if we are going to freeze this area." However, do not exceed the maximum safe dosage of the local anesthetic solution for both blocks. If to reblock the patient the maximum safe dose of the local anesthetic solution must be exceeded, 45 minutes should elapse between blocks.

CHAPTER 18

Anterior (Paratracheal) Approach
for Block of the Stellate Ganglion

INDICATIONS

Surgical: None.

Diagnostic: Differentiation of varieties of vasospastic diseases, cardiac diseases, and asthmas. To determine the advisability of stellate ganglionectomy or thoracic sympathectomy.

Therapeutic

Relief of Vasospastic Diseases of the Arm, Brain, Face, and Lungs.—Vasospastic diseases which can be relieved are the result of: (1) arterial dysfunction, *e.g.*, Raynaud's or Buerger's disease, scalenus anticus syndrome, Volkmann's ischemic contracture, arterial injuries, crushing injuries of the upper extremity, or embolisms and thrombosis of the arm, brain, or lungs (Figure 67, page 124); (2) venous dysfunction, *e.g.*, chronic or acute thrombophlebitis and postphlebitic edema; and (3) combinations of venous and arterial dysfunction, *e.g.*, postoperative lymphedema of the arm following radical breast amputation and frostbite.

Treatment of Post-traumatic Dystrophies.—For example, atrophy of the bone, traumatic edema, traumatic osteoporosis, causalgia, and phantom limb pain.

Treatment of Miscellaneous Complaints that are Improved by Blocking the Sympathetic Chain.—For example, prolonged infections of the upper extremities with or without edema, unhealed ulcers, subacromial bursitis, the acute, early stage of herpes zoster, scars of the face, hyperhidrosis of the upper extremities, and joint stiffness.

Alleviation of Anginal and Cardiac Pain.—A left stellate ganglion block will relieve the pain of a coronary occlusion when narcotics fail to do so. The autonomic nervous system, itself, does not transmit pain impulses. But the nerve fibers which do transmit pain impulses often travel with the nerves of the autonomic nervous system. This may be why pain from occlusion of a coronary artery is relieved by block of the stellate ganglion.

Alleviation of Status Asthmaticus.—Stellate ganglion block may stop asthma when all other therapy fails. However, it is not definitive treatment and should be used only if other routine medical therapy fails.

Support of Surgical Plastic Reconstructions of the Upper Extremity, Neck, and Face.—When the blood supply is insufficient in these areas following surgery, it may often be increased by a series of stellate ganglion blocks (Figure 68, page 125).

ANATOMY

The stellate ganglion is formed by the complete or partial fusion of the inferior cervical and first thoracic sympathetic ganglia. Its shape may resemble a star (stellate) or a dumbbell, depending on the amount of fusion. The two ganglia are always close together, although in somewhat less than one-half of instances they have not fused together. When fusion has occurred, the stellate ganglion is usually 1 inch (2.5 cm.) x ⅜ inch (1 cm.) x ³⁄₁₆ inch (0.5 cm.), and is larger than the middle cervical sympathetic ganglion and the thoracic sympathetic ganglion but smaller than the superior cervical sympathetic ganglion The

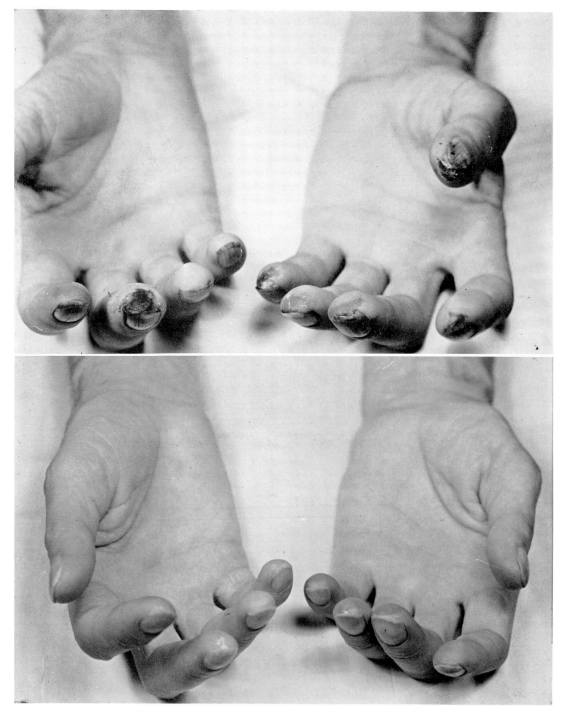

Figure 67. Results of stellate ganglion block for vascular insufficiency of the hands. A. *(Top)* Before block. B. *(Bottom)* Two weeks after a series of 20 stellate blocks were performed. The left side was blocked in the morning and the right side in the afternoon.

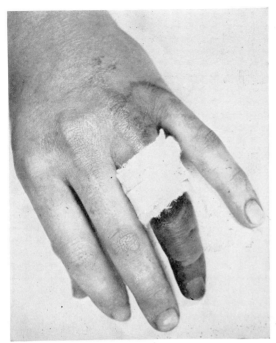

Figure 68. Shows the hand of a patient who partially amputated his ring finger. The finger was sewed in position and repeated stellate ganglion blocks administered in an attempt to help re-establish circulation. Finger had to be amputated at a later date.

stellate ganglion is situated between the base of the transverse process of the last cervical vertebra (seventh) and the neck of the first rib (Figure 69A and B, page 126). It lies behind the carotid sheath, ventral to the longus colli muscle, behind the vertebral artery, and slightly lateral to the body of the vertebra (Figure 70, page 126). The ganglion lies in close relationship to the subclavian artery, the inferior thyroid artery, the first intercostal artery, and the recurrent laryngeal nerve (Figure 69B, page 126). On the right side, the pleura is in close approximation to the ganglion, but on the left, the pleura is located ⅜ inch (1 cm.) to ¾ inch (2 cm.) below it. It sends gray rami to the seventh and eighth cervical nerves and to the first thoracic nerve. It is connected with the middle and superior cervical sympathetic ganglia via the cervical sympathetic trunk and the ansa subclavia. It sends peripheral branches to the cardiac plexus. Branches go to the cranial cavity along the vertebral arteries.

Other peripheral branches are contributed to the inferior thyroid plexus, the subclavian plexus, the internal mammary plexus, and occasionally a twig to the phrenic nerve.

PREMEDICATION

None is advised because: (1) attempts to elicit paresthesias, which may be painful, are not required for this block; (2) the procedure itself is not painful; and (3) most patients are treated on an outpatient basis.

If, however, the patient is particularly apprehensive, a barbiturate or opiate may be administered, i.e., 100 mg. (1½ gr.) to 200 mg. (3 gr.) of pentobarbital (Nembutal) orally or intravenously; or 10 mg. (⅙ gr.) to 15 mg. (¼ gr.) of morphine intramuscularly or intravenously.

DRUGS

Tetracaine (Pontocaine)

Dosage.—10 cc. to 20 cc. of 0.15 to 0.25 percent solution with or without 0.10 cc. of epinephrine (Adrenalin) 1:1000 in each 20 cc. of solution.*

Onset.—Horner's syndrome occurs in 2 to 15 minutes. Signs of vasodilatation of the upper extremity may not occur for 30 minutes.

Duration.—Horner's syndrome lasts 3½ to 6 hours, with stronger concentrations and solutions containing epinephrine giving the upper limits. While the signs of Horner's syndrome may clear in a few hours it is not unusual for the oscillometer readings in the arm to remain elevated for 24 to 48 hours.

Procaine (Novocain)

Dosage.—10 cc. to 20 cc. of 1.0 to 2.0 percent solution with or without 0.10 cc. of epinephrine (Adrenalin) 1:1000 in each 20 cc. of solution.*

---

*Optimal concentration of epinephrine is 1:200,000, that is, 0.1 cc. of epinephrine 1:1000 in 20 cc. of the local anesthetic solution (see page 39).

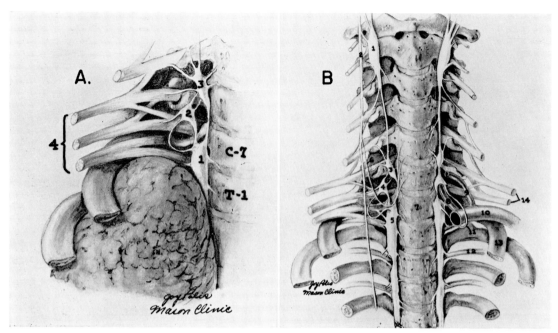

Figure 69. A. Anterior view of the relationship of the lung to the cervicothoracic portion of the sympathetic nervous system. 1. Stellate ganglion. 2. Intermediate ganglion. 3. Middle cervical ganglion. 4. Brachial plexus. B. Anterior view of the cervicothoracic portion of the sympathetic nervous system. 1. Superior cervical ganglion. 2. Vagus nerve. 3. Middle cervical ganglion. 4. Intermediate ganglion. 5. Stellate ganglion. 6. Recurrent laryngeal nerve. 7. Seventh cervical vertebra. 8. Vertebral artery. 9. Inferior thyroid artery. 10. Subclavian artery. 11. Ansa subclavia. 12. Second intercostal nerve. 13. First rib. 14. Part of the brachial plexus.

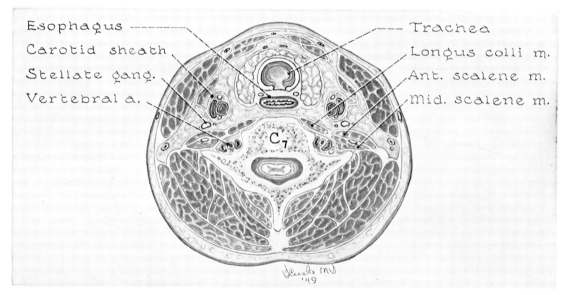

Figure 70. Cross section at the level of the seventh cervical vertebra showing the relationship of the stellate ganglia to the transverse processes, the longus colli muscles, and the carotid sheaths.

Onset.—Horner's syndrome occurs in 2 to 15 minutes. Signs of vasodilatation of the upper extremity may not occur for 30 minutes.

Duration.—Horner's syndrome lasts 1 to 1½ hours, with stronger concentrations and solutions containing epinephrine giving the upper limits. While the signs of a Horner's syndrome may clear in a few hours it is not unusual for the oscillometer readings in the arm to remain elevated for 24 to 48 hours.

Lidocaine (Xylocaine) or Mepivacaine (Carbocaine)

Dosage.—10 cc. to 20 cc. of a 1.0 to 1.5 percent solution with or without 0.10 cc. of epinephrine (Adrenalin) 1:1000 in each 20 cc. of solution.*

Onset.—Horner's syndrome occurs in 2 to 15 minutes. Signs of vasodilatation of the upper extremity may not occur for 30 minutes.

Duration.—Horner's syndrome lasts 1 to 3 hours, with stronger concentrations and solutions containing epinephrine giving the upper limits. While the signs of a Horner's syndrome may clear in a few hours, it is not unusual for the oscillometer readings in the arm to remain elevated for 24 to 48 hours.

MATERIALS

Regional tray (see Chapter 9, page 51) or:

1. One ¾-inch (2 cm.), 25-gauge Huber point security Lok-needle.

2. One 1½-inch (3.8 cm.), 22-gauge security Lok-needle, preferably with short bevel.

3. One 2-inch (5 cm.), 22-gauge security Lok-needle, preferably with short bevel.

4. One tuberculin Lok-syringe for measuring epinephrine.

5. One 10 cc. Lok-syringe, preferably with finger rings.

6. One graduated measuring cup, preferably stainless steel, for mixing solution.

7. One prep cup, preferably stainless steel.

8. Four sterile towels.

9. One sterilizer control.

TECHNIQUE

Position and Landmarks

1. The patient lies in the dorsal recumbent position without a pillow and with his arms at his sides.

2. The head is tilted backward so that the neck is in maximum extension (Figure 71, page 128 and Figure 72, page 128). This straightens the esophagus and makes the anatomical relationships in the neck constant.

3. An X is made 1¼ inches (3.2 cm.) to 1½ inches (3.8 cm.) lateral to the middle of the jugular notch of the sternum and 1¼ (3.2 cm.) to 1½ (3.8 cm.) inches above the clavicle. These distances may be approximately measured by the two-finger technique. The distance lateral to the jugular notch may be easily estimated by placing one finger in the jugular notch and then placing another finger beside it. The spot marked in this maneuver usually lies just lateral to the sternoclavicular joint. The distances above the clavicle may be approximately measured by measuring two finger-breadths above the clavicle (Figure 71, page 128; Figure 72, page 128; and Figure 73, page 129). This mark should lie over the transverse process of the seventh cervical vertebra and along the medial border of the sternocleidomastoid muscle (Figure 71, page 128; Figure 72, page 128; Figure 73, page 129; and Figure 74A, page 130).

4. The patient is now instructed to turn his head to the side opposite the one being blocked and Chassaignac's tubercle, the anterior tubercle of the transverse process of the sixth cervical vertebra, is located (Figure 74B, page

---

*Optimal concentration of epinephrine is 1:200,000, that is, 0.1 cc. of epinephrine 1:1000 in 20 cc. of the local anesthetic solution (see page 39).

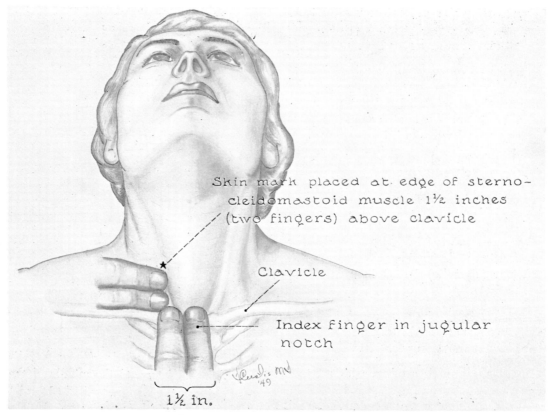

Figure 71. Method of locating the transverse process of the seventh vertebra.

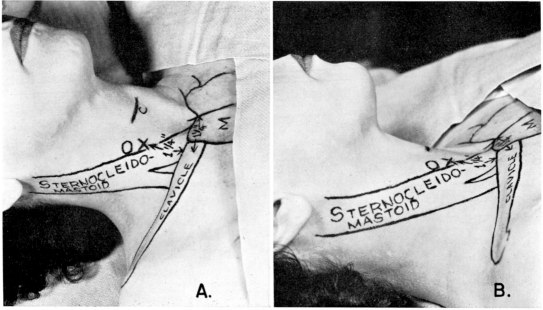

Figure 72. Patient in position for a stellate ganglion block by the anterior (paratracheal) approach. Note extension of the head. The topographical anatomy is indicated. X lies over the transverse process of the seventh cervical vertebra. O marks the sixth cervical transverse process, and the line marked C the cricoid cartilage. A. Anterolateral view. B. Lateral view.

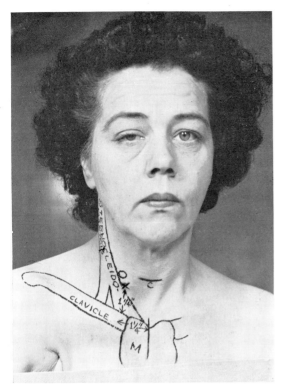

Figure 73. Landmarks for stellate ganglion block. Patient in sitting position following block. Note Horner's syndrome of patient's right eye.

130).* This is easily done by placing the fingers behind the lateral border of the sternocleidomastoid muscle and feeling for the most prominent anterior tubercle of the lower cervical transverse processes (Figure 74C, page 130). An O is placed on the skin overlying the the sixth transverse process along the medial border of the sternocleidomastoid muscle (Figure 72, page 128 and Figure 73, page 129). The cricoid cartilage is palpated and marked (Figure 72, page 128 and Figure 73, page 129). This usually lies at the level of the transverse process of the sixth cervical vertebra, the exception being a thin, long-necked patient—then the cricoid cartilage may be at the level of the fifth cervical vertebra. These two anatomical structures—the transverse process of the sixth cervical vertebra and the cricoid car-

*Chassaignac's tubercle is the anterior tubercle on the transverse process of the sixth cervical vertebra. This tubercle is easily felt, since it is the most prominent anterior tubercle of the cervical transverse processes.

tilage—serve as a check on the seventh transverse process, which was marked with an X and which should be approximately ½ inch (1.3 cm.) below the O and the cricoid cartilage marking the sixth transverse process (Figure 72, page 128; Figure 73, page 129; and Figure 74A, page 130).

Precautions

Check Landmarks.—A careful check of the landmarks should be carried out so as to be sure that they are not more than 1¼ inch (3.2 cm.) to 1½ inch (3.8 cm.) from the midline of the jugular notch of the neck.

Keep Head Extended.—The head should be fully extended at all times while carrying out the procedure. This maneuver straightens the slight normal curve of the esophagus to the left.

Patient Must Not Talk, Cough, or Move.—The patient should be instructed not to talk, cough, or move while the injection is being made. These instructions should be repeated as the needle is being inserted.

Keep Full Syringe Attached to Needle.—The full 10 cc. syringe should at all times during the procedure be securely attached to the Lok-needle so as to facilitate injection and to prevent possible dislodging of the needle.

Aspirate.—Careful aspiration for blood or spinal fluid is imperative.

Procedure

1. The sterilizer control is checked to be sure the equipment has been sterilized.

2. The area is aseptically prepared and draped.

3. The anesthetist stands at the side of the patient to be blocked, facing the side of the cart (Figure 75, page 131).

4. An intradermal wheal is raised at the determined X with the ¾-inch (2 cm.), 25-gauge Huber point security Lok-needle.

5. If the anesthetist is right-handed, the full 10 cc. Lok-syringe with the 1½-inch (3.8 cm.) or the 2-inch (5 cm.) security Lok-needle

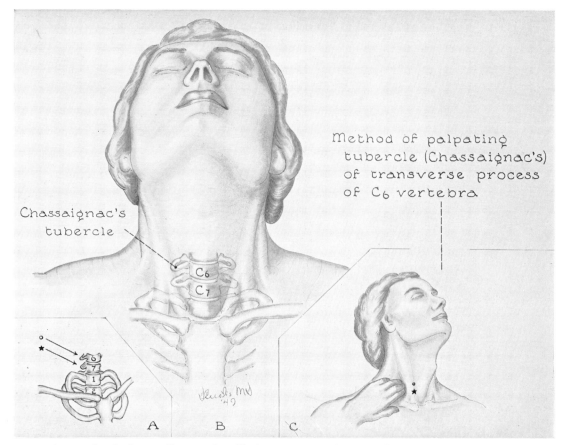

Chassaignac's
tubercle

Method of palpating
tubercle (Chassaignac's)
of transverse process
of C₆ vertebra

C₆
C₇

A   B   C

Figure 74. Landmarks for a stellate ganglion block. A. Position of the O and the X. B. Position of the cervical transverse process in relationship to the topographical anatomy of the neck. C. Palpation of the tubercle of the transverse process of the sixth cervical vertebra.

attached is held in the right hand while the index and middle fingers of the left hand straddle the X mark on the neck (Figure 75, page 131).

6. Downward and lateral pressure is exerted with the fingers of the left hand so that the sternocleidomastoid muscle and carotid sheath are pulled laterally (Figure 76, page 132). *The pulsation of the carotid artery should be felt on the lateral side of the depressing fingers.* The left hand holds this position until the block is completed. No attempt should be made at this time to palpate the transverse processes with either the index or middle (long) finger of the left hand. The straddling fingers act merely as retractors to pull the carotid sheath and sternocleidomastoid muscle laterally (Figure 77, page 132).

7. The needle is then inserted through the X perpendicular to the skin in all planes and pushed slowly posteriorly until it impinges on the transverse process of the seventh cervical vertebra (Figure 76, page 132; Figure 78, page 133; and Figure 79, page 133). The exact depth varies with the depression of the skin by the index and middle fingers of the left hand as well as with the build of the patient. However, it is seldom necessary to insert the needle more than 1½ inches (3.8 cm.).

8. If, however, the needle does not impinge on bone or if paresthesias of the brachial plexus are elicited, the needle should be withdrawn and reinserted so that the point is more medial. If bone is still missed, then the needle should be pointed either caudally

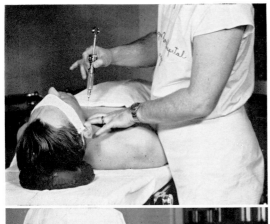

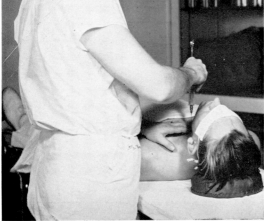

Figure 75. Position of the patient and the right-handed anesthetist for a stellate ganglion block. A. *(Top)* Right side. B. *(Bottom)* Left side.

or cephalad until it impinges on the transverse process. It is seldom necessary to readjust the needle.

9. After the needle rests on the transverse process of the seventh cervical vertebra, it should be withdrawn ⅛ inch (0.3 cm.) to free it from the substance of the muscles which lie over the transverse process (Figure 80, page 134).

10. A careful aspiration test is performed.

11. One to 2 cc. of the local anesthetic solution is injected and 15 to 30 seconds allowed to pass. If after this period no reaction occurs, the contents of the syringe are discharged. The needle is then withdrawn. The test dose of 1 to 2 cc. is injected because occasionally, even though no blood is obtained when per-

forming the aspiration test, the point of the needle may rest in the vertebral artery (Figure 69B, page 126). If this is true, 1 to 2 cc. of the blocking agent will produce dizziness, the feeling of "blacking out," and nausea within this time, because of the cerebral manifestations of the drug. When 1 to 2 cc. of the drug is not exceeded, serious complications with loss of consciousness seldom occur. If the above signs and symptoms are elicited, the injection should be stopped and the needle should be adjusted before this injection is made. These points are stressed because intravascular injection is the only serious complication of this approach which has been seen occasionally by us.

EFFECTS

Horner's Syndrome and Sympathetic Block of Chest, Axilla, and Upper Extremity: If a successful block has been accomplished a Horner's syndrome and evidence of a sympathetic block in the arm on the blocked side will result. These are characterized by the following signs and symptoms which are limited to the blocked side: (1) ptosis of the eyelid with narrowed palpebral fissure, (2) constricted pupil, (3) enophthalmus, (4) injected conjunctiva, (5) increased lacrimation, (6) increased temperature of the arm and face, (7) anhydrosis of the face and arm on the affected side, and (8) stuffiness of the nose.

Signs of Horner's Syndrome: A Horner's syndrome by definition is characterized by ptosis of the eyelid, constricted pupil, and enophthalmus (Figure 73, page 129). The involvement of the arm is not a part of the syndrome.

COMPLICATIONS

Pneumothorax: This occurs in less than one percent of the cases following this approach to the stellate ganglion. See Chapter 30, page 237.

Toxic Reactions (intravascular injections, etc.): See Chapter 3, page 19.

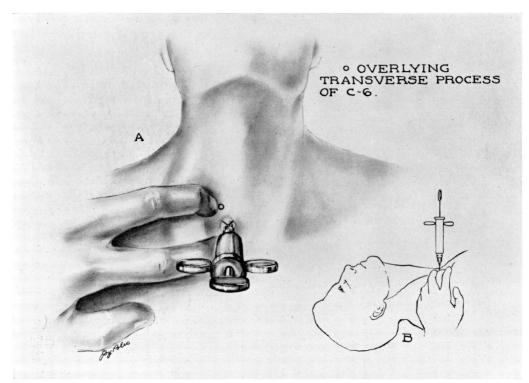

Figure 76. Method of "hooking" fingers over sternocleidomastoid muscle so that they may act as a retractor. A. Anterior view. B. Lateral view.

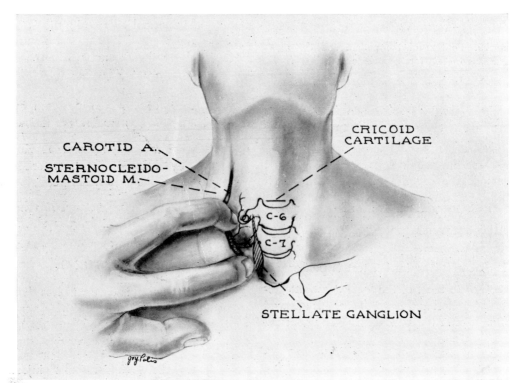

Figure 77. Index finger and middle finger being used as retractors to pull the sternocleidomastoid muscle and the carotid sheath laterally.

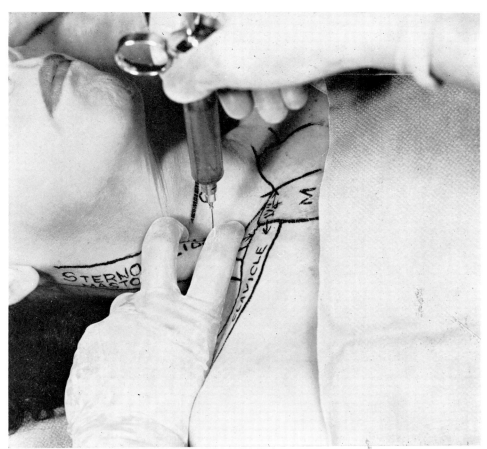

Figure 78. Anterolateral view of needle as it is being inserted perpendicular to the skin over the seventh cervical transverse process. Note position of index and middle fingers pulling the sterno-cleidomastoid and carotid sheath with its vessels and nerves laterally.

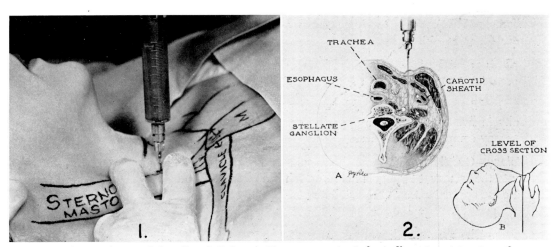

Figure 79. (1) Lateral view of the 1½-inch (3.8 cm.), 22-gauge security Lok-needle as its point rests on the transverse process of the seventh cervical vertebra. Note depth to which it has been inserted. (2) A. Cross section of the neck showing the retractor effect of the index finger and middle finger. Note that when the needle rests on the transverse process it lies in the substance of the longus colli muscles. Therefore, before injecting it should always be withdrawn slightly from this position. B. Level of cross section.

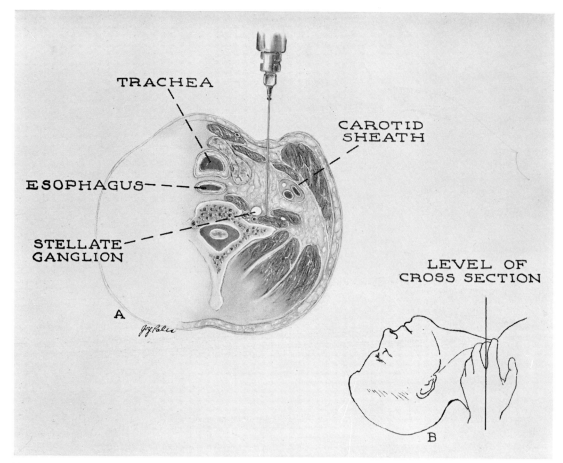

TRACHEA

CAROTID SHEATH

ESOPHAGUS----

STELLATE GANGLION

LEVEL OF CROSS SECTION

A

B

Figure 80. A. Cross section of the neck showing the needle's position after it was withdrawn ⅛ inch (0.3 cm.) from the transverse process of the seventh cervical vertebra. B. Level of cross section.

Subarachnoid Injection: Rarely occurs. See Chapter 43, page 353.

Paralysis of the Recurrent Laryngeal Nerve: This occurs in 5 to 8 percent of the cases.

Signs and Symptoms.—These are hoarseness, difficulty in swallowing, and an apprehensive patient may complain of dyspnea.

Etiology.—Overflow of the anesthetic solution onto the recurrent laryngeal nerve, which lies in close approximation to the stellate ganglion (Figure 69, page 126).

Course.—The recurrent laryngeal nerve recovers as the anesthesia dissipates itself.

Treatment.—None.

Paralysis of Part or All of the Brachial

Plexus: This occurs in approximately 5 percent of the cases following the use of the anterior approach.

Signs and Symptoms. — See Chapter 30, Distribution of Analgesia, page 235.

Etiology.—Overflow of the anesthetic solution.

Course.—The paralysis clears as the block dissipates itself.

Treatment.—None.

Asthmatic Attacks: Very infrequent. We have not observed this complication in over 3000 blocks.

Signs and Symptoms.—Those associated with asthmatic breathing and hypoxia.

Etiology.—Unknown, but usually occurs in patients who have an allergic or sensitive diathesis.

Course.—Depends on the effectiveness of the treatment.

Treatment.—Oxygen should be administered by bag and mask. Theophylline-ethylenediamine (Aminophylline), 500 mg. (7½ gr.), is given intravenously slowly by the single injection technique and repeated at 10 minute intervals if necessary, or 1000 mg. (15 gr.) may be added to 500 or 1000 cc. of 5 percent dextrose in water and given by the drip technique.

Epinephrine (Adrenalin) 1:1000, 0.10 cc. intravenously and repeated at 10 minute intervals or 0.25 cc. intramuscularly, may be administered. Therapy with theophylline is usually the more satisfactory of the two drug treatments.

REMARKS

Approach of Choice: The anterior (paratracheal) method of stellate ganglion block is the approach of choice because of its simplicity from the standpoint of both the patient and the anesthetist.

Definition of Term "Stellate Ganglion Block": The term "stellate ganglion block" is now used merely because the needle is inserted in the region of the ganglion. The block which results, provided the needle point is correctly placed and 10 cc. to 15 cc. of the agent injected, is actually a block of the upper four thoracic sympathetic ganglia, the middle cervical ganglion, the stellate ganglion, and the cords joining these ganglia, *i.e.*, a unilateral block of the entire cervicothoracic sympathetic nervous system.

Avoid Bilateral Block: Both stellate ganglia should not be blocked at the same time because of the following reasons. First, the cardiac accelerator nerves may be anesthetized, with the possibility of a resulting vagal cardiac arrest. When a unilateral block is performed, change in pulse rate and blood pressure is seldom noted. Should a bilateral block be considered imperative, then large doses

of atropine, 0.8 mg. (⅟₇₅ gr.) should be administered intravenously or intramuscularly in an attempt to block the vagus nerves.

Second, overflow of the local anesthetic solution and resulting bilateral paralysis of either the vagus nerves, the inferior laryngeal nerves, the brachial plexus, or the phrenic nerve may cause serious complications.

Lastly, the possibility of a bilateral pneumothorax must always be considered. *Therefore, if a bilateral block is anticipated, time should be allowed for the first block to wear off in order to avoid cardiac difficulties and note complications.* One side may be done in the morning and the other side in the afternoon (Figure 67, page 124). Although often no difficulty will occur from injecting both the stellate ganglia concurrently, the occasional complication argues against a bilateral block which is not warranted by a particular disease.

Care of the Outpatient: A large majority of the patients to whom this block is applicable may be treated as outpatients. They should be adequately instructed so that they do not become alarmed by the Horner's syndrome or complications such as hoarseness or anesthesia of part or all the upper extremity. As with any outpatients, they should be observed for at least one hour before leaving the office.

Omit or Use Small Amounts of Epinephrine (Adrenalin): Since many of the patients leave the office following the block, the epinephrine should either be omitted from the solutions or a very small amount employed. Epinephrine reactions occur relatively frequently and are uncomfortable.

Significance of Horner's Syndrome: If the sympathetic chain is effectively blocked at any place in the neck, a Horner's syndrome appears, but the stellate ganglion may not have been blocked. This makes little difference if the block was performed as a cerebral sympathetic block but if it was executed for disease in the upper extremity, no benefit will be derived. This point is stressed because all too often the anesthetist believes that he has successfully executed a stellate block if the facial signs of a Horner's syndrome appear. A careful check of the upper arm should always be made for the signs of a sympathetic block, *i.e.,* increase in skin temperatures, dryness, and vasodilatation of the peripheral veins. If these are not present and the block was performed to correct a deficiency of the upper extremity, it should be repeated after a recheck of the landmarks. However, at least 15 to 30 minutes should elapse before the block is repeated. It is not uncommon for the facial signs of a Horner's syndrome to appear in 2 to 5 minutes after the block has been completed, but it may take 15 to 30 minutes for the arm to show signs of an adequate sympathetic block. This is true as it often takes the local anesthetic solution injected at C7 this length of time to diffuse. The solution will diffuse as far caudad as the fourth thoracic vertebra if the local anesthetic solution has been placed in the correct fascial plane.

Explain Complications to Patient: If a patient is to have a series of stellate blocks and one of the complications occurs during the series, this is not a sign to discontinue the injections since it is very unlikely that the complication will present itself again. This should be impressed on the patient so that he will continue with the treatment.

Use Block Therapy Early—Not as Last Resort and Do a Series: Often in diseases where stellate block has proven its value, it is tried as a last resort when all other medical and surgical therapy has been exhausted. This neglect is to be condemned. When problems in which a stellate block is known to be of value arise, it should be used immediately. The results should not be evaluated according to the benefit derived from the first block. It is often necessary to perform a series of blocks, *i.e.,* seven to ten, before dramatic improvement occurs.

Misplacement of Needle: If the needle is placed too far laterally or advanced too far posteriorly when contact with the seventh cervical transverse process is being attempted, the physician will note the following. First, the needle seems to advance into fibrinous tissue, although bone may be encountered as the needle progresses to a greater depth. The

bone encountered is not the seventh cervical transverse process. Normally, the needle slips through the tissues to the seventh cervical transverse process with little or no resistance. Therefore, when partial resistance to the forward progress of the needle is met, it can be assumed the needle is in a fibrous type of tissue, *i.e.,* periosteum, ligaments, etc. Second, in order to contact bone the needle has been advanced deeper than is anticipated for the size of the patient. Finally, stimulation of the nerves of the brachial plexus may occur.

Results of Injecting Solution Through a Misplaced Needle: If the physician injects the local anesthetic solution with the needle placed too far laterally or too far posteriorly, he will note one or all of the following. First, the solution is not easily discharged from the syringe. Second, the signs of Horner's syndrome as well as those of a sympathetic block of the upper extremity are absent. Third, the pupil will dilate or remain normal instead of constricting. Lastly, the patient not infrequently complains of pain between the scapulae or in the region of the angle of the scapula. This pain may persist for a day or two and then disappear without any other complication.

Block Correct Side: In cerebral accidents, remember that the stellate ganglion on the side opposite the paralysis or paresis of the extremities should be blocked because of the decussation of the nerve fibers in the medulla. Blocks other than those for cerebral accidents should be performed on the same side as those for the disease or therapeutic or diagnostic problem.

Use of Stellate Ganglion Block Together with Anticoagulant Drug Therapy: Often physicians may wish to use stellate ganglion block in conjunction with anticoagulant therapy to correct vascular insufficiencies of the upper extremity.

At the present time, there are two aims in the therapy of abnormal vascular spasm from thrombosis or embolism. One is to reduce the spasm itself by sympathetic block, and the other is to prevent further clotting by anticoagulant drug administration. Obviously, the treatment of choice is to use both simultaneously. However, because of the reports of uncontrollable hemorrhage following the use of anticoagulants and sympathetic blocks concomitantly, one of these types of therapy but not both is usually decided upon. In spite of these reports, such fears are unfounded provided the physicians using the anticoagulant drugs and performing the sympathetic blocks are well acquainted with their usage. Serious and fatal hemorrhages have been blamed on anticoagulant drugs, when lack of skill on the part of the person administering them was the true cause. As with other therapeutic modalities, the safety of anticoagulant drugs, as well as sympathetic nerve blocks, used singly or in combination, depends entirely on the ability and knowledge of the person who is administering them. If due precautions are exercised, these two complementary forms of therapy can be used together safely for the benefit of the patient.

To date, it has been the author's experience that stellate ganglion blocks can be executed along with anticoagulant therapy without causing uncontrollable hemorrhage. Likewise, the chances of hemorrhage following stellate ganglion block during anticoagulant therapy is not as great as during lumbar sympathetic block because the vessels in the neck which are usually punctured are arteries and are not as easily torn as the vena cava. If hemorrhage occurs when these two complementary forms of therapy are being used, the effects of the anticoagulant drug must be reversed.

Puncture of Thyroid Gland: With the anterior approach, the needle must at times pierce the thyroid gland. However, complications from this puncture do not seem to occur.

Recover Broken Needle(s): All needles should be tested before use. If a needle breaks, every effort to recover it, including surgery, should be made. Unremoved needles have a tendency to migrate and may cause permanent injuries as well as medicolegal complications.

Repeat Block When Analgesia Is Inadequate: If the desired results from the first block attempt are unsatisfactory, do not hesitate to reblock the patient if time permits. Most patients will think nothing about being reblocked if the second attempt is prefaced by a statement such as: "Well, I guess we will have to inject a little more medicine if we are are going to freeze this nerve."

CHAPTER 19

Phrenic Nerve Block

INDICATIONS

Surgical: To arrest diaphragmatic action during a surgical procedure. This block is usually executed during chest surgery and can be done with more accuracy by the surgeon after the chest is opened.

Diagnostic: To help predict the effect of phrenic crush or section.

Therapeutic: Alleviation of persistent hiccups when other methods fail and phrenic crush by operation is not indicated.

ANATOMY

The phrenic nerve arises chiefly from the fourth cervical nerve but receives a branch from the third cervical nerve and another from the fifth cervical nerve. It descends to the root of the neck, running obliquely across the front of the anterior scalenus muscle and beneath the sternocleidomastoid muscle to descend in the thorax (Figure 81, page 138).

PREMEDICATION

None is advised because attempts to elicit paresthesias, which may be painful, are not required for this block and the procedure itself is not painful.

If, however, the patient is particularly apprehensive, a barbiturate or opiate may be administered, *i.e.*, 100 mg. (1½ gr.) to 200 mg. (3 gr.) pentobarbital (Nembutal) orally or intravenously or 10 mg. (⅙ gr.) to 15 mg. (¼ gr.) of morphine intramuscularly or intravenously.

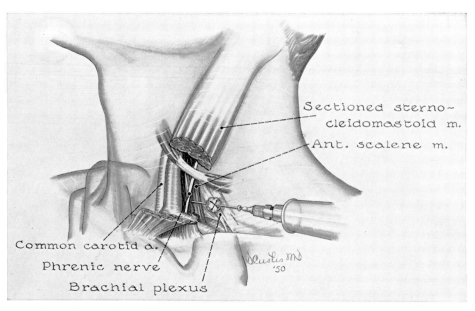

Figure 81. Anatomy of the phrenic nerve as it lies on the anterior scalenus muscles.

DRUGS

Tetracaine (Pontocaine)

Dosage.—15 cc. to 30 cc. of a 0.15 to 0.25 percent solution with or without 0.1 cc. of epinephrine (Adrenalin) 1:1000 in each 20 cc. of solution.*

Onset.—Phrenic nerve block is established in 5 to 15 mintues.

Duration.—Block lasts 4 to 6 hours, with stronger concentrations and solutions containing epinephrine giving the upper limits.

Procaine (Novocain)

Dosage.—15 cc. to 30 cc. of a 1.0 to 2.0 percent solution with or without 0.1 cc. of epinephrine (Adrenalin) 1:1000 in each 20 cc. of solution.*

Onset.—Phrenic nerve block is established in 5 to 15 minutes.

Duration.—Block lasts ¾ to 1½ hours, with stronger concentrations and solutions containing epinephrine giving the upper limits.

Lidocaine (Xylocaine) or Mepivacaine (Carbocaine)

Dosage.—15 cc. to 30 cc. of a 1.0 to 1.5 percent solution with or without 0.1 cc. of epinephrine (Adrenalin) 1:1000 in each 20 cc. of solution.*

Onset.—Phrenic nerve block is established in 5 to 15 minutes.

Duration.—Block lasts 1¼ to 3 hours, with stronger concentrations and solutions containing epinephrine giving the upper limits.

MATERIALS

Regional tray (see Chapter 9, page 51) or:

1. One ¾-inch (2 cm.), 25-gauge, Huber point security Lok-needle.

2. One 1½-inch (3.8 cm.), 22-gauge, security Lok-needle, preferably with a short bevel.

---

*Optimal concentration of epinephrine is 1:200,000, that is, 0.1 cc. of epinephrine 1:1000 in 20 cc. of the local anesthetic solution (see page 39).

3. One tuberculin Lok-syringe for measuring epinephrine.

4. One 10 cc. Lok-syringe, preferably with finger rings.

5. One graduated measuring cup, preferably stainless steel, for mixing solution.

6. One prep cup, preferably stainless steel.

7. Four sterile towels.

8. Six sterile sponges.

9. One sterilizer control.

TECHNIQUE

Position and Landmarks

1. The patient lies in the dorsal recumbent position without a pillow, his arms at his sides, and his head turned to the side opposite the one being blocked (Figure 82, page 140).

2. The patient is then instructed to raise his head 2 inches (5 cm.), approximately 30 degrees, off the table (Figure 138, page 226).

3. The lateral border of the clavicular head of the sternocleidomastoid muscle is located and marked with an X, 1 inch (2.5 cm.) above the clavicle (Figure 81, page 138). The muscle immediately lateral and posterior to this point, *i.e.*, the anterior scalenus, is palpated.

Precaution: *Aspirate.*—The neck is very vascular and careful aspiration tests are essential.

Procedure

1. The sterilizer control is checked to be sure the equipment is sterile.

2. If the anesthetist is right-handed, he stands at the head of the table facing the patient's feet for a right phrenic block and at the patient's side facing the head of the table for a left phrenic block (Figure 82, page 140). If the anesthetist is left-handed these positions are reversed.

3. The area is aseptically prepared and draped.

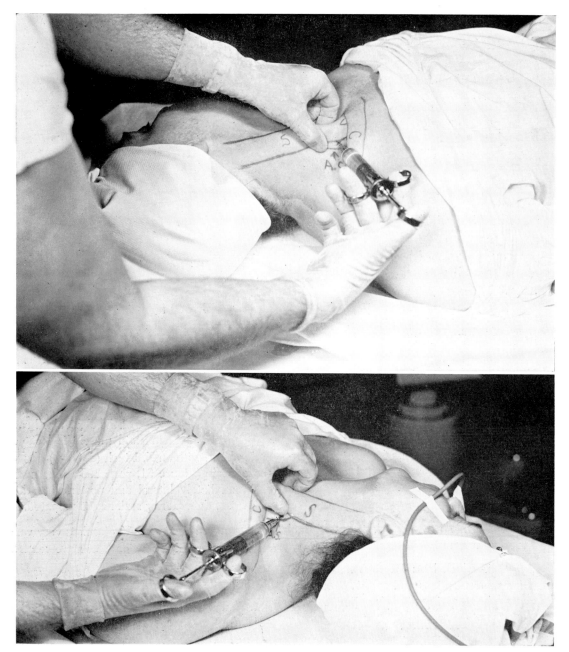

Figure 82. Method of injecting the phrenic nerve. S. sternocleidomastoid muscle; C. clavicle; A.S. anterior
scalenus muscle. A. *(Top)* Right phrenic block. B. *(Bottom)* Left phrenic block.

4. A skin wheal at the lateral border of the clavicular head of the sternocleidomastoid muscle at the X is made with the ¾-inch (2 cm.), 25-gauge Huber point security Lok-needle.

5. If the anesthetist is right-handed, the sternocleidomastoid muscle is grasped between the index finger and thumb of the left hand and pulled away from the neck (Figure 83, page 141). This maneuver actually pulls

the carotid sheath away from the phrenic nerve (Figure 84, page 141).

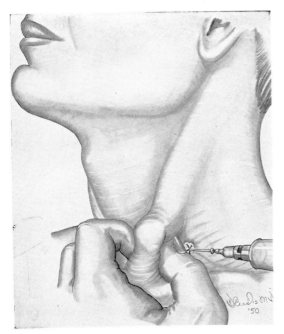

Figure 83. Method of holding sternocleidomastoid muscle while inserting needle for phrenic block.

6. The 1½-inch (3.8 cm.), 22-gauge, security Lok-needle attached to the full 10 cc. syringe is introduced through the skin wheal and advanced slowly for 1¼ inches (3.2 cm.) underneath the sternocleidomastoid muscle and parallel to the cross section of the body (Figure 82, page 140). Care must be exerted so that the needle point does not pass as far medially as the esophagus or trachea. By palpation on the medial side of the sternocleidomastoid muscle with the fingers of the hand pulling that muscle, the needle point may often be felt and the distance the needle point is from the trachea or esophagus easily ascertained.

7. The needle should lie within the cleavage plane between the sternocleidomastoid and anterior scalenus muscles.

8. 10 to 15 cc. of anesthetic solution is injected as the needle is slowly withdrawn.

EXTENT OF ANALGESIA

The only evidence of a successful phrenic block is cessation of diaphragmatic motion.

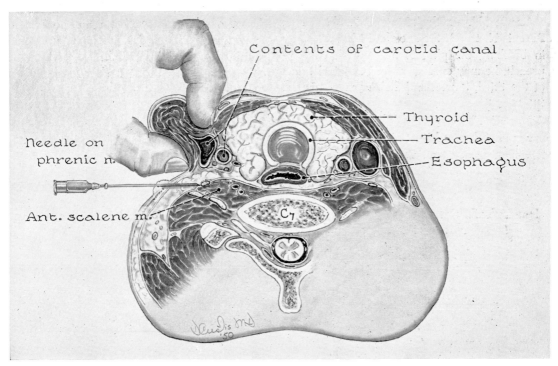

Figure 84. Cross section showing the effects of lifting the sternocleidomastoid muscle. Note the tendency to lift the carotid sheath away from the course of the needle.

This may be established by observation of the chest and abdomen as the patient is instructed to take a deep breath, or fluoroscopy may be done.

COMPLICATIONS

Occur very infrequently.

Toxic Reactions (intravascular injections, etc.): See Chapter 3, page 19.

Pneumothorax: See Chapter 30, page 237.

Horner's Syndrome: See Chapter 18, page 131.

Paralysis of the Recurrent Laryngeal Nerve: See Chapter 18, page 134.

REMARKS

Indication for Bilateral Block: Usually in cases of persistent hiccups a bilateral block is required. However, before doing the second side an interval of 15 to 30 minutes should elapse so that the effects of the initial block may be evaluated.

Cervical Nerve Block May Be Used to Block Phrenic Nerve: If the anesthetist has difficulty in blocking the phrenic nerve with this approach, he may execute a deep cervical block of the third, fourth, and fifth cervical nerves.

In this way he will block the fibers from which the phrenic nerve arises. The phrenic nerve derives its main component from the fourth cervical nerve and receives only small branches from the other two cervical nerves mentioned. Therefore, in some cases a block of the fourth cervical nerve alone may effect the desired results.

Recover Broken Needle(s): All needles should be tested before use. If a needle breaks, every effort to recover it, including surgery, should be made. Unremoved needles have a tendency to migrate and may cause permanent injuries as well as medicolegal complications.

Repeat Block When Result Is Inadequate: If the desired results from the first block attempt are unsatisfactory, do not hesitate to reblock the patient if time permits. Most patients will think nothing about being reblocked if the second attempt is prefaced by the statement: "Well, I guess we will have to inject a little more medicine if we are going to freeze this nerve."

However, do not exceed the maximum safe dosage of the local anesthetic solution for both blocks. If to reblock the patient the maximum safe dose of the local anesthetic solution must be exceeded, 45 minutes should elapse between blocks.

PART II

PERIPHERAL NERVE BLOCK ANESTHESIA

SECTION II

TRUNK (CHEST, ABDOMEN, AND PERINEUM)

CHAPTER 20

Intercostal Nerve Block Combined with Celiac Plexus (Splanchnic) Block

INDICATIONS

Surgical: Operations on the upper abdominal wall and its viscera, *i.e.*, gallbladder, stomach, duodenum, jejunum, small intestine, ascending and transverse colon, spleen, liver, ventral hernias, and eviscerations.

Diagnostic: Diagnosis of undifferentiated pain problems of the abdomen. Pain from abdominal wall is relieved by intercostal nerve block, and pain from the viscera is relieved by celiac plexus (splanchnic) block.

Therapeutic

Intercostal Nerve Block.—See Chapter 21, page 163.

Celiac Plexus (Splanchnic) Block.—(1) Relief of upper abdominal visceral pain, *i.e.*, pancreatic pain, etc., and (2) alleviation of the "dumping syndrome" (rapid emptying of the stomach) following gastric resections and other gastrointestinal anastomoses.

ANATOMY

Intercostal Nerves: The intercostal nerves are the anterior rami of the first eleven thoracic spinal nerves and are situated between the ribs (Figure 85, page 146). The anterior ramus of the twelfth thoracic nerve lies along the lower border of the twelfth rib and is anatomically not classified as an intercostal nerve. However, during this discussion it will be considered one. Except for a small branch, the first intercostal nerve is a part of the brachial plexus. The other intercostal nerves together with the intercostal vessels lie in the inter-costal spaces. The nerve lies a little below the blood vessels. The intercostal nerves lie between the pleura and the posterior intercostal membrane, proximal to the angles of the ribs. In the region of the angles of the ribs, they come to lie between the two laminae of the internal intercostal muscle, the innermost of which is known as the intercostalis internus. They continue forward in this relationship toward the front of the thorax (Figure 85A, B, page 146). The lower six intercostal nerves at the anterior ends of the intercostal spaces pass behind the costal cartilages and between the transversus abdominis muscle and the internal oblique muscle to reach the sheath of the rectus abdominis muscle, which they pierce. The terminal ends of both groups often pass the midline to the opposite side to a slight degree.

The most important branch of each intercostal nerve from the standpoint of regional block is the lateral cutaneous branch (Figure 85, page 146 and Figure 95, page 156). It branches from the intercostal nerves midway between the spine and the sternum, usually just anterior to the midaxillary line. It pierces the external intercostal muscles and the anterior serratus muscle and divides into anterior and posterior cutaneous branches (Figure 95, page 156). Therefore, if the intercostal nerves are not blocked posteriorly or along the posterior axillary line, it is very easy to miss this branch and not establish adequate analgesia.

The rib at its angle is approximately ¼ inch (0.6 cm.) thick.

Celiac Plexus (Solar or Splanchnic Plexus): The celiac plexus is situated at the level of the

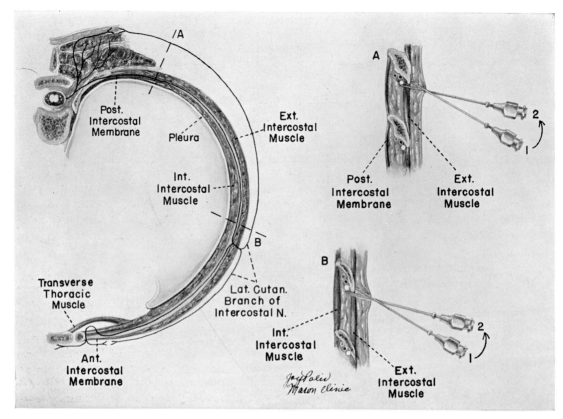

Figure 85. Anatomical sections of the chest wall showing the different locations of the intercostal nerves at the two points most frequently used for an intercostal nerve block. A. Sagittal section at approximately angles of ribs. B. Sagittal section at approximately midaxillary line.

upper part of the first lumbar vertebra and is composed of a right and left celiac ganglion and a dense network of nerve fibers connecting them (Figure 86 A, B, page 147). It surrounds the celiac artery and the base of the superior mesenteric artery (Figure 86B, page 147). It lies in areolar tissue behind the peritoneum, the stomach, and the omental bursa; in front of the crura of the diaphragm and the commencement of the abdominal aorta; and between the suprarenal glands. The plexus and ganglia receive the greater and lesser splanchnic nerves of both sides and some filaments from the right vagus. The plexus gives off secondary plexuses to the diaphragm, liver, spleen, stomach, suprarenal gland, kidney, spermatic cord, abdominal aorta, and the mesentery.

PREMEDICATION

No attempts to elicit paresthesias are made. Nevertheless, light premedication and supplementary analgesia with 0.6 percent thiopental (Pentothal) during the block procedure and very light general anesthesia during surgery is advocated for the surgical patient. Postoperative depression may be eliminated to a considerable extent by this method. When this block is used for therapeutic and diagnostic procedures the same technique of premedication may be employed. However, it is seldom necessary to use the intravenous thiopental, provided careful infiltration of the skin, subcutaneous tissue, and muscle layers is performed.

Light Premedication: The average patient (age 20 to 50, weight 150 pounds or over,

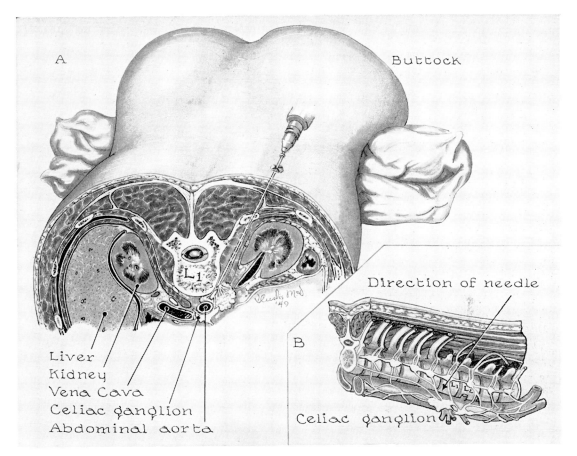

Figure 86. Anatomy in the region of the celiac plexus and the direction of the celiac needles. A. Cross section. B. Lateral view.

height 5 feet, 5 inches or over, and good physical status) receives:

1. 200 mg. (3 gr.) pentobarbital (Nembutal) by mouth at hour of sleep on the night prior to surgery.

2. No preoperative pentobarbital.

3. 15 mg. (¼ gr.) of morphine and 0.6 mg. (1/100 gr.) of atropine intramuscularly ¾ to 1 hour before estimated *block* time. Atropine is preferred to scopolamine because it more effectively decreases vagal reflexes which are sensitized by thiopental.

Reduction of Premedication: It is seldom necessary to increase this premedication irrespective of the over-all size of the patient until the patient arrives in either the anesthesia or operating room. However, it is very common to reduce this medication under various circumstances; for example, for the geriatric patient, the adolescent patient or child, the debilitated or cachectic patient, and for patients whose surgery is complicated by other disease, *e.g.,* myxedema, diabetes, heart disease, etc. In these patients, the barbiturate for sleep the night before surgery is reduced to 50 mg. (¾ gr.) or omitted and the preoperative morphine reduced to 8 mg. (⅛ gr.). *Always err on the light side.*

DRUGS

Tetracaine (Pontocaine): Tetracaine is the drug of choice for this block primarily because of its long duration (see page 16).

Dosage

INTERCOSTAL NERVE BLOCK: 100 cc. or less of 0.1 percent solution with or without 0.2 cc. of epinephrine (Adrenalin) 1:1000.*

CELIAC PLEXUS BLOCK: 50 cc. of 0.05 percent solution with or without 0.2 cc. of epinephrine 1:1000.*

Hyaluronidase 150 TRU is incorporated in the 50 cc. to effect a wider spread of anesthetic solution. When hyaluronidase is employed, epinephrine must be added to the anesthetic solution or the duration of anesthesia will be markedly shortened.

A 0.05 percent solution is easily made. 125 cc. of 0.1 percent tetracaine solution is mixed in the large graduated measuring cup and 25 cc. of normal saline is placed in a prep cup. Then 25 cc. of the 0.1 percent tetracaine solution is added to the 25 cc. of normal saline in the prep cup, giving a 0.05 percent solution. The specified amount of epinephrine (0.2 cc.) and 150 TRU of hyaluronidase are added to the prep cup. Hyaluronidase is not necessary for a successful block, but it does effect a wider spread of the solution in the prevertebral space.

Onset.—Operating analgesia is established in 15 to 45 minutes, with an average of 25 minutes.

Duration.—Operating analgesia lasts 3½ to 6 hours, with solutions containing epinephrine giving the upper limits.

Procaine (Novocain)

Dosage

INTERCOSTAL NERVE BLOCK: 80 cc. or less of 1.0 percent solution with or without 0.2 cc. of epinephrine (Adrenalin) 1:1000.*

CELIAC PLEXUS BLOCK: 50 cc. of 0.50 percent solution with or without 0.2 cc. of epinephrine 1:1000.*

Hyaluronidase 150 TRU is incorporated in the 50 cc. to effect a wider spread of the anesthetic solution. When hyaluronidase is employed, epinephrine must be added to the

local anesthetic solution or the operating time will be markedly shortened. Hyaluronidase is not necessary for a successful block.

Onset.—Operating analgesia is established in 5 to 15 minutes, with an average of 10 minutes.

Duration.—Operating analgesia lasts 1 to 1½ hours, with solutions containing epinephrine giving the upper limits.

Lidocaine (Xylocaine) or Mepivacaine (Carbocaine)

INTERCOSTAL NERVE BLOCK: 80 cc. or less of 0.5 percent solution with or without 0.2 cc. of epinephrine (Adrenalin) 1:1000.*

CELIAC PLEXUS BLOCK: 50 cc. of 0.25 percent solution with or without 0.2 cc. of epinephrine 1:1000.*

Hyaluronidase 150 TRU is incorporated in the 50 cc. to effect a wider spread of the anesthetic solution. When hyaluronidase is employed, epinephrine must be added to the local anesthetic solution or the operating time will be markedly shortened. Hyaluronidase is not necessary for a successful block.

Onset.—Operating analgesia is established in 5 to 15 minutes.

Duration.—Operating analgesia lasts 1¼ to 3 hours, with solutions containing epinephrine giving the upper limits.

Alcohol

Dosage

INTERCOSTAL NERVE BLOCK: Placement of alcohol on intercostal nerves is not advised—incidence of neuritis is high.

CELIAC PLEXUS BLOCK: 50 cc. of 50 percent alcohol.

Onset.—Analgesia is established in 1 to 3 minutes.

---

*This is the only block in which more than 0.25 cc. of epinephrine 1:1000 is used. The patient is usually heavily sedated or lightly anesthetized and he does not complain of palpitation, etc., from the epinephrine (see page 39).

Duration.—Sensory analgesia lasts three weeks to six months or longer.

MATERIALS

Regional tray plus celiac needles (see Chapter 9, page 51) or:

1. One ¾-inch (2 cm.), 25-gauge Huber point security Lok-needle.

2. One 1½-inch (3.8 cm.), 22-gauge security Lok-needle, preferably short bevel.

3. Two 4-inch (10 cm.), 20-gauge security Lok-needles, preferably short bevel.

4. Two 5-inch (12.5 cm.), 20-gauge security Lok-needles, preferably short bevel.

5. Two 6-inch (15 cm.), 20-gauge security Lok-needles, preferably short bevel.

6. One tuberculin Lok-syringe for measuring epinephrine.

7. One 10 cc. Lok-syringe, preferably with finger rings.

8. One graduated measuring cup, preferably stainless steel, 250 cc. size for mixing solution.

9. Two prep cups, preferably stainless steel.

10. Six sterile sponges.

11. Four sterile towels.

12. One sterilizer control.

TECHNIQUE

Position and Landmarks: The patient is placed in the prone position, his arms hanging off the operating room cart or table and a pillow under the abdomen between the ribs and the iliac crests. The pillow helps to straighten the lumbar curvature (Figure 87, page 149).

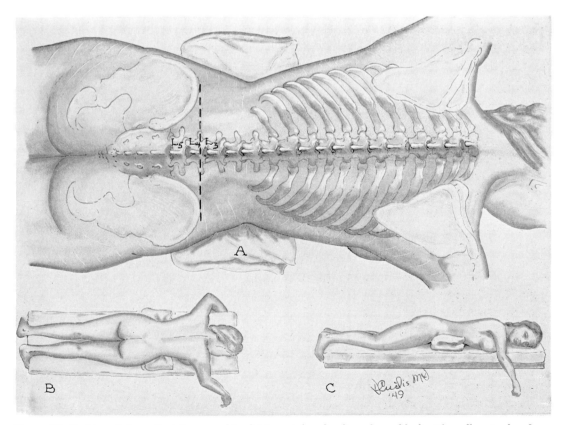

Figure 87. Position of the patient for a combined intercostal and celiac plexus block. The pillow is placed under the abdomen. A and B. Posterior view. C. Lateral view.

Intercostal Nerve Block

1. Draw two lines parallel to each other and to the spines along the thoracic cage on both sides 2½ inches (6.3 cm.) to 3 inches (7.5 cm.) from the spines of the vertebrae. The lines should lie in the region of the angles of the ribs just lateral to the sacrospinalis group of muscles (Figure 88, page 150).

2. Along these lines the ribs are easily felt and marked with X's. The distances between the twelfth and the eleventh ribs may be wide in comparison to the other intercostal interspaces as the twelfth rib is not fixed to the sternum anteriorly (Figure 88, page 150).

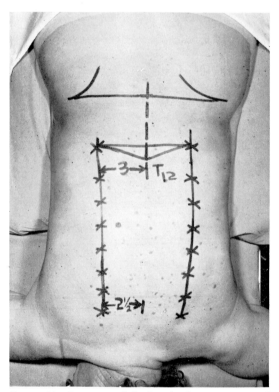

Figure 88. Position and landmarks for an intercostal and celiac plexus block for an upper abdominal operation. Note the pillow placed under the abdomen to straighten the lumbar curve. The arms hang off the operating table so as to widen the space between scapulae and spinous processes of vertebrae. Even so, the scapulae limit the distance the line can be drawn from the upper spinous processes of the vertebrae. The line between the iliac crests crosses the spinous process of the fourth lumbar vertebra. The X's mark the lower borders of the fifth through the twelfth ribs. The line from the X's at the twelfth rib to the cephalad edge of the spinous process of the first lumbar vertebra marks the path traveled by the needles on their way to the celiac plexus.

Celiac Plexus Block

1. The iliac crests are palpated and a line drawn between them (Figure 88, page 150). This line crosses the spine of the fourth lumbar vertebra or the interspace between the fourth and fifth lumbar vertebrae (Figure 88, page 150).

2. The index finger of the right hand is placed in the third lumbar interspace and the index finger, the middle (long) finger, and the ring finger of the left hand in the interspaces between the second and third lumbar vertebrae, the first and second lumbar vertebrae, and the twelfth thoracic and first lumbar vertebrae respectively (Figure 89, page 151).

In this manner, the spines of the twelfth thoracic and first lumbar vertebrae are determined accurately. The celiac plexus lies in the *prevertebral space* at the level of the cephalad edge of the spine of the first lumbar vertebra (Figure 86, page 147). To check the twelfth thoracic and first lumbar spinous processes, one should feel the spinous process of the first thoracic vertebra and count down.

3. The spine of the twelfth thoracic vertebra and the spine of the first lumbar vertebra are marked (Figure 88, page 150).

4. Lines are drawn between the X's of the twelfth ribs and the cephalad edge of the spine of the first lumbar vertebra (Figure 88, page 150). This should complete a triangle which usually is flat but may vary, depending on the position of the twelfth rib (Figure 88, page 150 and Figure 90, page 151). The sides of the triangle represent the pathway traveled by the long celiac needles on their way to the celiac plexus.

Precautions

Remove Contents of Stomach.—The anesthetist should be sure that the stomach has been completely aspirated before the anesthesia is started if a suction tube is in place. Often prior to surgery while the patient is being prepared in his room for the trip to the operating room, the Levin tube will be clamped, allowing gastric secretions to accumulate.

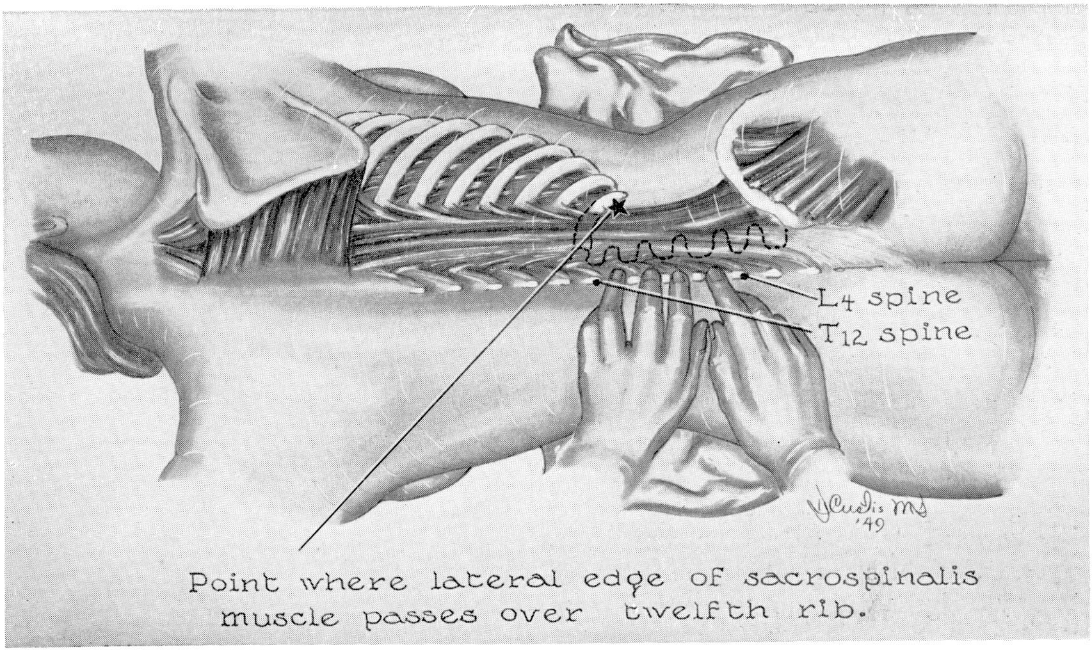

L4 spine
T12 spine
Point where lateral edge of sacrospinalis muscle passes over twelfth rib.
'49

Figure 89. Anatomy and method of determining the landmarks for a celiac plexus block. Note the position of the hands of a right-handed anesthetist when locating the interspace between the twelfth thoracic vertebra and the first lumbar vertebra—index finger of right hand palpates third lumbar interspace; index finger of left hand, second lumbar interspace; middle (long) finger of left hand, first lumbar interspace; and ring finger of left hand, the interspace between the twelfth thoracic and first lumbar vertebrae.

T12 vertebral spine
Twelfth rib
Sacrospinalis m.
'49

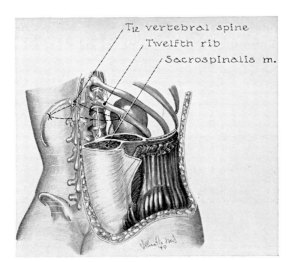

Figure 90. Landmarks for a celiac plexus block with the underlying anatomical considerations. Note the flat triangle which is formed by the lines drawn between the superficial bony landmarks.

Avoid Puncturing Pleura.—When performing intercostal nerve block, care should be exercised not to pierce the pleura.

Aspirate.—Aspiration tests should be made before injecting, especially in the celiac plexus region because there are many large blood vessels in this area.

Stop Block and Slow Thiopental Drip If Coughing Occurs.—If the patient starts to cough after the 0.6 percent thiopental is started, slow the drip until the episode passes. Also, stop the block since the reflexes from the periosteum of the ribs may be an inciting factor. When coughing has stopped, resume the block.

Treat Laryngospasm.—If laryngospasm occurs, turn patient on back and treat laryngospasm.

Block Upper Intercostal Nerves Along Posterior Axillary Line.—As many as possible of the intercostal nerves to be blocked should be blocked from the posterior approach. However, if landmarks are not easily found in the region of the scapulae, do not proceed blindly; wait until the patient is returned to the supine position. Then block the upper intercostal nerves along the posterior axillary line (Figure 95, page 156).

Maintain Asepsis.—When the side away from the operation is being intercostally blocked, a sterile towel should cover the back on the side nearest the anesthetist to prevent contamination.

Procedure

1. The sterilizer control is checked to be sure the equipment has been sterilized.

2. The patient receives a rapid drip of 0.6 percent thiopental until the lid reflex is lost. Then the drop is slowed. If the thiopental has been given wisely, the patient should be awake at the end of the block and may be tested for sensory analgesia with an Allis forceps.

3. The back is aseptically prepared and draped.

Intercostal Nerve Block

1. If the anesthetist is right-handed, he stands at the left side of the prone patient for the intercostal nerve block of both sides and vice versa (Figure 91, page 152). *It is easier to reach across the midline than change sides of the table and work back-handed.* The side where the incision will be made should be blocked first.

2. When the anesthetist is right-handed, the full 10 cc. Lok-syringe with the 1½-inch (3.8 cm.) security Lok-needle attached is held in the right hand while the index finger of the left hand palpates the inferior border of the rib at the X (Figure 91, page 152).

Skin wheals are not made with a ¾-inch (2 cm.), 25-gauge Huber point needle in the unconscious patient—to do so only prolongs block time. However, if the patient is not given intravenous anesthesia prior to the block, skin wheals should be made at the X's.

3. The index finger of the left hand pulls the skin which overlies the inferior border of the rib up and over the rib (Figure 92, page 153).

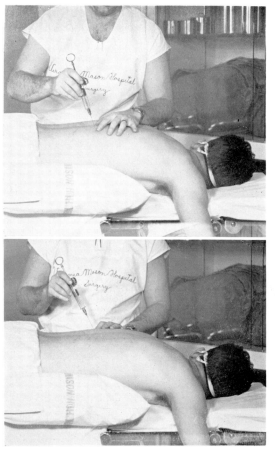

Figure 91. Position of the patient and right-handed anesthetist for an intercostal nerve block from the posterior approach. A. (*Top*) Right side. B. (*Bottom*) Left side.

4. The needle is introduced through the X on the skin at the tip of the index finger of the left hand. The hub of the needle is inclined caudad so that the shaft of the needle forms an 80-degree angle with the skin (Figure 92B, page 153 and Figure 93A, page 154). The needle is then slowly advanced until the point comes to rest on the lower border of the rib.

5. The index finger of the left hand releases the skin which had been pulled up and over the rib (Figure 92C, page 153).

6. Now the hub of the needle is held between the thumb and index finger of the left hand, and the middle (long) finger of the left hand rests against the shaft of the needle. *The left hand rests on the patient's back.* By

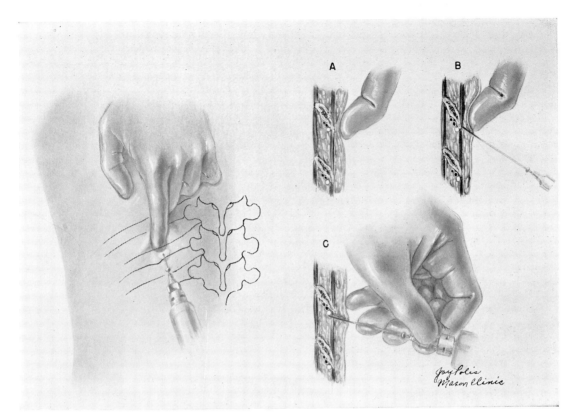

Figure 92. Method of blocking an intercostal nerve. Anterior view of the skin being pulled up and over the rib by the index finger. A. Cross-sectional view of the palpation of the rib prior to pulling the skin up and over the rib. B. Cross-sectional view of the skin being pulled up and over the rib with the needle being inserted just off the tip of the finger onto the lower border of the rib. C. Needle has been walked off the rib by the middle (long) and ring fingers.

exerting gentle pressure against the shaft of the needle, the middle (long) finger of the left hand then walks the needle off the lower edge of the rib. By holding the hub of the needle firmly between the thumb and index finger of the left hand *while the left hand rests on the patient's back,* the anesthetist has perfect control of the needle (Figure 93B, page 154 and Figure 94 A, B, page 155).

7. As the needle loses contact with the rib, the left hand resting on the back freezes the needle in place (Figure 93B, page 154 and Figure 94 A, B, page 155).

8. The needle is then slowly advanced about ⅛ inch (0.3 cm.). Now as the needle is jiggled forward and backward about ¹⁄₁₆ inch (0.15 cm.) guided by the thumb and index finger of the left hand, 5 cc. of the anesthetic solution is deposited. This technique is repeated on the lower seven or eight intercostal nerves. The jiggling of the needle guarantees that a part of the solution will be deposited between the internal intercostal muscles and the posterior intercostal membranes where the nerve lies (Figure 85A, page 146). If the needle were fixed outside the compartment bound by the internal intercostal muscle and the posterior intercostal membranes, no analgesia would result. Jiggling the needle also tends to minimize intravascular injections.

9. Since the lower seven or eight inter-

costal nerves should be blocked for upper abdominal surgery and since it is often difficult to palpate more than the lower six or seven intercostal nerves from the posterior approach, the anesthetist should proceed with the celiac plexus block. After it has been completed, the thiopental is stopped, the patient turned slowly into the supine position, his chest bared, and his hands placed behind his head. The intercostal nerves which were not done posteriorly should be blocked along the posterior axillary line (Figure 95A, page 156).

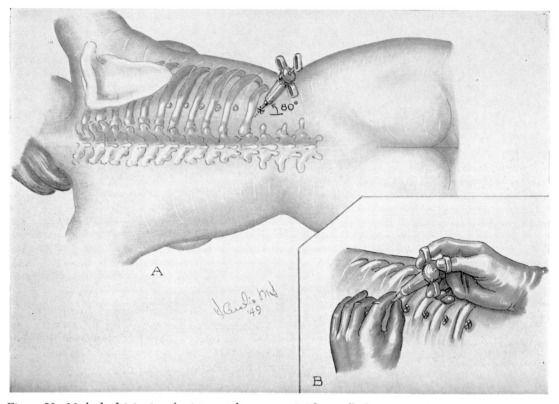

Figure 93. Method of injecting the intercostal nerves.   A. The needle forms an 80-degree angle with the skin so that it can slip under the inferior edge of the rib. B. Thumb, index finger, and middle finger of the left hand holding hub and shaft of needle while the hand rests on the patient's back.

Figure 94. Injection of the intercostal nerves. The right-handed anesthetist should reach across the midline to execute the intercostal nerve block on the right side. Note the angle of the syringe and needle as well as the method of holding the needle. It can be seen that the thumb and index finger of the left hand grip the hub of the needle and that the middle finger exerts pressure on the shaft of the needle and guides its direction. The side of the left hand rests on the patient's back to prevent too deep insertion of the needle if the patient moves. A. Posterior view. B. Lateral view

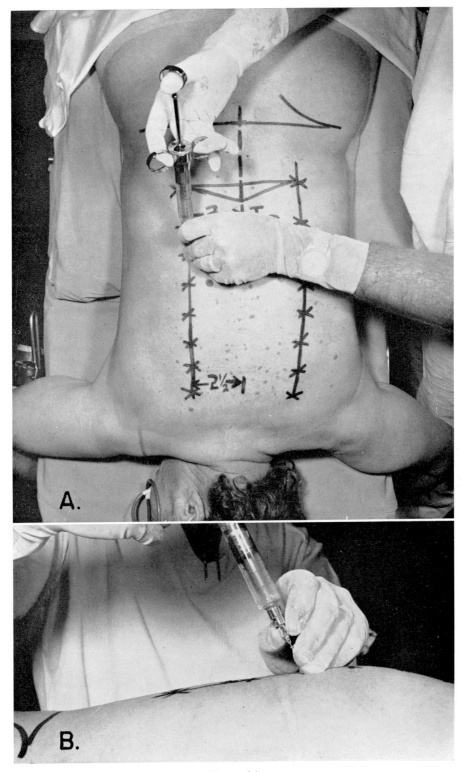

Figure 94.

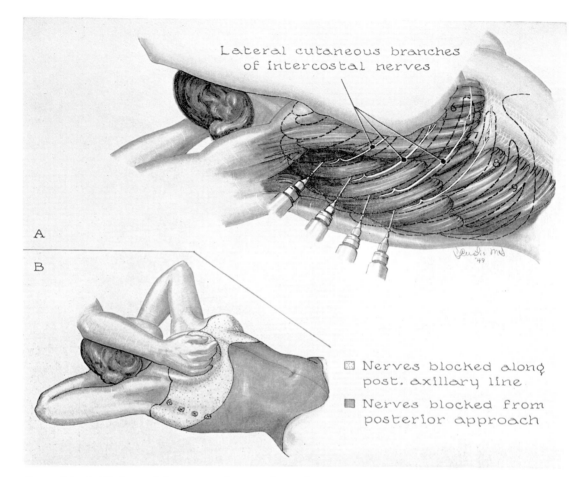

Figure 95. A. Blocking of the intercostal nerves from the anterior approach in the posterior axillary line. B. Position of the female patient for the approach with hands behind her head and breast supported by nurse. Variations in the shaded areas indicate areas of skin analgesia resulting from the different approaches.

In a female the breasts should be retracted medially (Figure 95B, page 156).

Celiac Plexus

1. The anesthetist stands by the patient at the side to be blocked (Figure 96, page 157).

2. In the average patient the 4-inch (10 cm.) or 5-inch (12.5 cm.) 20-gauge security Lok-needle will be sufficient. It is introduced through the X at the lower edge of the twelfth rib at a 45-degree angle to the skin and slowly advanced along the line of the side of the marked triangle until contact is made with the cephalad part of the body of the first lumbar vertebra (Figure 97, page 157 and Figure 98, page 158). The depth of the needle is noted.

3. The needle is withdrawn and the angle between its shaft and the skin increased slightly, i.e., to 60 degrees. Then it is reinserted to the bone. This maneuver is repeated, increasing the angle slightly each time until the needle is felt to slip off the body of the vertebra (Figure 98, page 158). The needle is now advanced ½ inch (1.3 cm.). It should lie in prevertebral areolar tissue which contains the celiac plexus. In the average patient the

distance from the skin to the celiac plexus is usually between 3½ inches (8.8 cm.) and 4 inches (10 cm.) when the above approach is used (Figure 99, page 158 and Figure 100, page 159).

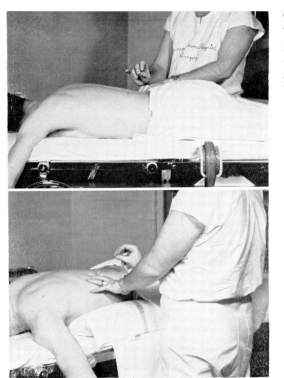

← —————————————————————

Figure 96. Position of the patient and the right-handed anesthetist for the celiac plexus block. A. *(Top)* Right side. B. *(Bottom)* Left side.

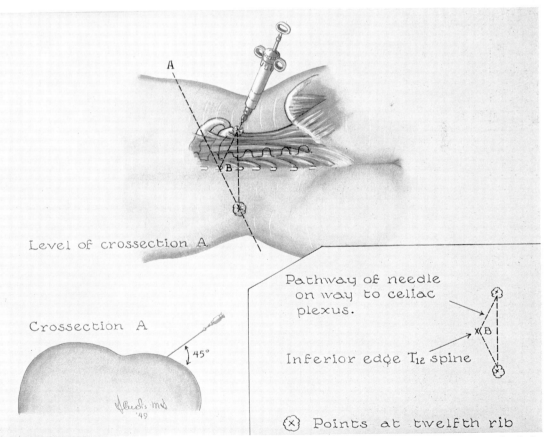

Level of crossection A.

Crossection A

45°

Pathway of needle on way to celiac plexus.

Inferior edge T₁₂ spine

Points at twelfth rib

Figure 97. Schematic drawing showing the 45 degree angle of the needle to the skin and the path of the long celiac needle as it seeks the body of the first lumbar vertebra.

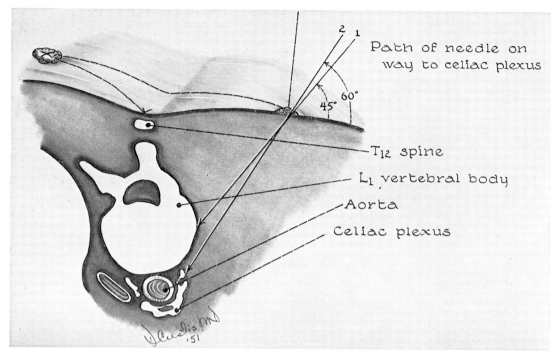

Figure 98. Oblique sectional schematic drawing showing the method used to place the needle in the region of the celiac ganglion.

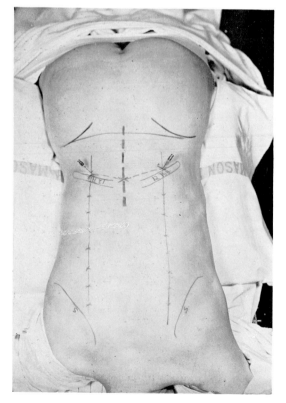

4. The hub of the needle is securely held by the thumb and index finger of the free hand as the hand rests on the back (Figure 101, page 159). The syringe is attached to the needle. The aspiration test is executed and 25 cc. of the diluted anesthetic solution is injected. When the needle is correctly placed there is no resistance to the injection of the anesthetic solution, and the anesthetist has the feeling he is injecting intravenously.

5. The other side is blocked in the same way.

EXTENT OF ANALGESIA

Intercostal Nerve Block: Somatic analgesia exists from approximately the nipple line to the pubic symphysis (Figure 102, page 159).

←———————————————

Figure 99. (Posterior view) 4-inch (10 cm.) needles in place for the execution of the celiac plexus block. Note the direction of the needles as they course along the line from the twelfth rib to the superior edge of the spinous process of the first lumbar vertebra. Also the 60 degree angle formed by the shaft of the needles and the skin.

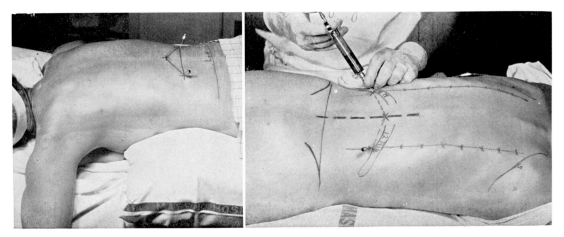

Figure 100. *(Left)* Lateral view showing the needles in place for the celiac plexus block. The straight line between the iliac crests passes through the interspace between the spinous processes of the third and fourth lumbar vertebrae.

Figure 101. *(Right)* Method of holding the celiac plexus needle while injecting the local anesthetic solution. Left hand rests on patient's back.

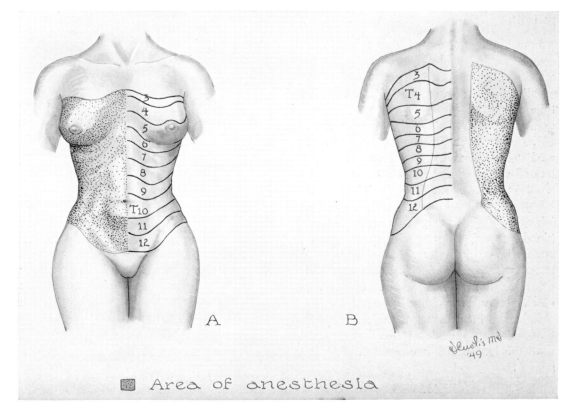

Figure 102. Skin analgesia resulting from the usual intercostal nerve block used in combination with a celiac block for abdominal procedures. A. Anterior. B. Posterior.

Celiac Plexus: Anesthesia of the viscera of the abdomen ensues, with the exception of the pelvic viscera, *i.e.*, sigmoid colon, rectum, bladder, and reproductive organs, which will react to pain and traction stimuli.

COMPLICATIONS

Pneumothorax: See Chapter 30, page 237.

Toxic Reactions (intravascular injections, etc.): See Chapter 3, page 19.

Subarachnoid Injections: See Chapter 43, page 353. When placing the needles for celiac plexus block, an incorrectly placed needle may enter the subarachnoid space. This has occurred to us. In all cases, the spinal fluid dripped from the 20-gauge needle, the needle was withdrawn, and placed correctly in the prevertebral space. No cases of total spinal block have occurred in our series of over 3,000 patients.

Low Blood Pressure: Either following the completion of the block or more frequently after the opening of the abdomen, there is usually a marked drop in systolic and diastolic blood pressure. The systolic drop is greater than the diastolic. This drop occurs in 80 percent of the patients and if treated immediately, causes little concern. It may be treated satisfactorily by using the usual vasoconstrictor drugs intravenously. The most satisfactory method is to use a phenylephrine (Neo-Synephrine) drip (see page 36). If blood loss occurs during surgery, it should be replaced by blood transfusions, even if the phenylephrine maintains an adequate blood pressure. After the abdomen is closed the blood pressure usually stabilizes at a reasonable level. If it does not, there is no objection to continuing the slow phenylephrine drip until the local anesthetic agent is dissipated.

REMARKS

Use Light Premedication: Premedication should not be heavy. The outstanding feature of this block is the fact that postoperatively the patient is awake and cooperative. A pa-

tient who is free from pain the first few hours postoperatively will be able to clear his bronchi and trachea of secretions that have accumulated during surgery and thus avoid respiratory complications. Since the patient is free from pain for three to six hours after surgery when tetracaine (Pontocaine) is employed, heavy premedication often would depress his respiration as well as render him stuporous.

Aspirate Stomach: All patients having upper abdominal operations performed under intercostal-celiac plexus block should have a Levin tube "sunk" in their stomachs before the block is attempted. While this is not mandatory *except in gastric surgery*, it is a valuable precaution and of great aid to the anesthetist. It allows him to empty the stomach prior to execution of the block and allows him to keep it empty during the operative and immediate postoperative periods. This simple prophylactic treatment will often avoid aspiration of gastric contents.

Advantages of Thiopental (Pentothal) During Block: 0.6 percent thiopental is administered during the execution of the block to avoid heavy premedication, to quiet respirations, and to keep the patient from moving. If the latter two conditions are not assured, the chances of a pneumothorax and intravascular or subarachnoid injection are greatly increased.

Block at Least Lower Seven or Eight Intercostal Nerves: The lower seven or eight intercostal nerves should always be blocked to assure that the anesthesia level is just below the nipple line. Otherwise, overlap of the intercostal nerves as well as an extension of an incision may render the block unsatisfactory (Figure 102, page 159).

Indications to Block Lumbar Nerves: If there is a possibility that the incision will be carried into the lower abdomen, it is often best also to block the first and second lumbar nerves paravertebrally (see Chapter 28, page 206).

Lightly Anesthetize the Surgical Patient: During extensive surgery, *e.g.*, gastric resection or cholecystectomy, under these blocks, it is best to lightly anesthetize the patient with a sleep dose of thiopental (125-250 mg.) and then maintain him with light anesthesia, e.g., halothane (Fluothane) 0.5 percent and oxygen (2 L.)—nitrous oxide (2 L.). This assures adequate oxygenation and allows the surgeon to explore the pelvic region as well as the diaphragmatic region. These two regions are not anesthetized by the block since the phrenic nerves supply the diaphragm and the lumbar nerves and hypogastric plexus innervate the pelvis. Also, during gastric resection uncomfortable traction reflexes are transmitted through the esophagus when the surgeon pulls the stomach.

Other methods of providing light anesthesia may be equally satisfactory.

Avoid Puncture of the Pleura: To avoid puncture of the pleura in an intercostal nerve block, the anesthetist must remember that at the angle the rib is only ¼ inch (0.6 cm.) thick and if he advances his needle off the edge with care as described, there is little chance of puncturing the pleura.

Wrap Legs: The legs should be wrapped from the foot to the thigh as described in Chapter 1, page 7.

Do Not Use These Blocks if Diagnosis is Questionable: Emergencies where the diagnosis cannot definitely be established or where the bowel is markedly distended, are best done under inhalation or spinal analgesia. This regional block technique is best limited to elective procedures where adequate preoperative preparation may be carried out.

Prone Position Advantageous for Executing Block: The prone position is preferred for this block because:

1. It entails minimal moving of the patient.

2. It is a very satisfactory position for the execution of the celiac plexus block.

3. It assures a complete block of the intercostal nerves. If the intercostal nerves are blocked at the angles of the ribs, i.e., approximately 2½ inches (6.3 cm.) to 3 inches (7.5

cm.) from the spinous processes of the thoracic vertebra, a complete block of each nerve ensues. However, if the supine position is used and the intercostal nerves are blocked along the axillary line, it is not uncommon for the lateral cutaneous branches of the intercostal nerves, particularly the lower four, to be missed. This is true because the lateral cutaneous nerves branch from the intercostal nerves near the anterior axillary line. The lateral cutaneous nerves innervate the skin over the abdomen and sides so that a block of the intercostal nerve must be performed posterior to the branching of the lateral cutaneous nerve to assure adequate analgesia of the skin (Figure 85, page 146 and Figure 95A, page 156).

Puncture of Kidney or Viscera: The question has often arisen as to whether or not the needles used in the celiac plexus block ever puncture the kidney or abdominal viscera. Irrespective of the ability of the anesthetist, at times they surely must. However, complications resulting from their puncture must be minimal and go unrecognized. Bloody urine, peritonitis, or hemoperitoneum from a celiac plexus block has not been seen by the author in his practice or noted in the literature.

Avoid Celiac Plexus Block in Patients of Poor Physical Status: Patients who are in shock should not have a celiac plexus block, since it will tend to lower their blood pressure. However, an intercostal nerve block may be given a patient in shock to decrease the amount of inhalation or intravenous anesthetic agents necessary without affecting the patient's blood pressure to any great degree.

In other patients with a compromised or poor physical status in whom a fall in blood pressure may be detrimental, e.g., the geriatric, debilitated, or cachectic patient, bilateral intercostal nerve block *without* celiac plexus block is used by us in preference to a muscle relaxant to obtain relaxation of the abdominal musculature. Thiopental is not used when the intercostal nerve block is executed, but skin wheals are made with a ¾-inch (2 cm.) 25-gauge Huber point needle and adequate local infiltration done as the 1½-inch (3.8 cm.) needle is inserted to locate the ribs.

Often the intercostal nerve block is the only anesthesia necessary for the surgery, *e.g.*, repair of a dehiscence of a previous abdominal incision or establishment of a feeding gastrostomy. If the block alone is not adequate, and if additional anesthesia is necessary, light general anesthesia may be used as described under Lightly Anesthetize the Surgical Patient (page 160).

Celiac Plexus Can Be Blocked from Either Left or Right Side: When performing the celiac plexus block only one needle need be placed. Either the right or left side may be chosen. If the needle is correctly placed in the prevertebral space the local anesthetic solution will diffuse so as to involve the whole plexus, providing an adequate volume, 50 cc. to 60 cc., is injected. Nevertheless the author prefers to block the celiac plexus by the bilateral approach as a means of insuring a quicker onset and a complete block.

For Gastric Surgery, Intubate Patients: In gastric surgery the author always intubates the patient because gastric contents are often regurgitated when the surgeon manipulates the stomach.

If the physical status of a patient is poor or if the patient is edentulous, the endotracheal tube is inserted while the patient is awake but "groggy" from the thiopental injected during the block procedure. The pharynx, larynx, and trachea in these patients are anesthetized topically by either transtracheal injection (see Chapter 39, page 321) or by the direct spray technique. Once the endotracheal tube, lubricated with a 2 percent dibucaine (Nupercaine) or 5 percent lidocaine (Xylocaine) ointment, has been in place for a few seconds the patient tolerates it ex-

tremely well without coughing or straining. The patient is then carried with oxygen (2 L.) —nitrous oxide (2 L.). If this is inadequate intermittent use of a more potent agent, *e.g.*, cyclopropane, halothane (Fluothane), etc., may be employed.

On the other hand, if the patient's physical status is good or if he is not edentulous, the endotracheal tube is inserted after the intravenous administration of 40 mg. of succinylcholine (Anectine). When the patient is awake but "groggy" from the thiopental injected during the block procedure, he will have no memory of the short period of paralysis (4-5 min.) from the succinylcholine. Once the patient is intubated, he is given artificial respiration with oxygen until the effects of the succinylcholine have been dissipated. Then anesthesia is administered as described under Lightly Anesthetize the Surgical Patient (page 160).

Use Alcohol with Care: Before using alcohol for celiac plexus block, consult Chapter 41, page 329.

Recover Broken Needle(s): All needles should be tested before use. If a needle breaks, every effort to recover it, including surgery, should be made. Unremoved needles have a tendency to migrate and may cause permanent injuries as well as medicolegal complications.

Repeat Block when Analgesia is Inadequate: If the desired results from the first block attempt are unsatisfactory, do not hesitate to reblock the patient if the time permits.

However, do not exceed the maximum safe dosage of the local anesthetic solution for both blocks. If to reblock the patient the maximum safe dose of the local anesthetic solution must be exceeded, 45 minutes should elapse between blocks.

CHAPTER 21

Intercostal Nerve Block

INDICATIONS

Surgical: Operations on the superficial structures of the back, chest, and abdomen may be performed. The block may be used to supplement general anesthesia in abdominal surgery, thereby reducing the amount of the general anesthetic agent (see page 161).

Diagnostic: Differentiation of somatic from sympathetic pain. Often arthritic root pain of the intercostal nerves may be mistaken for anginal pain.

Therapeutic: Relief of intercostal pain caused by fractured ribs, pleurisy, and undiagnosed neuritic conditions. The acute pain of herpes zoster may temporarily be relieved, but block of the sympathetic ganglia is considered definitive treatment. Postoperative intercostal nerve block in abdominal procedures will alleviate muscle spasm and incisional pain and facilitates the stir-up regime, *i.e.*, voluntary coughing, deep breathing, and early ambulation. This is one of the most outstanding uses for this block.

ANATOMY

(See Anatomy, Chapter 20, page 145.)

PREMEDICATION

No attempts to elicit paresthesias are made. Therapeutic and diagnostic block patients need not be medicated since the execution of the block is not painful if a skin wheal is made and local infiltration is carefully executed.

Surgical patients are usually heavily medicated to avoid restlessness during the operation.

Heavy Premedication: The average patient (age 20 to 50, weight 150 pounds or over, approximate height 5 feet, 5 inches or over, and good physical status) receives:

1. 200 mg. (3 gr.) of pentobarbital (Nembutal) by mouth at hour of sleep the night before surgery.

2. 200 mg. (3 gr.) of pentobarbital by mouth 1½ to 2 hours before the estimated *block* time.

3. 15 mg. (¼ gr.) of morphine and 0.6 mg. (¹⁄₁₀₀ gr.) of scopolamine intramuscularly ¾ to 1 hour before the estimated *block* time.

Reduction of Premedication: It is seldom necessary to increase this premedication irrespective of the over-all size of the patient until the patient arrives in either the anesthesia or operating room. However, it is very common to reduce this medication under various circumstances; for example, for the geriatric patient, the adolescent patient or child, the debilitated or cachectic patient, and for patients whose surgery is complicated by other disease, *e.g.*, myxedema, diabetes, heart disease, etc. In the patient over 60 years of age, barbiturates and especially scopolamine may often cause disorientation. Therefore, in these patients atropine is usually substituted for scopolamine and the dosage of the barbiturate omitted or greatly reduced, *i.e.*, to 50 mg. (¾ gr.) or less. *Always err on the light side.*

Inadequate Premedication: If medication is inadequate either for the block or for the surgical procedure, intravenous pentobarbital 50 mg. (¾ gr.) to 100 mg. (1½ gr.), or intravenous morphine 8 mg. (⅛ gr.) to 15 mg. (¼ gr.), may be given slowly. Judicious use of added sedation is extremely important. Often small supplementary doses of morphine or pentobarbital will make a block successful, especially when a patient interprets touch and motion as pain.

DRUGS

Tetracaine (Pontocaine)

Dosage.—10 cc. to 100 cc. (depending on the number of intercostal nerves to be blocked) of 0.15 percent solution with or without 0.25 cc. of epinephrine (Adrenalin) 1:1000 in 50 cc. to 100 cc. of solution.*

Onset.—Operating analgesia is established in 15 to 45 minutes, with an average of 20 minutes. Pain may disappear within 5 minutes after a therapeutic or diagnostic block.

Duration.—Operating analgesia lasts 3½ to 6 hours, with solutions containing epinephrine giving the upper limits.

Procaine (Novocain)

Dosage.—10 cc. to 100 cc. (depending on the number of intercostal nerves to be blocked) of 1.0 percent solution with or without 0.25 cc. of epinephrine (Adrenalin) 1:1000 in 50 cc. to 100 cc. of solution.*

Onset.—Operating analgesia is established in 5 to 15 minutes, with an average of 10 minutes. Pain may disappear within 5 minutes after a therapeutic or diagnostic block.

Duration.—Operating analgesia lasts 1 to 1¼ hours, with solutions containing epinephrine giving the upper limits.

Lidocaine (Xylocaine) or Mepivacaine (Carbocaine)

Dosage.—10 cc. to 100 cc. (depending on the number of intercostal nerves to be blocked) of 0.5 to 1.5 percent solution with or without 0.25 cc. of epinephrine (Adrenalin) 1:1000 in

---

*Optimal concentration of epinephrine is 1:200,000, that is, 0.1 cc. of epinephrine 1:1000 in 20 cc. of the local anesthetic solution. Do not exceed 0.25 cc. of epinephrine 1:1000 even if amount of local anesthetic solution exceeds 50 cc. (see page 39).

50 cc. to 100 cc. of solution.* Do not exceed 35 cc. of a 1.5 percent solution or 500 mg. (0.5 gm.) of lidocaine or mepivacaine.

Onset.—Operating analgesia is established in 5 to 15 minutes. Pain may disappear within 1 to 3 minutes after a therapeutic or diagnostic block.

Duration.—Operating analgesia lasts 1¼ to 3 hours, with stronger concentrations and solutions containing epinephrine giving the upper limits.

MATERIALS

Regional tray (see Chapter 9, page 51) or:

1. One ¾-inch (2 cm.), 25-gauge Huber point security Lok-needle.

2. One 1½-inch (3.8 cm.), 22-gauge security Lok-needle, preferably with short bevel.

3. One tuberculin Lok-syringe for measuring epinephrine.

4. One 10 cc. Lok-syringe, preferably with finger rings.

5. One 250 cc. graduated cup, preferably stainless steel, for mixing solution.

6. One prep cup, preferably stainless steel.

7. Four sterile towels.

8. Six sterile sponges.

9. One sterilizer control.

TECHNIQUE

Position and Landmarks

1. Usually, the patient is placed in the lateral decubitus position (side). His upper arm is pulled forward and cephalad so that his scapula is rotated upward and outward from the vertebral column (Figure 103, page 165).

However, when the block is used to relieve the pain from fractured ribs, the sitting position with a pillow held across the abdomen and with a nurse supporting the patient may be more comfortable (Figure 228, page 346).

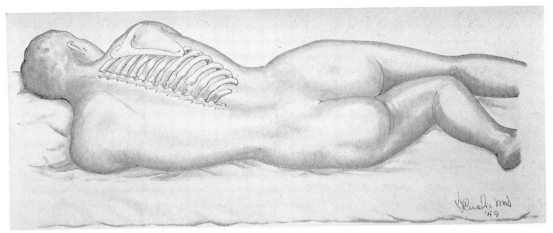

Figure 103. Position of the patient for a therapeutic or diagnostic intercostal block.

2. The lower borders of the ribs of the intercostal nerves to be blocked are palpated and marked 2½ inches (6.3 cm.) to 3 inches (7.5 cm.) from the spines of the vertebrae, or immediately lateral to the sacrospinalis group of muscles. This is usually in the region of the angles of the ribs.

Precautions

Avoid Pneumothorax. — When performing this block, care should be exercised not to pierce the pleura.

Aspirate.—Aspiration test should be made before injecting.

Procedure

1. The sterilizer control is checked to be sure the equipment has been sterilized.

2. The skin is aseptically prepared and draped.

3. Skin wheals are raised at the determined points.

4. When the anesthetist is right-handed, the full 10 cc. Lok-syringe with the 1½-inch (3.8 cm.) security Lok-needle attached is held in the right hand while the index finger of the left hand palpates the inferior border of the rib.

5. The index finger of the left hand pulls the skin which overlies the inferior border of the rib up and over the rib (Figure 92, page 153).

6. The needle is introduced through the skin at the tip of the index finger of the left hand so that its point comes to rest on the lower border of the rib (Figure 92, page 153).

7. The index finger of the left hand releases the skin which had been pulled up and over the rib (Figure 92 page 153).

8. Now the hub of the needle is held between the thumb and index finger of the left hand, and the middle finger of the left hand rests against the shaft of the needle. *The left hand rests on the patient's back.* By exerting gentle pressure against the shaft of the needle, the middle finger of the left hand walks the needle off the lower edge of the rib. By holding the hub of the needle firmly between the thumb and index finger of the left hand *while the left hand rests on the patient's back,* the operator has perfect control of the needle (Figure 93B, page 154 and Figure 94 A, B, page 155).

9. As the needle loses contact with the rib, the left hand resting on the back freezes the needle in place (Figure 93B, page 154 and Figure 94 A, B, page 155).

10. The needle is then slowly advanced about ⅛ inch (0.3 cm.). Now, as the needle is jiggled forward and backward about ¹⁄₁₆ inch

(0.15 cm.), guided by the left hand, 5 cc. of the anesthetic solution is deposited. This technique is repeated on the intercostal nerves to be blocked. The jiggling of the needle is very important as its assures the anesthetist that at least a part of the injected solution will be deposited between the internal intercostal muscle and the posterior intercostal membrane where the nerve lies (Figure 85, page 146). If the needle were fixed outside the compartment bound by the internal intercostal muscle and the posterior intercostal membrane, no analgesia would result. Jiggling the needle also tends to minimize intravascular injections (Figure 85, page 146).

EXTENT OF ANALGESIA

Analgesia over the distribution of the intercostal nerves anesthetized (Figure 102, page 159).

COMPLICATIONS

Pneumothorax: See Chapter 30, page 237.

Toxic Reactions (intravascular injections, etc.): See Chapter 3, page 19.

REMARKS

Perform Block Posterior to Axillary Line: From the standpoint of the anesthetist, the most important branch of the intercostal nerve is the lateral cutaneous nerve. It has its origin in most instances anterior to the midaxillary line. Therefore, to include this branch in an intercostal nerve block, the local anesthetic solutions should be placed at or posterior to the axillary line (Figure 95, page 156).

Use Lateral Position: The lateral decubitus position is the easiest on the patient as well as the anesthetist when the intercostal nerve block is not combined with a celiac plexus block, because: (1) a postoperative patient cannot easily lie on his abdomen or sit up; (2) if he remains in the supine position and if the injection is executed along the midaxillary line, there is a definite possibility that the lateral cutaneous branch of the lower four intercostal nerves will not be anesthetized; (3) a patient in the sitting position will have a tendency to

pull away from the anesthetist's needle; and (4) it has been shown that premedicated patients placed upright may faint when the block is performed.

Block First Four Intercostal Nerves with Paravertebral Approach: When it is necessary to block the first four intercostal nerves and when the first four ribs cannot be palpated between the spines of the vertebrae and the border of the scapula, one should resort to a paravertebral block of these nerves (Chapter 27, page 200). One should never probe blindly for a rib.

When Peritoneum Is To Be Stimulated Do a Celiac Plexus Block: Large hernias of the abdominal wall often cannot be repaired under intercostal nerve block alone. If the peritoneum is to be vigorously manipulated, the peritoneum should be anesthetized with a celiac plexus block, or supplementary general anesthesia will have to be administered.

Postherpetic Pain Not Improved with Intercostal Nerve Block: While the acute pain of herpes zoster may be improved by intercostal nerve blocks, postherpetic neuritis responds poorly.

Recover Broken Needle(s): All needles should be tested before use. If a needle breaks, every effort to recover it, including surgery, should be made. Unremoved needles have a tendency to migrate and may cause permanent injuries as well as medicolegal complications.

Repeat Block When Analgesia Is Inadequate: If the desired results from the first block attempt are unsatisfactory, do not hesitate to reblock the patient if time permits. Most patients will think nothing about being reblocked if the second attempt is prefaced by a statement such as: "Well, I guess we will have to inject a little more medicine if we are going to freeze this area."

However, do not exceed the maximum safe dosage of the local anesthetic solution for both blocks. If to reblock the patient the maximum safe dose of the local anesthetic solution must be exceeded, 45 minutes should elapse between blocks.

CHAPTER 22

Block of the Inguinal Region

INDICATIONS

Surgical: Operations in the inguinal region.

Therapeutic: None.

Diagnostic: None.

ANATOMY

The inguinal region, which includes the inguinal canal, spermatic cord, and surrounding soft structures, receives its sensory innervation from the eleventh and twelfth thoracic nerves and the first and second lumbar nerves (Figure 104, page 168). The spermatic sympathetic plexus contains the sensory fibers for the testes. The eleventh and twelfth thoracic nerves lie between the internal oblique and transversalis muscles and continue anteriorly to the sheath of the rectus muscle which they pierce (Figure 104, page 168). They supply filaments to the internal and external oblique muscles, the transversus muscle, the rectus sheath, the rectus muscle, and the pyramidalis muscle. The ilioinguinal and iliohypogastric nerves are formed by branches of T12 and L1. The iliohypogastric nerve passes between the internal oblique and transversalis muscles. The ilioinguinal nerve runs subperitoneally at first and then pierces the transversus abdominis muscle as did the iliohypogastric nerve. The ilioinguinal nerve and iliohypogastric nerve gradually pierce the internal oblique muscle and lie between it and the external oblique muscles as they near the internal inguinal ring. They are occupants of the inguinal canal, lying on the anterior surface of the spermatic cord (Figure 104, page 168). The genitofemoral nerve (L1 and 2) enters the inguinal canal through the internal inguinal ring and lies on the posterior aspect of the spermatic cord (Figure 104, page 168). Branches of the genital division of the genitofemoral nerve are distributed to the scrotal skin and cremaster muscle, to the anterior portion of the labium majus in the female, and occasionally a communicating branch to the ilioinguinal nerve. The femoral division passes into the thigh to supply the skin and fascia of Scarpa's triangle.

PREMEDICATION

No attempts to elicit paresthesias are made and heavy preoperative medication is advised.

Heavy Premedication: The average patient (age 20 to 50, weight 150 or over, height 5 feet, 5 inches or over, and good physical status) receives:

1. 200 mg. (3 gr.) of pentobarbital Nembutal) by mouth at hour of sleep on night previous to surgery.

2. 200 mg. (3 gr.) of pentobarbital with one ounce of water by mouth 1½ to 2 hours before the estimated *block* time.

3. 15 mg. (¼ gr.) of morphine and 0.6 mg. (¹⁄₁₀₀ gr.) of scopolamine intramuscularly ¾ to 1 hour before the estimated *block* time.

Reduction of Premedication: It is seldom necessary to increase this premedication irrespective of the over-all size of the patient until the patient arrives in either the anesthesia or operating room. However, it is very common to reduce this medication under various circumstances; for example, for the geriatric patient, the adolescent patient or child, the de-

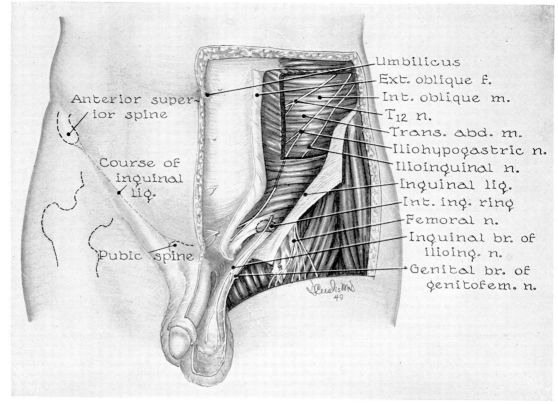

Figure 104. Anatomy of the inguinal region.

bilitated or cachectic patient, and for patients whose surgery is complicated by other disease, *e.g.*, myxedema, diabetes, heart disease, etc. In the patient over 60 years of age, barbiturates and especially scopolamine may often cause disorientation. Therefore, in these patients atropine is usually substituted for scopolamine and the dosages of the barbiturate omitted or greatly reduced, *i.e.*, to 50 mg. (¾ gr.) or less. *Always err on the light side.*

Inadequate Premedication: If medication is inadequate either for the block or for the surgical procedure, intravenous pentobarbital 50 mg. (¾ gr.) to 100 mg. (1½ gr.) or intravenous morphine 8 mg. (⅛ gr.) to 15 mg. (¼ gr.), may be given slowly. Judicious use of added sedation is extremely important. Often small supplementary doses of morphine or pentobarbital will make a block successful, especially when a patient interprets touch and motion as pain.

DRUGS

Tetracaine (Pontocaine)

Dosage.—100 cc. of 0.1 or 0.15 percent solution with or without 0.25 cc. of epinephrine (Adrenalin) 1:1000.*

Onset.—Operating analgesia is established in 15 to 45 minutes with an average of 20 minutes.

Duration.—Operating analgesia lasts 3½ to 6 hours, with solutions containing epinephrine giving the upper limits.

Procaine (Novocain)

Dosage.—100 cc. of 1.0 percent solution with or without 0.25 cc. of epinephrine (Adrenalin) 1:1000.*

---

*Although the optimal concentration of epinephrine is 1:200,000, that is, 0.1 cc. of epinephrine 1:1000 in 20 cc. of the local anesthetic solution, do not exceed 0.25 cc. of epinephrine 1:1000 (see page 39).

Onset.—Operating analgesia is established in 5 to 15 minutes, with an average of 10 minutes.

Duration.—Operating analgesia lasts ¾ to 1½ hours, with solutions containing epinephrine giving the upper limits.

Lidocaine (Xylocaine) or Mepivacaine (Carbocaine)

Dosage.—100 cc. of a 0.5 percent solution with or without 0.25 cc. of epinephrine (Adrenalin 1:1000.*

Onset.—Operating analgesia is established in 5 to 15 minutes, with an average of 10 minutes.

Duration.—Operating analgesia lasts 1¼ to 3 hours, with solutions containing epinephrine giving the upper limits.

Hyaluronidase: Hyaluronidase, 150 TRU, added to the solutions will prove valuable in this block by effecting a wider spread of the anesthetic solution. When hyaluronidase is employed, epinephrine must be added to the local anesthetic solution or the operating time will be markedly shortened. Hyaluronidase is not necessary for a successful block.

MATERIALS

Regional block tray (see Chapter 9, page 51) or:

1. One ¾-inch (2 cm.), 25-gauge Huber point security Lok-needle.

2. One 1½-inch (3.8 cm.) or 2-inch (5 cm.), 22-gauge security Lok-needle, preferably with short bevel.

3. One 3-inch (7.5 cm.), 22-gauge security Lok-needle, preferably with short bevel.

4. One 4-inch (10 cm.), 22-gauge security Lok-needle, preferably with short bevel.

---

*Although the optimal concentration of epinephrine is 1:200,000, that is, 0.1 cc. of epinephrine 1:1000 in 20 cc. of the local anesthetic solution, do not exceed 0.25 cc. of epinephrine 1:1000 (see page 39).

5. One tuberculin Lok-syringe for measuring epinephrine.

6. One 10 cc. Lok-syringe, preferably with finger rings.

7. One graduated measuring cup, preferably stainless steel, for mixing solution.

8. One prep cup, preferably stainless steel.

9. Four sterile towels.

10. Six sterile sponges.

11. One sterilizer control.

TECHNIQUE

Position and Landmarks

1. The patient lies in the dorsal recumbent position with or without a pillow and his hands behind his head.

2. The anterior superior iliac spine is palpated and marked with an O (Figure 105A, page 170).

3. A line is drawn from the anterior superior iliac spine to the umbilicus (Figure 105A, page 170).

4. On this line 1 inch (2.5 cm.) from the anterior superior spine a 1 is marked on the skin (Figure 105A, page 170). This point lies approximately over the ilioinguinal and iliohypogastric nerves.

5. The tubercle of the pubic bone is palpated and the overlying skin is marked with a 2 (Figure 105A, page 170).

6. The femoral artery is located and ¼ inch (0.6 cm.) lateral to it, a 3 is marked on the overlying skin ½ inch (1.3 cm.) to 1 inch (2.5 cm.) below the ilioinguinal (Poupart's) ligament (Figure 105A, page 170). The 3 lies approximately over the femoral nerve.

7. A line is drawn on the skin in the groin from the edge of the scrotum to the lateral border of the anterior superior spine (Figure 105A, page 170). This line lies just below the ilioinguinal ligament (Poupart's ligament).

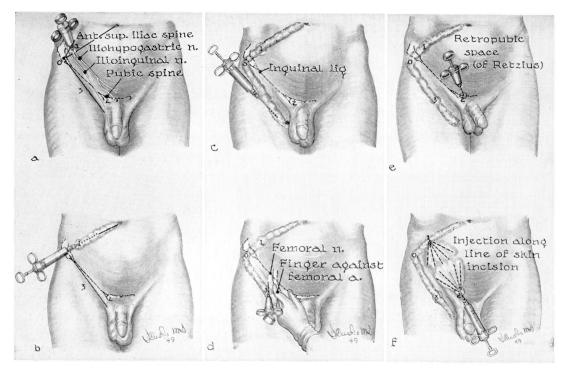

Figure 105. Technique and method of blocking the inguinal region. A. and B. Establishing of a wall of anesthesia from the anterior superior spine of the iliac bone to the umbilicus and from the peritoneum to the skin. C. Blocking of the gluteal nerves and some branches of the femoral nerve by subcutaneous infiltration ½-inch (1.3 cm.) caudad to the ilioinguinal ligament. D. Blocking the femoral nerve. E. Injection of the retropubic space. F. Intradermal and subcutaneous infiltration along the line of incision to obtain immediate onset of skin and subcutaneous analgesia.

Precautions

Avoid Intravascular Injection.—Care should be taken when injecting near the femoral vessels to avoid intra-arterial injections. If no solution is deposited in these vessels, their puncture is of small consequence. An arteriovenous shunt is a highly unlikely possibility.

Procedure

1. The sterilizer control is checked to be sure the equipment has been sterilized.

2. A wide area is aseptically prepared and draped.

3. The anesthetist stands facing the side to be blocked.

4. Intradermal wheals are raised at the 1, 2, and 3 with a 25-gauge Huber point security Lok-needle.

5. The 1½-inch (3.8 cm.) or 2-inch (5 cm.), 22-gauge security Lok-needle, depending on the size of the individual, is connected with the full Lok-syringe and inserted through the wheal at 1 (Figure 105A, page 170). The needle is advanced downward and slightly lateral so as to contact the inside shelf of the iliac bone (Figure 106, page 171). 5 to 10 cc. of the local anesthetic solution is deposited along the inside shelf of the iliac bone as the needle moves in and out. The needle is now withdrawn to the subcutaneous tissue and with a slight medial slant reinserted slowly. Local anesthetic solution is injected as the needle advances. If the needle is advanced slowly, it may be felt to penetrate the fascia covering the external oblique muscle, the internal oblique muscle, and the transversalis muscle. When the internal layer of the fascia covering the transversalis muscle is punctured, 3 cc. of the local anesthetic solution should be

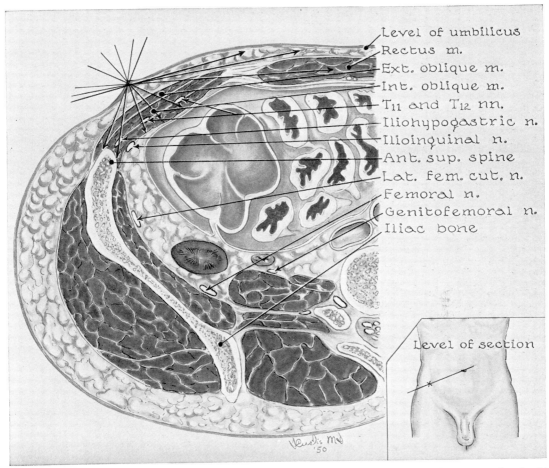

Figure 106. Cross section through the body from the umbilicus to the anterior superior iliac spine. This should emphasize the need for careful, thorough infiltration in this area if all the nerves in this area are to be blocked. The arrows represent the course of the needle as it deposits the anesthetic solution.

injected as the needle is slowly withdrawn. By repeating this maneuver 5 times, directing the needle point ¼ inch (0.6 cm.) more medially each time, the ilioinguinal and iliohypogastric nerves are anesthetized (see Figure 106, page 171).

6. The 3-inch (7.5 cm.) or 4-inch (10 cm.) 22-gauge security Lok-needle, depending upon the size of the individual, is connected with the full Lok-syringe, and inserted through the wheal at 1 (Figure 105B, page 170). The local anesthetic solution is distributed carefully intradermally, subcutaneously, and intramuscularly from just lateral to the anterior superior spine to the umbilicus. This requires approximately 25 cc. of the anesthetic solution. This

injection should anesthetize thoracic nerve ten, which may supply the skin by overlap, and thoracic nerves eleven and twelve (Figure 106, page 171).

7. With 20 cc. of solution, intradermal and subcutaneous injections are made parallel to and below the ilioinguinal (Poupart's) ligament from O along the patient's groin (Figure 105C, page 170). The index finger of the left hand should be palpating the femoral vessels during these injections to prevent their puncture. This injection should control overlapping branches of the lateral femoral cutaneous and lumboinguinal nerves.

8. A femoral nerve block is now executed. The open 1½-inch (3.8 cm.), 22-gauge security

Lok-needle is passed through wheal 3 as close to the femoral artery as possible, and 10 cc. of solution is deposited in a fan-wise direction laterally as described in Chapter 33, Femoral Nerve Block, page 281. This will block any fibers from the femoral nerve which might course back over the abdomen (Figure 105D, page 170).

9. The needle is then passed through wheal 2 and deep injections are made along the superior ramus of the pubis, on each side of the spermatic cord, into the rectus muscle attachment to the pubis, and the space of Retzius, i.e., the space between the bladder and the pubic bone. 15 cc. of solution is required for this maneuver (Figure 105E, page 170).

10. Superficial infiltration of the skin and subcutaneous tissue over the line of the incision from points 1 and 2 is performed, using a total of 10 cc. (Figure 105F, page 170).

11. No attempt is made to inject the spermatic sympathetic plexus at the external ring or the genitofemoral nerve or peritoneum at the internal ring. If the anesthetist should prod these structures, unnecessary hematomas which may complicate the surgeon's field are likely to occur. Therefore the surgeon should be warned to inject these structures under direct vision as they are exposed.

DISTRIBUTION OF ANALGESIA

The abdominal wall in the inguinal region, the skin over the lateral anterior aspect of the scrotum, and the distribution of the femoral nerve in the leg are anesthetized (Figure 107, page 172).

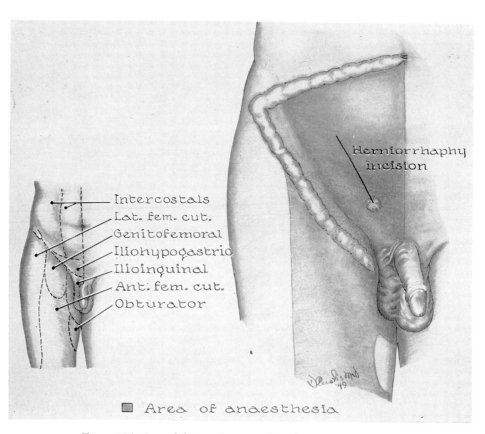

Figure 107. Area of skin analgesia resulting from a hernia block.

COMPLICATIONS

Toxic Reactions (intravascular injections, etc.): See Chapter 3, page 19.

REMARKS

Use Block for Reducible Hernia: This block is adequate for reducible hernias in the inguinal region in slight- and medium-built patients.

Avoid Block in Hernias Which May Be Difficult to Repair: Sliding hernias, femoral hernias, scrotal hernias, recurrent hernias, and irreducible hernias are best repaired under spinal (subarachnoid) or epidural (peridural) analgesia, because excessive manipulation of the intestine and peritoneum causes the patient discomfort in spite of an adequate block.

Avoid Block in Obese Patient: In obese patients, spinal or epidural analgesia is preferred because these patients require excessive amounts of local anesthetic agents and correct placement of solutions in the muscle layers is difficult. In these patients, if a block is mandatory, paravertebral block of the last three thoracic nerves and the first three lumbar nerves is easier to perform and more satisfactory both to the surgeon and the anesthetist.

Be Meticulous: To assure an adequate hernial block, injections should be slow, steady, and continuous as the needles are inserted and withdrawn from the various layers of the abdominal wall.

Surgeon Must Be Gentle: It must be remembered that even if the peritoneal sac is anesthetized under direct vision, rough handling and excessive pull on it will give rise to pain referred to the parietal peritoneum beyond the anesthetized area.

Avoid Bilateral Hernia Block: Bilateral hernias may be repaired by bilateral inguinal block, but here again, because of the large amount of local anesthetic agent required, spinal or epidural analgesia is preferred.

Recover Broken Needle(s): All needles should be tested before use. If a needle breaks, every effort to recover it, including surgery, should be made. Unremoved needles have a tendency to migrate and may cause permanent injuries as well as medicolegal complications.

Use Local Infiltration When Analgesia is Inadequate: When this block is inadequate, small amounts of the local anesthetic solution should be injected into the sensitive area by the surgeon.

CHAPTER 23

Block of the Penis

INDICATIONS

Surgical: Operations on the penis and all its structures, *i.e.*, prepuce, urethra, glans, and corpora cavernosa.

Diagnostic: None.

Therapeutic: None.

ANATOMY

The penis proper is innervated by the left and right dorsal nerves of the penis which are the deeper divisions of the pudendal nerves (S2, 3, 4) in the perineum. Just after each dorsal nerve of the penis passes under the pubic bone, it divides so that the main branch runs along the dorsal surface of the penis and the several smaller branches pass on to the under surface. The main branches of the dorsal nerves of the penis supply the dorsum of the penis and the glans while its smaller branches supply the underside of the penis and frenulum (Figure 108, page 174). The skin around the base of the penis is innervated by the ilioinguinal nerve (L1) and occasionally a branch of the genitofemoral (L1, 2) (Figure 108, page 174).

PREMEDICATION

No attempts to elicit paresthesias are made. If the block is performed on an outpatient for a minor operation, it is not necessary to give premedication providing infiltration is carefully executed as the needle advances.

Hospitalized patients who are to undergo surgical procedures should be heavily sedated.

Heavy Premedication: The average patient

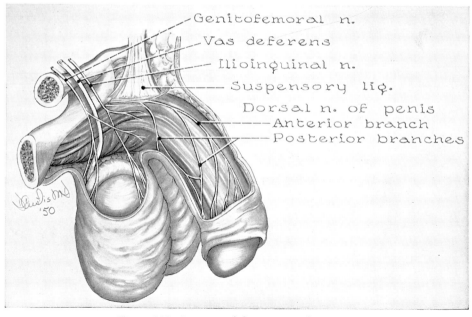

Figure 108. Anatomy of the nerves to the penis.

(age 20 to 50, weight 150 pounds or over, height 5 feet, 5 inches or over, and good physical status) receives:

1. 200 mg. (3 gr.) of pentobarbital (Nembutal) by mouth at hour of sleep on the day previous to surgery.

2. 200 mg. (3 gr.) of pentobarbital by mouth with one ounce of water 1½ to 2 hours before the estimated *block* time.

3. 15 mg. (¼ gr.) of morphine and 0.6 mg. (1/100 gr.) of scopolamine intramuscularly ¾ to 1 hour before the estimated *block* time.

Reduction of Premedication: It is seldom necessary to increase this premedication irrespective of the over-all size of the patient until the patient arrives in either the anesthesia or operating room. However, it is very common to reduce this medication under various circumstances; for example, for the geriatric patient, the adolescent patient or child, the debilitated or cachectic patient, and for patients whose surgery is complicated by other disease, *e.g.*, myxedema, diabetes, heart disease, etc. In the patient over 60 years of age, barbiturates and especially scopolamine may often cause disorientation. Therefore, in these patients atropine is usually substituted for scopolamine and the dosage of the barbiturate is greatly reduced, *i.e.*, to 50 mg. (¾ gr.) or less. *Always err on the light side.*

Inadequate Premedication: If the medication is inadequate for either the anesthetic or surgical procedure, intravenous pentobarbital 50 mg. (¾ gr.) to 100 mg. (1½ gr.) or intravenous morphine 8 mg. (⅛ gr.) to 15 mg. (¼ gr.) may be given slowly. Judicious use of added sedation is extremely important. Often small supplementary doses of morphine or pentobarbital will make a block successful, especially when a patient interprets touch and motion as pain.

DRUGS

Tetracaine (Pontocaine)

Dosage.—50 cc. of 0.15 to 0.25 percent solu-

tion with or without 0.25 cc. of epinephrine (Adrenalin) 1:1000.*

Onset.—Operating analgesia is established in 5 to 20 minutes.

Duration.—Operating analgesia lasts 3½ to 6 hours, with stronger concentrations and solutions containing epinephrine giving the upper limits.

Procaine (Novocain)

Dosage.—50 cc. of 1.0 to 2.0 percent solution with or without 0.25 cc. of epinephrine (Adrenalin) 1:1000.*

Onset.—Operating analgesia is established in 5 to 15 minutes.

Duration.—Operating analgesia lasts 1 to 1½ hours, with stronger concentrations and solutions containing epinephrine giving the upper limits.

Lidocaine (Xylocaine) or Mepivacaine (Carbocaine)

Dosage.—50 cc. of 1.0 percent solution with or without 0.25 cc. of epinephrine (Adrenalin) 1:1000.*

Onset.—Operating analgesia is established in 5 to 15 minutes.

Duration.—Operating analgesia lasts 1¼ to 3 hours, with solutions containing epinephrine giving the upper limits.

MATERIALS

Regional tray (see Chapter 9, see page 51) or:

1. One ¾-inch (2 cm.), 25-gauge Huber point security Lok-needle.

2. One 3-inch (7.5 cm.), 22-gauge security Lok-needle, preferably with short bevel.

3. One tuberculin Lok-syringe for measuring epinephrine.

---

*Optimal concentration of epinephrine is 1:200,000, that is, 0.1 cc. of epinephrine 1:1000 in 20 cc. of the local anesthetic solution (see page 39).

4. One 10 cc. Lok-syringe, preferably with finger rings.

5. One graduated measuring cup, preferably stainless steel, for mixing solution.

6. One prep cup, preferably stainless steel.

7. Four sterile towels.

8. Six sterile sponges.

9. One sterilizer control.

TECHNIQUE

Position and Landmarks

1. The patient lies in the dorsal recumbent position with or without a pillow, and his hands behind his head.

2. The tubercles of the pubic bone are palpated and ½ inch (1.3 cm.) caudad and ½ inch (1.3 cm.) medial to them, X's are marked on the overlying skin (Figure 109, page 176 and Figure 110, page 177).

3. An O is marked on the median raphe of the scrotum at the base of the penis (Figure 109, page 176 and Figure 110, page 177).

Precautions

Use Aqueous Solution to Prepare Skin.— Aqueous solutions should be used in the prep so as not to burn the patient.

Aspirate.—Aspirate carefully for blood before injecting the local anesthetic solution.

Procedure

1. The sterilizer control is checked to be sure the equipment has been sterilized.

2. The area is aseptically prepared and draped.

3. The anesthetist stands first at one side of the patient, then at the other in order to facilitate the block.

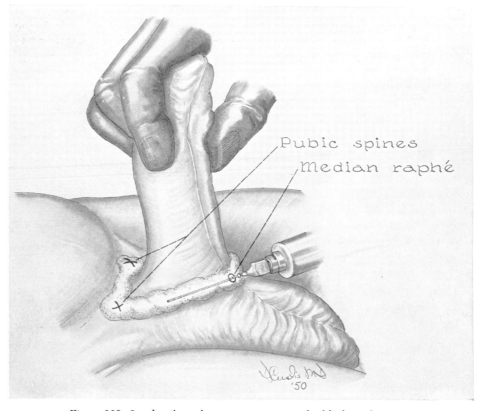

Figure 109. Landmarks and necessary injections for blocking the penis.

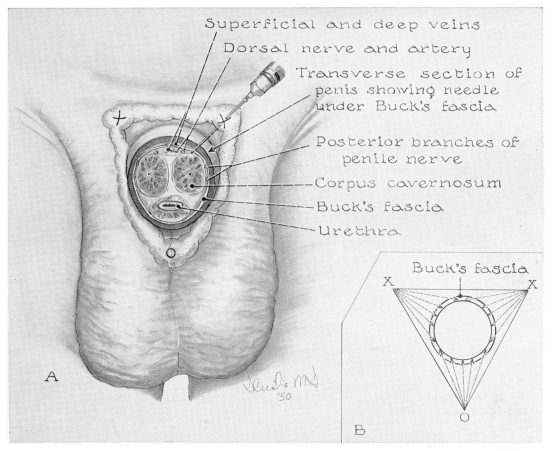

Figure 110. A. Cross section of the base of the penis. B. Schematic drawing emphasizing that Buck's fascia must be pierced to assure a satisfactory block of the penis.

4. Intradermal wheals are raised at the two X's using the ¾-inch (2 cm.) 25-gauge Huber point security Lok-needle (Figure 109, page 176 and Figure 110, page 177).

5. The two X's are connected by means of slow, careful, intradermal and subcutaneous infiltration with a 3-inch (7.5 cm.), 22-gauge security Lok-needle from the skin to the pubic bone (Figure 109, page 176 and Figure 110, page 177). This requires 10 cc. of solution.

6. Intradermal and subcutaneous infiltration with the 3-inch (7.5 cm.), 22-gauge security Lok-needle is now carried out between the X's and the O. 20 cc. of anesthetic solution is used in the maneuver (Figure 109, page 176 and Figure 110, page 177).

7. If steps 5 and 6 are carried out care-fully, the ilioinguinal and genitofemoral nerves should be adequately blocked.

8. The penis is now held in a vertical position by the anesthetist or his assistant (Figure 109, page 176).

9. The 3-inch (7.5 cm.), 22-gauge security Lok-needle with full syringe attached is passed in succession through the X's and the O and anesthetic solution deposited fanwise in intradermal and subcutaneous tissue from the X's to the base of the penis. Great care must be taken to see that the needle point passes as far as the corpus cavernosum each time and that a ring of anesthetic solution is deposited around the base of the penis between the corpora cavernosa and the deep penile fascia (Buck's) (Figure 110, page

177). This requires approximately 20 cc. of solution.

EXTENT OF ANALGESIA

The penis and triangular area around the base of the penis are analgesic.

COMPLICATIONS

Toxic Reactions (intravascular injections, etc.): See Chapter 3, page 19.

REMARKS

Avoid Block of Prepuce: Slough following infiltration of the prepuce, *per se,* occurs with enough frequency to discourage use of the block of the prepuce. Therefore, the block described in this chapter is usually preferred.

Inject Meticulously: Great care must be exercised in placing the anesthetic solution around the corpora cavernosa at the base of the penis; otherwise, the small nerve filaments which innervate the posterior lateral sides of the penis and the frenulum will not be anesthetized (Figure 108, page 174). This point is stressed because failure of this block to produce adequate analgesia for circumcision, amputation of the penis, or urethral exploration is usually caused by pain at the frenulum or the underside of the penis.

Impotency Following Block: The block of the penis at its base should not be used without consideration of the fact that a few reports have appeared attributing impotency to the placement of local anesthetic solutions under the deep penile fascia (Buck's fascia). This block has been used in over 200 cases by the author and his associates with no untoward results.

Recover Broken Needle(s): All needles should be tested before use. If a needle breaks, every effort to recover it, including surgery, should be made. Unremoved needles have a tendency to migrate and may cause permanent injuries as well as medicolegal complications.

Repeat Block When Analgesia Is Inadequate: If the desired results from the first block attempt are unsatisfactory, do not hesitate to reblock the patient if time permits. Most patients will think nothing about being reblocked if the second attempt is prefaced by a statement such as: "Well, I guess we will have to inject a little more medicine if we are going to freeze this area."

However, do not exceed the maximum safe dosage of the local anesthetic solution for both blocks. If to reblock the patient the maximum safe dose of the local anesthetic solution must be exceeded, 45 minutes should elapse between blocks.

CHAPTER 24

Paracervical (Uterosacral) Block

INDICATIONS

Surgical: Paracervical block is frequently administered for relief of the pain of the first stage of labor, but it is seldom used for operations.

Operations.—Bilateral block may be used for dilatation of the cervix and uterine curettage. Occasionally, it may be combined with pudendal nerve block and local infiltration to perform a vaginal hysterectomy.

Vaginal Delivery.—Bilateral paracervical block alleviates the pain of the first stage of labor, and this is the most frequent use of this block. Combined with bilateral pudendal nerve block, it will relieve the pain of the second and third stages of labor. The block is usually performed when the cervix is approximately 5 cm. dilated in the woman who is delivering her first child, and when the cervix is 3 cm. dilated in the woman who has delivered one or more children.

Therapeutic: Relief of severe dysmenorrhea.

Diagnostic: Differentiation of severe dysmenorrhea from other similar complaints which may be associated with menstruation.

ANATOMY

Pain from the uterus passes in sequence through: (1) the uterine plexus; (2) the pelvic ganglia and plexus; (3) the hypogastric nerve; (4) the superior hypogastric plexus; (5) the lumbar and lower thoracic sympathetic chain; and (6) the white rami communicans, associated with the eleventh and twelfth nerves. Then, the pain stimuli pass through the posterior roots of these spinal nerves (T11 and T12) to enter the spinal cord. (Figure 111, page 180).

Paracervical block interrupts this pain pathway at the pelvic (inferior hypogastric) ganglia and plexus which is located in the uterosacral ligament on each side of the cervix at the depth of approximately ½ inch (1.3 cm.) to ⅗ inch (1.5 cm.) beneath the mucosa of the lateral fornices of the vagina. (Figure 111, page 180).

PREMEDICATION

No attempt to elicit paresthesias is made. In the surgical patient, heavy medication is used. In the obstetrical patient, light medication is advised.

Heavy Premedication: The average patient (age 20 to 50, weight 150 or over, height 5 feet, 5 inches or over, and good physical status) receives:

1. 200 mg. (3 gr.) of pentobarbital (Nembutal) by mouth at hour of sleep on night previous to surgery.

2. 200 mg. (3 gr.) of pentobarbital with one ounce of water by mouth 1½ to 2 hours before estimated *block* time.

3. 15 mg. (¼ gr.) of morphine and 0.6 mg. (¹⁄₁₀₀ gr.) of scopolamine intramuscularly ¾ to 1 hour before the estimated *block* time.

Light Premedication: The parturient (woman in labor), during the early part of the first stage of labor, often receives barbiturates, narcotics, belladonna derivatives, and tranquilizers, or combinations of these drugs to alleviate pain, allay apprehension, promote

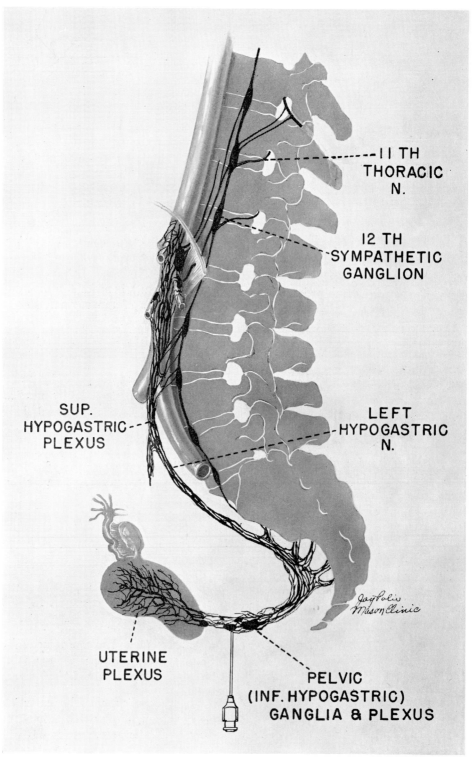

Figure 111. Anatomy of sensory (pain) pathway of the uterus.

amnesia, or effect a combination of these conditions. If these drugs are effective, further premedication when the block is to be started is not indicated.

If no medication has been given the parturient prior to the block, then 50 mg. of meperidine (Demerol) together with 25 mg. of promethazine (Phenergan) may be given. If the optimal effect of such medication is to be obtained, it should be given intramuscularly at least forty-five minutes prior to the block, or intravenously fifteen minutes prior to the block.

Reduction of Premedication: It is seldom necessary to increase this premedication irrespective of the over-all size of the patient. However, in the surgical patient, it is very common to reduce the previously stated heavy premedication under various circumstances; for example, for the geriatric patient, the debilitated or cachectic patient, and for patients whose surgery is complicated by other disease, *e.g.*, myxedema, diabetes, heart disease, etc. In the patient over 60 years of age, barbiturates and especially scopolamine may often cause disorientation. Therefore, in these patients atropine is usually substituted for scopolamine and the dosages of the barbiturate omitted or greatly reduced, *i.e.*, to 50 mg. (¾ gr.) or less. *Always err on the light side.*

Inadequate Premedication: If, in the surgical patient, medication is inadequate either for the block or for the operation, intravenous pentobarbital 50 mg. (¾ gr.) to 100 mg. (1½ gr.) or intravenous morphine 8 mg. (⅛ gr.) to 15 mg. (¼ gr.) may be given slowly. Judicious use of added sedation is extremely important. Often, small supplementary doses of morphine or pentobarbital will make a block successful, especially when the patient interprets touch and motion as pain.

Prior to ordering additional sedation for the parturient, the effects of any previously administered drug must be evaluated. Most drugs given to the mother during labor will pass the placental barrier, will equilibrate in the infant in about the same time as in the mother, and may cause fetal depression.

DRUGS

Tetracaine (Pontocaine)

Dosage.—20 to 40 cc. of 0.15 to 0.25 percent solution with or without 0.1 cc of epinephrine (Adrenalin) 1:1000 in each 20 cc. of solution.* Omit or reduce amount of epinephrine when block is performed in parturient (see page 186).

Onset.—Operating analgesia is established in 15 to 45 minutes, with an average of 20 minutes.

Duration.—Operating analgesia lasts 3½ to 6 hours, with stronger concentrations and solutions containing epinephrine giving the upper limits.

Procaine (Novocain)

Dosage.—20 to 40 cc. of 1.0 to 2.0 percent solutions with or without 0.1 cc of epinephrine (Adrenalin) 1:1000 in each 20 cc. of solution.* Omit or reduce amount of epinephrine when block is performed in parturient (see page 186).

Onset.—Operating analgesia is established in 5 to 15 minutes with an average of 10 minutes.

Duration.—Operating analgesia lasts 1 to 1½ hours, with stronger concentrations and solutions containing epinephrine giving the upper limits.

Lidocaine (Xylocaine) or Mepivacaine (Carbocaine)

Dosage.—20 to 40 cc. of 1.0 to 1.5 percent solution with or without 0.1 cc. epinephrine (Adrenalin) 1:1000 in each 20 cc. of solution.* *Do not exceed 35 cc. of a 1.5 percent solution, i.e., 500 mg. (0.5 gm.) of lidocaine or mepivacaine.* Omit or reduce amount of epinephrine when block is performed in parturient (see page 186).

---

*Optimal concentration of epinephrine is 1:200,000, that is, 0.1 cc. of epinephrine 1:1000 in 20 cc. of the local anesthetic solution (see page 39).

Onset.—Operating analgesia is established in 5 to 15 minutes.

Duration.—Operating analgesia lasts 1½ to 3 hours, with stronger concentrations and solutions containing epinephrine giving the upper limits.

MATERIALS

Regional block tray (see Chapter 9, page 51) plus a needle guide. The Iowa trumpet, Kobak instrument, a plastic straw, or a variation of these is used as a guide for the placement of the needle. The Iowa trumpet is so constructed that when the 20-gauge, 6-inch (15 cm.) needle is placed through it, the point of the needle extends approximately 1 inch (2.5 cm.) beyond the end of the guide (Figure 112, page 183). The Kobak instrument is so constructed that when the needle is advanced through it, the point of the needle extends approximately ½ inch (1.3 cm.) beyond the end of the guide (Figure 113, page 184). When the plastic straw is used, it is cut so that the needle extends ½ inch (1.3 cm.) to ⅝ inch (1.5 cm.) beyond its end (Figure 114, page 185).

If a regional block tray is not available, then the following equipment is needed:

1. One needle guide and a 5-inch (12.5 cm.) or a 6-inch (15 cm.), 20-gauge security Lok-needle, preferably with short bevel.

2. One tuberculin Lok-syringe to measure epinephrine.

3. One 10 cc. Lok-syringe, preferably with finger rings.

4. One graduated measuring cup, preferably stainless steel, for mixing solution.

5. One prep cup, preferably stainless steel.

6. Four sterile towels.

7. Six sterile sponges.

8. One sterilizer control.

TECHNIQUE

Position and Landmarks: The patient is placed in the supine position with her legs apart and partially in the lithotomy position. The injection is made in the lateral fornices of the vagina.

Precautions: *Aspirate.*—Carefully aspirate for blood. The uterine blood vessels lie in close approximation to the nerves and in the pregnant patient, the size of the vessels is markedly increased.

Procedure

1. pHisoHex, aqueous benzalkonium chloride (Zephiran), or both, may be used to prepare the vagina, but whether they reduce the bacterial count and the possibility of infection is open to debate.

2. The needle guide is directed into the lateral fornix of the vagina by the index and middle fingers of the physician (Figure 115, page 186).* It should rest against the wall of the vagina at the 3 o'clock position as related to the cervix (Figure 115, page 186).

3. The needle is then inserted through the guide and advanced until contact with the mucosal wall of the vagina is made.

4. Then, the needle is advanced into the uterosacral ligament for a distance of ½ inch (1.3 cm.) to ⅝ inch (1.5 cm.).

5. *Careful aspiration for blood must be performed.* If blood is obtained, the needle is either slightly withdrawn or advanced until no blood is obtained.

6. Then 10 to 15 cc. of the local anesthetic solution is injected.

7. The needle is removed, the guide redirected to the other side of the cervix at the 9 o'clock position, and the injection repeated.

EXTENT OF ANALGESIA

Painful stimuli from the uterus are interrupted. The block does not alter uterine contractions unless the local anesthetic solution

---

*When the Kobak instrument is used, the guide and needle are inserted as a unit (Figure 113, page 184).

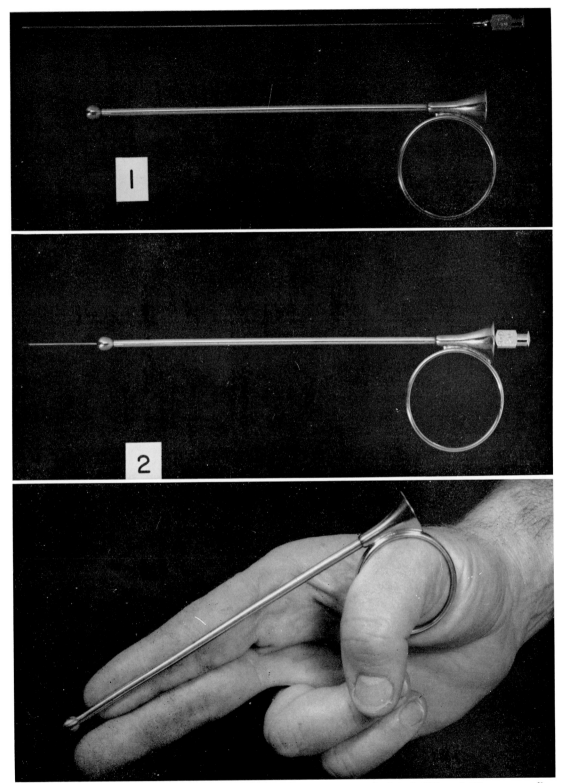

Figure 112. 1. 6-inch (15 cm.), 20-gauge needle and Iowa trumpet. 2. 6-inch (15 cm.), 20-gauge needle inserted through Iowa trumpet—needle point extends 1 inch (2.5 cm.) beyond end of guide. With this guide, the needle's forward progress is not automatically stopped at the ½ inch (approximately 1.3 cm.) depth usually recommended for its insertion into the uterosacral ligament. A 5½-inch (13.8 cm.) needle would be the correct size to use with this guide, but this is not a standard needle size and it is not easy to obtain. (Bottom) Method of holding Iowa trumpet. The Iowa trumpet may be obtained from the Iowa Medical Supply Company, Fort Dodge, Iowa.

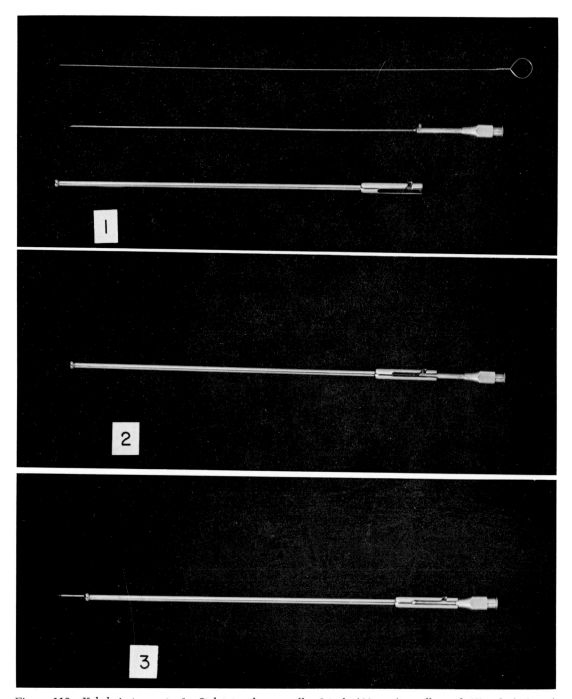

Figure 113. Kobak instrument. 1. Stylet to clean needle, 8-inch (20 cm.) needle, and 6¾-inch (17 cm.) guide. 2. Needle and guide assembled for placement in lateral fornix of vagina. 3. Needle's point extending ½ inch (1.3 cm.) beyond end of guide—the recommended distance the needle should be inserted into the utero-sacral ligament. The Kobak instrument may be obtained from V. Mueller and Company, Chicago, Illinois.

The principle of the Freeman and the Brittain transvaginal needle guides is the same as the needle guides described herein, i.e., they limit the distance the needle can be inserted into the tissues. The Freeman needle guide may be obtained from Becton, Dickinson and Company, Rutherford, New Jersey; and the Brittain needle guide may be obtained from Brittain Industries, Incorporated, Hawthorne, California.

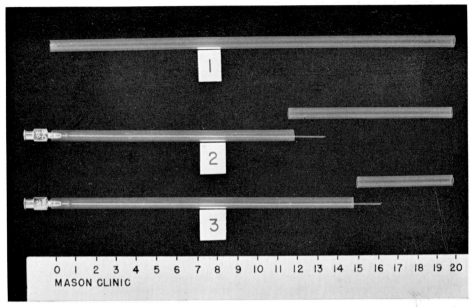

Figure 114. Plastic drinking straw. 1. 8-inch (20 cm.) straw. 2. Straw cut to accommodate 5-inch (12.5 cm.), 20-gauge needle—needle's point extends ½ inch (approximately 1.3 cm.) beyond end of guide, *i.e.*, the recommended distance that it should be inserted into the uterosacral ligament. 3. Straw cut to accommodate 6-inch (15 cm.), 20-gauge needle—needle's point extends ½ inch (approximately 1.3 cm.) beyond end of guide, *i.e.*, the recommended distance that it should be inserted into the uterosacral ligament.

contains epinephrine (see page 186). Neither the peritoneum nor the bladder is anesthetized.

COMPLICATIONS

Systemic Toxic Reactions (intravascular injections, etc.): See Chapter 3, page 19.

Block, Neuritis, or Both of the Sciatic Nerves: Following paracervical block, neuritis, temporary paralysis, or both of the sciatic nerves has occurred. They may be a result of the needle being inserted further than ⅝ inch (1.5 cm.) beyond the vaginal mucosa, the use of too great a volume of local anesthetic solution, or a combination of these. If it is due to the anesthetic solution, it will automatically be corrected as the solution's effects are dissipated. If it is due to trauma from the needle, the neuritis will usually disappear in a week or two, but in some cases may last as long as six months.

When a neuritis develops the question arises: Did the block cause the neuritis? The sciatic nerve can be traumatized by the head of the fetus and it is not uncommon to see the patient's leg twitch as the head of the fetus is rotated by the forceps. Therefore, when a neuritis results, it does not seem just to condemn the anesthetic technique automatically without a careful investigation of all of the factors that may result in this type of complication.

Hematoma of the Parametrium: This occurs from trauma to a blood vessel during the execution of the block. Usually, it requires no treatment other than watchful waiting, but, on occasion, it may require incision and drainage.

Fetal Distress, Bradycardia, Deaths, and Low Apgar Scores: These have been reported following paracervical block. The causes are open to debate and may or may not be associated with the block.

REMARKS

Paracervical or Uterosacral Block: Paracervical and uterosacral blocks are identical pro-

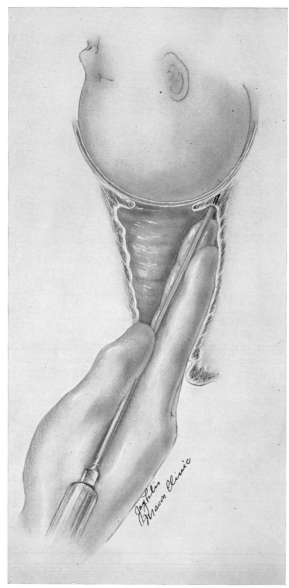

Figure 115. Paracervical block. Method of placement of guide (plastic straw) and needle into lateral fornix of vagina. Needle point rests in uterosacral ligament.

cedures and the local anesthetic solution bathes the same plexus and ganglia. If the solution is deposited at the 3 and 9 o'clock positions, the block is termed paracervical, and if the solution is deposited at the 4 and 8 o'clock positions, the block is termed uterosacral. The pelvic (inferior hypogastric) ganglia and plexus are anesthetized when this block is executed.

The 9 and 3 O'clock Positions or the 8 and 4 O'clock Positions for Performing the Block: Some authors recommend that the 4 and 8 o'clock positions be used for inserting the needle rather than the 3 and 9 o'clock positions. Other authors recommend a compromise, they insert the needle between the 3 and 4 o'clock positions and the 8 and 9 o'clock positions. This discrepancy occurs in an effort to avoid failures from misplacement of the solution too deep or into the peritoneal cavity because of the downward angulation of the birth canal which results during pregnancy.

Addition of Epinephrine to the Local Anesthetic Solution May Slow Labor: When epinephrine is added to the local anesthetic solution in a concentration of 1:200,000 for paracervical block, uterine contractions may slow or temporarily stop. Therefore, some physicians advise against the use of epinephrine in this block. However, others believe it may be employed without slowing or stopping contractions, provided, the amount does not exceed 1.2 minims (0.076 cc.) of epinephrine 1:1000.

If epinephrine is used and if labor is slowed, the uterus will respond normally to oxytocic drugs.

Severe Hypertension May Result from the Use of an Oxytocic Drug, a Vasoconstrictor Drug, or Both: See Chapter 5, page 41.

Continuous Paracervical Block Technique: One of the drawbacks of paracervical block is that it may have to be repeated. To avoid repeating a paracervical block when labor is long, continuous techniques for paracervical block have been introduced and further study will prove whether a continuous technique is a practical method.

Addition of Tetracaine (Pontocaine) to a Solution of Lidocaine (Xylocaine) or Mepivacaine (Carbocaine): Tetracaine may be added to these solutions to prolong the duration of action of the solution (see page 18).

Advantages of the Use of the Plastic Straw as a Needle Guide: The plastic straw is a very effective needle guide and it has the following advantages: (1) a plastic straw used for drinking liquids is easily obtainable; (2) it is disposable; (3) it is 8 inches (20 cm.) long; (4) it can be cut so that it can accommodate either a 5-inch (12.5 cm.) or a 6-inch (15 cm.) 20-gauge needle and allow the needle to extend only ⅗ inch (⅕ cm.) beyond the end of the straw—this is the distance the needle should be inserted into the tissues for either a paracervical or a transvaginal pudendal nerve block; (5) it is flexible and can be bent to conform to the topography of the vagina; (6) the plastic is a soft material and will not penetrate or damage the mucosa of the vagina; (7) it can be sterilized in the gas autoclave or by other cold sterilization techniques; and (8) it is inexpensive.

Recover Broken Needle(s): All needles should be tested before use. If a needle breaks, every effort to recover it, including surgery, should be made. Unremoved needles have a tendency to migrate and may cause permanent injuries as well as medicolegal complications.

Repeat Block When Analgesia Is Inadequate: If the desired results from the first block attempt are unsatisfactory, do not hesitate to reblock the patient if time permits. Most patients will think nothing about being reblocked if the second attempt is prefaced by a statement such as: "Well, I guess we will have to inject a little more medicine if we are going to freeze this area."

However, do not exceed the maximum safe dosage of the local anesthetic solution for both blocks. If to reblock the patient the maximum safe dose of the local anesthetic solution must be exceeded, 45 minutes should elapse between blocks.

CHAPTER 25

Perineal Pudendal Nerve Block

INDICATIONS

Surgical: It may be used in rectal operations and in perineal operations in both sexes but its most frequent use is for anesthesia of the female perineum during uncomplicated obstetrical deliveries. For deliveries the transvaginal approach is used more than the perineal approach (Chapter 26, page 194).

Diagnostic: Differentiation of perianal pain.

Therapeutic: Relief of pain and itching of the perineum, alleviation of pain caused from carcinoma of the vulva, or metastasis from carcinoma of the cervix.

ANATOMY

The pudendal nerve derives its fibers from the ventral branches of the second, third, and fourth sacral nerves. It leaves the pelvis through the lower part of the greater sciatic foramen, passes behind the spine of the ischium and re-enters the pelvis (infralevator portion) through the lesser sciatic foramen (Figure 116, page 189). It accompanies the internal pudendal vessels upward and forward along the lateral wall of the ischiorectal fossa, being contained in a sheath of the obturator fascia known as Alcock's canal. Alcock's canal lies close to the medial surface of the ischium in the region between the ischial spine and the tuberosity (Figure 116, page 189). Its branches are the inferior hemorrhoidal nerve, the perineal nerve, and the dorsal nerve of the penis or clitoris (Figure 116, page 189).

The pudendal branch of the posterior femoral cutaneous nerve curves forward somewhat anterior to the ischial tuberosity to unite with the posterior labial branches of the perineal nerve which is one of the branches of the pudendal nerve in the female, or with the posterior scrotal branches of the pudendal nerve in the male (Figure 117, page 190).

The ilioinguinal (L1) and genitofemoral (L1, 2) nerves supply the skin and subcutaneous tissue over the mons pubis and anterior portions of the labium majus or the scrotum (Figure 116, page 189).

PREMEDICATION

No attempt to elicit paresthesias is made. In the surgical patient, heavy medication is used. In the obstetrical patient, light medication is advised.

Heavy Premedication: The average patient (age 20 to 50, weight 150 or over, height 5 feet, 5 inches or over, and good physical status) receives:

1. 200 mg. (3 gr.) of pentobarbital (Nembutal) by mouth at hour of sleep on night previous to surgery.

2. 200 mg. (3 gr.) of pentobarbital with one ounce of water by mouth 1½ to 2 hours before estimated *block* time.

3. 15 mg. (¼ gr.) of morphine and 0.6 mg. (¹⁄₁₀₀ gr.) of scopolamine intramuscularly ¾ to 1 hour before the estimated *block* time.

Light Premedication: The parturient (woman in labor), during the early part of the first stage of labor, often receives barbiturates, narcotics, belladonna derivatives, and tranquilizers, or combinations of these drugs to alleviate pain, allay apprehension, promote amnesia, or effect a combination of these conditions. If these drugs are effective, further pre-

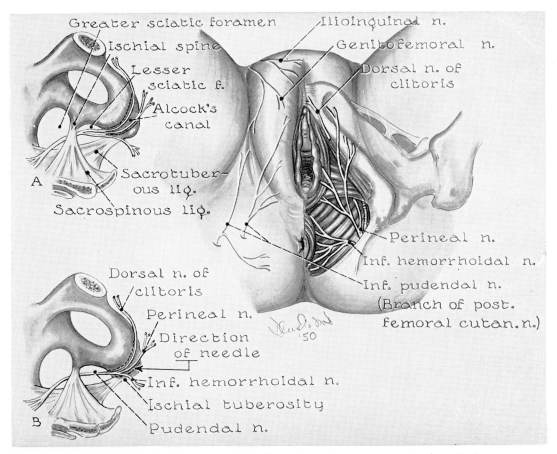

Figure 116. Anatomy of the female perineum. A. Shows the pudenal nerve passing beneath the sacrospinous ligament and branching in the ischiorectal fossa before it reaches the tuberosity of the ischium. B. Shows the pudenal nerve passing beneath the sacrospinous ligament, coursing through the ischiorectal fossa, and branching at the tuberosity of the ischium.

medication when the block is to be started is not indicated.

If no medication has been given the parturient prior to the block, then 50 mg. of meperidine (Demerol) together with 25 mg. of promethazine (Phenergan) may be given. If the optimal effect of such medication is to be obtained, it should be given intramuscularly at least forty-five minutes prior to the block or intravenously fifteen minutes prior to the block.

Reduction of Premedication: It is seldom necessary to increase this premedication irrespective of the over-all size of the patient. However, in the surgical patient, it is very common to reduce this medication under various circumstances; for example, for the geri-atric patient, the debilitated or cachectic patient, and for patients whose surgery is complicated by other disease, e.g., myxedema, diabetes, heart disease, etc. In the patient over 60 years of age, barbiturates and especially scopolamine may often cause disorientation. Therefore, in these patients atropine is usually substituted for scopolamine and the dosages of the barbiturate omitted or greatly reduced, i.e., to 50 mg. (¾ gr.) or less. *Always err on the light side.*

Inadequate Premedication: If, in the surgical patient, medication is inadequate either for the block or for the operation, intravenous pentobarbital 50 mg. (¾ gr.) to 100 mg. (1½ gr.) or intravenous morphine 8 mg. (⅛ gr.) to 15 mg. (¼ gr.) may be given slowly. Judi-

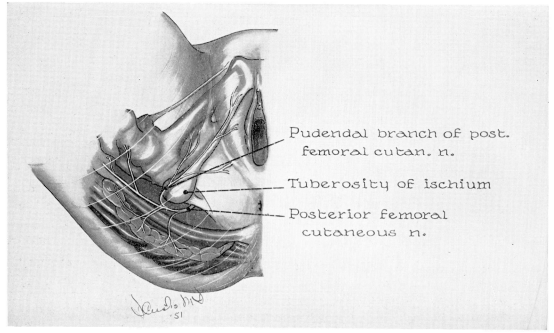

Figure 117. Course of the pudendal branch of the posterior femoral cutaneous nerve. N.B. This is not the same nerve as the perineal nerve, which is a terminal branch of the pudendal nerve.

cious use of added sedation is extremely important. Often, small supplementary doses of morphine or pentobarbital will make a block successful, especially when the patient interprets touch and motion as pain.

Prior to ordering additional sedation for the parturient, the effects of any previously administered drug must be evaluated. Most drugs given to the mother during labor will pass the placental barrier, will equilibrate in the infant in about the same time as in the mother, and may cause fetal depression.

DRUGS

Tetracaine (Pontocaine)

Dosage.—50 cc. to 100 cc. of 0.15 percent solution with or without 0.25 cc. of epinephrine (Adrenalin) 1:1000.* When using tetracaine, do not exceed 1 mg. per pound of body weight (see page 17).

Onset.—Operating analgesia is established in 5 to 25 minutes.

Duration.—Operating analgesia lasts 3½ to

6 hours, with solutions containing epinephrine giving the upper limits.

Procaine (Novocain)

Dosage.—50 cc. to 100 cc. of 1.0 percent solution with or without 0.25 cc. of epinephrine (Adrenalin) 1:1000.*

Onset.—Operating analgesia is established in 5 to 15 minutes.

Duration.—Operating analgesia lasts 1 to 1½ hours, with solutions containing epinephrine giving the upper limits.

Lidocaine (Xylocaine) or Mepivacaine (Carbocaine)

Dosage.—50 cc. to 100 cc. of 0.5 to 1.0 percent solution with or without 0.25 cc. of epinephrine (Adrenalin) 1:1000.* Do not exceed

---

*Optimal concentration of epinephrine is 1:200,000, that is, 0.1 cc. of epinephrine 1:1000 in 20 cc. of the local anesthetic solution. Do not exceed 0.25 cc. of epinephrine 1:1000 even if amount of local anesthetic solution exceeds 50 cc. (see page 39).

50 cc. of a 1.0 percent solution, *i.e.,* 500 mg. (0.5 gm.) of lidocaine or mepivacaine.

Onset.—Operating analgesia is established in 5 to 15 minutes.

Duration.—Operating analgesia lasts 1¼ to 3 hours, with stronger concentrations and solutions containing epinephrine giving the upper limits.

MATERIALS

Regional tray (see Chapter 9, page 51) or:

1. One ¾-inch (2 cm.), 25-gauge Huber point security Lok-needle.

2. One 1½-inch (3.8 cm.), 22-gauge security Lok-needle, preferably with short bevel.

3. Two 3-inch (7.5 cm.), 22-gauge security Lok-needles, preferably with short bevel.

4. Two 4-inch (10 cm.), 22-gauge security Lok-needles, preferably with short bevel.

5. One tuberculin Lok-syringe for measuring epinephrine.

6. One 10 cc. Lok-syringe, preferably with finger rings.

7. One stainless steel ruler.

8. One graduated measuring cup, preferably stainless steel, for mixing solution.

9. One prep cup, preferably stainless steel.

10. Four sterile towels.

11. Six sterile sponges.

12. One sterilizer control.

TECHNIQUE

Position and Landmarks

1. The patient is placed in the lithotomy position with shoulder braces in place and the hands in restraint cuffs along the side. The straps of the stirrups are made snug.

2. The tuberosity of the ischium is located and an X marked on the skin overlying its

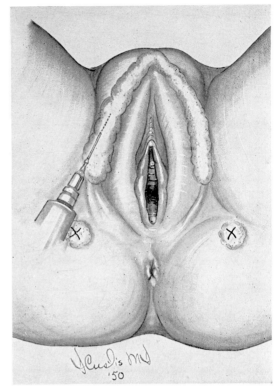

Figure 118. Method of blocking the ilioinguinal and genitofemoral nerves to the labia.

medial inferior border (Figure 118, page 191).

Precautions

Avoid Puncture of Rectum.—When advancing the needle past the tuberosity of the ischium into the ischiorectal fossa, do not puncture the rectum.

Aspirate.—The pudendal nerve is accompanied in Alcock's canal by the pudendal artery and vein. Aspiration tests must be carried out carefully to prevent intravascular injection.

Double Glove.—The vagina instead of the rectum may be used for the palpation of the landmarks so as to eliminate contamination of the palpating hand. However, the finger in the rectum is usually preferred—only then can the anesthetist be certain that the needle point does not enter the rectum. If the obstetrician is his own anesthetist he should double glove the hand which is placed in the rectum at the start of the block. Then when the block is completed, the extra glove may be removed.

Procedure

1. The sterilizer control is checked to be sure the equipment has been adequately sterilized.

2. A small area the size of a silver dollar is prepared around the X with alcoholic antiseptic solutions, or the whole perineum is prepared with aqueous antiseptic solutions. If the perineum is prepared prior to the block with alcoholic solutions, it will cause the patient great discomfort.

3. An intradermal wheal is raised at the X with a ¾-inch (2 cm.), 25-gauge Huber point security Lok-needle (Figure 118, page 191).

4. If the anesthetist is right-handed, the in-dex finger of the left hand is placed in the rectum. If the anesthetist is left-handed, the other hand is used (Figure 119, page 192).

5. The 3-inch (7.5 cm.) or 4-inch (10 cm.) security Lok-needle, depending on the size of the patient, with the full 10 cc. syringe attached is inserted through the wheal perpendicular to the skin.

6. The needle is slowly advanced, injecting small amounts of anesthetic solution before it.

7. The left index finger guides the needle point to the tuberosity of the ischium (Figure 119A, page 192). This usually lies at a depth of 1 inch (2.5 cm.) to 1½ inches (3.8 cm.) from the skin, depending on the size of the patient. Five to 10 cc. of the local anesthetic solution is deposited around the lateral (anterior) side and under the tuberosity to anesthetize the inferior pudendal nerve, which is the pudendal branch of the posterior femoral

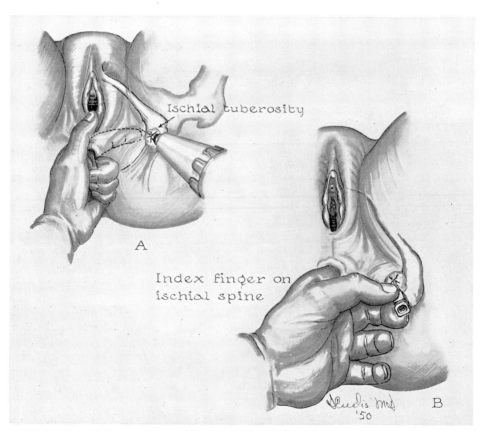

Ischial tuberosity

A

Index finger on ischial spine

B

Figure 119. A. Method of palpating landmarks for block of the female perineum. B. Method of holding needle while injecting.

cutaneous nerve (Figure 116, page 189 and Figure 117, page 190).

8. The syringe is detached, refilled, and reattached to the needle. This maneuver is easily performed as the left hand is merely rotated without removing the index finger from the rectum so the hub of the needle may be grasped between the middle finger and the thumb of the left hand (Figure 119B, page 192).

9. The needle point is then guided to the medial side of the tuberosity and 10 cc. of the local anesthetic solution is deposited at this point as the needle is moved forward and backward. Branches of the pudendal nerve often lie in this spot.

10. The syringe is refilled and 10 cc. more of the local anesthetic solution injected as the needle is advanced 1 inch (2.5 cm.) past the tuberosity into the ischiorectal fossa (space between tuberosity and spine of the ischium) (Figure 116A, B, page 189). Alcock's canal, in which the pudendal nerve lies, usually courses through this spot.

11. The point of the needle should now be guided posterior (underneath) to the spine of the ischium with the index finger of the hand which rests in the rectum, and it should pierce the sacrospinous ligament (Figure 116A, B, page 189). The needle point "pops" through this ligament, giving much the same feeling as when a spinal needle pierces the dura. The sacrospinous ligament itself can be felt by the finger in the rectum. The needle is now advanced ¼ inch (0.6 cm.) and 5 to 10 cc. of the local anesthetic solution is deposited. This is the best location to anesthetize the pudendal nerve before it branches (Figure 116A, B, page 189). The needle is now withdrawn.

12. If the block is to be bilateral, the other side is done at this time.

13. The anesthetist then either regloves or if he was double gloved, he removes the glove from the hand which was in the rectum. Using the clean 3-inch (7.5 cm.) needle, he infiltrates

the area ½ inch (1.3 cm.) lateral and parallel to the labia majorum from the middle of the labia majorum to the mons pubis bilaterally. This maneuver anesthetizes the fibers of the iliohypogastric, ilioinguinal, and genitocrural nerves, which course over the anterior part of the labia (Figure 118, page 191).

EXTENT OF ANALGESIA

The female genitalia, the rectal area, and inner aspect of the thighs are rendered analgesic (Figure 120, page 193).

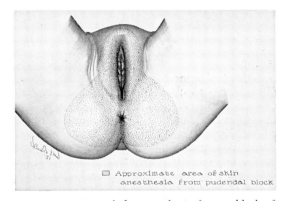

Figure 120. Area of skin anesthesia from a block of the female perineum.

COMPLICATIONS

Toxic Reactions (intravascular injections, etc.): See Chapter 3, page 19.

Puncture of the Rectum with the Needle Point: This is not serious and when detected by the finger in the rectum, the needle should be discarded. Fistulas, etc., following puncture of the rectum during this block are extremely infrequent.

Ecchymosis of the Perineum and Buttocks: This is not serious and requires no treatment.

REMARKS

Remarks applicable to pudendal nerve block by either the perineal approach or the transvaginal approach are similar (see Chapter 26, page 197).

Transvaginal Approach for
Block of the Pudendal Nerve

INDICATIONS

Surgical: This approach for block of the pudendal nerve is applicable only in the female. It is used primarily for vaginal deliveries and infrequently for operations.

Operations.—It may be used for perineal and vaginal operations. Occasionally, it may be combined with paracervical block and local infiltration to perform a vaginal hysterectomy.

Vaginal Deliveries.—Bilateral pudendal nerve block relieves the pains of the second stage of labor that are caused by the distention of the lower birth canal, vulva, and perineum. This block does not relieve the pains of the first stage of labor caused by the contractions of the uterus, and, therefore, it is often combined with paracervical block for vaginal delivery. Pudendal nerve block permits an episiotomy to be made and the use of low forceps. Intra-uterine manipulations and midforceps applications usually cause discomfort.

Diagnostic: Differentiation of perianal pain.

Therapeutic: Relief of pain and itching of the perineum.

ANATOMY

The pudendal nerve derives its fibers from the ventral branches of the second, third, and fourth sacral nerves. It leaves the pelvis through the lower part of the greater sciatic foramen, passes behind the spine of the ischium and re-enters the pelvis (infralevator portion) through the lesser sciatic foramen

(Figure 116, page 189). It accompanies the internal pudendal vessels upward and forward along the lateral wall of the ischiorectal fossa, being contained in a sheath of the obturator fascia known as Alcock's canal. Its branches are the inferior hemorrhoidal nerve, the perineal nerve, and, in the female, the dorsal nerve of the clitoris (Figure 116, page 189).

PREMEDICATION

No attempt to elicit paresthesias is made. In the surgical patient, heavy medication is used. In the obstetrical patient, light medication is advised.

Heavy Premedication: The average patient (age 20 to 50, weight 150 or over, height 5 feet, 5 inches or over, and good physical status) receives:

1. 200 mg. (3 gr.) of pentobarbital (Nembutal) by mouth at hour of sleep on night previous to surgery.

2. 200 mg. (3 gr.) of pentobarbital with one ounce of water by mouth 1½ to 2 hours before estimated *block* time.

3. 15 mg. (¼ gr.) of morphine and 0.6 mg. (¹⁄₁₀₀ gr.) of scopolamine intramuscularly ¾ to 1 hour before the estimated *block* time.

Light Premedication: The parturient (woman in labor), during the early part of the first stage of labor, often receives barbiturates, narcotics, belladonna derivatives, and tranquilizers, or combinations of these drugs to alleviate pain, allay apprehension, promote amnesia, or effect a combination of these conditions. If these drugs are effective, further premedication when the block is to be started is not indicated.

If no medication has been given the parturient prior to the block, then 50 mg. of meperidine (Demerol) together with 25 mg. of promethazine (Phenergan) may be given. If the optimal effect of such medication is to be obtained, it should be given intramuscularly at least forty-five minutes prior to the block or intravenously fifteen minutes prior to the block.

Reduction of Premedication: It is seldom necessary to increase this premedication irrespective of the over-all size of the patient. However, in the surgical patient, it is very common to reduce this medication under various circumstances; for example, for the geriatric patient, the debilitated or cachectic patient, and for patients whose surgery is complicated by other disease, e.g., myxedema, diabetes, heart disease, etc. In the patient over 60 years of age, barbiturates and especially scopolamine may often cause disorientation. Therefore, in these patients atropine is usually substituted for scopolamine and the dosages of the barbiturate omitted or greatly reduced, i.e., to 50 mg. (¾ gr.) or less. *Always err on the light side.*

Inadequate Premedication: If, in the surgical patient, medication is inadequate either for the block or for the operation, intravenous pentobarbital 50 mg. (¾ gr.) to 100 mg. (1½ gr.) or intravenous morphine 8 mg. (⅛ gr.) to 15 mg. (¼ gr.) may be given slowly. Judicious use of added sedation is extremely important. Often, small supplementary doses of morphine or pentobarbital will make a block successful, especially when the patient interprets touch and motion as pain.

Prior to ordering additional sedation for the parturient, the effects of any previously administered drug must be evaluated. Most drugs given to the mother during labor will pass the placental barrier, will equilibrate in the infant in about the same time as in the mother, and may cause fetal depression.

DRUGS

Tetracaine (Pontocaine)

Dosage.—20 to 40 cc. of 0.15 to 0.25 percent solution with or without 0.1 cc. of epinephrine (Adrenalin) 1:1000 in each 20 cc. of solution.*

Onset.—Operating analgesia is established in 15 to 45 minutes, with an average of 20 minutes.

Duration.—Operating analgesia lasts 3½ to 6 hours, with stronger concentrations and solutions containing epinephrine giving the upper limits.

Procaine (Novocain)

Dosage.—20 to 40 cc. of 1.0 to 2.0 percent solution with or without 0.1 cc. of epinephrine (Adrenalin) 1:1000 in each 20 cc. of solution.*

Onset.—Operating analgesia is established in 5 to 15 minutes with an average of 10 minutes.

Duration.—Operating analgesia lasts 1 to 1½ hours, with stronger concentrations and solutions containing epinephrine giving the upper limits.

Lidocaine (Xylocaine) or Mepivacaine (Carbocaine)

Dosage.—20 to 40 cc. of a 1.0 to 1.5 percent solution with or without 0.1 cc. of epinephrine (Adrenalin) 1:1000 in each 20 cc. of solution.* *Do not exceed 35 cc. of a 1.5 percent solution, i.e., 500 mg. (0.5 gm.) of lidocaine or mepivacaine.*

Onset.—Operating analgesia is established in 5 to 15 minutes.

Duration.—Operating analgesia lasts 1½ to 3 hours, with stronger concentrations and solutions containing epinephrine giving the upper limits.

---

*Optimal concentration of epinephrine is 1:200,000, that is, 0.1 cc. of epinephrine 1:1000 in 20 cc. of the local anesthetic solution (see page 39).

MATERIALS

Regional block tray (see Chapter 9, page 51) plus a needle guide. The Iowa trumpet, Kobak instrument, a plastic straw, or a variation of these is used as a guide for the placement of the needle. The Iowa trumpet is so constructed that when the 20-gauge, 6-inch (15 cm.) needle is placed through it, the point of the needle extends approximately 1 inch (2.5 cm.) beyond the end of the guide (Figure 112, page 183). The Kobak instrument is so constructed that when the needle is advanced through it, the point of the needle extends approximately ½ inch (1.3 cm.) beyond the end of the guide (Figure 113, page 184). When the plastic straw is used, it is cut so that the needle extends ½ inch (1.3 cm.) to ⅝ inch (1.5 cm.) beyond its end (Figure 114, page 185).

If a regional block tray is not available, then the following equipment is needed:

1. One needle guide and a 5-inch (12.5 cm.) or a 6-inch (15 cm.), 20-gauge security Lok-needle, preferably with short bevel.

2. One tuberculin Lok-syringe to measure epinephrine.

3. One 10 cc. Lok-syringe, preferably with finger rings.

4. One graduated measuring cup, preferably stainless steel, for mixing solution.

5. One prep cup, preferably stainless steel.

6. Four sterile towels.

7. Six sterile sponges.

8. One sterilizer control.

TECHNIQUE

Position and Landmarks

1. The patient is placed in the lithotomy position with shoulder braces in place and her wrists in restraint cuffs. The straps of the stirrups are made snug.

2. The ischial spine is the landmark (Figure 116, page 189).

Precautions

Aspirate.—Carefully aspirate for blood. The pudendal blood vessels lie in close approximation to the nerves and in the pregnant patient, the size of the vessels is markedly increased.

Palpate Spine of Ischial Bone.—Be sure the spine of the ischium, not its tuberosity, is palpated—the spine is posterior to the tuberosity (Figure 116, page 189).

Procedure

1. pHisoHex, aqueous benzalkonium chloride (Zephiran), or both, may be used to prepare the vagina, but whether they reduce the bacterial count and the possibility of infection is open to debate.

2. The physician places his index and middle fingers in the vagina and palpates the spine of the ischium (Figure 121, page 197).

3. The needle guide (Iowa trumpet, Kobak instrument, or plastic straw) is inserted just posterior (underneath) to the spine.* The guide is directed to this position by the index and middle fingers which rest in the vagina (Figure 121, page 197).

4. The 20-gauge, 5-inch (12.5 cm.) or 6-inch (15 cm.) needle, depending on the length of the guide, is threaded through the guide until its point rests on the vaginal mucosa.

5. It is then slowly advanced through the mucosa; it pierces the sacrospinous ligament with a "pop" and is advanced to a total depth of ½ inch (1.3 cm.) to ⅝ inch (1.5 cm.) from the mucosa (Figure 121, page 197).

6. *After careful aspiration for blood,* 10 cc. of the local anesthetic solution is injected. The pudendal vessels lie in close proximity to the nerve at this point; if blood is obtained the needle is either withdrawn or advanced slightly until no blood is obtained, then the solution is injected and the needle and guide withdrawn.

---

*When the Kobak instrument is used, the guide and needle are inserted as a unit (Figure 113, page 184).

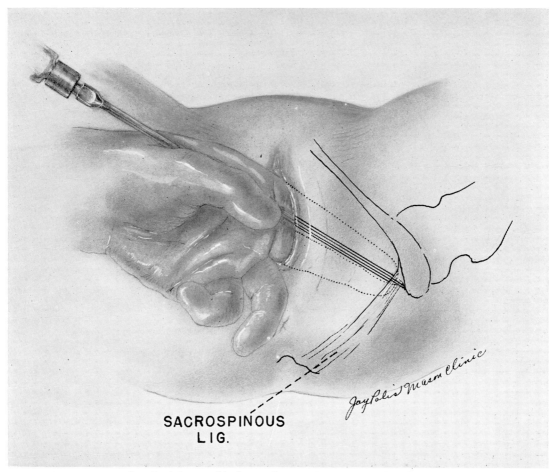

SACROSPINOUS
LIG.

Figure 121. Transvaginal pudendal nerve block. Method of placing the guide (plastic straw) on mucous membrane of the vagina just lateral to the tip of ischial spine and over sacrospinous ligament. The needle has been inserted into the tissues ½ inch (approximately 1.3 cm.). Needle point rests approximately ¼ inch (0.6 cm.) underneath sacrospinous ligament in close proximity to the pudendal nerve. Be sure the ischial spine, not the tuberosity, is palpated—the spine is posterior to the tuberosity (Figure 116A and B, page 189).

EXTENT OF ANALGESIA

Analgesia of the vagina, rectum, anus, and skin immediately adjacent to these structures ensues.

COMPLICATION

Systemic Toxic Reactions (intravenous injections, etc.): See Chapter 3, page 19.

Puncture of the Rectum with the Needle Point: This seldom occurs with this technique.

Hematoma of the Parametrium: See page 185.

Sciatic Nerve Block: See page 284.

REMARKS

For Vaginal Deliveries, Transvaginal Approach Preferred to Perineal Approach: For vaginal deliveries this is the approach most often employed because: (1) the tissue traversed by the needle is not more than ⅝ inch (1.5 cm.) as compared to the 2 inches (5 cm.) to 3 inches (7.5 cm.) via the perineal route; (2) less anesthetic solution is required; (3) it is quicker; (4) ecchymosis of the perineum and buttocks, which is often seen with the perineal route, is avoided; and (5) puncture of the rectum is less likely.

Do Not Exceed Toxic Dose of Local Anesthetic Drug When Paracervical Block Is Com-

bined with Pudendal Nerve Block: If pudendal nerve block is combined with paracervical
block and if a systemic toxic reaction from
overdosage of the local anesthetic agent is to
be avoided, one of the following two precautions must be observed. First, a minimum of
thirty to forty-five minutes should elapse between the completion of the paracervical
block and the start of the pudendal nerve
block. Or, second, the total volume of the
local anesthetic solution employed for both
blocks must not exceed the maximum safe
dose of the agent, *e.g.*, no more than 50 cc. of
a 1.0 percent solution of lidocaine or mepivacaine should be used for both blocks. Furthermore, the solution used for the pudendal nerve
block should contain epinephrine in the concentration of 1:200,000.

Pudendal Nerve Block May Slow Labor:
Following execution of this block, labor may
slow or stop for fifteen to twenty minutes. Administration of an oxytocic drug will correct
this.

**Severe Hypertension May Result from Use
of an Oxytocic Drug, a Vasoconstrictor Drug,
or Both:** See Chapter 5, page 41.

Vaginal Delivery is Principal Use of Block:
Since this block is employed primarily for obstetrical delivery, the following should be
emphasized. First, small doses of meperidine
(Demerol) instead of morphine are preferred
in obstetrics. Second, episiotomies and outlet
forceps are the only operative obstetrics that
can be performed under this block. The ac-
coucheur's hand may not be placed in the
uterus without pain to the patient, unless a
paracervical block also is executed. Third, this
block does not give the marked relaxation that
is afforded by a saddle or caudal block. Fourth,
uterine contractions do not occur without pain
as with spinal or caudal analgesia unless a
paracervical block also is done. Lastly, if the
patient is rapidly moving the baby down the
birth canal and it is imperative that anesthesia
be established immediately, a "saddle block"
or low spinal block is usually a more satisfactory type of regional anesthetic procedure.

**Underneath (Posterior) to the Ischial Spine
Is Most Satisfactory Location to Block Pudendal Nerve:** At this location the pudendal nerve
(S1, 2, 3) and the posterior femoral cutaneous
nerve (S1, 2, 3) are in close approximation and
the local anesthetic solution usually will bathe
both nerves (Figure 122, page 199). The posterior femoral cutaneous nerve, as well as the
pudendal nerve, must be blocked to obtain satisfactory anesthesia of the perineum. The
perineal branch of the posterior femoral cutaneous nerve innervates the posterior portion of
the labia majorum (Figure 116, page 189).

**Block of the Ilioinguinal Nerve and the
Genitofemoral Nerve Is Not a Necessity for
Vaginal Delivery:** Local infiltration of the labia
majorum from the middle of the labia majorum to the mons pubis to block the ilioinguinal and genitofemoral nerves need not be done
(Figure 116, page 189 and Figure 118, page
191). When local infiltration of the labia majorum from the middle of the labia majorum
anteriorly is omitted, the patient may have
slight discomfort as the head of the infant
passes the labia. In most instances, if the patient has received moderate sedation, 50 mg.
of meperidine (Demerol) with 25 mg. of
promethazine (Phenergan)), she will not complain of pain, or if she does, the discomfort is
usually minimal. On the other hand, the physician should not be misled that with the transvaginal pudendal nerve block he has blocked
all of the nerves of the female perineum.

Restrain Patient: The patient should be adequately restrained, and the shoulder brace
in particular should be applied. This prevents
the patient from pulling away from the anesthetist during the block.

**Epidural, Caudal, and Spinal Blocks Pre-
ferred for Surgery:** For procedures other than
obstetrical deliveries, most physicians prefer
a caudal block, a spinal block, or an epidural
block as the resulting anesthesia is usually
more satisfactory, and these procedures are
less time-consuming and more easily executed.

Recover Broken Needle(s): All needles
should be tested before use. If a needle breaks,

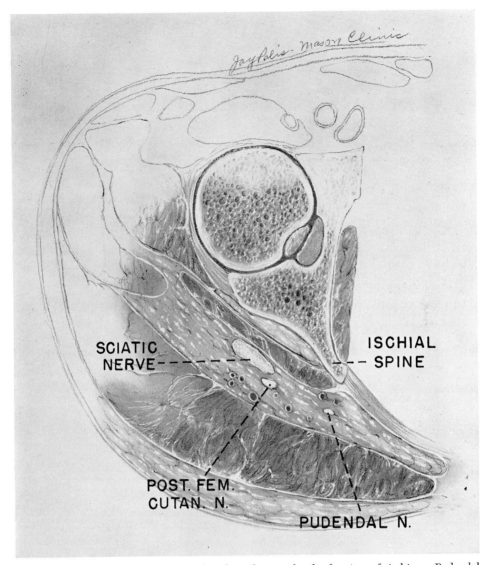

Figure 122. Cross section through female pelvis at level of spine of ischium. Pudendal nerve, posterior femoral cutaneous nerve, and sciatic nerve lie in same fascial plane and in close proximity. This explains why posterior femoral cutaneous nerve usually is anesthetized along with the pudendal nerve and why sciatic nerve block is at times a complication of this block.

every effort to recover it, including surgery, should be made. Unremoved needles have a tendency to migrate and may cause permanent injuries as well as medicolegal complications.

Repeat Block When Analgesia Is Inadequate: If the desired results from the first block attempt are unsatisfactory, do not hesitate to reblock the patient if time permits. Most patients will think nothing about being reblocked if the second attempt is prefaced by a statement such as: "Well, I guess we will have to inject a little more medicine if we are going to freeze this area."

However, do not exceed the maximum safe dosage of the local anesthetic solution for both blocks. If to reblock the patient the maximum safe dose of the local anesthetic solution must be exceeded, 45 minutes should elapse between blocks.

CHAPTER 27

Paravertebral Thoracic Somatic Nerve Block

INDICATIONS

Surgical: Operations on the thoracic and abdominal walls.

Diagnostic: Differentiation and localization of intercostal neuralgias, causalgias, and cardiac pain.

Therapeutic: Relief of intercostal neuralgias and causalgias caused by the acute phase of herpes zoster, fractured ribs, and undiagnosed conditions. Relief of postoperative abdominal incisional pain.

ANATOMY

In the thoracic region, the spinous process of one vertebra lies in a line with the transverse processes of the vertebra immediately below it. For example, the superior edge of the tip of the spinous process of the eighth thoracic vertebra lies in a line with the transverse processes of the ninth thoracic vertebra (Figure 124A, page 203).

The long downward slope of the thoracic spinous processes tends to decrease caudally as the spinous processes become heavier, so that the spinous process of the eleventh thoracic vertebra lies in line with the space between the transverse processes of the eleventh thoracic and twelfth thoracic vertebrae, and the spinous process of the twelfth thoracic vertebra lies in line with the space between the transverse processes of the twelfth thoracic and first lumbar vertebrae.

The thoracic nerves emerge from the intervertebral foramina and are divided into anterior and posterior primary divisions. The posterior division supplies the muscles and skin of the upper portion of the back. The anterior division, after giving off the ramus communicans, passes laterally to lie midway between the transverse processes, e.g., the anterior division of the ninth thoracic nerve lies midway between the transverse processes of the ninth and tenth thoracic vertebrae (Figure 124A, page 203). The nerve then approaches the rib just above it to enter the intercostal groove.

PREMEDICATION

No attempts to elicit paresthesias are made. If the block is performed on an outpatient for diagnosis, therapy, or a minor operation, it is not necessary to give premedication, providing infiltration is adequate as the needle advances.

Hospitalized patients who are to undergo surgical procedures should be heavily medicated.

Heavy Premedication: The average patient (age 20 to 50, approximate weight 150 pounds or over, height 5 feet, 5 inches, and good physical status) receives:

1. 200 mg. (3 gr.) of pentobarbital (Nembutal) by mouth at hour of sleep on the day previous to surgery.

2. 200 mg. (3 gr.) of pentobarbital by mouth with one ounce of water 1½ to 2 hours before the estimated *block* time.

3. 15 mg. (¼ gr.) of morphine and 0.6 mg. (¹⁄₁₀₀ gr.) of scopolamine intramuscularly ¾ to 1 hour before the estimated *block* time.

Reduction of Premedication: It is seldom necessary to increase this premedication irrespective of the over-all size of the patient until the patient arrives in either the anesthesia or operating room. However, it is very common to reduce this medication under various circumstances; for example, for the geriatric patient, the adolescent patient or child, the debilitated or cachectic patient, and for patients whose surgery is complicated by other disease, e.g., myxedema, diabetes, heart disease, etc. In the patient over 60 years of age, barbiturates and especially scopolamine may often cause disorientation. Therefore, in these patients atropine is usually substituted for scopolamine and the dosages of the barbiturates omitted or greatly reduced, i.e., to 50 mg. (¾ gr.) or less. *Always err on the light side.*

Inadequate Premedication: If the medication is inadequate, either for the block or surgical procedure, intravenous pentobarbital 50 mg. (¾ gr.) to 100 mg. (1½ gr.) or intravenous morphine 8 mg. (⅛ gr.) to 15 mg. (¼ gr.) may be given slowly. Judicious use of added sedation is extremely important. Often small supplementary doses of morphine or pentobarbital will make a block successful, especially when a patient interprets touch and motion as pain.

DRUGS

Tetracaine (Pontocaine)

Dosage.—10 cc. to 100 cc. of 0.15 percent solution with or without 0.25 cc. of epinephrine (Adrenalin) 1:1000 in 50 cc. of solution.*

Onset.—Operating analgesia is established in 5 to 30 minutes.

Duration.—Operating analgesia lasts 3½ to 6 hours, with solutions containing epinephrine giving the upper limits.

Procaine (Novocain)

Dosage.—10 cc. to 100 cc. of 1.0 percent solution with or without 0.25 cc. of epinephrine (Adrenalin) 1:1000 in 50 cc. of solution.*

Onset.—Operating analgesia is established in 5 to 15 minutes.

Duration.—Operating analgesia lasts 1 to 1½ hours, with solutions containing epinephrine giving the upper limits.

Lidocaine (Xylocaine) or Mepivacaine (Carbocaine)

Dosage.—10 cc. to 100 cc. of 0.5 percent solution with or without 0.25 cc. of epinephrine (Adrenalin) solution 1:1000 in 50 cc. of solution.* *Do not exceed 500 mg. (0.5 gm.) of lidocaine or mepivacaine.*

Onset.—Operating analgesia is established in 5 to 15 minutes.

Duration.—Operating analgesia lasts 1¼ to 3 hours, with solutions containing epinephrine giving the upper limits.

MATERIALS

Regional tray (see Chapter 9, page 51) or:

1. One ¾-inch (2 cm.), 25-gauge Huber point security Lok-needle.

2. One 1½-inch (3.8 cm.), 22-gauge security Lok-needle, preferably with short bevel.

3. Three 3-inch (7.5 cm.), 22-gauge security Lok-needles, preferably with short bevel.

4. One tuberculin Lok-syringe for measuring epinephrine.

5. One 10 cc. Lok-syringe, preferably with finger rings.

6. One stainless steel ruler.

7. One graduated measuring cup, preferably stainless steel, for mixing solution.

8. One prep cup, preferably stainless steel.

9. Four sterile towels.

10. Six sterile sponges.

11. One sterilizer control.

TECHNIQUE

Position and Landmarks

1. The patient lies in the prone position

---

*Optimal concentration of epinephrine is 1:200,000, that is, 0.1 cc. of epinephrine 1:1000 in 20 cc. of the local anesthetic solution. Do not exceed 0.25 cc. of epinephrine 1:1000 even if amount of local anesthetic solution exceeds 50 cc. (see page 39).

with a pillow under his abdomen and his arms hanging over the table (Figure 128, page 213). If the upper thoracic nerves are to be blocked, it is best to have the patient's head hanging off the end of the table and supported by an assistant. This makes it easier to palpate the landmarks.

2. The appropriate spinous processes which align with the intercostal nerves to be blocked are determined and marked. This is done by locating the space between the spinous processes of the seventh cervical and the first thoracic vertebrae and counting caudad. The spinous process of the seventh cervical vertebra is the first prominent spinous process in the neck and it has a small V in it, differentiating it from the spinous process of the first thoracic vertebra, which has no groove. Always check the selected spinous processes by locating the spinous process of the fourth lumbar vertebra and counting cephalad—a line drawn between the iliac crests crosses the spinous process of the fourth lumbar vertebra or the space between the spinous processes of the fourth and fifth lumbar vertebrae (Figure 125, page 208).

3. Horizontal lines are drawn through the superior edge of the spinous processes and extended laterally (Figure 123, page 202).

4. A vertical line, parallel and 1¼ inches (3.2 cm.) to 1½ inches (3.8 cm.), depending on the size of the patient, lateral to the spinous processes, is drawn along the back (Figure 123, page 202).

5. The points of crossing of the lines drawn in steps 3 and 4 mark spots overlying the transverse processes (Figure 123, page 202).

Precautions

Carefully Check Landmarks.—The vertical line usually should not be more than 1½ inches (3.8 cm.) or less than 1 inch (2.5 cm.) from the spinous processes because: (1) the transverse processes slant toward the back in an anteroposterior direction and the more lateral the mark, the greater the distance from the process to the nerve (Figure 124A, page 203);

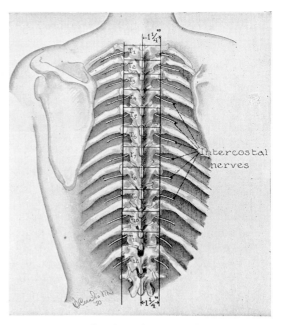

Figure 123. Landmarks and anatomy for a paravertebral thoracic block.

(2) if the mark is too far lateral, instead of contacting the transverse process with the needle point, the anesthetist may be feeling the rib, and as he advances the needle it may enter the pleura (Figure 123, page 202); and (3) if the mark is too close to the spine, the anesthetist will feel the lamina of the arch of the vertebra and as he advances the needle, it may enter the epidural space or puncture the dura (Figure 123, page 202).

Aspirate.—Careful aspiration for spinal fluid and blood should always be carried out.

Avoid Pneumothorax.—If the patient coughs, remove the needle immediately. The pleura has probably been either stimulated or entered.

Procedure

1. The sterilizer control is checked to be sure the equipment has been sterilized.

2. The area is aseptically prepared and draped.

3. The anesthetist stands at the side of the patient to be blocked, facing the side of the table or cart (Figure 128, page 213).

4. Intradermal wheals are raised over the selected transverse processes with the ¾-inch (2 cm.), 25-gauge Huber point security Lok-needle. Remember that, with the exception of the eleventh and twelfth vertebrae, where the determined spots lie over the spaces between the respective transverse processes, the determined spots overlie the transverse proc-esses of the vertebra below the one through whose spinous process the horizontal line was drawn, not its homologous transverse process-es, *i.e.*, the horizontal line through the spinous process of the eighth thoracic vertebra over-lies the transverse processes of the ninth tho-racic vertebra (Figure 124, page 203).

5. Infiltration is then carried deeper with a

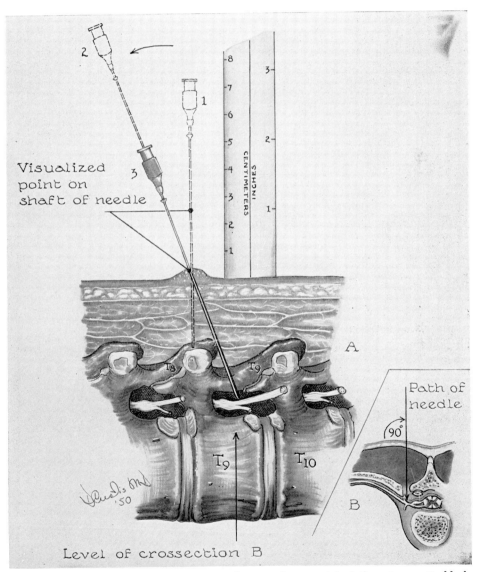

Figure 124. A. Sagittal section showing technique of paravertebral thoracic somatic block. 1. Needle rests on the transverse process of the ninth vertebra. 2. Needle withdrawn slightly and directed caudad to the transverse process of the ninth vertebra. 3. Needle inserted to the visualized depth on the shaft of the needle and coming in close proximity to the ninth thoracic nerve. The needle passes caudad to the transverse process of the ninth vertebra. B. Relation-ship of needle to the cross section of the body.

1½-inch (3.8 cm.), 22-gauge security Lok-needle. In a medium sized patient this needle may be sufficiently long to feel the transverse process.

6. The 3-inch (7.5 cm.), 22-gauge security Lok-needle without syringe is advanced perpendicularly in all planes to the skin (Figure 124 A, B, page 203) through the skin wheal, until it impinges on the transverse process. This is usually 1 inch (2.5 cm.) to 1¼ inches (3.2 cm.) below the skin. In a muscular or obese patient this distance may be 2 inches (5 cm.). If a marker is to be used, it should be set at the above determined distance (Figure 124A, page 203).

7. With the stainless steel ruler ¾ inch (2 cm.) to 1 inch (2.5 cm.) is measured up from the skin on the shaft of the needle. If a marker is being employed, reset it at this distance. If not, the anesthetist should visualize the distance from the ¾ inch (2 cm.) or 1 inch (2.5 cm.) mark to the security bead (Figure 124A, page 203).

8. The needle is slightly withdrawn and inclined caudad until it is felt to slide off the caudad edge of the transverse process, and then it is inserted either to the marker or the visualized mark. A depth of ¾ inch (2.0 cm.) to 1 inch (2.5 cm.) is required since the transverse process is about ¼ inch (0.6 cm.) thick and the nerve lies ¼ inch (0.6 cm.) to ½ inch (1.3 cm.) below it (Figure 124A, page 203).

9. Whether paresthesias do or do not occur, 10 cc. of anesthetic solution is deposited so as to flood the space adequately.

EXTENT OF ANALGESIA

This depends on the number of thoracic nerves injected and whether or not the block is bilateral or unilateral. The first thoracic nerve is part of the brachial plexus and the distribution of the second is covered by the cervical plexus fibers. The third through sixth thoracic nerves innervate the chest wall from just above the nipple line to the xiphoid process, the seventh through the tenth innervate the lateral side of the thoracic wall and ab-dominal wall from the xiphoid to the umbilicus, and the tenth through the twelfth the lower portion of the thoracic wall and the abdominal wall from the umbilicus to the pubic bone (Figure 242, page 354).

COMPLICATIONS

Toxic Reactions (intravascular injections, etc.): See Chapter 3, page 19.

Subarachnoid Injections: Rare occurrence. See Chapter 43, page 353.

Pneumothorax: See Chapter 30, page 237.

REMARKS

Pneumothorax is Possible Sequela: The danger of pneumothorax is a real one if the needle is inserted deeper than 1 inch (2.5 cm.) past the transverse process. This is why paravertebral thoracic *sympathetic* ganglion block is not included in this book. Even in the hands of the specialist, thoracic sympathetic ganglion block yields a higher percentage of pneumothoraces, not to mention the fact that if it is performed for cardiac pain, the percentage of deaths may be high. Besides, if the needle point lies close to the spinal nerve as it emerges from the intervertebral foramen, a block of the gray and white rami communicans occurs and an effective block of the sympathetics follows, even though no attempt has been made to place the local anesthetic solution in the region of the thoracic sympathetic ganglia.

Overlap of Intercostal Nerves Is Extensive: The cutaneous ipsilateral overlap of the intercostal nerves is extensive and therefore the nerve innervating the dermatome above and below the area to be anesthetized must be blocked to assure analgesia. Also, anesthesia does not extend to the midline, because of the slight overlap of the nerves from the other side.

Indication to Block Cervical Nerves: If operations are to be performed on the upper chest wall, this block must be supplemented by local infiltration to block the nerves of the superficial cervical plexus.

Indication to Block Lumbar Nerves: If operations on the abdominal wall below the umbilicus are to be performed, it is best also to block the first and second lumbar nerves paravertebrally.

Pleura Not Anesthetized: Operations on the pleura or its contents cannot be performed under paravertebral thoracic somatic nerve block because: (1) the visceral pleura is not adequately anesthetized by this block; and (2) collapse of the lung and mediastinal shift, which are associated with the opening of the pleura, are best handled with positive pressure anesthetic techniques.

Peritoneum Not Anesthetized: The abdominal peritoneum usually cannot be entered or manipulated without discomfort to the patient unless the celiac plexus is also blocked or the surgeon is gentle.

Use of Block for Herpes Zoster: While the active lesion of herpes zoster may be definitely improved by paravertebral thoracic somatic nerve block, postherpetic neuritis responds poorly and surgical root section is a more satisfactory treatment.

Recover Broken Needle(s): All needles should be tested before use. If a needle breaks, every effort to recover it, including surgery, should be made. Unremoved needles have a tendency to migrate and may cause permanent injuries as well as medicolegal complications.

Repeat Block When Analgesia Is Inadequate: If the desired results from the first block attempt are unsatisfactory, do not hesitate to reblock the patient if time permits. Most patients will think nothing of being reblocked if the second attempt is prefaced by by a statement such as: "Well, I guess we will have to inject a little more medicine if we are going to freeze this area."

However, do not exceed the maximum safe dosage of the local anesthetic solution for both blocks. If to reblock the patient the maximum safe dose of the local anesthetic solution must be exceeded, 45 minutes should elapse between blocks.

CHAPTER 28

Paravertebral Lumbar Somatic Nerve Block

INDICATIONS

Surgical: Operations on the lower abdominal wall and parts of the leg. In practically all instances it must be combined with sacral block or paravertebral somatic block of the thoracic region to produce adequate anesthesia.

Diagnostic: Differentiation and localization of pain of the inguinal region and legs as well as low back pain.

Therapeutic: Relief of pain referable to the dermatomes innervated by the lumbar somatic plexus (Figure 242, page 354).

ANATOMY

In the lumbar region, the superior edge of the spinous process lies in a line with its homologous transverse processes (Figure 125, page 208). The distance between the transverse processes of any two lumbar vertebrae is usually ¾ inch (2 cm.).

The lumbar nerves emerge from intervertebral foramina and divide into an anterior and posterior primary division. The posterior division supplies the muscles and skin of the lower portion of the back. The anterior divisions of the first four lumbar nerves together with a branch of the twelfth thoracic nerve form the lumbar plexus. The branches of the lumbar plexus are the iliohypogastric (L1), the ilioinguinal (L1), the genitofemoral (L1, 2), the lateral femoral cutaneous (L2, 3), the femoral (L2, 3, 4), the obturator (L2, 3, 4), the accessory obturator (L3, 4), when present, and muscular rami to the psoas and quadratus lumborum muscles (Figure 187, page 277).

PREMEDICATION

No attempts to elicit paresthesias are made.

If the block is performed on an outpatient for therapy, diagnosis or minor operations, it is not necessary to give premedication if infiltration is performed as the needle advances.

Hospitalized patients who are to undergo surgical procedures should be heavily sedated.

Heavy Premedication: The average patient (age 20 to 50, weight 150 pounds or over, height 5 feet, 5 inches, and good physical status) receives:

1. 200 mg. (3 gr.) of pentobarbital (Nembutal) by mouth at hour of sleep on the day previous to surgery.

2. 200 mg. (3 gr.) of pentobarbital by mouth with one ounce of water 1½ to 2 hours before the estimated *block* time.

3. 15 mg. (¼ gr.) of morphine and 0.6 mg. (¹⁄₁₀₀ gr.) of scopolamine intramuscularly ¾ to 1 hour before the estimated *block* time.

Reduction of Premedication: It is seldom necessary to increase this premedication irrespective of the over-all size of the patient until the patient arrives in either the anesthesia or operating room. However, it is very common to reduce this medication under various circumstances; for example, for the geriatric patient, the adolescent patient or child, the debilitated or cachectic patient, and for patients whose surgery is complicated by other disease, *e.g.*, myxedema, diabetes, heart disease, etc. In the patient over 60 years of age, barbiturates and especially scopolamine often cause disorientation. Therefore, in these patients atropine is usually substituted for scopolamine and the dosages of the barbiturate omitted or greatly reduced, *i.e.*, 50 mg. (¾ gr.) or less. *Always err on the light side.*

Inadequate Premedication: If the medication is inadequate for either the block or the surgical procedure, intravenous pentobarbital 50 mg. (¾ gr.) to 100 mg. (1½ gr.) or intravenous morphine 8 mg. (⅛ gr.) to 15 mg. (¼ gr.) may be given slowly. Judicious use of added sedation is extremely important. Often small supplementary doses of morphine or pentobarbital will make a block successful, especially when a patient interprets touch and motion as pain.

DRUGS

Tetracaine (Pontocaine)

Dosage.—10 cc. to 100 cc. of 0.15 percent solution with or without 0.25 cc. of epinephrine (Adrenalin) 1:1000 in 50 cc. of solution.*

Onset.—Operating analgesia is established in 5 to 30 minutes.

Duration.—Operating analgesia lasts 3½ to 6 hours, with solutions containing epinephrine giving the upper limits.

Procaine (Novocain)

Dosage.—10 cc. to 100 cc. of 1.0 percent solution with or without 0.25 cc. of epinephrine (Adrenalin) 1:1000 in 50 cc. of solution.*

Onset.—Operating analgesia is established in 5 to 15 minutes.

Duration.—Operating analgesia lasts 1 to 1½ hours, with solutions containing epinephrine giving the upper limits.

Lidocaine (Xylocaine) or Mepivacaine (Carbocaine)

Dosage.—10 cc. to 100 cc. of a 0.5 to 1.0 percent solution with or without 0.25 cc. of epinephrine (Adrenalin) 1:1000 in 50 cc. of solution.* *Do not exceed 500 mg. (0.5 gm.) of lidocaine or mepivacaine.*

---

*Optimal concentration of epinephrine is 1:200,000, that is, 0.1 cc. of epinephrine 1:1000 in 20 cc. of the local anesthetic solution. Do not exceed 0.25 cc. of epinephrine 1:1000 even if amount of local anesthetic solution exceeds 50 cc. (see page 39).

Onset.—Operating analgesia is established in 5 to 15 minutes.

Duration.—Operating analgesia lasts 1¼ to 3 hours, with stronger concentrations and solutions containing epinephrine giving the upper limits.

MATERIALS

Regional tray (see Chapter 9, page 51) or:

1. One ¾-inch (2 cm.), 25-gauge Huber point security Lok-needle.

2. One 1½-inch (3.8 cm.), 22-gauge security Lok-needle, preferably with short bevel.

3. Three 3-inch (7.5 cm.), 22-gauge security Lok-needles.

4. One tuberculin Lok-syringe for measuring epinephrine.

5. One 10 cc. Lok-syringe, preferably with finger rings.

6. One stainless steel ruler.

7. One graduated measuring cup, preferably stainless steel, for mixing solution.

8. One prep cup, preferably stainless steel.

9. Four sterile towels.

10. Six sterile sponges.

11. One sterilizer control.

TECHNIQUE

Position and Landmarks

1. The patient lies in the prone position with his arms hanging off the cart (Figure 128, page 213).

2. A pillow is placed under the abdomen between the ribs and the crest of the iliac bones so as to flatten the lumbar curvature of the vertebrae (Figure 128, page 213).

3. The iliac crests are palpated and a line drawn between them (Figure 125, page 208). This line usually crosses the spine of the fourth lumbar vertebra or the interspace be-

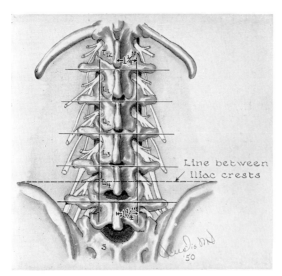

Figure 125. Landmarks and anatomy for a paravertebral lumbar somatic block.

tween the spines of the fourth and fifth lumbar vertebrae (Figure 125, page 208).

4. The spines of the lumbar vertebrae are identified and marked (Figure 125, page 208).

5. Horizontal lines are drawn through the cephalad edge of the tip of the spinous processes and projected laterally (Figure 125, page 208). Each line overlies the caudad edge of the transverse processes of its homologous vertebra.

6. A vertical line, parallel and 1¼ inches (3.2 cm.) to 1½ inches (3.8 cm.) depending on the size of the patient, lateral to the spines of the vertebrae, is drawn on the skin (Figure 125, page 208).

7. The points of crossing of the lines made in steps 5 and 6 mark the approximate positions of the transverse processes of the lumbar vertebrae (Figure 125, page 208).

Precaution

Aspirate.—Careful aspiration for spinal fluid and blood should be made in this region.

Procedure

1. The sterilizer control is checked to be sure the equipment has been sterilized.

2. The area is aseptically prepared and draped.

3. The anesthetist stands at the side of the patient to be blocked facing the side of the table or cart (Figure 128, page 213).

4. Intradermal wheals are raised over the transverse processes of the nerves to be blocked with a ¾-inch (2 cm.), 25-gauge Huber point security Lok-needle. It must be remembered that in the lumbar region the lumbar nerves emerge from the intervertebral foramina of the vertebra whose homologous spinous process was used for a landmark.

5. Infiltration is then carried deeper with a 1½-inch (3.8 cm.), 22-gauge security Lok-needle. In a thin patient this needle may be sufficiently long to feel the transverse process.

6. The 3-inch (7.5 cm.), 22-gauge security Lok-needle without syringe attached is advanced perpendicularly in all planes to the skin through the skin wheal until it impinges on the transverse process (Figure 126 A, B, page 209). This is usually 1½ inches (3.8 cm.) to 2 inches (5 cm.) below the skin (Figure 127, page 212). In an obese patient, it may be deeper. If a marker is to be used, it should be set at the above determined distance.

7. With the stainless steel ruler, 1 inch (2.5 cm.) to 1¼ inches (3.2 cm.) is measured up from the skin on the shaft of the needle. If a marker is being used, it should be reset at this distance. If not, the anesthetist should visualize the distance from the 1-inch (2.5 cm.) or 1¼-inch (3.2 cm.) mark to the security bead (Figure 126A, page 209).

8. The needle is slightly withdrawn and inclined caudally until it is felt to slide off the caudad edge of the transverse process; it is then inserted to the marker or the visualized depth (Figure 126A, page 209).

9. Whether paresthesias do or do not occur, 10 cc. of anesthetic solution is deposited so as to flood the space adequately.

EXTENT OF ANALGESIA

This depends on the number of lumbar nerves injected and whether or not the block

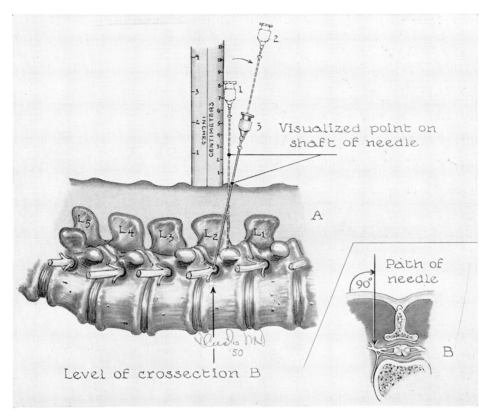

Figure 126. A. Sagittal section showing the technique of paravertebral lumbar somatic block. 1. Needle rests on the transverse process of the second lumbar vertebra. 2. Needle withdrawn slightly and directed caudad. 3. Needle inserted to the visualized depth on the shaft of the needle and coming in close proximity to the second lumbar nerve. The needle passes caudad to the transverse process of the second lumbar vertebra. B. Path of needle in relationship to the cross section of the body.

is bilateral or unilateral. Analgesia occurs over the innervation of the nerves blocked (Figure 242, page 354).

COMPLICATIONS

Toxic Reactions (intravascular injections, etc.): See Chapter 3, page 19.

Subarachnoid Injections: Occasional occurrence. See Chapter 43, page 353.

REMARKS

Block of Lumbar Nerves Usually Used in Conjunction with Block of Other Nerves: For operating analgesia, the lumbar nerves must be blocked in conjunction with other peripheral nerves because of overlapping of nerves.

For example, in herniorrhaphy the last three thoracic nerves and the first four lumbar nerves must be included in the block to assure adequate analgesia of the abdominal wall. Even then, the peritoneum must be infiltrated if it is to be opened.

Anesthesia Does Not Extend to Midline: Anesthesia does not extend to the midline because of overlapping of the nerves from the other side.

Puncture of Peritoneum and Organs Is Not Serious: Even if the needles are incorrectly placed, puncture of the peritoneum and abdominal or retroperitoneal organs is not a serious complication. They must be occasionally punctured by the specialist without his recognizing the fact or having a complication arise.

Recover Broken Needle(s): All needles should be tested before use. If a needle breaks, every effort to recover it, including surgery, should be made. Unremoved needles have a tendency to migrate and may cause permanent injuries as well as medicolegal complications.

Repeat Block When Analgesia Is Inadequate: If the desired results from the first block attempt are unsatisfactory, do not hesitate to reblock the patient if time permits.

Most patients will think nothing about being reblocked if the second attempt is prefaced by a statement such as: "Well, I guess we will have to inject a little more medicine if we are going to freeze this area."

However, do not exceed the maximum safe dosage of the local anesthetic solution for both blocks. If to reblock the patient the maximum safe dose of the local anesthetic solution must be exceeded, 45 minutes should elapse between blocks.

CHAPTER 29

Paravertebral Lumbar Sympathetic Ganglion Block

INDICATIONS

Surgical: None.

Diagnostic: To prognosticate the advisability of lumbar sympathectomy in vascular deficiencies of the lower extremity and to differentiate varieties of vasospastic diseases.

Therapeutic

Relief of Vasospastic Diseases of the Lower Extremities.—Vasospastic diseases which can be relieved are the result of: (1) arterial dysfunction, *e.g.*, Buerger's disease, cast contractures, arterial injuries, crushing injuries, embolisms, and thromboses; (2) venous dysfunction, *e.g.*, chronic or acute thrombophlebitis and postphlebitic edema; and (3) combinations of venous and arterial dysfunction, *e.g.*, frostbite, trench foot, and immersion foot.

Treatment of Post-traumatic Dystrophies.—For example, atrophy of bone, traumatic osteoporosis, causalgia, traumatic edema, and phantom limb pain.

Treatment of Miscellaneous Complaints That Are Improved by Blocking the Sympathetic Chain.—For example, prolonged infection, unhealed ulcer, hyperhidrosis, and joint stiffness.

Relief of Pain of Acute Pancreatitis.—Pain in acute pancreatitis may be dramatically relieved by blocking the first lumbar sympathetic ganglion unilaterally or bilaterally. The reason for this may be that the solution spreads in the areolar tissue of the prevertebral space and involves the celiac plexus.

ANATOMY

The lumbar portion of the sympathetic trunk lies along the vertebral column on the anterolateral surface of the bodies of the lumbar vertebrae and medial to the border of the psoas muscle (Figure 131, page 215). The ganglia are small in size. The depth from the transverse processes to the ganglia is 1½ inches (3.8 cm.) to 2 inches (5 cm.) (Figure 131, page 215). This distance is fairly constant since the anteroposterior dimension of the body of the lumbar vertebrae varies less than ¼ inch (0.6 cm.) irrespective of the patient's build. However, the distance from the skin to the transverse process varies widely, depending on size and obesity of the patient (Figure 127, page 212). The ganglia send branches to the aortic and hypogastric plexus as well as to the iliac vessels. Gray rami communicans pass to the nerves of the lumbar plexuses. Usually lumbar ganglia two, three, and four control the sympathetic impulses to the lower extremity, with the second being predominant.

PREMEDICATION

Most patients are treated as outpatients and no premedication is necessary because no attempt to elicit paresthesias is made and the block is not painful.

If, however, the patient is particularly apprehensive, a barbiturate or opiate or combination of the two may be administered, *i.e.*, 100 mg. (1½ gr.) of pentobarbital (Nembutal) orally or intravenously or 10 mg. (⅙ gr.) to 15 mg. (¼ gr.) of morphine intramuscularly or intravenously.

DRUGS

Tetracaine (Pontocaine)

Dosage.—40 cc. to 50 cc. of 0.15 to 0.25 percent solution with or without 0.1 cc. of epi-

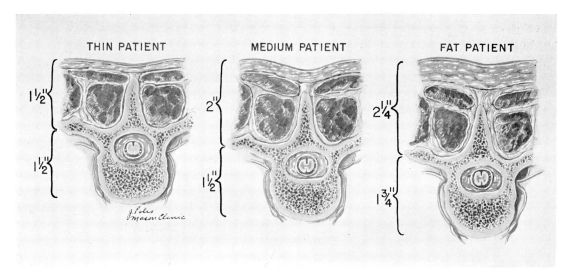

Figure 127. Variations in the distance from the skin to the transverse process in different sized individuals.

nephrine (Adrenalin) 1:1000 in each 20 cc. of solution.*

Onset.—Signs of vasodilatation occur in 5 to 30 minutes.

Duration.—Block lasts 3½ to 6 hours, with stronger concentrations and solutions containing epinephrine giving the upper limits. While signs of vasodilatation may disappear in a relatively short time, the oscillometric readings may remain elevated for 24 to 48 hours.

Procaine (Novocain)

Dosage.—40 cc. to 50 cc. of 1.0 to 2.0 percent solution with or without 0.1 cc. of epinephrine (Adrenalin) 1:1000 in each 20 cc. of solution.*

Onset.—Signs of vasodilatation occur in 5 to 20 minutes.

Duration.—Block lasts 1 to 1½ hours, with stronger concentrations and solutions containing epinephrine giving the upper limits. While signs of vasodilatation may disappear in a relatively short time, the oscillometric readings may remain elevated for 24 to 48 hours.

Lidocaine (Xylocaine) or Mepivacaine (Carbocaine)

Dosage.—40 cc. to 50 cc. of 0.5 to 1.0 percent solution with or without 0.1 cc. of epi-

nephrine (Adrenalin) 1:1000 in each 20 cc. of solution.*

Onset.—Signs of vasodilatation occur in 5 to 20 minutes.

Duration.—Block lasts 1¼ to 3 hours, with stronger concentrations and solutions containing epinephrine giving the upper limits. While signs of vasodilatation may disappear in a relatively short time, the oscillometric readings may remain elevated for 24 to 48 hours.

MATERIALS

Regional block tray plus 4-inch (10 cm.), 20-gauge security Lok-needles (Chapter 9, page 51).

1. One ¾-inch (2 cm.), 25-gauge Huber point security Lok-needle.

2. One 1½-inch (3.8 cm.), 22-gauge security Lok-needle, preferably with short bevel.

3. Three 4-inch (10 cm.) 20- or 22-gauge security Lok-needles, preferably with short bevels.

---

*Optimal concentration of epinephrine is 1:200,000, that is, 0.1 cc. of epinephrine 1:1000 in 20 cc. of the local anesthetic solution (see page 39).

4. One tuberculin Lok-syringe for measuring epinephrine.

5. One 10 cc. Lok-syringe, preferably with finger rings.

6. One graduated measuring cup, preferably stainless steel, for mixing solution.

7. One stainless steel ruler.

8. One prep cup, preferably stainless steel.

9. Four sterile towels.

10. Six sterile sponges.

11. One sterilizer control.

TECHNIQUE

Position and Landmarks

1. The patient lies in the prone position with his arms hanging off the cart or table (Figure 128, page 213).

2. A pillow is placed under the abdomen between the ribs and the crests of the iliac bones so as to flatten the lumbar curvature of the vertebrae (Figure 128, page 213).

3. The iliac crests are palpated and a line drawn between them. This line usually crosses the spine of the fourth lumbar vertebra or the interspace between the spines of the fourth and fifth lumbar vertebrae (Figure 129, page 213 and Figure 130, page 214).

4. The spines of the lumbar vertebrae are identified and marked (Figure 130, page 214).

5. The caudad portion of the transverse processes of each lumbar vertebra lies opposite the cephalad tip of its spinous process (Figure 131 A, page 215). Contact with the transverse process is made during the procedure only to determine the depth from the skin to the transverse process. In this technique one should try to avoid hitting the transverse process as much as possible, since periosteal stimulation makes the block more painful.

6. Horizontal lines are drawn through the middle of the spines of the lumbar vertebrae whose ganglia are to be blocked. These lines should extend over the spaces between the respective transverse processes (Figure 129, page 213 and Figure 130, page 214).

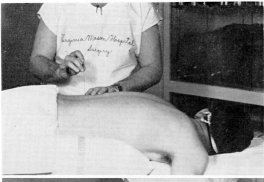

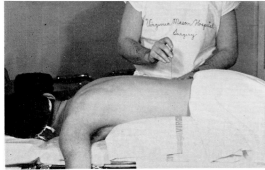

Figure 128. Position of patient and right-handed anesthetist for a lumbar sympathetic ganglion block. A. (Top) Left side. B. (Bottom) Right side.

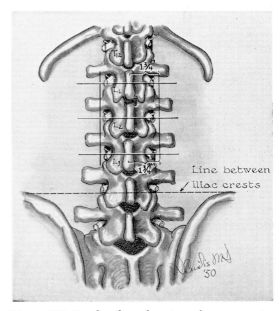

Figure 129. Landmarks and anatomy for a paravertebral lumbar sympathetic block.

7. A vertical line is now drawn parallel and 1¾ inches (4.5 cm.) to 2 inches (5 cm.), depending on the size of the patient, lateral to the spines of the vertebrae (Figure 129, page 213 and Figure 130, page 214). This line

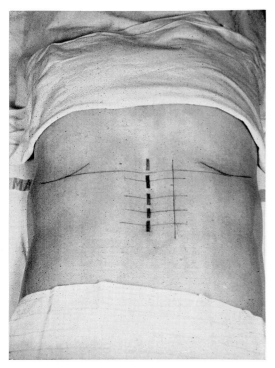

Figure 130. Determining the landmark for the lumbar sympathetic block. The straight line between the iliac crests passes through the interspace between the spine of the fourth and fifth lumbar vertebrae. A horizontal line is drawn through the middle of each of the spinous processes of the fourth, third, second, and first lumbar vertebrae respectively. A vertical line 1¾ inches (4.5 cm.) lateral and parallel to the spinous processes is drawn through the previously drawn horizontal lines. The point where the horizontal and vertical lines cross on the skin lies over a point between the lumbar transverse process just lateral to the body of the vertebra. Note that the patient is in the supine position with a pillow under his abdomen between the iliac crests and the twelfth rib.

should lie just lateral to the topographical anatomy of the body of the vertebra in question, and cross the horizontal lines drawn through the middle of the spines of the lumbar vertebrae whose ganglia are to be blocked.

8. The intersections of the lines made in

steps 6 and 7 mark the points of insertion of the needles.

Precautions

Aspirate.—Careful aspiration for spinal fluid and blood should be made in this region as the dura, vena cava, and abdominal aorta may be punctured.

Instruct Patient Not to Move.—The patient is instructed not to move. The back muscles are extremely strong, and coupled with the leverage of the bone, they may easily break a needle.

Procedure

1. The sterilizer control is checked to be sure the equipment has been sterilized.

2. The area is aseptically prepared and draped.

3. The anesthetist stands at the side of the patient to be blocked, facing the side of the cart or table (Figure 128, page 213).

4. Intradermal wheals are raised with a ¾-inch (2 cm.), 25-gauge Huber point security Lok-needle at the junction of the horizontal and vertical lines marking the lumbar sympathetic ganglia to be blocked.

5. Infiltration is then carried deeper with a 1½-inch (3.8 cm.), 22-gauge security Lok-needle. Should a longer needle be employed, a paravertebral block of the somatic nerve may be executed. This is to be avoided.

6. A 4-inch (10 cm.), 22- or 20-gauge security Lok-needle is then passed through the wheal opposite the middle of the spine of one of the lumbar vertebra whose ganglion is to be blocked, after the relationship of the markings on the hub of the needle to the bevel of the needle have been established. The point of the needle is inclined cephalad so that the shaft forms a 45-degree angle with the skin. The needle is then advanced until the transverse process of the lumbar vertebra is contacted. This is usually 1½ inches (3.8 cm.) to 2 inches (5 cm.) below the skin (Figure 131A, page 215). If a marker is used

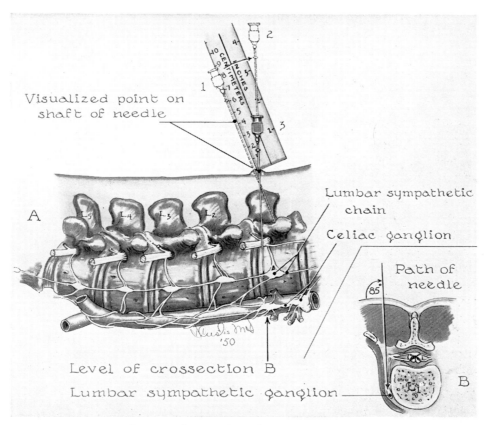

Figure 131. A. Sagittal section showing the technique of paravertebral lumbar sympathetic block. 1. Needle rests on the transverse process of the first lumbar vertebra. 2. Needle slightly withdrawn and directed caudad. Needle inserted to the visualized depth on the shaft of the needle and coming in close proximity to the lumbar sympathetic ganglion. The needle passes caudad to the transverse process of the first lumbar vertebra. B. Path of the needle in relationship to the cross section of the body.

on the needle, it should be set at that distance previous to the insertion of the needle. It is important to remember that this distance varies with the physique of the individual (Figure 127, page 212) and that it is often necessary to make two or three attempts at inserting the needle before the transverse process is located.

7. With the stainless steel ruler the anesthetist then measures 1¾ inches (4.5 cm.) to 2 inches (5 cm.) from the skin toward the hub of the needle (Figure 131A, page 215). The distance from this mark to the hub is visualized and remembered. If the depth marker is used, it should be reset to this point.

8. The needle point is now withdrawn to the subcutaneous tissue and tilted so that the shaft is parallel to the transverse plane of the body at an angle of 85 degrees to the skin in the sagittal plane of the body (Figure 131A, B, page 215). With the needle in this position, its point should pass caudally to the caudad edge of the transverse process (Figure 131A, page 215). The needle is rotated so that the opening in the needle faces the vertebra. With a quick thrust the needle is inserted to the visualized point on the needle (Figure 131A, page 215 and Figure 132A, B, page 216). If periosteum or bone of the body of the vertebra is encountered, the needle is partially withdrawn and reinserted with the shaft inclined a little more medially, i.e., perpendicular to the skin (90 degree angle), so the point slips off the body of the vertebra (Figure 131B, page 215).

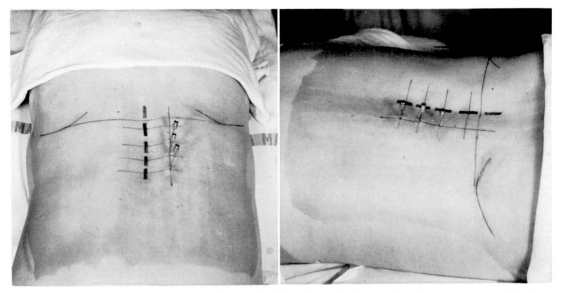

Figure 132. Same patient as Figure 130, the 4-inch (10 cm.) needles lie in place for the injection of the first, second, and third lumbar sympathetic ganglia. A. *(Left)* Front view. B. *(Right)* Lateral view.

9. After adequate aspiration tests, 10 cc. of the anesthetic solution is injected.

10. Two cc. of air is then pushed through the needle as it is withdrawn. This maneuver prevents anesthetic solution from being deposited on the sensory and motor nerves as the needle is withdrawn.

11. Needles are now inserted at the mark opposite the middle of the spines of the other lumbar vertebrae whose ganglia are to be blocked, as directed in 6 to 8 (Figure 132A, B, page 216). It is not necessary to locate the transverse process of the other lumbar vertebrae whose ganglia are to be blocked because the depth determined for one is satisfactory for the others. This means that a quick thrust of the needle to the visualized point is all that is necessary to place the other needles.

12. When the needles are in place the local anesthetic solution is injected and the needles withdrawn, as described in steps 9 and 10.

EFFECTS

If a successful block has been performed, the signs of vasodilatation of the lower extremities appear. These are: (1) increase in skin temperature; (2) absence of sweating of the skin; (3) redness of the skin; and (4) vascular dilatation.

Sensory or motor anesthesia should not result unless the lumbar somatic nerves have been anesthetized.

COMPLICATIONS

Toxic Reactions (intravascular injections, etc.): See Chapter 3, page 19.

Subarachnoid Injections: Rare occurrence. See Chapter 43, page 353.

Paralysis of Lumbar Nerves

Signs and Symptoms.—Partial or complete sensory and motor loss of the lower extremity.

Etiology.—Overflow of anesthetic solution onto the lumbar nerve due to faulty technique.

Course.—Disappears as anesthetic dissipates itself.

Treatment.—None.

REMARKS

Block Is Easy To Perform: This approach to the lumbar sympathetic ganglia is simple, easy, and causes the patient little discomfort. Serious complications are rare.

Block May Be Used in Outpatients: A large majority of the patients in whom this block is applicable may be treated as outpatients. Following the block they should be observed for at least one hour to see if any paralysis of the lumbar nerves occurs.

Omit or Use Small Amounts of Epinephrine (Adrenalin): Since most of these patients leave the office following the block, the epinephrine should either be omitted from the solution or a very small amount employed. Epinephrine reactions occur relatively frequently and are uncomfortable.

Measure Depth of Ganglia Once: The depth of the transverse process from the skin should be measured for one ganglion only. Stimulation of the periosteum of the transverse process is painful and it should be done only once. Where patients are to have a series of blocks, this measured distance should be marked on the chart and anesthetic record so that future blocks may be carried out without repeating this step.

Facts To Remember When Performing Diagnostic Block: When performing a diagnostic lumbar sympathetic block to prognosticate surgical results, the following should be remembered.

First, anesthesia of the lumbar nerves should be avoided.

Second, an unsuccessful block may be of no significance in prognosticating the outcome of a lumbar sympathectomy because: (1) the block technique may be faulty—a repeat of the sympathetic block on another day should be attempted to help rule out faulty block technique; and (2) fibers from the sympathetic chain on the opposite side may cross over. Because of these, some anesthetists prefer to administer a caudal or spinal block rather than a lumbar sympathetic block when dealing with therapeutic problems in hospitalized patients.

Third, when a block is unsuccessful, it should be checked with a spinal block to at least the ninth thoracic dermatome. If after the spinal block, signs of block of the sympathetic ganglion occur, i.e., increase in temperature, change in color of the extremities, etc., the anesthetist may assume one of the causes listed above influenced the first block. If after spinal block no signs of block of the sympathetic ganglion occur, then it is highly probable that surgery is not indicated.

Lastly, a successful block is very significant as the surgeon then can be fairly certain of his results.

Do Not Anesthetize Lumbar Somatic Nerves: When a therapeutic block is being performed on an outpatient, great care should be taken to avoid anesthetizing the lumbar nerves, since the patient will not be able to leave the office under his own power if this occurs.

Needle Point Should Pierce Fascia of Psoas Muscle: Anatomically, it is not necessary to place the needle right next to the body of the vertebra to have a successful block. As long as the needle has pierced the fascia surrounding the psoas muscle, it will lie in the same loose areolar tissue in which the lumbar sympathetic ganglion lies. Therefore, the anesthetic solution will by diffusion reach the ganglion.

Use Block Therapy Early—Not as Last Resort and Do a Series: Often in diseases where lumbar sympathetic ganglion block has proven its value, it is tried as the last resort when all other medical and surgical therapy has been exhausted. This is to be condemned. When problems in which a lumbar sympathetic ganglion block is known to be of value arise, it should be used immediately. The results should not be evaluated on the benefit derived from the first block. It is often necessary to perform a series of blocks, i.e., 7 to 10, before dramatic improvement occurs.

Puncture of Peritoneum and Organs Is Not Serious: Even if the needles are incorrectly placed, puncture of the peritoneum and abdominal or retroperitoneal organs is not a serious complication. These organs must be punctured occasionally by the specialist without his recognizing the fact or having a complication arise.

Indications for Spinal, Caudal, and Epidural Block in Preference to Lumbar Sympathetic Ganglion Block: When acute vascular emergencies of the lower extremities arise, and proficiency at lumbar sympathetic blocking has not been acquired, spinal, epidural, or caudal block should be considered as it may save part or all of an extremity.

When prolonged lumbar sympathetic block is indicated in the treatment of a vascular insufficiency of the extremity in a hospitalized patient, a continuous epidural, spinal, or caudal block should be considered. If these procedures are instituted, care of the bladder and rectum are of prime importance and should be anticipated.

Second, Third, and Fourth Lumbar Sympathetic Ganglia Control Circulation of Lower Extremity: The second, third, and fourth lumbar sympathetic ganglia are the most important of the lumbar sympathetic ganglia because to a large extent they control the circulation of the lower extremities. Many physicians feel that the second lumbar sympathetic ganglion is the most important in controlling the circulation to the lower extremities and only block that ganglion for vascular deficiency. However, in most instances a block of all three ganglia is a more satisfactory procedure.

Use of Anticoagulant Therapy and Lumbar Sympathetic Ganglia Block Concomitantly: Often physicians may wish to use lumbar sympathetic block in conjunction with anticoagulant therapy to correct vascular insufficiencies of the lower extremity.

At the present time, there are two aims in the therapy of abnormal vascular spasm from thrombosis or embolism. One is to reduce the spasm itself by sympathetic block, and the other is to prevent further clotting by anticoagulant drug administration. Obviously, the treatment of choice is to use both simultaneously. However, because of the reports of uncontrollable hemorrhage following the use of anticoagulants and sympathetic blocks con-

comitantly, one of these types of therapy but not both is usually decided upon. In spite of these reports, such fears are unfounded provided the physicians using the anticoagulant drugs and performing the sympathetic blocks are well acquainted with their usage. Serious and fatal hemorrhages have been blamed on anticoagulant drugs, when lack of skill on the part of the person administering them was the true cause. As with other therapeutic modalities, the safety of anticoagulant drugs, as well as sympathetic nerve blocks, used singly or in combination, depends entirely on the ability and knowledge of the person who is administering them. If due precautions are exercised, these two complementary forms of therapy can be used together safely for the benefit of the patient.

To date, it has been the author's experience that lumbar sympathetic blocks can be executed along with anticoagulant therapy without causing uncontrollable hemorrhage. If hemorrhage occurs when these two complementary forms of therapy are being used, the effects of the anticoagulant drug must be reversed.

Recover Broken Needle(s): All needles should be tested before use. If a needle breaks, every effort to recover it, including surgery, should be made. Unremoved needles have a tendency to migrate and may cause permanent injuries as well as medicolegal complications.

Repeat Block When Block Is Inadequate: If the desired results from the first block attempt are unsatisfactory, do not hesitate to reblock the patient if time permits. Most patients will think nothing about being reblocked if the second attempt is prefaced by a statement such as: "Well, I guess we will have to inject a little more medicine if we are going to freeze these nerves."

However, do not exceed the maximum safe dosage of the local anesthetic solution for both blocks. If to reblock the patient the maximum safe dose of the local anesthetic solution must be exceeded, 45 minutes should elapse between blocks.

PART II

PERIPHERAL NERVE BLOCK
ANESTHESIA

SECTION III

EXTREMITIES

CHAPTER 30

Supraclavicular Approach for Block of the Brachial Plexus

INDICATIONS

Surgical: Operations or manipulations of the shoulder joint, arm, forearm, and hand. Infection in the upper extremity, particularly if it is below the elbow, and the patient is on chemotherapy or an antibiotic, is not a contra-indication to the use of a brachial plexus block. The increased circulation of the extremity following the brachial plexus block may actually be beneficial in promoting healing (Figure 157, page 243).

Diagnostic: To differentiate central pain from peripheral pain.

Therapeutic: Severe pain of the upper extremity such as that caused by acute bursitis or herpes zoster may be relieved by a brachial plexus block when suprascapular nerve block and stellate ganglion block are not completely effective (Figure 133, page 221). Also, it may be used to block the sympathetic nerves when stellate ganglion block is contraindicated.

ANATOMY

The brachial plexus is formed by the union of the anterior rami of the lower cervical nerves (C5, 6, 7, 8) and the greater part of the anterior division of the first thoracic nerve (Figure 134, page 222). The fourth cervical and the second thoracic nerves usually send a small branch to the plexus. The plexus emerges from the neck together with the subclavian artery between the anterior and middle scalenus muscles (Figure 135, page 223 and Figure 136, page 224). The rami form three trunks (upper, middle, and lower), which

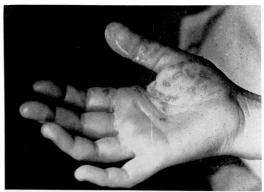
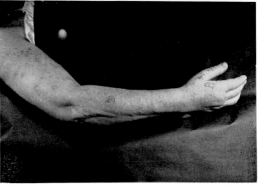

Figure 133. Herpes zoster of the brachial plexus which appears to be limited to the radial nerve. The patient was treated with three brachial blocks with immediate alleviation of pain and drying of the lesions after stellate ganglion block gave no relief.

split under the clavicle into anterior and posterior divisions. Therefore, the plexus passes over the first rib as divisions. These divisions reunite with each other to form cords in the region of the second part of the axillary artery. From these cords come the various nerves which innervate the shoulder joint, the outer surface of the upper arm, the forearm, and the hand (Figure 134, page 222).

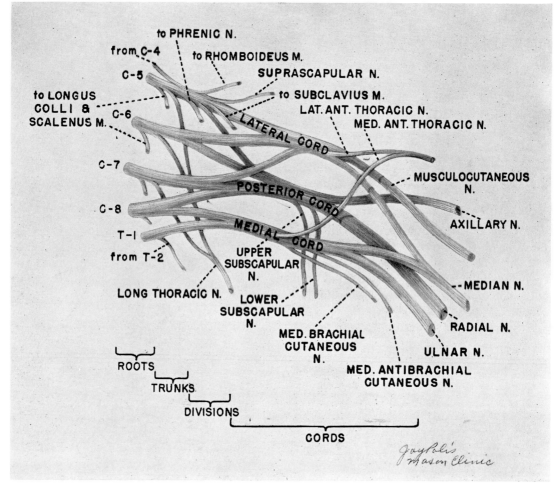

to PHRENIC N.
from C-4
C-5
to RHOMBOIDEUS M.
SUPRASCAPULAR N.
to LONGUS COLLI & SCALENUS M.
C-6
to SUBCLAVIUS M.
LAT. ANT. THORACIC N.
MED. ANT. THORACIC N.
LATERAL CORD
C-7
POSTERIOR CORD
MUSCULOCUTANEOUS N.
C-8
MEDIAL CORD
AXILLARY N.
T-1
from T-2
UPPER SUBSCAPULAR N.
LONG THORACIC N.
LOWER SUBSCAPULAR N.
MEDIAN N.
MED. BRACHIAL CUTANEOUS N.
RADIAL N.
ULNAR N.
MED. ANTIBRACHIAL CUTANEOUS N.
ROOTS
TRUNKS
DIVISIONS
CORDS

Figure 134. Anatomy of the brachial plexus. The divisions of the brachial plexus pass between the first rib and the clavicle.

PREMEDICATION

Paresthesias are always sought. Therefore, light premedication is advised.

Light Premedication: The average patient (age 20 to 50, weight 150 pounds, or over, height 5 feet, 5 inches or over, and good physical status) receives:

1. 200 mg. (3 gr.) of pentobarbital (Nembutal) by mouth at hour of sleep the night before surgery.

2. 100 mg. (1½ gr.) of pentobarbital by mouth with one ounce of water 1½ to 2 hours before estimated *block* time. This dose of barbiturate is omitted if there is a possibility that the patient will be too heavily sedated to give *an immediate response* when paresthesias are obtained .

3. 10 mg. (⅙ gr.) of morphine and 0.4 mg. (1/150 gr.) of scopolamine intramuscularly *on call* to surgery.

Reduction of Premedication: It is seldom necessary to increase this premedication irrespective of the over-all size of the patient until the patient arrives in either the anesthesia or operating room. However, it is very common to reduce this medication under various circumstances; for example, in the case of the geriatric patient, the adolescent patient or child, the debilitated or cachectic patient,

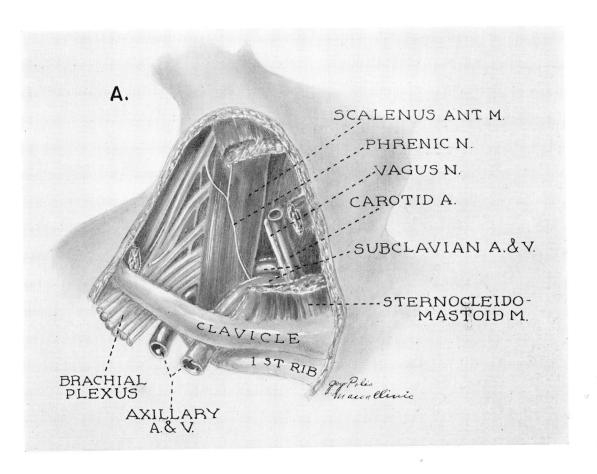

A.

SCALENUS ANT. M.

PHRENIC N.

VAGUS N.

CAROTID A.

SUBCLAVIAN A. & V.

STERNOCLEIDO-
MASTOID M.

CLAVICLE

1 ST RIB

BRACHIAL
PLEXUS

AXILLARY
A. & V.

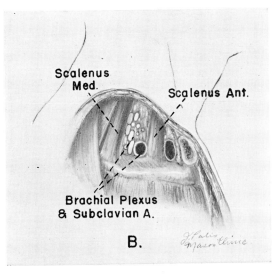

Scalenus
Med.

Scalenus Ant.

Brachial Plexus
& Subclavian A.

B.

Figure 135. A. Anatomy of the brachial plexus.
While in a drawing the brachial plexus is often
shown as lying in a straight line parallel to the
first rib, this relationship is not so. B. The plexus
when seen in a sagittal section lies in a random pattern one above another or one next to another.

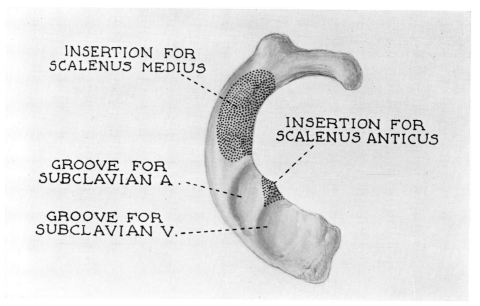

Figure 136. Anatomy of the first rib. Brachial plexus emerges between the anterior and medial scalenus muscles along with the subclavian artery. The artery lies in the groove between the insertion of these two muscles. The subclavian groove lies at the point on the rib where it starts to curve posteriorly.

and for those whose surgery is complicated by other disease, *e.g.*, myxedema, diabetes, heart disease, etc. In the patient over 60 years of age, barbiturates and especially scopolamine often cause disorientation. Therefore, in these patients atropine is usually substituted for scopolamine and the dosages of the barbiturate omitted or greatly reduced, *i.e.*, to 50 mg. (¾ gr.) or less. *Always err on the light side.*

Inadequate Premedication: If medication is inadequate either for the block or surgical procedure, intravenous pentobarbital 50 mg. (¾ gr.) to 100 mg. (1½ gr.) or intravenous morphine 8 mg. (⅛ gr.) to 15 mg. (¼ gr.) may be given *slowly.* Judicious use of added sedation is extremely important. Often small supplementary intravenous doses of morphine or pentobarbital will make a block successful, especially when a patient interprets touch and motion as pain.

DRUGS

Tetracaine (Pontocaine)

Dosage

Including half ring of arm, but *not* block of

superficial cervical plexus: 30 cc. to 50 cc. of 0.15 to 0.25 percent solution with or without 0.25 cc. of epinenephrine (Adrenalin) 1:1000 in each 50 cc. of solution.*

Including block of superficial cervical plexus: 60 cc. to 90 cc. of 0.15 percent solution with or without 0.25 cc. of epinephrine 1:1000.*

Onset.—Operating analgesia is established in 15 to 45 minutes, with an average of 20 minutes.

Duration.—Operating analgesia lasts 3½ to 6 hours, with stronger concentrations and solutions containing epinephrine giving the upper limits.

Procaine (Novocain)

Dosage

Including half ring of arm, but *not* block of superficial cervical plexus: 30 cc. to 50 cc. of

---

*Optimal concentration of epinephrine is 1:200,000 that is, 0.1 cc. of epinephrine 1:1000 in 20 cc. of the local anesthetic solution. Do not exceed 0.25 cc. of epinephrine 1:1000 even if amount of local anesthetic solution exceeds 50 cc. (see page 39).

1.0 to 2.0 percent solution with or without 0.25 cc. of epinephrine (Adrenalin) 1:1000 in each 50 cc. of solution.*

Including block of superficial cervical plexus: 60 cc. to 90 cc. of 1.0 percent solution with or without 0.25 cc. of epinephrine 1:1000.*

Onset.—Operating analgesia is established in 5 to 15 minutes.

Duration.—Operating analgesia lasts 1 to 1½ hours, with stronger concentrations and solutions containing epinephrine giving the upper limits.

Lidocaine (Xylocaine) or Mepivacaine (Carbocaine)

Dosage

Including half ring of arm, but *not* block of the superficial cervical plexus: 30 cc. to 50 cc. of 1.0 percent solution with or without 0.25 cc. of epinephrine (Adrenalin) 1:1000 in each 50 cc. of solution.*

Including block of the superficial cervical plexus: 60 cc. to 90 cc. of a 0.5 percent solution with or without 0.25 cc. of epinephrine 1:000.*

Onset.—Operating analgesia is established in 5 to 15 minutes.

Duration.—Operating analgesia lasts 1½ to 3 hours, with stronger concentrations and solutions containing epinephrine giving the upper limits.

Hyaluronidase: The use of 150 TRU of hyaluronidase in the local anesthetic solution does not insure a higher incidence of satisfactory brachial plexus block. But, it does prevent hematoma formation by hastening the absorption of blood from the tissues if the subclavian artery is inadvertently punctured. Prior to the use of hyaluronidase in brachial plexus block, we had a hematoma the size of

a chicken egg form from trauma to the subclavian artery after a brachial plexus block in one patient. It persisted without causing pain for six months before disappearing, and during this time the patient's only complaint was of swelling. X-ray studies revealed small areas of calcium in the hematoma but this was eventually absorbed. Now, hyaluronidase is incorporated in all the local anesthetic solutions used for supraclavicular brachial plexus blocks and no such complication has been observed. Before using hyaluronidase, see page 43.

MATERIALS

Regional tray (see Chapter 9, page 51) or:

1. One ¾-inch (2 cm.), 25-gauge Huber point security Lok-needle.

2. One 1½-inch (3.8 cm.), 22-gauge security Lok-needle, preferably with short bevel.

3. One 2-inch (5 cm.), 22-gauge security Lok-needle, preferably with short bevel.

4. One tuberculin Lok-syringe for measuring epinephrine.

5. One 10 cc. Lok-syringe, preferably with finger rings.

6. One graduated measuring cup, preferably stainless steel, for mixing solution.

7. One prep cup, preferably stainless steel.

8. Four sterile towels.

9. Six sterile sponges.

10. One sterilizer control.

TECHNIQUE

Position and Landmarks

1. The patient lies in the dorsal recumbent position without a pillow, his arms at his sides, and his head turned to the side opposite the one being blocked (Figure 137, page 226).

2. The patient is then instructed to raise his head 2 inches (5 cm.), approximately 20 degrees, off the table, putting strain on the neck muscles (Figure 138, page 226).

---

*Optimal concentration of epinephrine is 1:200,000 that is, 0.1 cc. of epinephrine 1:1000 in 20 cc. of the local anesthetic solution. Do not exceed 0.25 cc. of epinephrine 1:1000 even if amount of local anesthetic solution exceeds 50 cc. (see page 39).

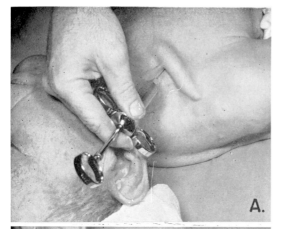

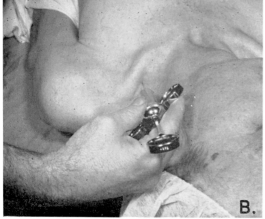

Figure 137. Position of the patient and the right-handed anesthetist for a brachial plexus block. A. Right side. B. Left side.

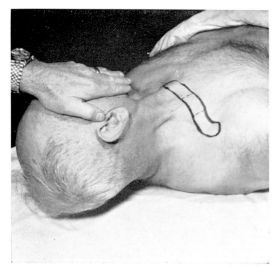

Figure 138. Patient raises his head off table against slight pressure from the anesthetist's hand. This allows easy identification of clavicular head of sternocleido-mastoid muscle.

3. The lateral border of the clavicular head of the sternocleidomastoid muscle is located and the muscle lateral to this, the anterior scalenus, is palpated. The patient is now instructed to lower his head and to keep it turned to the side opposite the one to be blocked. The brachial plexus makes its exit at the distal (lateral) border of the anterior scalenus muscle (Figure 135, page 223) and at this point, immediately above the clavicle, the skin is marked with an X (Figure 142, page 229). Usually, but not always, this point lies approximately at the middle of the clavicle and ½ inch (1.3 cm.) to ¾ inch (2 cm.) from the lateral border of the clavicular head of the sternocleidomastoid muscle (Figure 142, page 229). Furthermore, it lies over the rib at the groove for the subclavian artery—this is where the rib starts to turn posterior (Figure 136, page 224).

4. The subclavian artery should be located by palpation since it emerges along with the brachial plexus just lateral to the anterior scalenus muscle—this serves as a check on the other landmarks (Figure 135, page 223).

A sandbag may be placed under the patient's shoulder to permit his head to tilt posterior (Figure 140, page 228 and Figure 141, page 228). The tilting of the head makes it easier for the anesthetist to place the needle correctly.

Precautions

Do Not Puncture Jugular Vein.—One should avoid puncture of the jugular vein. If the mark for insertion of the needle lies over it, the determined point should be moved medially or laterally.

Keep Control of Needle at All Times.—The forward advance of the needle must be controlled constantly by the anesthetist firmly holding the hub of the needle between the index finger and thumb while the hand rests against the neck and shoulder (Figure 139, page 227). With the exception of Figure 139, page 227, the index finger and thumb were purposely removed from their usual mandatory position holding the hub of the needle. This

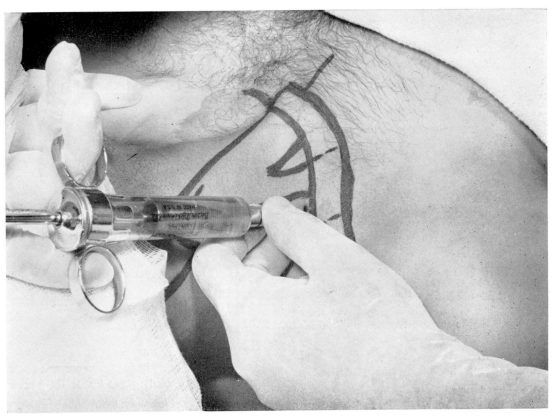

Figure 139. When the anesthetist is right-handed, the thumb and index finger of the left hand hold the hub of the needle while the hand rests against the neck and shoulder, giving the physician full control of the needle at all times. In this figure; Figure 138, page 226; Figure 140, page 228; and Figure 141, page 228; the clavicle was divided into thirds to emphasize that the spot for insertion of the needle is not at the junction of the inner two thirds and the outer third; but, usually, closer to the midpoint of the clavicle as shown in the other figures.

was done so that the direction of the needle could be demonstrated.

Keep Syringe on Needle.—Keep a full syringe on the end of the needle at all times when searching for the brachial plexus to permit immediate injection when a paresthesia occurs and to maintain the correct direction of the needle (Figure 139, page 227).

Rest the Needle on the Rib When Refilling the Syringe.—When refilling the syringe, be sure the needle point rests on or above the first rib, not in the pleura or lung substance.

Aspirate.—Before injecting, always aspirate to determine if the needle is inserted intravascularly or subarachnoidally. The latter is highly unlikely unless the dura has continued out with the nerve roots beyond an intervertebral foramen.

If blood is aspirated, do not become alarmed or discontinue the procedure. Withdraw the needle slowly until it is no longer in the vessel, keeping in mind its direction so that the needle may be reinserted in a slightly lateral direction. The chances are good that the needle was in the subclavian artery, an excellent landmark because the brachial plexus lies immediately lateral to it (Figure 140, page 228).

Withdraw Needle If Patient Coughs.—If the patient coughs, the needle should be withdrawn immediately since the pleura may have been stimulated or entered. This warning of pleural irritation is occasional. The usual signs

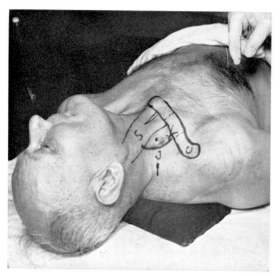

Figure 140. Needle rests in subclavian artery and a valuable landmark has been located. Blood is dripping from hub of needle. The syringe was removed from the needle to show that the bevel of the needle rests inside the artery.

that the pleura has been invaded are those of a pneumothorax.

A cough is no indication to discontinue the block. But, it does indicate that the point of the needle may be near the pleura and that it should be withdrawn and redirected.

Procedure

1. The sterilizer control is checked to be sure the equipment has been sterilized.

2. The area is aseptically prepared and draped.

3. The author prefers to stand at the side of the patient who is to be blocked, facing the head of the table (Figure 137, page 226 and Figure 141A, page 228). Because of the direction of the initial insertion of the needle, some anesthetists prefer to stand at the head of the patient, facing the foot of the table (Figure 141B, page 228).

4. An intradermal wheal is raised at the determined point with the ¾-inch (2 cm.), 25-gauge Huber point security Lok-needle (Figure 142, page 229).

5. A depth marker of rubber or cork may be set 1 inch (2.5 cm.) from the point of the needle. However, this is not necessary if the anesthetist is careful not to insert the needle more than 1 inch (2.5 cm.) at the start.

6. If the anesthetist is right-handed, the full 10 cc. Lok-syringe with the 1½-inch (3.8 cm.) or 2-inch (5 cm.), 22-gauge security Lok-needle

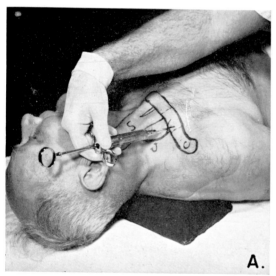

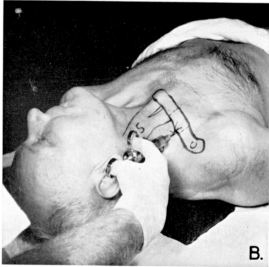

Figure 141. Position of the right-handed anesthetist for a brachial plexus block. The anesthetist may stand either at the patient's side (A) or at the head of the table (B). The author prefers to stand at the patient's side facing the head of the table. Sandbag under patient's shoulder allows head to tilt backward, permitting needle to be placed perpendicular to skin. Finger ring of syringe lies at tragus of ear for initial insertion.

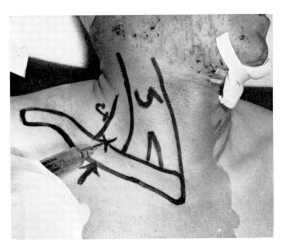

Figure 142. S. sternocleidomastoid muscle. J. jugular vein. Skin wheal is being raised at the X which is located at: (1) the midpoint of the clavicle—marked by the black arrow; (2) the cephalad border of the clavicle; and (3) the lateral border of the anterior scalenus muscle. This illustration and illustration A. in Figures 143, 146, 148, 149, and 150 were obtained by placing the camera in the position in which the anesthetist's eyes normally would be located. This is why the illustrations are in an upright position—this is the way the anesthetist standing at the side of the patient views the patient.

attached is held in the right hand (Figure 139, page 227 and Figure 141, page 228).

7. The patient is instructed to say *"Now"* and not move as soon as he feels a "tingle" or electric shock go down his arm. *Paresthesias of the brachial plexus are characterized by sharp, spraying, electric shock sensations which radiate down the arm to the fingertips. Since it is possible to stimulate the various divisions of the plexus, the paresthesias may radiate to the various parts of the hand but for assurance of a good block they should be elicited in all fingers as well as the thumb.*

8. The needle is inserted through the skin wheal and advanced *slowly* caudad, slightly mediad and slightly backward. *When the initial attempt to contact the first rib is made, the shaft of the needle and the syringe should be almost parallel to the patient's head and the right-handed anesthetist's right hand should rest or almost rest against the patient's head* (Figure 137, page 226; Figure 141, page 228; and Figure 143, page 229). The needle should

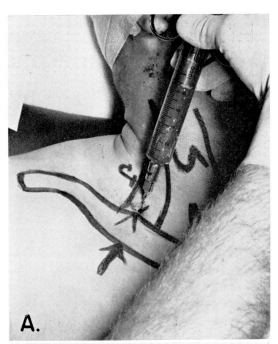

A.

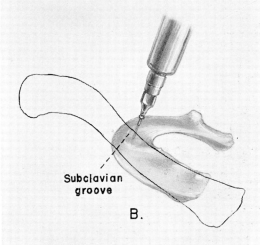

Subclavian groove

B.

Figure 143. A. S, sternocleidomastoid muscle. J, external jugular vein, and black arrow middle of clavicle. The 2-inch (5 cm.) needle is inserted at X, which marks the lateral border of the anterior scalenus muscle. The needle has just contacted the first rib and elicited a paresthesia in a 210 pound, 6-foot, 2-inch patient. The left hand has been removed from its usual position holding the hub of the needle (Figure 139) so that the direction of the syringe and the needle can be better viewed by the reader. The anesthetist's hand almost rests against the patient's head. The ring on the syringe lies at about the tragus of the ear. B. Schematic drawing showing that the needle rests on the first rib approximately in the groove for the subclavian artery. This is the point where the rib starts to turn toward the first thoracic vertebra.

be guided close to the subclavian artery, to which the plexus lies laterally. At no time when seeking the rib should the needle point be directed too mediad or cephalad. Otherwise, it will slip over the first rib and may pierce the pleura and lung substance. The index finger and thumb of the left hand firmly hold the hub of the needle and control the movement of the needle at all times (Figure 139, page 227).

This direction of placing the needle has also been described as vertically downward and inwards.

9. If paresthesias should occur before the first rib is encountered, the anesthetist freezes the needle and injects one-half the contents of the syringe after the aspiration test. Then the needle and syringe are rotated 180 degrees and the remaining solution is injected after the aspiration test (Figure 144, 1, page 230).

10. The point of the needle with empty syringe attached is advanced without changing the direction until the point of the needle is brought to rest on the first rib (Figure 144, 2, page 230).

11. The needle is held securely against the rib with the left hand and the syringe is detached, refilled, and reattached. Then as the needle is withdrawn slowly to the skin, the content of the syringe is discharged (Figure 144, 3, page 230).

12. The syringe is refilled, reattached to the needle, and the needle reinserted until it contacts the rib. Now the anesthetist should seek additional paresthesias by walking the needle forward, backward, and toward the vertebral column on the first rib as described in steps 14, 15, 16, and 17.

13. If no paresthesia occurs and if the first rib is not encountered after a redirection and

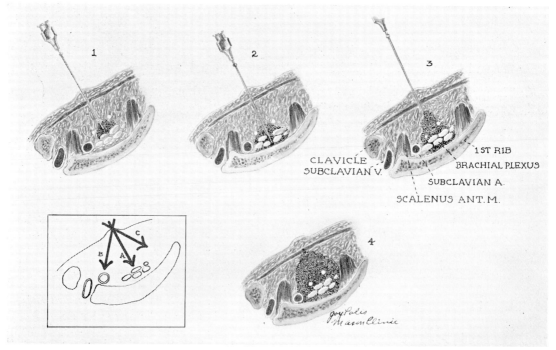

CLAVICLE
SUBCLAVIAN V.

1ST RIB
BRACHIAL PLEXUS

SUBCLAVIAN A.

SCALENUS ANT. M.

Figure 144. Method of injecting the plexus to assure a complete block. 1. Needle fixed when a paresthesia occurs and the syringe contents emptied. 2. Needle is pushed onto the rib and the syringe refilled. 3. The content of the syringe is discharged as the needle is withdrawn. 4. Shows the end results which may be accomplished if injection as described in 1, 2, and 3 are carried out as shown in this insert. C. ½-inch (1.3 cm.) posterior to arrow A. and B. ½-inch (1.3 cm.) anterior to arrow A. The insert assumes that arrow A. represents the initial paresthesia.

reinsertion of the needle at a 1-inch (2.5 cm.) depth, one should slowly advance the needle until the first rib is located. The depth of the first rib from the skin may vary from ¾ inch (2 cm.) to 2 inches (5 cm.) depending on the build of the individual and the depression of the skin by the needle's security bead. In most instances the brachial plexus lies just above the first rib. If the anesthetist will not advance his needle more than ¾ inch (2 cm.) to 1 inch (2.5 cm.) from the skin, many blocks will be missed (Figure 145, page 231 and Figure 143, page 229).

The distance from the skin to the first rib should be carefully noted and it should be used as a guide for all further insertions of the needle. As the needle is walked forward, backward, and toward the vertebral column (posteriorly) on the rib and the local anesthetic solution injected, the needle may have to be inserted slightly deeper, i.e., ¼ inch (0.6 cm.) to ⅜ inch (1.0 cm.) in order to contact the first rib. But, under no circumstances should the needle be advanced deeper. Otherwise the chance of producing a pneumothorax is greatly increased. The need for inserting the needle ¼ inch (0.6 cm.) to ⅜ inch (1.0 cm.) deeper is caused by: (1) the moving of the needle a greater distance away from the point of the initial insertion—the shortest distance from the skin to the rib usually occurs with the initial insertion of the needle; (2) an increase in distance between the skin and first rib from injecting the local anesthetic solution or from puncturing a blood vessel with extravasation of blood; or (3) a combination of these.

14. After the rib is encountered, the anesthetist, by gently tapping the point of the nee-

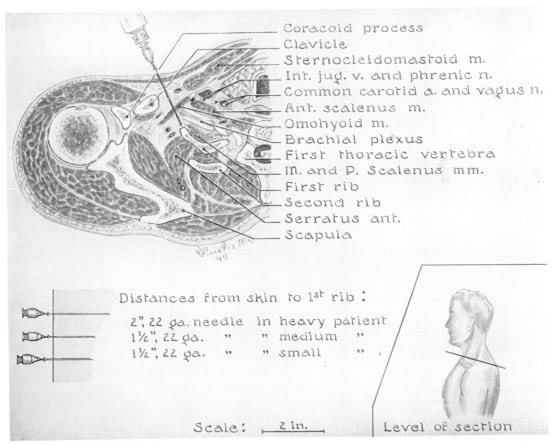

Coracoid process
Clavicle
Sternocleidomastoid m.
Int. jug. v. and phrenic n.
Common carotid a. and vagus n.
Ant. scalenus m.
Omohyoid m.
Brachial plexus
First thoracic vertebra
M. and P. Scalenus mm.
First rib
Second rib
Serratus ant.
Scapula

Distances from skin to 1st rib :

2", 22 ga. needle in heavy patient
1½", 22 ga.   "   " medium   "
1½", 22 ga.   "   " small   " .

Scale: 2 in. | Level of section

Figure 145. Scale drawing showing the depth to which the needle must be inserted from the skin in order to reach the first rib in patients of various builds.

dle, walks it forward (anteriorly) along the rib for approximately ½ inch (1.3 cm.), maintaining the *initial plane of direction* of the needle and seeking paresthesias (Figure 146A,

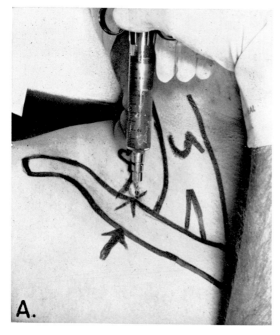

A.

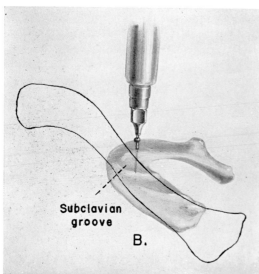

Subclavian groove

B.

Figure 146. A. Needle has been walked anteriorly (forward) on rib ½ inch (1.3 cm.). Note direction of hand and syringe and compare it with Figure 143, page 229. Hand is still close to head, finger ring of syringe is now posterior to tragus of ear, and is in same directional plane as original insertion. B. Schematic drawing showing needle resting at anterior edge of the groove for the subclavian artery.

page 232). He should keep in mind the anatomy of the first rib and conform with it (Figure 146 B, page 232). *The needle must not be walked the width of the rib instead of the length of the rib or a pneumothrorax may occur (Figure 147, page 233).*

With each thrust of the needle, aspiration tests should be made to see that the needle point is not in the subclavian artery. But if it is, the anesthetist should not become alarmed; he has found a valuable landmark (Figure 140, page 228). By withdrawing the needle ½ inch (1.3 cm.) and reinserting it ⅛ inch (0.3 cm.) laterally to the subclavian artery, paresthesias will usually be elicited as the needle is slowly advanced.

15. Then, the needle is walked backward beyond the point where the original insertion was made maintaining the same *plane of direction* until the needle is walked off the rib (Figure 148, page 233). This is the point where the rib starts to turn posterior to connect to the vertebra (Figure 148, page 233). No pneumothorax will occur from walking the needle off the rib in this direction because the needle point passes to the outside of the rib cage.

16. The needle's point is now replaced on the first rib (Figure 149, page 234).

17. *Now and only now* can the needle be walked posteriorly on the rib toward the first vertebra being certain that the needle will not enter the lung—this is done for ½ inch (1.3 cm.) (Figure 150, page 234).

18. If at any time while walking the rib from the lateral border of the anterior scalenus muscle to the anterior border of the medial scalenus muscle (steps 14, 15, 16, and 17) paresthesias are obtained, the needle should be frozen and 5 cc. to 8 cc. of the anesthetic solution injected. If the rib is walked from the lateral border of the anterior scalenus muscle to the anterior border of the medial scalenus muscle and if injections are carried out as described in steps 9, 10, 11, and 12 when paresthesias are elicited, all the divisions of the brachial plexus should be anesthetized with the

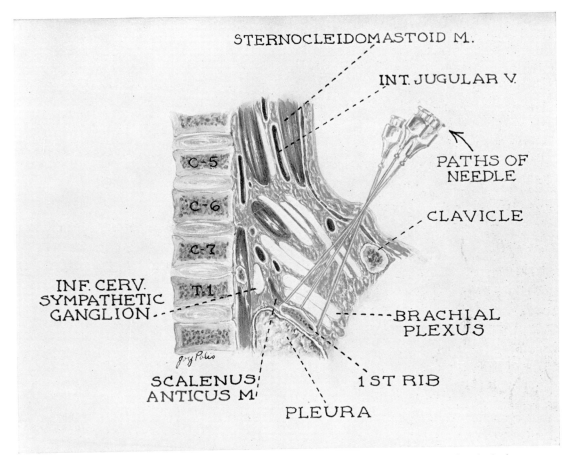

STERNOCLEIDOMASTOID M.

INT. JUGULAR V.

C-5

C-6

C-7

T-1

PATHS OF
NEEDLE

CLAVICLE

INF. CERV.
SYMPATHETIC
GANGLION

BRACHIAL
PLEXUS

SCALENUS
ANTICUS M.

1ST RIB

PLEURA

Figure 147. Incorrect method of "walking" the rib with the needle when performing a brachial plexus nerve block. "Walking" the width of the rib as shown in this drawing rather than the length of the rib as shown in Figure 146, page 232 and Figures 148 through 150, pages 233 to 234, will result in a high incidence of pneumothoraces.

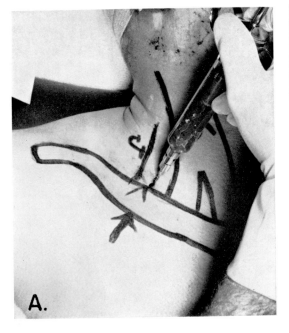

A.

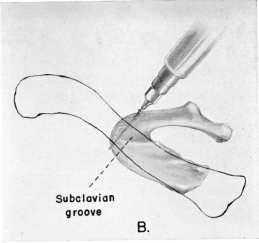

Subclavian
groove

B.

Figure 148. A. Needle has been walked backward on the rib maintaining its original directional plane until it no longer contacts the rib—finger ring of syringe is now anterior to tragus of ear. B. Schematic drawing showing needle's position off rib.

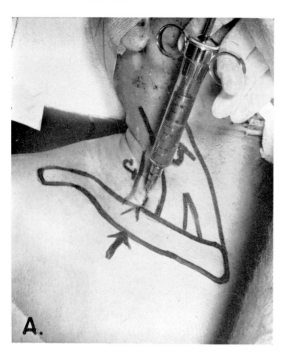

A.

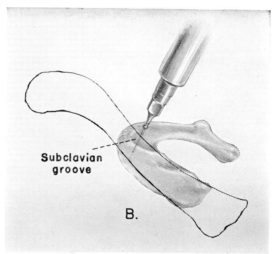

Subclavian
groove

B.

Figure 149. A. Needle has been replaced on the rib. B. Schematic drawing of needle's location on rib. Now and only now should the point of the needle be directed medially toward the vertebral column in an attempt to walk it posteriorly on the rib.

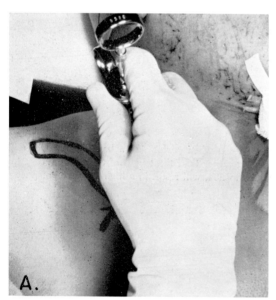

A.

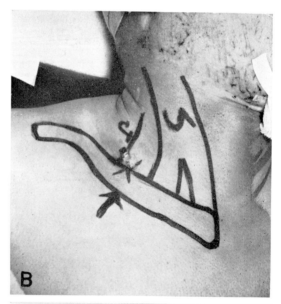

B

Figure 150. A. The needle has been walked posteriorly on the rib. With the camera located as noted in Figure 142, page 229, only the hand can be seen. B. Syringe removed to show direction of needle. With the position of the camera, the anesthetist is actually looking down the lumen and shaft of the needle when it is in this position. C. Schematic drawing showing point where needle contacts rib approximately at anterior border of insertion of medial scalenus muscle on the first rib.

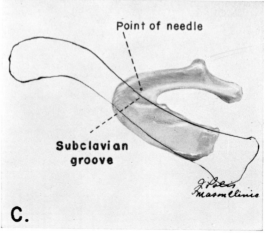

Point of needle

Subclavian
groove

C.

exception of the medial brachial cutaneous and the intercostal brachial nerves.

19. After the block has been executed, pressure and massage over the intradermal wheal will help spread the solution.

DISTRIBUTION OF ANALGESIA

Nerves and Areas Anesthetized: Operations on the lower arm, hand, fingers, and the upper outer arm below the insertion of the deltoid may be performed. Dislocated shoulders may be reduced. Skin analgesia exists over the upper outer arm, the forearm, and the hand (Figure 151, page 235).

The nerves of the brachial plexus, which innervate the arm and are anesthetized by this block, are the axillary nerve, the medial an-

tebrachial cutaneous nerve, the musculocutaneous nerve, the radial nerve, the ulnar nerve, and the median nerve. The skin distribution of these nerves is shown in Figure 152, page 236.

Additional Nerves Which Must Be Blocked to Eliminate Tourniquet Pain: When a tourniquet is to be applied to the upper arm, additional intradermal and subcutaneous local infiltration is necessary in the axilla to block the intercostobrachial (T2) and the medial brachial cutaneous (T1 and T2) nerves. This need only be a half ring (Figure 153B, page 237).

Additional Nerves Which Must Be Blocked for Operations on Inner Upper Forearm, Elbow, or Upper Arm: When brachial plexus

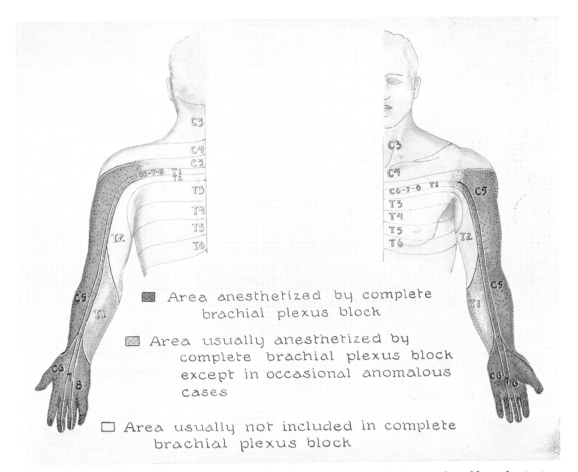

Figure 151. Skin anesthesia created by a complete brachial block. It clearly shows why additional injections are needed for operations on the shoulder and upper inner arm.

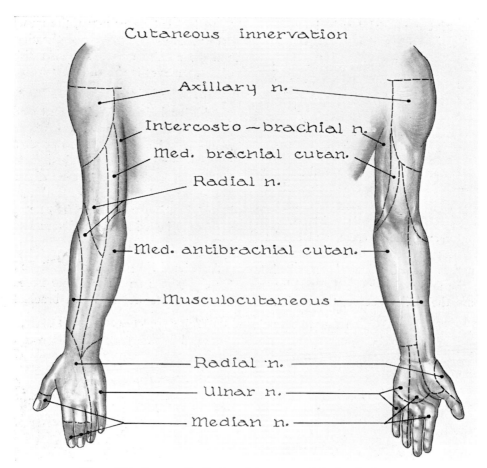

Cutaneous innervation

Axillary n.

Intercosto-brachial n.

Med. brachial cutan.

Radial n.

Med. antibrachial cutan.

Musculocutaneous

Radial n.

Ulnar n.

Median n.

Figure 152. Sensory distribution of the nerves of the brachial plexus.

block is used for operations on the elbow, or on the inner upper arm, additional intradermal and subcutaneous local infiltration is necessary in the axilla. This need only be a half ring (Figure 153B, page 237). If this is not done, the intercostobrachial (T2) and the medial brachial cutaneous (T1 and 2) nerves will not permit surgical incision (Figure 151, page 235 and Figure 152, page 236).

Additional Nerves Which Must Be Blocked for Operations on Shoulder: When brachial plexus block is employed for open surgical operations on the shoulder, additional intradermal and subcutaneous infiltrations are necessary to anesthetize the superficial cervical plexus, the intercostobrachial nerve, and the medial brachial cutaneous nerve. Two methods will accomplish this, depending on the type of incision. The first consists of a block

of the superficial cervical plexus by intradermal and subcutaneous local infiltration along the clavicle and border of the trapezius combined with the half ring of the axilla (Figure 153A, page 237). And, the alternate method consists of an intradermal and subcutaneous ring of local infiltration around the arm starting at the coracoacromial junction (Figure 153C, page 237).

COMPLICATIONS

Serious ones ensue very infrequently.

Horner's Syndrome (Stellate Ganglion Block): Occurs in approximately 70 to 90 percent of brachial blocks when 50 cc. or more of the local anesthetic solution is injected (Figure 73, page 129).

Signs and Symptoms.—Occur on the blocked

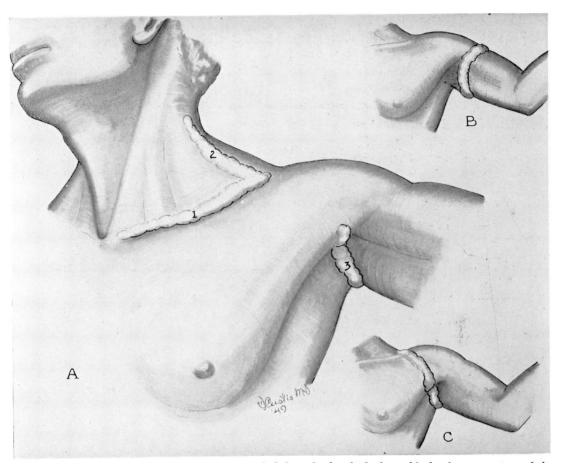

Figure 153. Method of anesthetizing areas not included in the brachial plexus block when operations of the shoulder and upper inner arm are undertaken. A. 1 and 2. Field block of the superficial cervical plexus by injection along the clavicle and border of the trapezius muscle. 3. Block of the intercostobrachial and medial brachial cutaneous nerves. B. ½ ring block of the intercostobrachial and medial brachial cutaneous nerves. C. Ring block of the superficial cervical plexus and intercostobrachial and medial brachial cutaneous nerves.

side so the signs and symptoms are unilateral and consist of flushed face, constricted pupil, ptosis of eyelid, vascular engorgement of the conjunctiva, enophthalmus, narrowed palpebral fissure, increase in skin temperature on affected side of the face, anhydrosis of face of affected side, and stuffiness of nose.

Etiology.—The anesthetic solution spreads so that it involves the stellate ganglion (Figure 69, page 126).

Course.—The syndrome clears as the block is dissipated.

Treatment.—No treatment is necessary and the appearance of this complication should cause the anesthetist little concern. The signs and symptoms should be explained to the patient with assurance that they will disappear as the block dissipates. This is essential to avoid unnecessary alarm in the average patient.

Pneumothorax: Frequency of occurrence is approximately 0.5 to 4 percent, and decreases as the anesthetist becomes more skilled. The *tall, thin* patient, who characteristically has a high apical pleura, usually accounts for the greater number of pneumothoraces.

Signs and Symptoms.—Occur on the blocked side and depend on the severity of the pneumothorax. The first indication is pain in the chest, accentuated by deep breathing. This may be the only sign that the pleura and lung have been invaded. Initial x-ray, auscultation, and percussion may not reveal the cause (Figure 154, page 238). They should be repeated in six hours if pain persists. It is not uncommon for x-ray signs not to become positive until hours after the block has been performed (Figure 154, page 238). Some cases have not complained of pain until 12 hours following the block. When the pneumothorax is greater than 20 percent, the following are present: (1) increase in resonance to percussion; (2) absent or decreased breath sounds; (3) lag of expansion on the affected side in comparison to the unaffected side; and (4) the patient

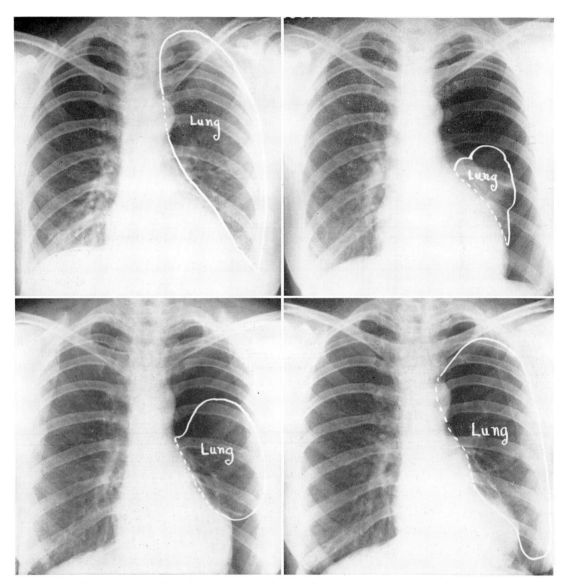

Figure 154. This patient complained of pain in her chest at the time of the brachial block. A. *(Top left)* X-ray taken six hours after the block had been performed and the surgery completed shows no evidence of pneumothorax. The difference in density of the left chest in this x-ray is caused by the shadow of the scapula, not air in the chest. B. *(Top right)* X-ray taken the following day shows an almost complete pneumothorax. Following this film 1000 cc. of air were withdrawn from the chest. C. *(Bottom left)* X-ray taken four days following film B after repeated withdrawal of 1000 cc. of air from the chest on successive days. D. *(Bottom right)* X-ray taken two days after film C shows lung 80 percent expanded.

complains of difficulty in "getting his breath" when he lies on the affected side.

Dyspnea usually occurs initially and then may subside. There may or may not be a change in the blood pressure, indicating respiratory embarrassment or shift of the mediastinum. At times air may be felt in the tissue at the site of the insertion of the needle. Occasionally a marked subcutaneous and mediastinal emphysema may occur (Figure 155, page 239).

Etiology.—Some physicians have attributed the pneumothorax which occasionally accompanies this block to the piercing of the pleura with air entering through the needle. However, this seems unlikely for a number of reasons: (1) it has been proven a difficult maneuver in tuberculosis sanitariums where therapeutic pneumothoraces are performed; (2) many of the pneumothoraces which are seen following a block do not occur for two to six hours following the procedure (Figure 154, page 238); and (3) a syringe is kept on the end of the needle at all times while seeking paresthesias, and it is removed only when the needle rests on or above the rib.

It is felt by the author that most pneumothoraces are caused by the piercing of the lung substance proper by a misplaced needle. If this is not rectified immediately, inhalation and exhalation occur, and the lung surface is torn by the needle point. The pneumothorax that occurs is then caused by air escaping from the lung, not entering through the needle.

Treatment.—Symptomatic treatment of the dyspnea with oxygen and the pain with intra-

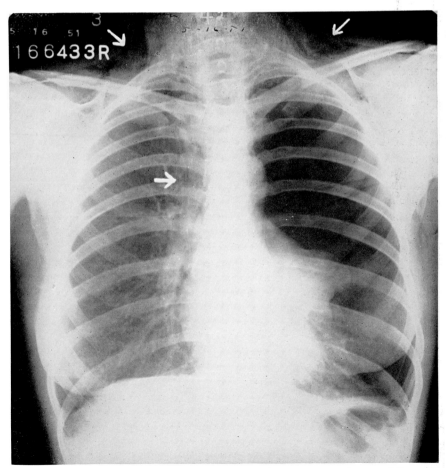

Figure 155. Pneumothorax with mediastinal and subcutaneous emphysema following a brachial block. Arrows mark areas of emphysema.

venous opiates should be instituted immediately if the initial discomfort is marked. The patient's anxiety should be soothed by assuring him that everything will be all right. A 6-foot x-ray should be taken immediately if surgery is cancelled or after surgery is completed to ascertain the extent of the pneumothorax. If no pneumothorax is found, the x-ray should be repeated in six hours (Figure 154, page 238). *Bedside x-rays are misleading, uncertain, cause improper treatment, and are a waste of the x-ray department's time and the patient's money, and should not be taken.*

If the pneumothorax is slight, *i.e.*, 20 percent or less, no treatment is necessary because the lung will re-expand. Codeine and aspirin may be given for pain and discomfort. If the pneumothorax exceeds 20 percent, then aspiration of air from the pleural cavity is indicated. Re-expansion of the lung by positive pressure may be used but it may tend to keep the hole in the lung open. X-rays of the chest should be taken at one- to two-day intervals to be sure expansion is proceeding. After the lung shows progressive expansion, the patient should have a chest x-ray at least once a week until complete re-expansion has taken place.

Block of the Phrenic Nerve: This complication occurs in 40 to 60 percent of the cases (Figure 156, page 240).

Signs and Symptoms.—Usually none. Close observation of the chest during inspiration and expiration may reveal no diaphragmatic action on the side or sides which have been blocked. However, if a bilateral block is performed on a patient with an underlying chest disease, particularly an old marked emphysema, and a bilateral phrenic block occurs, signs of an oxygen want, *i.e.*, dyspnea, cyanosis, increased blood pressure and pulse, and restlessness may result (Figure 156, page 240).

Etiology.—Spread of the anesthetic solution over the anterior surface of the anterior scalenus muscle (Figure 135A, page 223).

Course.—Clears as the block dissipates itself.

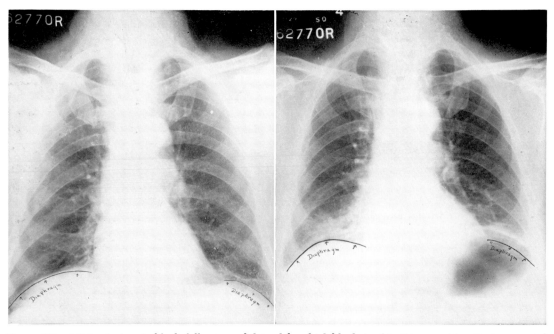

Figure 156. Bilateral phrenic block following a bilateral brachial block in this 75 year old patient presented the signs and symptoms of acute oxygen want because of the marked emphysema and fixed ribs. His distress lasted six hours until the block dissipated itself. During this time an oxygen tent was necessary. A. *(Left)* Chest x-ray previous to surgery. B. *(Right)* Chest x-ray two hours postoperatively. Note the bilateral elevation of the diaphragm.

Treatment.—None is usually necessary. If signs of oxygen want occur, oxygen under pressure should be given by bag and mask, or other forms of oxygen therapy may suffice (Figure 156, page 240).

Toxic Reactions (intravascular injections, etc.): See Chapter 3, page 19.

Subarachnoid Injection: Rarely occurs. See Chapter 43, page 353.

Neurological Complications: These occur very infrequently and when they do, they are usually due to faulty position of the anesthetized arm rather than due to the block.

Signs and Symptoms.—Those typical of a nerve injury.

Etiology.—The most frequent reason for neurological complications is faulty positioning of the anesthetized arm during surgery or in the immediate postoperative period. All pressure points should be padded to avoid this. Improperly applied casts to the anesthetized arm should be avoided with particular care as the patient will not be cognizant of pressure with the arm in this state.

Occasional trauma by the needle, prolonged ischemia of the nerve due to the vasoconstrictor drug, or a too concentrated anesthetic solution may be the offender.

Course.—Usually, time cures these injuries in days to months.

Treatment.—Large doses of thiamine chloride should be given, *i.e.*, 100 mg. t.i.d. by mouth or intramuscularly. Physiotherapy by trained technicians and exercise at home are invaluable in the prevention of atrophy.

A neurologic consultation should be obtained to establish the level, extent, and treatment of the lesion as well as to avoid and protect against medicolegal action (see page 11).

Arteriovenous Fistula Following Brachial Plexus Block: This complication following supraclavicular brachial plexus block from puncture of the subclavian artery and vein is unlikely because the subclavian artery is separated from the subclavian vein by the anterior scalenus muscle (Figure 135, page 223 and Figure 136, page 224). In over 2,500 supraclavicular brachial plexus blocks, we have not seen this complication.

REMARKS

Elicit Paresthesias: Paresthesias which radiate to the hand should be elicited if at all possible to assure adequate block. Remember the dictum, *"No paresthesias, no anesthesia"* and the failures will be minimal. When the anesthetist seeks paresthesias the patient may complain of pain in the chest. In the greater number of cases this is usually due to stimulation of the long thoracic nerve, but the anesthetist should consider the possibility of pleural irritation.

When performing a brachial plexus block on a child under basal narcosis, a heavily medicated adult, or a stoic patient, the anesthetist should give particular attention to facial expressions as well as to the arm and hand of the side being blocked. Even if the patient will not verbally indicate that a paresthesia has occurred, his arm or hand will suddenly twitch or move, or he will wince when the brachial plexus is stimulated.

There is no contraindication to using a large volume of anesthetic agent in the region of the brachial plexus. 50 cc. or more may be injected, providing the maximum toxic dosage is not exceeded; however, large amounts will not give better or longer analgesia than small amounts. *No matter how great the volume, the anesthetic solution must be placed correctly, and this requires eliciting paresthesias.*

Is It Mandatory To Locate the First Rib? Prior to exploring for paresthesias, we always attempt to locate the first rib because once it is contacted we know how to direct the needle and not puncture the lung.

However, if paresthesias are elicited before contacting the first rib, injection of the local anesthetic solution will result in satisfactory anesthesias—the eliciting of paresthesias is essential.

Brachial Block with Supraclavicular Ap-

proach Most Satisfactory Method of Blocking Upper Extremity: It is the author's opinion that from the standpoint of the patient, surgeon, and anesthetist brachial plexus block using the supraclavicular approach is the most satisfactory of all regional procedures for anesthetizing the upper extremity.

Comparison of Supraclavicular Approach and Axillary Approach for Blocking of the Brachial Plexus: See Chapter 31, pages 255 and 256.

Beginner Should Not Attempt Bilateral Block: Since bilateral pneumothorax is a serious problem, bilateral brachial plexus block with the supraclavicular approach should not be attempted by the beginner.

Preservation of Motor Function Is Difficult: If motor function is to be preserved while sensory fibers are blocked, a very weak concentration of the local anesthetic solution must be employed, and even then motor function usually will not be preserved.

Swelling of Arm Can Be Avoided or Reduced by Block: If marked swelling of the arm exists from an injury, or if it is wise to avoid marked swelling following an operation or manipulation, brachial plexus block is the anesthesia of choice since it tends to reduce whatever swelling is present and often prevents more.

Etiology of and Relief of Tourniquet Pain: Often nerve fibers of the autonomic nervous system, *e.g.*, Kuntz's nerves, will accompany the blood vessels to the arm and will not be anesthetized by the brachial plexus block. Also, it is possible that every nerve fiber in the plexus is not anesthetized. This is especially true of the large nerves. About forty-five minutes after the tourniquet is inflated, the ischemia may occasionally cause these small unanesthetized nerves to send out painful stimuli which are usually interpreted as aching. This aching may be relieved by: (1) small intravenous doses of an opiate; (2) releasing and reapplying the tourniquet; or (3) a half ring of local infiltration just distal to the axilla when the block is executed (Figure 153B, page 237).

Recover Broken Needle(s): All needles should be tested before use. If a needle breaks, every effort to recover it, including surgery, should be made. Unremoved needles have a tendency to migrate and may cause permanent injuries as well as medicolegal complications.

Repeat Block When Analgesia Is Inadequate: Since the brachial plexus is divided into divisions as it passes over the first rib, it is possible to have excellent anesthesia of one division and no anesthesia of the others. If this occurs, do not hesitate to reblock the patient if time permits. Most patients will think nothing about being reblocked if the second attempt is prefaced with a statement such as: "Well, I guess we will have to inject a little more medicine if we are going to freeze this area."

However, do not exceed the maximum safe dosage of the local anesthetic solution for both blocks. If to reblock the patient the maximum safe dose of the local anesthetic solution must be exceeded, 45 minutes should elapse between blocks.

CHAPTER 31

Axillary Approach for Block of the Brachial Plexus

INDICATIONS

Surgical: Operations or manipulations of the arm, forearm, and hand. Infection in the upper extremity, particularly if it is below the elbow, and the patient is on chemotherapy or an antibiotic, is not a contraindication to the use of a brachial plexus block (Figure 157,

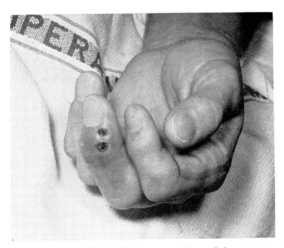

Figure 157. Axillary block was performed for incision and drainage of finger in this outpatient.

page 243). The increased circulation of the extremity following the brachial plexus block may actually be beneficial in promoting healing.

Diagnostic: To differentiate central pain from peripheral pain.

Therapeutic: Severe pain of the upper extremity such as that caused by acute bursitis or herpes zoster may be relieved by a brachial plexus block when suprascapular nerve block and stellate ganglion block are not completely effective (Figure 133, page 221). Also, it may be used to block the sympathetic nerves when stellate ganglion block is contraindicated.

ANATOMY

The brachial plexus is formed by the union of the anterior rami of the lower cervical nerves (C5, 6, 7, 8) and the greater part of the anterior division of the first thoracic nerve (Figure 134, page 222). The fourth cervical and the second thoracic nerves usually send a small branch to the plexus. The plexus emerges from the neck together with the subclavian artery between the anterior and middle scalenus muscles (Figure 135, page 223). The rami form three trunks (upper, middle, and lower), which split under the clavicle into anterior and posterior divisions.

The subclavian artery becomes the axillary artery at the outer border of the first rib and the axillary artery becomes the brachial artery at the lower border of the teres major muscle (Figure 158, page 244). For description purposes, the axillary artery is divided into three parts, the first lies above, the second behind, and the third part below the pectoralis minor muscle (Figure 158, page 244).

In the axilla, the divisions of the brachial plexus lie lateral to the first part of the axillary artery and they reunite with each other to form cords in the region of the second part of the axillary artery—the medial cord lies medial to the artery, the lateral cord lies lateral to it, and the posterior cord, posterior to it. At approximately the third part of the axillary artery, the cords form the three major nerves of the upper arm, forearm, and hand. The radial nerve lies behind the axillary artery; the median nerve lies in front and slightly above it; and the ulnar nerve lies in front and slightly below it (Figure 159, page 245 and Figure 160, page 246).

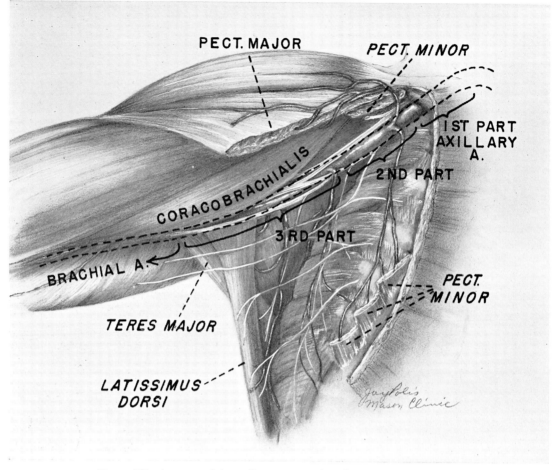

Figure 158. Anatomy of the axillary artery and its division into three parts.

The musculocutaneous nerve arises from the lateral cord of the brachial plexus at the lower border of the pectoralis minor muscle. It pierces the coracobrachialis muscle and passes obliquely to the lateral side of the forearm as the lateral antibrachial cutaneous nerve (Figure 160, page 246). The intercostobrachial nerve arises from the second intercostal nerve and it innervates the skin of the upper half of the medial and posterior part of the arm (Figure 159, page 245). These two nerves are not in as close approximation to the lower part of the axillary artery (the landmark for the axillary approach) as the other nerves and are the ones which may not be anesthetized (Figure 159, page 245).

The medial brachial cutaneous nerve arises from the eighth cervical and first thoracic nerves. In the axilla, it lies behind, and then medial to the axillary vein and usually it is blocked with the median, ulnar, and radial nerves.

PREMEDICATION

When paresthesias are elicited and the patient can describe their exact location, the incidence of successful block is slightly higher than when they are not elicited at all or when eliciting them depends on watching for twitching of the arm, hand, or both (see page 248). Therefore, we prefer light premedication but do not hesitate to use heavy premedication when an axillary brachial plexus block is the anesthesia of choice and when the patient will not cooperate.

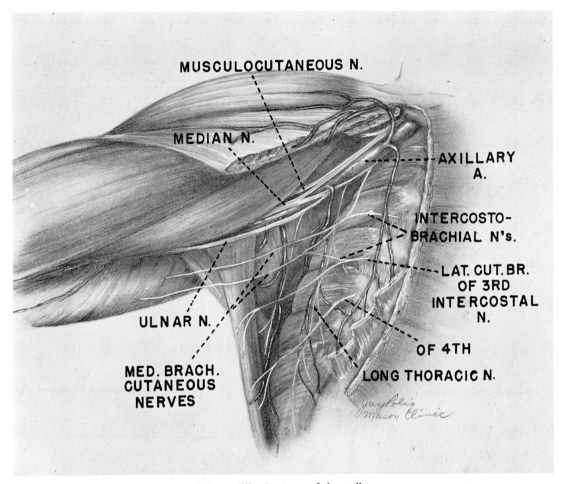

Figure 159. Anatomy of the axilla.

Light Premedication: The average patient (age 20 to 50, weight 150 pounds or over, approximate height 5 feet, 5 inches or over, and good physical status) receives:

1. 200 mg. (3 gr.) of pentobarbital (Nembutal) by mouth at hour of sleep the night before surgery.

2. 100 mg. (1½ gr.) of pentobarbital by mouth with one ounce of water 1½ to 2 hours before estimated *block* time. This dose of barbiturate is omitted if there is a possibility that the patient will be too heavily sedated to give *an immediate response* when paresthesias are obtained.

3. 10 mg. (⅙ gr.) of morphine and 0.4 mg. (1/150 gr.) of scopolamine intramuscularly *on call* to surgery.

Heavy Premedication: The average patient (age 20 to 50, weight 150 pounds or over, approximate height 5 feet, 5 inches or over, and good physical status) receives:

1. 200 mg. (3 gr.) of pentobarbital (Nembutal) by mouth at hour of sleep the night before surgery.

2. 100 mg. (1½ gr.) to 200 mg. (3 gr.) of pentobarbital with one ounce of water by mouth 1½ to 2 hours before estimated *block* time.

3. 15 mg. (¼ gr.) of morphine and 0.6 mg. (1/100 gr.) of scopolamine intramuscularly ¾ to 1 hour before estimated *block* time.

Reduction of Premedication: It is seldom necessary to increase this premedication irre-

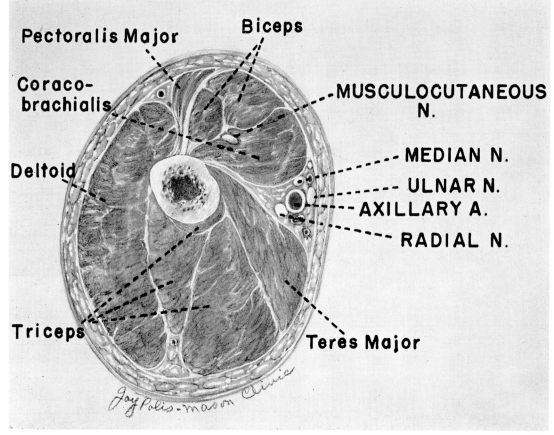

Figure 160. Cross-sectional anatomy of the upper arm at approximately the point where the block is executed. Note position of musculocutaneous nerve.

spective of the over-all size of the patient until the patient arrives in either the anesthesia or the operating room. However, it is very common to reduce this medication under various circumstances; for example, in the case of the geriatric patient, the adolescent patient or child, the debilitated or cachectic patient, and for those whose surgery is complicated by other disease, e.g., myxedema, diabetes, heart disease, etc. In the patient over 60 years of age, barbiturates and especially scopolamine often cause disorientation. Therefore, in these patients, atropine is usually substituted for scopolamine and the dosages of the barbiturate omitted or greatly reduced, i.e., to 50 mg. (¾ gr.) or less. *Always err on the light side.*

Inadequate Premedication: If medication is inadequate either for the block or surgical procedure, intravenous pentobarbital 50 mg.

(¾ gr.) to 100 mg. (1½ gr.) or intravenous morphine 8 mg. (⅛ gr.) to 15 mg. (¼ gr.) may be given *slowly.* Judicious use of added sedation is extremely important. Often small supplementary doses of pentobarbital or morphine will make a block successful when a patient interprets touch and motion as pain.

Premedication in Children: Of all the peripheral nerve blocks, this block is the one used most frequently in children 12 years of age or younger. For regional block in children, two types of premedication are employed by us—rectal thiopental (Pentothal) or meperidine (Demerol) and scopolamine.

Rectal Thiopental.—This is used for basal anesthesia. It is administered only in the induction area under direct supervision of the anesthetist and in doses of 15 to 20 mg. per pound of body weight 20 to 30 minutes prior to the estimated *block* time. The total dose of thiopental never exceeds 1000 mg. regardless of body weight.

Meperidine and Scopolamine.—These two drugs are given intramuscularly in the patient's room by the floor nurse in dosages of 1 mg. of meperidine per pound of body weight with 0.1 mg. (1/600 gr.) to 0.6 mg. (1/100 gr.) of scopolamine ¾ to 1 hour before estimated *block* time. If this sedation is inadequate, it may be supplemented in the induction area prior to the block with 10 mg. of rectal thiopental per pound of body weight or additional intravenous meperidine.

DRUGS

Lidocaine (Xylocaine) or Mepivacaine (Carbocaine): These are the two local anesthetic agents of choice for this approach. Tetracaine (Pontocaine) 1 to 2 mg. may be added to each 1 cc. of lidocaine or mepivacaine to prolong the duration of the local anesthetic solution approximately 30 to 50 percent. Tetracaine or procaine (Novocain) alone is not recommended for this block because the incidence of satisfactory block is significantly less.

To obtain satisfactory anesthesia in over 90 percent of the cases, 40 to 50 cc. of the local anesthetic solution should be injected in the adult and 10 to 30 cc. in the child. This block is employed infrequently for surgery above the elbow. If it is, local infiltration to block the intercostobrachial nerve, the superficial cervical plexus and/or the medial brachial cutaneous nerve may be necessary (Figure 153, page 237).

Dosage.—In adults, 10 cc. to 50 cc. of 1.0 to 1.5 percent solution with or without 0.1 cc. of epinephrine (Adrenalin) 1:1000 in each 20 of solution.* Do not exceed 35 cc. of a 1.5 percent solution or 500 mg. (0.5 gm.) of lidocaine or mepivacaine. This is a maximum dose even if it is necessary to ring the upper arm.

In children, do not exceed 3 to 5 mg. of the local anesthetic agent per pound of body weight. For example, a 50-pound child would receive no more than 25 cc. of a 1.0 percent

solution or 15 cc. of a 1.5 percent solution with epinephrine 1:200,000.* When a child weighs 100 pounds or more, then the adult dosage may be used.

Onset.—Operating analgesia is established in 20 to 45 minutes. Onset of operating analgesia usually is not as rapid with the axillary approach as compared with the supraclavicular approach.

Duration.—Operating analgesia lasts 1½ to 3 hours, with stronger concentrations and solutions containing epinephrine giving the upper limits.

MATERIALS

Regional tray (see Chapter 9, page 51) and a rubber tourniquet, *i.e.*, 12 to 18 inches (30 to 45 cm.) of ⅞ inch (2.3 cm.) Penrose drain or:

1. One ¾-inch (2 cm.), 25-gauge Huber point security Lok-needle.

2. One 1½-inch (3.8 cm.), 22-gauge security Lok-needle, preferably with short bevel.

3. One tuberculin Lok-syringe to measure epinephrine.

4. One 10 cc. Lok-syringe, preferably with finger rings.

5. One graduated measuring cup, preferably stainless steel, for mixing solutions.

6. One prep cup, preferably stainless steel.

7. Four sterile towels.

8. Six sterile sponges.

9. One sterilizer control.

10. One rubber tourniquet, *i.e.*, 12 to 18 inches (30 to 45 cm.) of ⅞-inch (2.3 cm.) Penrose drain.

TECHNIQUE

Position and Landmarks

1. The patient lies in the dorsal recumbent position with or without a pillow.

---

*Optimal concentration of epinephrine is 1:200,000, that is, 0.1 cc. of epinephrine 1:1000 in 20 cc. of the local anesthetic solution (see page 39).

2. The upper extremity is abducted to a 90-degree angle with the body. The forearm is flexed at a 90-degree angle to the arm. And the upper extremity is rotated 180 degrees at the shoulder girdle so that the arm, forearm, and hand rest on the cart, table, or pillow (Figure 161, page 249).

3. An X is marked on the skin overlying the third part of the axillary artery approximately 1½ inches (3.8 cm.) cephalad (medial) to the lateral border of the teres major muscle and just below the coracobrachialis muscle (Figure 161, page 249). The X should lie in the axillary fold.

4. A tourniquet (Penrose drain) is placed tightly on the arm 2 inches (5 cm.) to 3 inches (7.5 cm.) below the X to prevent spread of the local solution peripherally (Figure 162, page 250). It is removed 5 to 10 minutes after the block is completed.

Precautions

Landmark Should Be In Axilla But Not Too High.—Do not place the landmark too high in the axilla. Otherwise, if the needle is too long, misdirected, or both, the point of the needle may enter the pleura (Figure 161, page 249).

Fix Artery Against Humerus.—When inserting the needle, the artery should be fixed against the humerus by the index finger of the left hand of the right-handed physician (Figure 163, page 250).

Observe Arm for Paresthesias.—In the heavily medicated patient who will not respond verbally when a paresthesia is obtained, watch for jerky movements of the arm, forearm, hand, and/or fingers when placing the needle in the vicinity of the artery. Such movements usually indicate that the needle's point has stimulated the radial, median, or ulnar nerves.

Puncture of Axillary Artery Is No Sign to Discontinue Block.—If the axillary artery is entered, as evidenced by aspirating blood, do not withdraw the needle from the arm—a valuable landmark has been located (Figure 167, page 253).

Procedure

1. The sterilizer control is checked to be sure the equipment has been sterilized.

2. The area is aseptically prepared and draped.

3. The anesthetist stands at the side of the patient who is to be blocked, facing the head of the table (Figure 163, page 250).

4. An intradermal wheal is raised at the determined point with the ¾-inch (2 cm.), 25-gauge Huber point security Lok-needle (Figure 163, page 250).

5. Although paresthesias are always sought by us, they may not be obtained. In the heavily medicated patient, they are evidenced by jerking of the fingers or arms. A cooperative patient who is lightly medicated is instructed to say *"Now"* and not move as soon as he feels a "tingle" or electric shock go down his arm. *Paresthesias of the brachial plexus are characterized by sharp, spraying, electric shock sensations which radiate down the arm to the fingertips. Since it is possible to stimulate the radial, median, and ulnar nerves, the paresthesias may radiate to the various parts of the hand, but for assurance of a good block they should be elicited in all fingers as well as the thumb.*

6. If the anesthetist is right-handed, the index finger (forefinger) or middle finger of the left hand palpates the axillary artery and fixes it and the neurovascular bundle between the skin and subcutaneous tissue and the humerus (Figure 163, page 250).

7. Now one of four methods may be used to effect the block: (1) infiltration of the area from the humerus to the skin on each side of the artery with no attempt to elicit paresthesias; (2) obtaining of paresthesias; (3) obtaining blood from the artery and then injecting perivascularly; or (4) a combination of these. We prefer to elicit paresthesias and aspirate blood when executing this block and only use the infiltration technique when neither of these can be obtained.

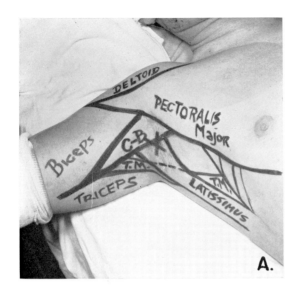

Figure 161. A. Landmarks for upper extremity block by the axillary approach. B. Anatomy of the landmarks.

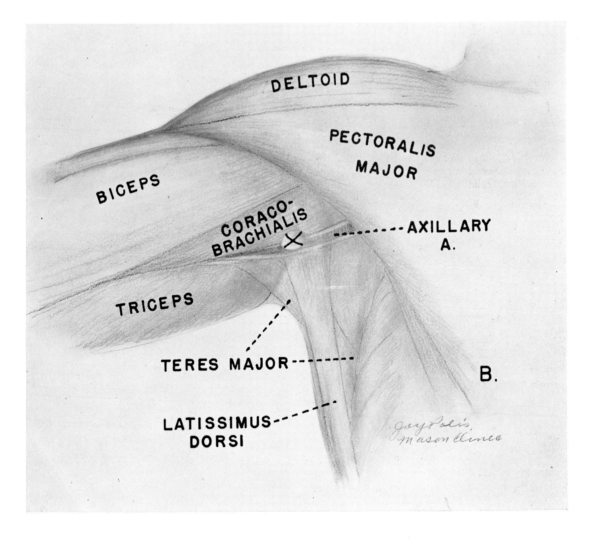

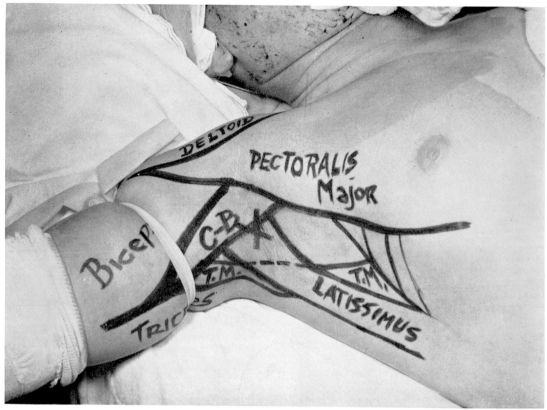

Figure 162. ⅞ inch (2.3 cm.) wide Penrose drain is in position 2 inches (5 cm.) to 3 inches (7.5 cm.) below site of injection of local anesthetic solution. The tourniquet is used in an effort to encourage the spread of the anesthetic solution cephalad inside the axillary sheath (Figure 170, page 255; and Remarks, page 254).

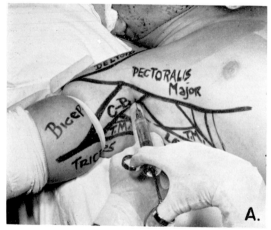

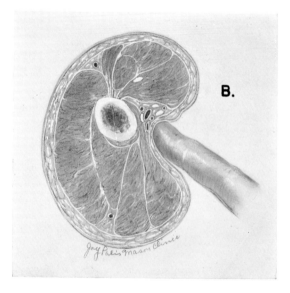

Figure 163. A. Middle finger palpates axillary artery and compresses neurovascular bundle against humerus. B. Cross section showing this maneuver.

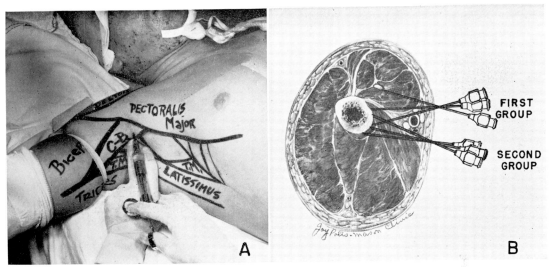

Figure 164. A. Needle inserted above artery and humerus contacted. B. (Needle group 1). Cross section showing this maneuver. Note that needle has also been inserted above humerus in an effort to block the musculocutaneous nerve.

8. Regardless of the technique selected, remove the Penrose tourniquet 5 to 10 minutes after completion of the block.

Infiltration Technique

1. The right-handed anesthetist holds the full 10 cc. Lok-syringe with the 1½-inch (3.8 cm.), 22-gauge security Lok-needle attached in his right hand (Figure 164A, page 251). The needle is inserted through the skin wheal at the tip of the palpating finger of the left hand (Figure 164A, page 251). Then, it is advanced toward the artery as 1 cc. of the local anesthetic solution is injected.

2. As the needle approaches the artery, its direction is changed slightly by moving the skin wheal and shaft of the needle with the finger which is palpating the artery so that the needle passes in close proximity to the upper side of the artery. The needle is advanced until its point contacts the humerus (Figure 164, page 251).

3. Then, 5 to 6 cc. of the local anesthetic solution is injected as the needle is withdrawn to the subcutaneous tissue.

4. This maneuver is repeated two or three times in a fanwise direction for about ½ inch (1.3 cm.) to ¾ inch (2 cm.) above the artery (Figure 164, first needle group, page 251). Then, an attempt to block the musculocutaneous nerve is made (Figure 164, first needle group, page 251).

5. The needle is withdrawn until the point rests in the subcutaneous tissue. Now, the palpating finger shifts the skin wheal and directs the needle to the lower side of the artery and the procedure is repeated (Figure 165, second needle group, page 252).

6. In this fashion, a wall of anesthesia is made on each side of the artery from the skin to the humerus.

Obtaining Paresthesias

1. The right-handed anesthetist holds the full 10 cc. Lok-syringe with the 1½-inch (3.8 cm.), 22-gauge security Lok-needle attached in his right hand (Figure 165A, page 252). The needle is inserted through the skin wheal at the tip of the palpating finger of the left hand (Figure 165A, page 252). Then, it is advanced toward

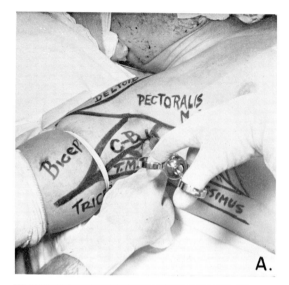

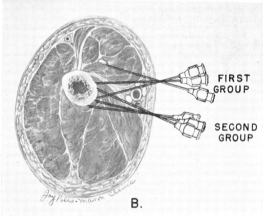

Figure 165. A. Needle inserted below artery and humerus contacted. B. (Needle group 2.) Cross section showing this maneuver.

the artery as 1 cc. of the local anesthetic solution is injected.

2. As the needle approaches the artery, its direction is changed slightly so that it passes in close proximity to one side of the artery. It is advanced until a paresthesia is obtained or it contacts the humerus (Fagure 166, page 252).

3. If the humerus is contacted without obtaining paresthesias, the needle is withdrawn and reinserted in a seeking manner until paresthesias are obtained.

4. When paresthesias are obtained, the advancement or withdrawal of the needle

is stopped and the local anesthetic solution is injected—10 to 20 cc. in the adult and 3 to 10 cc. in the child (Figure 166, page 252).

5. The needle is then passed to the other side of the artery, paresthesias obtained, and the injections repeated (Figure 166, page 252).

6. While paresthesias of the median and ulnar nerve are not difficult to elicit, paresthesias of the radial nerve are often unobtainable because usually the radial nerve is located behind the axillary artery (Figure 160, page 246).

Puncturing of the Artery

1. The right-handed anesthetist holds the full 10 cc. Lok-syringe with the 1½-inch (3.8 cm.), 22-gauge security Lok-needle attached in his right hand (Figure 165A, page 252). The needle is inserted through the skin wheal at the tip of the palpating finger of the left hand (Figure 165A, page 252). Then, it is advanced toward the artery as 1 cc. of the local anesthetic solution is injected.

2. Now, the bevel of the needle purposely is placed in the lumen of the axillary ar-

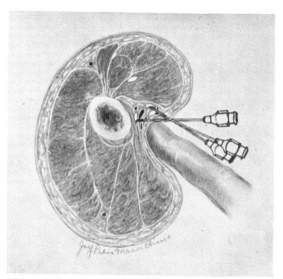

Figure 166. Cross section showing eliciting of paresthesias.

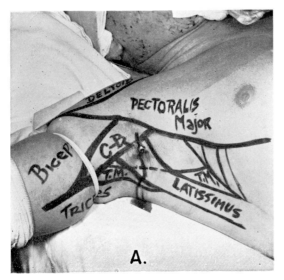
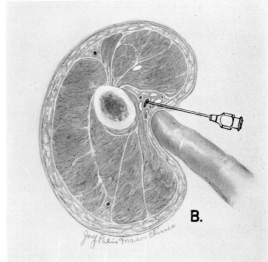

Figure 167. A. Needle in artery—note blood dripping from needle hub. The syringe was removed from the needle to demonstrate the blood. B. Cross section demonstrating needle's position.

tery and blood aspirated into the syringe (Figure 167, page 253).

3. The needle's point is then slowly withdrawn 1/16 inch (0.15 cm.) to 1/8 inch (0.3 cm.) until no blood is obtained on aspiration. It can now be presumed that the needle point lies outside the artery but still within or in close approximation to the neurovascular bundle (Figure 168, page 253).

4. Then, the local anesthetic solution is injected and the needle is withdrawn. In the adult 40 to 50 cc. is injected and in the child, depending on his weight, 10 to 30 cc.

DISTRIBUTION OF ANALGESIA

Analgesia of most of the nerves of the upper extremity ensues at least from the site of the block peripherally. If a tourniquet is used or operations on the arm at or above the elbow are performed, an intradermal and subcutaneous ring of local anesthesia around the inner one-half of the arm may be necessary to block the medial brachial cutaneous nerve, the intercostobrachial nerve, the superficial cervical plexus, or all three (Figure 153, page 237 and Figure 169, page 254).

With this approach, the musculocutaneous nerve may not be blocked consistently because of its distance from the site of the injection (Figure 160, page 246).

COMPLICATIONS

Systemic Toxic Reactions (intravascular injections, etc.): See Chapter 3, page 19.

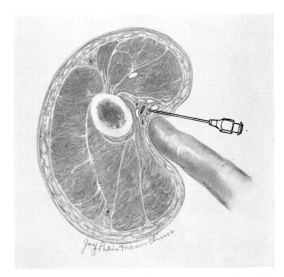

Figure 168. Cross section showing position of needle after its withdrawal from artery. The bevel of the needle lies in the neurovascular bundle or in close proximity to it.

Pneumothorax: With this approach correctly executed, pneumothoraces do not occur. If one does result, it is from an improper technique. For etiology, signs and symptoms, etc., see page 237.

Phrenic Nerve Block: Phrenic nerve block has not been observed by us with this technique.

Stellate Ganglion Block: Only one instance of stellate ganglion block has been observed by us in over 300 cases. For etiology, signs and symptoms, etc., see page 131.

Obliteration of Radial Pulse: Temporary compression of the axillary artery with obliteration of a palpable radial pulse from either bleeding or too great a volume of the local anesthetic solution has been observed in approximately 10 of 700 children. In these cases the pulse returned within 2 to 4 hours and no permanent sequelae resulted.

REMARKS

Embryonic Development of the Arm Bud: As the arm bud of the embryo develops, the spinal nerves and blood vessels move peripher-

ally in a tubular encasement of the prevertebral fascia, which in the axilla is called the axillary sheath (Figure 170, page 255). This sheath contains nerves, blood vessels, lymph nodes, and adipose tissue. Theoretically, a local anesthetic solution injected inside the axillary sheath should spread sufficiently centrad above the clavicle and block the entire brachial plexus. However, we have not observed this to occur consistently. It is more likely to result if: (1) 40 to 50 cc. is injected in the adult and 10 to 30 cc. is injected in a child; (2) a tourniquet is placed on the arm to prevent spread of the local anesthetic solution in the axillary sheath distal to the point of injection and facilitate its spread cephalad; (3) adequate time (30 to 45 minutes) is allowed for analgesia to establish; (4) paresthesias, blood from the axillary artery, or both, are sought when executing the block; (5) a local anesthetic solution with a rapid onset and spreading characteristics is employed; (6) the concentration of the local solution used is adequate, *e.g.*, 1.0 percent or greater; and (7) the injection is made at the level of the lower part of the axillary artery rather than at the level of the brachial artery.

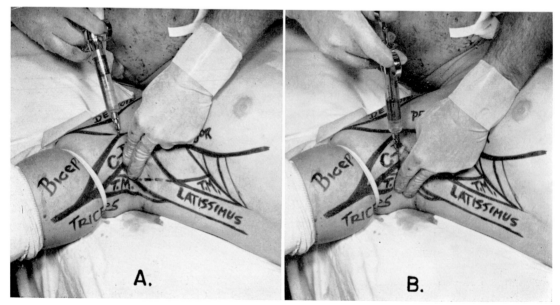

Figure 169. Local infiltration to block branches of intercostobrachial nerve. A. The 1½-inch (3.8 cm.) needle is infiltrating the upper one-half of inner surface of arm. B. Infiltration of lower half of arm.

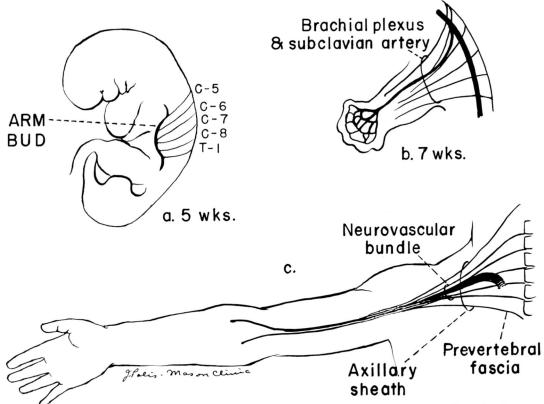

Figure 170. Schematic drawing of embryonic development of arm bud showing that axillary sheath is prolongation of prevertebral fascia, and that neurovascular bundle lies within axillary sheath.

Selection of the Axillary Approach or Supraclavicular Approach? *Axillary Approach.*—The author prefers the axillary approach for: (1) patients 12 years of age or under—children are often uncooperative, need heavy sedation, have small first ribs, and seldom require manipulations of, or surgery on, the shoulder girdle; (2) uncooperative patients of any age; (3) outpatients who cannot be carefully observed over a twenty-four hour period; and (4) patients with emphysema who rely on the phrenic nerve for air intake.

Supraclavicular Approach.—The author prefers to employ and *teach* the supraclavicular approach in all other patients because of the following reasons. First, it can be used to block the entire upper extremity when the extremity cannot be abducted and because anesthesia is consistently more satisfactory. Second, he does not consider the possibility of a pneumothorax to be a deterrent because

its incidence in our institution is very small (less than 0.5 percent), and if treated correctly and immediately, it seldom causes a permanent problem. Third, he does not consider stellate ganglion block or phrenic nerve block with alarm, since both are reversible when the effects of the local anesthetic agent are dissipated; and if hypoxia occurs from a phrenic nerve block, oxygen will alleviate the signs and symptoms. Fourth, with either approach, nerve damage which is the most disabling of all the complications of upper extremity block may result. Fifth, if the supraclavicular approach is not taught the resident physician in a training program, he may never learn the approach—the possibility of a pneumothorax may be too great a deterrent. Lastly, the supraclavicular approach, not the axillary approach, must be used when: (1) the upper extremity cannot be abducted; (2) operations or manipulations involve the shoulder girdle, the axilla, or the humerus, *e.g.*, dislocated shoulder, fractured humerus, or breast surgery; (3) movement of the shoulder girdle by the conscious patient may interfere with delicate surgery of the forearm and hand; and (4) the surgical procedure requires more than 2½ to 3 hours of anesthesia—of the commonly used local anesthetic agents, only tetracaine (Pontocaine) solutions freshly mixed from crystals provide 6 to 8 hours of anesthesia and only when tetracaine is used by the supraclavicular approach does it produce satisfactory brachial plexus anesthesia in over 95 percent of the cases.

Select Approach According to the Circumstances: Each approach for blocking the upper extremity has its own advantages, disadvantages, and indications. Selection of the approach should depend on: (1) the skill and experience of the physician performing the block; (2) the availability of direct personal supervision by a staff physician skilled in these two approaches when they are being learned; (3) the type of operation and its duration; (4) the age and cooperation of the patient; and (5) the physical status of the patient.

Are Paresthesias Essential When the Axillary Approach Is Employed? The answer is *NO*, but the incidence of successful block usually is higher when paresthesias are obtained.

Neurovascular Bundle is Superficial: Probably the most common mistake when performing a brachial plexus block with the axillary approach is placing the needle too deep. Often the neurovascular bundle can be entered with a needle that is no longer than ¾ inch (Figure 160, page 246).

Recover Broken Needle(s): All needles should be tested before use. If a needle breaks, every effort to recover it, including surgery, should be made. Unremoved needles have a tendency to migrate and may cause permanent injuries as well as medicolegal complications.

Repeat Block When Analgesia Is Inadequate. If the desired results from the first block attempt are unsatisfactory, do not hesitate to reblock the patient if time permits. Most patients will think nothing about being reblocked if the second attempt is prefaced with a statement such as: "Well, I guess we will have to inject a little more medicine if we are going to freeze this area."

However, do not exceed the maximum safe dosage of the local anesthetic solution for both blocks. If to reblock the patient the maximum safe dose of the local anesthetic solution must be exceeded, 45 minutes should elapse between blocks.

CHAPTER 32

Blocking of the Nerves of the Arm at the Elbow and Wrist

GENERAL CONSIDERATIONS

WHENEVER it might seem preferable to produce analgesia of part or all of the forearm and hand by blocking the individual nerves of the arm at the elbow or wrist rather than by producing complete analgesia of the upper extremity with a brachial plexus block, the following facts should be remembered.

Nerve Distribution Varies Markedly and the Nerves Overlap: With the exception of operations and manipulations of the little finger, it is rare to have a wound of the forearm or the hand that can be repaired or manipulated by a single block of either the ulnar, median, or radial nerves. The wide and varying distribution, as well as the overlapping of these three nerves, necessitates that either two of the three nerves or all of them must be anesthetized to produce adequate analgesia for most procedures. The anesthetist should have a knowledge of the surface and deep innervations of the radial, median, and ulnar nerves, but he should also realize that these innervations of the arm and hand often do not conform to the textbook illustrations.

Pneumatic Tourniquet Should Be Placed Above the Elbow: The most suitable region to place a pneumatic tourniquet on the upper extremity is between the elbow and shoulder. Therefore, if an elbow or wrist block is performed, this type of tourniquet cannot be employed since the pressure it exerts on the unanesthetized arm is extremely uncomfortable.

Additional Subcutaneous Infiltration Is Often Necessary: If an elbow or wrist block is performed to give total analgesia of the forearm or hand below the block, it is necessary to place an intradermal and subcutaneous ring of the local anesthetic solution around the elbow or the wrist. This is particularly true of the elbow block since the medial antebrachial cutaneous nerve (C8, T1) descends across the elbow level in the superficial fascia and is removed from the other major nerves which are blocked directly. The intercostobrachial nerve (T2) may also send a few twigs to the proximal part of the forearm.

Muscle Relaxation May Be Inadequate: Relaxation of all the muscles of the upper extremity is not complete. This is extremely important when suturing tendons or reducing a fracture. For example, if a tendon of the hand is to be repaired, a wrist block will produce adequate analgesia to work on the hand if a tourniquet is not employed. However, the muscles which control the tendons in the hand are in the forearm and if their nerve supply is not interrupted, it may be impossible to pull the retracted tendon into position for suturing.

Do Not Exceed Maximum Dose of Local Anesthetic Agent: The maximum dosage of the local anesthetic drug should not be exceeded for the procedure as a whole, *i.e.*, if 0.25 percent tetracaine (Pontocaine) solution is being employed, the total volume used in all three nerve blocks as well as the ring of the elbow or wrist should not exceed 50 cc. (125 mg.).

Use Hyaluronidase: Hyaluronidase, 150 TRU may be of aid in these blocks, particularly if definite paresthesias are not elicited. Before using hyaluronidase (see page 43).

Master Brachial Plexus Block First: *Because of the above-mentioned facts, blocks of the nerves of the arm at the elbow and wrist are* *relatively infrequently performed in most surgical cases when compared to the number of brachial plexus blocks. The beginner should master the brachial plexus block before attempting the procedures outlined in this chapter. Brachial plexus block produces complete analgesia of the upper extremity, which is adequate for any operation or manipulation of the upper extremity and meets most of the requirements of the surgeon.*

RADIAL NERVE BLOCK

INDICATIONS

Surgical: Operations and manipulations of the arm and hand limited to the innervation of the radial nerve.

Diagnosis: To localize pain problems of the upper extremity.

Therapeutic: To treat pain problems and vasospastic diseases of the arm and hand limited to radial nerve innervation. Such limitation is rare, for these conditions usually involve an area innervated by more than one nerve and therefore are best treated by stellate ganglion block.

ANATOMY

The radial nerve is the largest branch of the brachial plexus and its fibers are derived from the fifth, sixth, seventh, and eighth cervical and first thoracic nerves (Figure 134, page 222). It courses downward on the medial side of the humerus. It passes behind the third part of the axillary artery and the upper part of the brachial artery, and in front of the tendons of the latissimus dorsi and teres major muscles. It then courses from the medial to the lateral side of the humerus between the medial and lateral heads of the triceps muscle (Figure 171A, page 258). It pierces the lateral intermuscular septum, about 2½ inches (6.3 cm.) to 3 inches (7.5 cm.) above the external condyle and passes between the brachialis and brachioradialis muscles to the front of the lateral condyle, where it divides into four branches (Figure 171A, page 258). The mus-

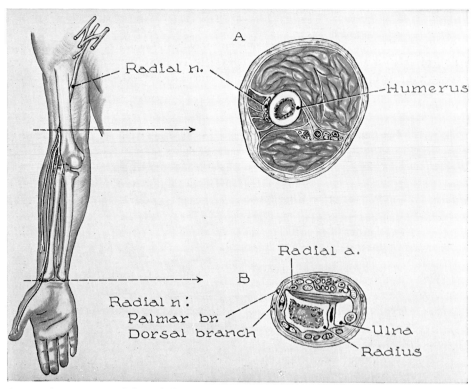

Figure 171. Anatomy of the radial nerve. A. Cross section above the elbow. B. Cross section at wrist.

cular, cutaneous, and deep branches innervate parts of the forearm and upper arm. The superficial branch follows the lateral side of the radial artery and has no branches in the upper forearm. It leaves the artery about 2½ (6.3 cm.) to 3 inches (7.5 cm.) above the wrist, passes beneath the tendon of the brachioradialis muscle to pierce the deep fascia, and enters the subcutaneous tissue. Then, it divides a little above the wrist into two branches to innervate part of the hand (Figure 171B, page 258).

PREMEDICATION

Paresthesias are not sought. However, the procedure is not painful and since paresthesias are sought in median and ulnar nerve blocks, which are frequently performed in conjunction with the radial to complete the desired analgesia, light premedication is advised.

Light Premedication: Average patient (age 20 to 50, weight 150 pounds or over, height 5 feet, 5 inches or over, and good physcial status) receives:

1. 200 mg. (3 gr.) of pentobarbital (Nembutal) by mouth at hour of sleep the night before surgery.

2. 100 mg. (1½ gr.) of pentobarbital by mouth with one ounce of water 1½ to 2 hours before estimated *block* time. If this block is to be combined with a block of the ulnar and/or median nerves, this dose of barbiturate is omitted if there is a possibility that the patient will be too heavily sedated to give *an immediate response* when paresthesias of the other nerves are obtained.

3. 10 mg. (⅙ gr.) of morphine and 0.4 mg. (¹⁄₁₅₀ gr.) of scopolamine intramuscularly *on call* to surgery.

Reduction of Premedication: It is seldom necessary to increase this premedication irrespective of the over-all size of the patient until the patient arrives in either the anesthesia or operating room. However, it is normal to reduce this medication under various circumstances; for example, for the geriatric patient,

the adolescent patient or child, the debilitated or cachectic patient, and for patients whose surgery is complicated by other disease, *e.g.,* myxedema, diabetes, heart disease, etc. In the patient over 60 years of age, barbiturates and especially scopolamine may often cause disorientation. Therefore, in these patients, atropine is usually substituted for scopolamine and the dosages of the barbiturate omitted or greatly reduced, *i.e.,* to 50 mg. (¾ gr.) or less. *Always err on the light side.*

Inadequate Premedication: If medication is not adequate either for the anesthesia or surgical procedure, intravenous pentobarbital 50 mg. (¾ gr.) to 100 mg. (1½ gr.) or intravenous morphine 8 mg. (⅛ gr.) to 15 mg. (¼ gr.) may be given *slowly.* Judicious use of added sedation is extremely important. Often small supplementary doses of morphine or pentobarbital will make a block successful, especially if the patient interprets touch and motion as pain.

DRUGS

Tetracaine (Pontocaine)

Dosage.—10 cc. to 20 cc. of 0.15 to 0.25 percent solution with or without 0.1 cc. of epinephrine (Adrenalin) 1:1000 in 20 cc. of solution.*

Onset.—Operating analgesia is established in 10 to 30 minutes, with an average of 20 minutes.

Duration.—Operating analgesia lasts 3 to 6 hours, with stronger concentrations and solutions containing epinephrine giving the upper limits.

Procaine (Novocain)

Dosage.—10 cc. to 20 cc. of 1.0 to 2.0 percent solution with or without 0.1 cc. of epinephrine (Adrenalin) 1:1000 in 20 cc. of solution.*

---

*Optimal concentration of epinephrine is 1:200,000, that is, 0.1 cc. of epinephrine 1:1000 in 20 cc. of the local anesthetic solution (see page 39).

Onset.—Operating analgesia is established in 5 to 15 minutes, with an average of 10 minutes.

Duration.—Operating analgesia lasts 1 to 1½ hours, with stronger concentrations and solutions containing epinephrine giving the upper limits.

Lidocaine (Xylocaine) or Mepivacaine (Carbocaine)

Dosage.—10 cc. to 20 cc. of a 1.0 to 1.5 percent solution with or without 0.1 cc. of epinephrine (Adrenalin) 1:1000 in 20 cc. of solution.*

Onset.—Operating analgesia is established in 5 to 15 minutes.

Duration.—Operating analgesia lasts 1¼ to 3 hours, with stronger concentrations and solutions containing epinephrine giving the upper limits.

MATERIALS

Regional tray (Chapter 9, page 51) or:

1. One ¾-inch (2 cm.), 25-gauge Huber point security Lok-needle.

2. One 2-inch (5 cm.), 22-gauge security Lok-needle, preferably with short bevel.

3. One tuberculin Lok-syringe for measuring epinephrine.

4. One 10 cc. Lok-syringe, preferably with finger rings.

5. One graduated measuring cup, preferably stainless steel, for mixing solution.

6. One prep cup, preferably stainless steel.

7. Four sterile towels.

8. Six sterile sponges.

9. One sterilizer control.

---

*Optimal concentration of epinephrine is 1:200,000, that is, 0.1 cc. of epinephrine 1:1000 in 20 cc. of the local anesthetic solution (see page 39).

TECHNIQUE OF RADIAL NERVE BLOCK AT THE ELBOW

Position and Landmarks

1. The patient lies in the dorsal recumbent position with or without a pillow, his arm partially abducted, and the forearm extended (Figure 176, page 265). The position is the same as for a median nerve block at the elbow.

2. The lateral epicondyle of the humerus is palpated and 2½ inches (6.3 cm.) to 3 inches (7.5 cm.), approximately four finger breadths, above it the skin overlying the lateral surface of the humerus is marked with an X (Figure 172, page 260). This X marks approximately the point where the radial nerve pierces the intermuscular septum and lies in close approximation to the humerus.

Precaution

Aspirate.—Careful aspiration for blood should be performed.

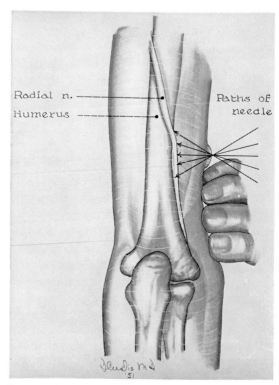

Radial n. ——————
Humerus ——————
Paths of needle

Figure 172. Posterior view of the landmarks and the method of blocking the radial nerve at or slightly above the elbow. The arrows represent the courses of the needle.

Procedure

1. The sterilizer control is checked to be sure the equipment has been sterilized.

2. The area is aseptically prepared and draped.

3. The anesthetist stands at the side to be blocked, facing the head of the patient (Figure 176, page 265).

4. An intradermal wheal is raised at the determined X with a ¾-inch (2 cm.), 25-gauge Huber point security Lok-needle (Figure 172, page 260).

5. The patient is instructed to say *"Now"* and not to move if typical paresthesias of the nerve are elicited. *Paresthesias of the radial nerve are characterized by the sharp, spraying, electric shock-like sensations to the thumb and back of the hand.*

6. The 2-inch (5 cm.) short beveled 22-gauge security Lok-needle with the full 10 cc. Lok-syringe attached is introduced through the wheal perpendicular to the skin. The needle is advanced until contact is made with the lateral surface of the humerus. 2 cc. to 3 cc. of the local anesthetic solution is injected as the needle is slowly withdrawn ½ inch (1.3 cm.) By repeating this maneuver and changing the direction of the needle so as to deposit a line of anesthetic solution along the long axis of the humerus for 1 inch (2.5 cm.) above and 1 inch (2.5 cm.) below the point of the initial injection, an excellent block of the radial nerve will usually ensue (Figure 172, page 260).

7. If at any time during this injection paresthesias are elicited, the needle should be fixed and 5 cc. of the anesthetic solution should be injected.

8. Approximately 20 cc. of the anesthetic solution will be adequate for this block.

TECHNIQUE OF RADIAL NERVE BLOCK AT THE WRIST

Position and Landmarks

1. The patient lies in a dorsal recumbent position with or without a pillow, his arm ab-ducted, forearm extended, and his hand partially supinated (Figure 173, page 261).

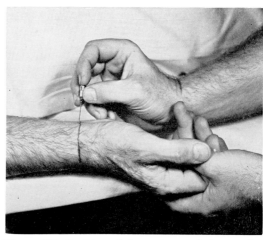

Figure 173. Position of the patient and the anesthetist for a block of the nerves at the wrist.

2. The styloid process of the ulnar bone is palpated and a line through it drawn around the wrist (Figure 174, page 262). On this line just lateral to the radial artery the skin is marked with an X (Figure 174, page 262).

Precaution

Aspirate.—Careful aspiration for blood should be performed.

Procedure

1. The sterilizer control is checked to be sure the equipment has been sterilized.

2. The area is aseptically prepared and draped.

3. The anesthetist stands at the side to be blocked, facing the wrist (Figure 173, page 261).

4. An intradermal wheal is raised at the determined X with a 25-gauge Huber point security Lok-needle (Figure 174, page 262).

5. The patient is instructed to say *"Now"* and not to move if typical paresthesias of the nerve are elicited. *Paresthesias of the radial nerve are characterized by sharp, spraying, electric shock-like sensations to the thumb and back of the hand.*

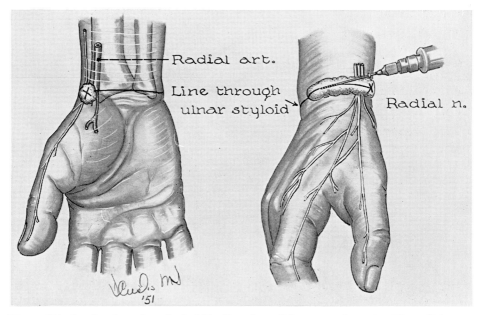

Figure 174. Landmarks and method of blocking the radial nerve at the wrist. The radial nerve divides at the wrist to innervate both lateral surfaces of the thumb as well as part of the back of the hand.

6. The 2-inch (5 cm.) short beveled 22-gauge security Lok-needle with the full 10 cc. Lok-syringe attached is introduced through the intradermal wheal. Intradermal and subcutaneous infiltration of the lateral side of the wrist from just lateral to the radial artery to the back of the radial half of the wrist is performed slowly and carefully along the line drawn through the styloid process of the ulnar bone (Figure 174, page 262). This requires 10 to 20 cc. of the anesthetic solution.

7. If radial nerve paresthesias occur at any point the needle should be fixed and 1 cc. to 2 cc. of the anesthetic solution should be injected.

DISTRIBUTION OF ANALGESIA

Analgesia of the area innervated by the radial nerve and its branches beyond the point of the block ensues (Figure 152, page 236).

COMPLICATIONS

Toxic Reactions (intravascular injections, etc.): See Chapter 3, page 19.

REMARKS

Block of Radial Nerve is Usually a Result of Diffusion of Local Anesthetic Solution: In most instances the radial nerve is anesthetized by *diffusion* of the anesthetic solution rather than by accurate placement of a small amount of solution.

Block of Radial Nerve at Elbow: Care must be taken when infiltrating fan-wise to deposit the anesthetic solution in close proximity to the humerus and not in the muscle; otherwise the block may fail.

Block of Radial Nerve at Wrist: Careful slow movement of the needle to insure an even distribution of the anesthetic solutions in subcutaneous tissue is essential. At the wrist, usually just above the "snuff box," the radial nerve divides and therefore it is possible to get two paresthesias, one to the thumb and the other to the back of the first three fingers (Figure 171B, page 258; and Figure 174, page 262).

Care should be taken to avoid puncture of the cephalic vein (Figure 209, page 308).

Recover Broken Needle(s): All needles

should be tested before use. If a needle breaks, every effort to recover it, including surgery, should be made. Unremoved needles have a tendency to migrate and may cause permanent injuries as well as medicolegal complications.

Repeat Block When Analgesia Is Inadequate: If the desired results from the first block attempt are unsatisfactory, do not hesitate to reblock the patient if time permits. Most patients will think nothing about being reblocked if the second attempt is prefaced by a statement such as: "Well, I guess we will have to inject a little more medicine if we are going to freeze this area."

MEDIAN NERVE BLOCK

INDICATIONS

Surgical: Operations and manipulations of the arm and hand limited to the innervation of the median nerve.

Diagnostic: To localize pain problems of the upper extremity.

Therapeutic: To treat pain problems and vasospastic disease of the arm and hand limited to median nerve innervation. Stellate block is more suitable for treatment of the latter conditions.

ANATOMY

The median nerve derives its fibers from the sixth, seventh, and eighth cervical and first thoracic nerves (Figure 134, page 222). At the elbow it lies a few millimeters medial to the brachial artery and is separated from the elbow joint by the brachialis muscle (Figure 175A, page 263). At the transverse carpal ligament (wrist), the median nerve lies behind and slightly to the radial side of the tendon of the palmaris longus muscle and is covered by the skin and fascia (Figure 175B, page 263). It is fairly common to find an absence of the palmaris longus muscle and ten-

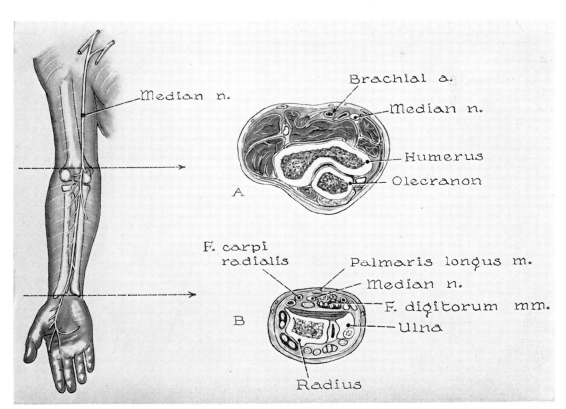

Figure 175. Anatomy of the median nerve. A. Cross section at elbow. B. Cross section at wrist.

don, and in these cases, the median nerve is situated between the flexor digitorum sublimis and flexor carpi radialis tendons (Figure 175B, page 263).

PREMEDICATION

Paresthesias are always sought and light premedication is advised.

Light Premedication: Average patient (age 20 to 50, weight 150 pounds or over, height 5 feet, 5 inches, and good physical status) receives:

1. 200 mg. (3 gr.) of pentobarbital (Nembutal) by mouth at hour of sleep the night before surgery.

2. 100 mg. (1½ gr.) of pentobarbital by mouth with one ounce of water 1½ to 2 hours before estimated *block* time. This dose of barbiturate is omitted if there is a possibility that the patient will be too heavily sedated to give *an immediate response* when paresthesias are obtained.

3. 10 mg. (⅙ gr.) of morphine and 0.4 mg. (¹⁄₁₅₀ gr.) of scopolamine intramuscularly *on call* to surgery.

Reduction of Premedication: It is seldom necessary to increase this premedication irrespective of the over-all size of the patient until the patient arrives in either the anesthesia or operating room. However, it is very common to reduce this medication under various circumstances; for example, in the case of the geriatric patient, the adolescent patient or child, the debilitated or cachectic patient, and for those whose surgery is complicated by other disease, *e.g.*, myxedema, diabetes, heart disease, etc. In the patient over 60 years of age, barbiturates and especially scopolamine may often cause disorientation. Therefore, in these patients atropine is usually substituted for scopolamine and the doses of the barbiturate omitted or greatly reduced, *i.e.*, to 50 mg. (¾ gr.) or less. *Always err on the light side.*

Inadequate Premedication: If medication is not adequate either for the block or surgical

procedure, intravenous pentobarbital 50 mg. (¾ gr.) to 100 mg. (1½ gr.) or intravenous morphine 8 mg. (⅛ gr.) to 15 mg. (¼ gr.) may be given *slowly.* Judicious use of added sedation is extremely important. Often small supplementary doses of morphine or pentobarbital will make a block successful, particularly when the patient interprets touch and motion as pain.

DRUGS

Tetracaine (Pontocaine)

Dosage.—10 cc. to 20 cc. of 0.15 to 0.25 cent solution with or without 0.1 cc. of epinephrine (Adrenalin) 1:1000 in 20 cc. of solution.*

Onset.—Operating analgesia is established in 10 to 30 minutes, with an average of 20 minutes.

Duration.—Operating analgesia lasts 3½ to 6 hours, with stronger concentrations and solutions containing epinephrine giving the upper limits.

Procaine (Novocain)

Dosage.—10 cc. to 20 cc. of 1.0 to 2.0 percent solution with or without 0.1 cc. of epinephrine (Adrenalin) 1:1000 in 20 cc. of solution.*

Onset.—Operating analgesia is established in 5 to 15 minutes, with an average of 10 minutes.

Duration.—Operating analgesia lasts 1 to 1½ hours, with stronger concentrations and solutions containing epinephrine giving the upper limits.

Lidocaine (Xylocaine) or Mepivacaine (Carbocaine)

Dosage.—10 cc. to 20 cc. of 1.0 to 1.5 percent solution with or without 0.1 cc. of epinephrine (Adrenalin) 1:1000 in 20 cc. of solution.*

---

*Optimal concentration of epinephrine is 1:200,000, that is, 0.1 cc. of epinephrine 1:1000 in 20 cc. of the local anesthetic solution (see page 39).

Onset.—Operating analgesia is established in 5 to 15 minutes.

Duration.—Operating analgesia lasts 1¼ to 3 hours, with stronger concentrations and solutions containing epinephrine giving the upper limits.

MATERIALS

Regional tray (Chapter 9, page 51) or:

1. One ¾-inch (2 cm.), 25-gauge Huber point security Lok-needle.

2. One 2-inch (5 cm.), 22-gauge security Lok-needle, preferably with short bevel.

3. One tuberculin Lok-syringe for measuring epinephrine.

4. One 10 cc. Lok-syringe, preferably with finger rings.

5. One graduated measuring cup, preferably stainless steel, for mixing solutions.

6. One prep cup, preferably stainless steel.

7. Four sterile towels.

8. Six sterile sponges.

9. One sterilizer control.

TECHNIQUE OF MEDIAN NERVE BLOCK AT THE ELBOW

Position and Landmarks

1. The patient lies in the dorsal recumbent position with or without a pillow, his arm abducted, the forearm extended, and the hand supinated (Figure 176, page 265).

2. The epicondyles of the humerus are located and a line drawn between them (Figure 177, page 266).

3. The brachial artery is palpated and its position indicated on the line by an O (Figure 177, page 266).

4. ¼ inch (0.6 cm.) medial to this O an X is made on the line. This mark should overlie the median nerve (Figure 177, page 266).

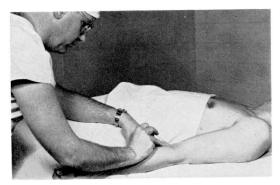

Figure 176. Position of the patient and anesthetist for block of the median and radial nerves at the elbow.

Precaution

Aspirate.—Care should be taken to avoid puncture of the brachial artery, the basilic vein, and the median cubital vein. Careful aspiration for blood should be performed.

Procedure

1. The sterilizer control is checked to be sure the equipment has been sterilized.

2. The area is aseptically prepared and draped.

3. The anesthetist stands at the side to be blocked facing the upper arm (Figure 176, page 265).

4. An intradermal wheal is raised 1 inch (2.5 cm.) below the determined X with a 25-gauge Huber point security Lok-needle (Figure 177, page 266).

5. The 2-inch (5 cm.) short beveled 22-gauge security Lok-needle with the full 10 cc. Lok-syringe attached is introduced through the wheal and slowly directed superiorly at a 20 degree angle to the skin so that the point pierces the lacertus fibrosus (Figure 177, page 266).

6. The patient is instructed to say *"Now"* and not to move when typical paresthesias of the nerve radiating to the hand and fingers are elicited. *Paresthesias of the median nerve are characterized by sharp, spraying electric shock-like sensations to the palm of the hand, index finger, middle (long) finger, and the radial side of the ring finger.*

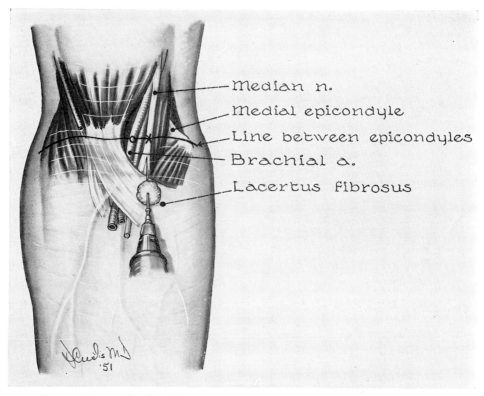

Figure 177.   Landmarks and anatomy for a median nerve block at the elbow.

7. The angle of the needle with the skin is then decreased to approximately 10 degrees and the needle is advanced parallel to the brachial artery for 1 inch (2.5 cm.), *i.e.*, until the needle point lies in the region of the X marking the median nerve (Figure 177, page 266). If no paresthesias of the median nerve are elicited, the needle is withdrawn until the point is just below the lacertus fibrosus. The direction of the needle is varied in a seeking manner, first laterally and then medially, being reinserted after each change in direction until paresthesias occur.

8. When paresthesias are encountered, after careful aspiration 5 to 10 cc. of the anesthetic drug is injected. Then another 5 to 10 cc. is deposited as the needle is gently moved backward and forward.

TECHNIQUE OF MEDIAN NERVE BLOCK AT THE WRIST

Position and Landmarks

1. The patient lies in the dorsal recumbent position with or without a pillow and his arm abducted.

2. The styloid process of the ulnar bone is palpated and a line through it drawn around the wrist (Figure 178, page 267 and Figure 179, page 268).

3. The patient is instructed to flex his fist on the wrist, the forearm at the elbow and tense the muscles of the arm (Figure 178, page 267). In this manner the palmaris longus tendon, or in its absence the flexor digitorum sublimis tendon, may be easily seen or palpated. The skin just lateral to the palmaris longus tendon, or in the absence the flexor digitorum sublimis tendon, is marked with an X on the line drawn in step 2 (Figure 179, page 268). The median nerve lies under or just lateral (the radial side) to the palmaris longus muscle. In the absence of the palmaris longus muscle the X is placed on the skin ¼ inch (0.6 cm.) lateral to the

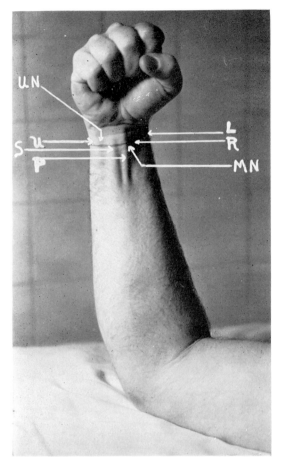

Figure 178. Topographical anatomy involved in locating the position of the median nerve at the wrist. L, line around the wrist through the styloid process of the ulnar bone. R, flexor carpi radialis. P, palmaris longus. S, flexor digitorum sublimis. U, flexor carpi ulnaris. U N, ulnar nerve. M N, median nerve.

flexor digitorum sublimis tendon as the median nerve will lie lateral to the radial side of this tendon (Figure 178, page 267).

4. The forearm and hand are now extended and the hand supinated so that they lie flat on the table or cart (Figure 173, page 261).

Precaution

Aspirate.—Careful aspiration for blood should be performed.

Procedure

1. The sterilizer control is checked to be sure the equipment has been sterilized.

2. The area is aseptically prepared and draped.

3. The anesthetist stands at the side to be blocked facing the wrist (Figure 173, page 261).

4. An intradermal wheal is made at the determined X with a ¾-inch (2 cm.), 25-gauge Huber point security Lok-needle (Figure 179, page 268).

5. The patient is instructed to say *"Now"* and not to move when typical paresthesias of the nerve are elicited. *Paresthesias of the median nerve are characterized by sharp, spraying, electric shock-like sensations to the palm of the hand, index finger, middle (long) finger, and the radial side of the ring finger.*

6. The 25-gauge Lok-needle used for the intradermal wheal with the full 10 cc. syringe attached is inserted perpendicular to the skin for ¾ inch (2 cm.) or until paresthesias occur. If paresthesias do not occur, the needle point should be withdrawn to the skin and reinserted in a fan-wise direction medially or laterally. This procedure should be repeated until paresthesias occur.

7. When paresthesias occur, the needle is fixed and 5 to 10 cc. of the anesthetic solution is injected.

DISTRIBUTION OF ANALGESIA

Analgesia of the area innervated by the median nerve and its branches beyond the point of the block ensues (Figure 152, page 236).

COMPLICATIONS

Toxic Reactions (intravascular injections, etc.): See Chapter 3, page 19.

REMARKS

Avoid Blood Vessels in Cubital Fossa: Care should be taken to avoid puncture of the several blood vessels in the cubital fossa.

Median Nerve May Lie Behind Flexor Carpi Radialis Tendon: At times the median

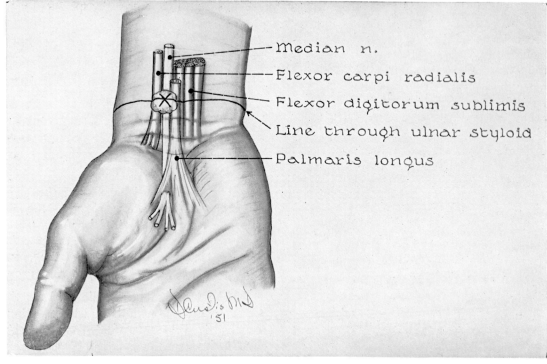

Figure 179. Landmarks and anatomy for a median nerve block at the wrist.

nerve lies behind the flexor carpi radialis tendon and when paresthesias in the usual locale are not elicited, this possibility should be considered.

Elicit Paresthesias: In these block procedures, paresthesias should be elicited. Remember the dictum *"No paresthesias, no anesthesia,"* and the failures will be minimal.

Recover Broken Needle(s): All needles should be tested before use. If a needle breaks, every effort, including surgery, should be made to recover it. Unremoved needles have a tendency to migrate and may cause permanent injuries as well as medicolegal complications.

Repeat Block When Analgesia Is Inadequate: If the desired results from the first block attempt are unsatisfactory, do not hesitate to reblock the patient if time permits. Most patients will think nothing about being reblocked if the second attempt is prefaced by a statement such as: "Well, I guess we will have to inject a little more medicine if we are going to freeze this area."

ULNAR NERVE BLOCK

INDICATIONS

Surgical: Operations and manipulations of the arm and hand limited to the little finger and fifth metacarpal bone.

Diagnostic: To localize pain problems of the upper extremity.

Therapeutic: To treat pain problems and vasospastic diseases of the arm and hand limited to the ulnar nerve. Stellate ganglion block is more suitable for the latter as vasospastic diseases are seldom limited to an area innervated by one nerve.

ANATOMY

The ulnar nerve derives its fibers from the eighth cervical and first thoracic nerves, but about 50 percent of ulnar nerves also receive fibers from the seventh cervical nerve. It lies along the medial side of the upper arm as far as the middle of the arm. Here it pierces the medial intermuscular septum, runs obliquely across the medial head of the triceps muscle and becomes superficial in the groove between the medial epicondyle of the humerus and the olecranon process of the ulna (Figure 180, page 269). It descends in the forearm, and about 2 inches (5 cm.) above the wrist it divides into a dorsal and a volar branch (Figure 180B, page 269; Figure 182, page 271; and Figure 183, page 273). The dorsal branch passes backward beneath the flexor carpi ulnaris tendon to supply the ulnar side of the dorsum of the little finger and the adjacent sides of the dorsum of the little and the ring fingers (Figure 152, page 236). The volar branch crosses the transverse carpal ligament on the lateral side of the pisiform bone, medial to and a bit behind the ulnar artery. It supplies the skin on the ulnar side of the hand and the skin of the little finger and ulnar side of the ring finger (Figure 152, page 236). It also supplies all the intrinsic muscles of the hand except the two radial lumbricals (I and II), the abductor pollicis brevis, the opponens pollicis and the superficial head of the flexor pollicis brevis.

PREMEDICATION

Paresthesias are always sought and light premedication is advised.

Light Premedication: Average patient (age 20 to 50, weight 150 pounds or over, height 5 feet, 5 inches or over, and good physical status) receives:

1. 200 mg. (3 gr.) of pentobarbital (Nembutal) by mouth at hour of sleep the night before surgery.

2. 100 mg. (1½ gr.) of pentobarbital by mouth with one ounce of water 1½ to 2 hours before estimated *block* time. This dose of barbiturate is omitted if there is a possibility that the patient will be too heavily sedated to give *an immediate response* when paresthesias are obtained.

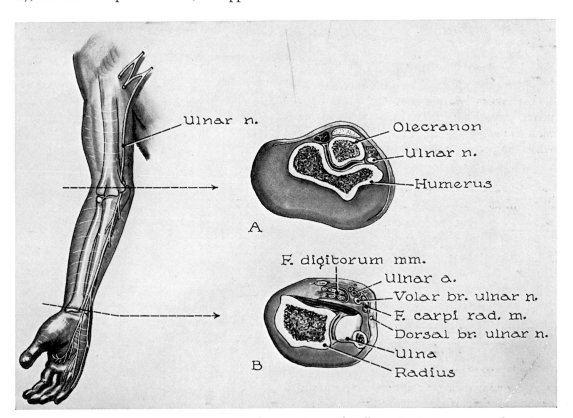

Figure 180. Anatomy of the ulnar nerve. A. Cross section at the elbow. B. Cross section at the wrist.

3. 10 mg. (⅙ gr.) of morphine and 0.4 mg. (¹⁄₁₅₀ gr.) of scopolamine intramuscularly *on call* to surgery.

Reduction of Premedication: It is seldom necessary to increase this premedication irrespective of the over-all size of the patient until the patient arrives in either the anesthesia or operating room. However, it is very common to reduce this medication under various circumstances; for example, in the case of the geriatric patient, the adolescent patient or child, the debilitated or cachectic patient, and for those whose surgery is complicated by other disease, *e.g.*, myxedema, diabetes, heart disease, etc. In the patient over 60 years of age, barbiturates and especially scopolamine may often cause disorientation. Therefore, in these patients atropine is usually substituted for scopolamine and the dosages of the barbiturate omitted or greatly reduced, *i.e.*, to 50 mg. (¾ gr.) or less. *Always err on the light side.*

Inadequate Premedication: If medication is not adequate either for the block or the surgical procedure, intravenous pentobarbital 50 mg. (¾ gr.) to 100 mg. (1½ gr.) or intravenous morphine 8 mg. (⅛ gr.) to 15 mg. (¼ gr.) may be given *slowly*. Judicious use of added sedation is extremely important. Often small supplementary doses of morphine or pentobarbital will make a block successful, particularly when the patient interprets touch and motion as pain.

DRUGS

Tetracaine (Pontocaine)

Dosage.—10 cc. to 20 cc. of 0.15 to 0.25 percent solution with or without 0.1 cc. of epinephrine (Adrenalin) 1:1000 in 20 cc. of solution.*

Onset.—Operating analgesia is established in 10 to 30 minutes, with an average of 20 minutes.

Duration.—Operating analgesia lasts 3½ to 6 hours, with stronger solutions and solutions containing epinephrine giving the upper limits.

Procaine (Novocain)

Dosage.—10 cc. to 20 cc. of 1.0 to 2.0 percent solution with or without 0.1 cc. of epinephrine (Adrenalin) 1:1000 in 20 cc. of solution.*

Onset.—Operating analgesia is established in 5 to 15 minutes, with an average of 10 minutes.

Duration.—Operating analgesia lasts 1 to 1½ hours, with stronger concentrations and solutions containing epinephrine giving the upper limits.

Lidocaine (Xylocaine) or Mepivacaine (Carbocaine)

Dosage.—10 cc. to 20 cc. of 1.0 to 1.5 percent solution with or without 0.1 cc. of epinephrine (Adrenalin) 1:1000 in 20 cc. of solution.*

Onset.—Operating analgesia is established in 5 to 15 minutes.

Duration.—Operating analgesia lasts 1¼ to 3 hours, with stronger concentrations and solutions containing epinephrine giving the upper limits.

MATERIALS

Regional tray (Chapter 9, page 51) or:

1. One ¾-inch (2 cm.), 25-gauge Huber point security Lok-needle.

2. One 2-inch (5 cm.), 22-gauge security Lok-needle, preferably with short bevel.

3. One tuberculin Lok-syringe for measuring epinephrine.

4. One 10 cc. Lok-syringe, preferably with finger rings.

5. One graduated measuring cup, preferably stainless steel, for mixing solutions.

6. One prep cup, preferably stainless steel.

7. Four sterile towels.

---

*Optimal concentration of epinephrine is 1:200,000, that is, 0.1 cc. of epinephrine 1:1000 in 20 cc. of the local anesthetic solution (see page 39).

8. Six sterile sponges.

9. One sterilizer control.

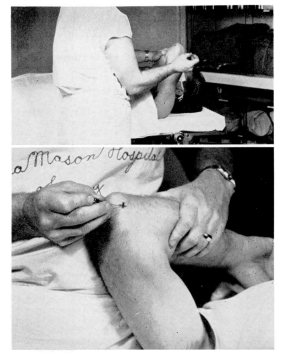

Figure 181. Position of the patient and the anesthetist for block of the ulnar nerve at the elbow. A. *(Top)* Left. B. *(Bottom)* Right.

TECHNIQUE OF ULNAR NERVE BLOCK AT THE ELBOW

Position and Landmarks

1. The patient lies in the dorsal recumbent position with or without a pillow, the upper extremity internally rotated and flexed at the humerus so that it is perpendicular to the table. The forearm is flexed at the elbow (Figure 181, page 271).

2. The groove between the medial epicondyle of the humerus and the olecranon process of the ulna is located. This is the ulnar groove and contains the ulnar nerve (Figure 182, page 271).

3. The exact location of the ulnar nerve may be found in the greater percentage of cases if the anesthetist will exert pressure in the ulnar groove with his thumb. The patient should be cautioned to say *"Now"* as soon as he feels tingling in his little finger or experiences the sensation which occurs when he hits his elbow ("crazy bone") inadvertently. The skin over this point should be marked with an X (Figure 182, page 271).

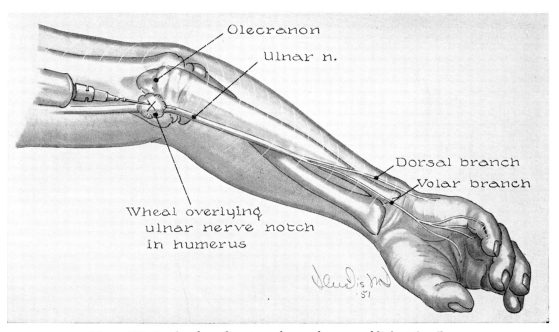

Figure 182. Landmarks and anatomy for an ulnar nerve block at the elbow.

4. If paresthesias cannot be elicited, an X should be marked midway between the tip of the olecranon process of the ulnar bone and the tip of the medial epicondyle of the humerus (Figure 182, page 271).

Precaution

Aspirate.—Careful aspiration for blood should be performed.

Procedure

1. The sterilizer control is checked to be sure the equipment has been sterilized.

2. The area is aseptically prepared and draped.

3. The anesthetist stands at the side to be blocked and faces the elbow (Figure 181, page 271).

4. An intradermal wheal is raised at the determined X with a ¾-inch (2 cm.), 25-gauge Huber point security Lok-needle (Figure 182, page 271).

5. The patient is instructed to say *"Now"* and not to move when typical paresthesias radiating to the little finger are elicited. *Paresthesias in the little finger should be characterized by sharp, spraying, electric shock-like sensations.*

6. The 2-inch (5 cm.), 22-gauge security Lok-needle with a full 10 cc. Lok-syringe attached is introduced in the direction of the nerve and almost parallel with it to a depth of ¼ inch (0.6 cm.) to ½ inch (1.3 cm.) below the skin (Figure 182, page 271). It should be advanced forward not more than 1 inch (2.5 cm.) or until paresthesias occur. If no paresthesias are found, the needle point should be withdrawn to the skin and reinserted in the same fashion fan-wise medial and lateral to the X until paresthesias occur.

7. When paresthesias occur, the needle is fixed and 5 to 10 cc. of the solution injected.

TECHNIQUE OF BLOCKING THE VOLAR AND DORSAL BRANCHES OF THE ULNAR NERVE AT THE WRIST

Position and Landmarks

1. The patient lies in the dorsal recumbent position with or without a pillow, his arm at his side and his hand supinated (Figure 173, page 261).

2. The styloid process of the ulnar bone is located and a line through it drawn around the wrist (Figure 183, page 273).

3. The flexor carpi ulnaris is located by having the patient flex his fist on the wrist, the forearm at the elbow, and tense the muscles of the arm (Figure 178, page 267). On its radial side an X is marked on the line through the ulnar processes (Figure 183, page 273). By careful palpation the ulnar artery may be felt just lateral to the X.

Precautions

Aspirate.—The volar branch of the ulnar nerve lies between the flexor carpi ulnaris tendon and the ulnar artery; if possible, puncture of the artery or of the joint spaces below should be avoided. Before injecting, aspirate carefully for blood.

Procedure

1. The sterilizer control is checked to be sure the equipment has been sterilized.

2. The area is aseptically prepared and draped.

3. The anesthetist stands at the side to be blocked at the hand and faces the patient's head (Figure 173, page 261).

4. An intradermal wheal is made at the determined X with a ¾-inch (2 cm.), 25-gauge Huber point security Lok-needle (Figure 183, page 273).

5. The patient is instructed to say *"Now"* and not to move when typical paresthesias are felt radiating to the little finger. *Paresthesias*

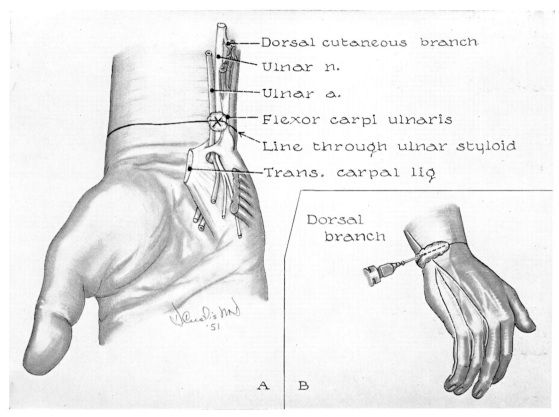

Figure 183. Landmarks and anatomy for an ulnar nerve block at the wrist. A. Volar branch. B. Dorsal branch

in the little finger should be characterized by sharp, spraying, electric shock-like sensations.

6. With the index finger of the left hand palpating the ulnar artery, the 25-gauge needle used to make the wheal, with the full 10 cc. Lok-syringe attached, is inserted perpendicular to the skin in close approximation to the artery for ¾ inch (2 cm.) or until paresthesias of the volar branch of the ulnar nerve or bone are felt (Figure 183, page 273). If paresthesias do not occur, the needle point should be withdrawn to the skin and reinserted in a fan-wise direction laterally until paresthesias are felt.

7. When paresthesias occur, the needle is fixed and 5 to 10 cc. of anesthetic solution injected.

8. The dorsal branch of the ulnar nerve is now anesthetized by intradermal and subcutaneous infiltration along the line drawn through the styloid process from the ulnar side of the flexor carpi ulnaris tendon to the middle of the back of the wrist (Figure 183, page 273).

DISTRIBUTION OF ANALGESIA

Analgesia of the area innervated by the ulnar nerve and its branches beyond the point of the block ensues (Figure 152, page 236).

COMPLICATIONS

Toxic Reactions (intravascular injections, etc.): See Chapter 3, page 19.

REMARKS

Block Ulnar Nerve at Elbow: Block of the ulnar nerve at the elbow is easier and produces more satisfactory analgesia than its block at the wrist. This is true because the ulnar nerve usually branches 2 inches (5 cm.) above the wrist into a dorsal and a volar branch, and unless a "garter" or ring of the anesthetic solution is put around the wrist to anesthetize the dorsal branch which lies in the subcutaneous tissue, only the volar branch will be blocked.

Elicit Paresthesias: In this block procedure, paresthesias should be elicited. Remember the dictum, *"No paresthesias, no anesthesia,"* and the failures will be minimal.

Recover Broken Needle(s): All needles should be tested before use. If a needle breaks, every effort to recover it, including surgery, should be made. Unremoved needles have a tendency to migrate and may cause permanent injuries as well as medicolegal complications.

Repeat Block When Analgesia Is Inadequate: If the desired results from the first block attempt are unsatisfactory, do not hesitate to reblock the patient if time permits. Most patients will think nothing about being reblocked if the second attempt is prefaced by a statement such as: "Well, I guess we will have to inject a little more medicine if we are going to freeze this area."

CHAPTER 33

Block of the Sciatic and Femoral Nerves

INDICATIONS

Surgical: Operations or manipulations on the leg and foot from 2 inches (5 cm.) beyond the inferior edge of the patella. Closed manipulations of the knee and thigh may be done but open operations cannot be performed unless the obturator and lateral femoral cutaneous nerves are also blocked. They supply part of the skin of the thigh and, usually, both nerves often send a twig to the knee joint.

Diagnostic: Localization of pain problems.

Therapeutic: Relief of neuralgias of the sciatic and femoral nerves. When block of the lumbar sympathetic ganglia is contraindicated, sciatic nerve block may be used to effect a block of most of the sympathetic nerves of the lower extremity.

ANATOMY

Sciatic Nerve: The sciatic nerve is formed by the union of the anterior rami of the fourth and fifth lumbar nerves and the first, second, and third sacral nerves (Figure 184, page 275). It is the largest nerve in the body, measuring ¾ inch (2 cm.) in width and passes out of the pelvis through the greater sciatic notch (Figure 185A, page 276). It descends between the tuberosity of the ischium and the

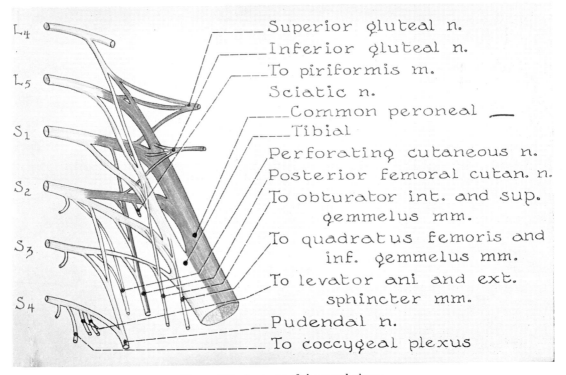

Figure 184. Anatomy of the sacral plexus.

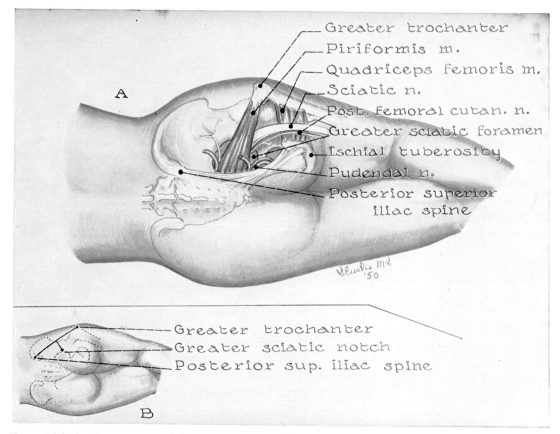

Figure 185. A. Deep anatomy of the sciatic nerve in relationship to the landmarks. B. Topographical anatomy of the landmarks for a sciatic block.

greater trochanter along the back of the leg (Figure 186, page 277). It divides into the tibial and common peroneal nerves, usually at about the lower third of the thigh (Figure 186, page 277).

Femoral Nerve: The femoral nerve is formed by the dorsal divisions of the anterior rami of the second, third, and fourth lumbar nerves (Figure 187, page 277). It emerges from the pelvis beneath the inguinal ligament just lateral to and ¼ inch (0.6 cm.) posterior to the femoral artery (Figure 188, page 278). This relationship to the femoral artery exists near the inguinal ligament, not after the nerve enters the thigh. As the nerve passes into the thigh, it divides into an anterior and a posterior division. The anterior division gives off anterior cutaneous and muscular branches to the sartorius muscle. The posterior division gives off the saphenous nerve which is the largest cutaneous branch of the femoral nerve, muscular branches, and articular branches.

PREMEDICATION

Paresthesias of the femoral nerve are never sought, but paresthesias of the sciatic nerve are always sought. Therefore, light premedication is advised until the sciatic nerve is blocked.

Light Premedication: Average patient (age 20 to 50, weight 150 pounds or over, height 5 feet, 5 inches or over, and good physical status) receives:

1. 200 mg. (3 gr.) of pentobarbital (Nembutal) by mouth at hour of sleep the night before surgery.

2. 100 mg. (1½ gr.) of pentobarbital by mouth 1½ to 2 hours before estimated *block*

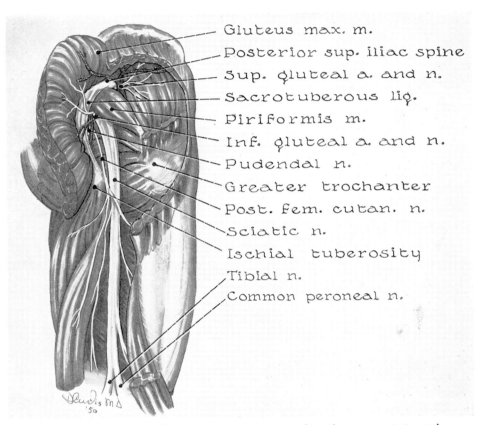

Gluteus max. m.

Posterior sup. iliac spine

Sup. gluteal a. and n.

Sacrotuberous lig.

Piriformis m.

Inf. gluteal a. and n.

Pudendal n.

Greater trochanter

Post. fem. cutan. n.

Sciatic n.

Ischial tuberosity

Tibial n.

Common peroneal n.

Figure 186. Anatomy of the sciatic nerve as it emerges from the greater sciatic notch.

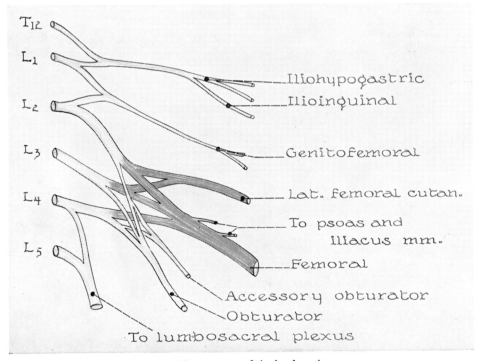

T_{12}

L_1

L_2

L_3

L_4

L_5

Iliohypogastric

Ilioinguinal

Genitofemoral

Lat. femoral cutan.

To psoas and
iliacus mm.

Femoral

Accessory obturator

Obturator

To lumbosacral plexus

Figure 187. Anatomy of the lumbar plexus.

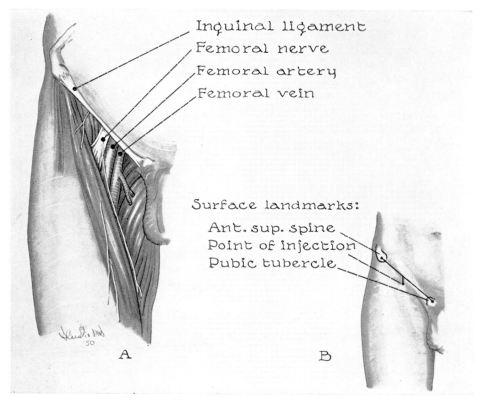

Figure 188. A. Deep anatomy involved in the blocking of the femoral nerve. B. Topographical anatomy involved in the blocking of the femoral nerve.

time. This dose of barbiturate is omitted if there is a possibility that the patient will be too heavily sedated to give *an immediate response* when paresthesias of the sciatic nerve are obtained.

3. 10 mg. (⅙ gr.) of morphine and 0.4 mg. (¹⁄₁₅₀ gr.) of scopolamine intramuscularly *on call* to surgery.

Reduction of Premedication: It is seldom necessary to increase this premedication irrespective of the over-all size of the patient until the patient arrives in either the anesthesia or operating room. However, it is very common to reduce this medication under various circumstances; for example, in the case of the geriatric patient, the adolescent patient or child, the debilitated or cachectic patient, and for those whose surgery is complicated by other disease, *i.e.*, myxedema, diabetes, heart disease, etc. In the patient over 60 years of age barbiturates and especially scopolamine

may often cause disorientation. Therefore, in these patients atropine is usually substituted for scopolamine and the dosages of the barbiturate omitted or greatly reduced, *i.e.*, to 50 mg. (¾ gr.) or less. *Always err on the light side.*

Inadequate Premedication: If medication is not adequate either for the block or surgical procedure, intravenous pentobarbital 50 mg. (¾ gr.) to 100 mg. (1½ gr.) or intravenous morphine 8 mg. (⅛ gr.) to 15 mg. (¼ gr.) may be given *slowly*. Judicious use of added sedation is extremely important. Often small supplementary doses of morphine or pentobarbital will make a block successful, especially when a patient interprets touch and motion as pain.

DRUGS

Tetracaine (Pontocaine)

Dosage.—50 cc. of 0.15 to 0.25 percent solution with or without 0.25 cc. of epinephrine (Adrenalin) 1:1000.*

Onset.—Operating analgesia is established in 15 to 45 minutes, with an average of 20 minutes.

Duration.—Operating analgesia lasts 3½ to 6 hours, with stronger concentrations and solutions containing epinephrine giving the upper limits.

Procaine (Novocain)

Dosage.—50 cc. of 1.0 to 2.0 percent solution with or without 0.25 cc. of epinephrine (Adrenalin) 1:1000.*

Onset.—Operating analgesia is established in 5 to 15 minutes, with an average of 10 minutes.

Duration.—Operating analgesia lasts 1 to 1½ hours, with stronger concentrations and solutions containing epinephrine giving the upper limits.

Lidocaine (Xylocaine) or Mepivacaine (Carbocaine)

Dosage.—50 cc. of a 1.0 percent solution with or without 0.25 cc. of epinephrine (Adrenalin) 1:1000.*

Onset.—Operating analgesia is established in 5 to 15 minutes, with an average of 10 minutes.

Duration.—Operating analgesia lasts 1¼ to 3 hours, with stronger concentrations and solutions containing epinephrine giving the upper limits.

MATERIALS

Regional tray (see Chapter 9, page 51) or:

1. One ¾-inch (2 cm.), 25-gauge Huber point security Lok-needle.

2. One 1½-inch (3.8 cm.), 22-gauge security Lok-needle, preferably with short bevel.

---

*Optimal concentration of epinephrine is 1:200,000, that is, 0.1 cc. of epinephrine 1:1000 in 20 cc. of the local anesthetic solution (see page 39).

3. One 3-inch (7.5 cm.), 22-gauge security Lok-needle, preferably with short bevel.

4. One 4-inch (10 cm.), 22-gauge security Lok-needle, preferably with short bevel.

5. One tuberculin Lok-syringe for measuring epinephrine.

6. One 10 cc. Lok-syringe, preferably with finger rings.

7. One graduated measuring cup, preferably stainless steel, for mixing solution.

8. One prep cup, preferably stainless steel.

9. Four sterile towels.

10. Six sterile sponges.

11. One sterilizer control.

TECHNIQUE OF SCIATIC NERVE BLOCK

When both the sciatic nerve and the femoral nerve are to be blocked, the sciatic nerve is anesthetized first and then the patient is turned supine for the femoral block.

Position and Landmarks

1. The patient lies on the side opposite the one to be blocked with the underneath leg straight and the hip joint of the uppermost extremity in 40 degrees of flexion, 20 to 30 degrees of abduction, and neutral as to rotation. The knee of the extremity to be blocked is flexed at a 90 degree angle (Figure 189, page 280).

2. The posterior superior iliac spine is palpated and the skin overlying it is marked with an X (Figure 189, page 280 and Figure 185B, page 276).

3. The greater trochanter is palpated and the skin overlying its superior border marked with an X (Figure 189, page 280 and Figure 185B, page 276). At this portion of the greater trochanter there is an impression for the insertion of the piriformis muscle (Figure 185A, page 276).

4. A straight line is drawn between the

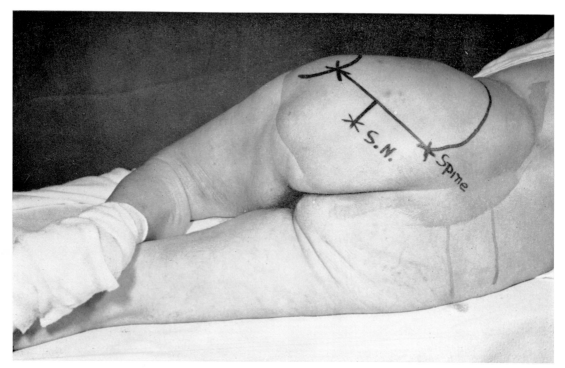

Figure 189. A. Patient in position for sciatic nerve block. Note position of legs and position of X's. Anesthetic administered for removal of metatarsal bone. S. N., point of insertion of needle for sciatic nerve block.

two determined points (Figure 189, page 280 and Figure 185A, page 276).

5. The midpoint of this line is determined and a line perpendicular to it at this point is drawn in a downward direction (Figure 189, page 280 and Figure 185B, page 276).

6. 1½ inches (3.8 cm.) to 2 inches (5 cm.) below the base line, an X is made (Figure 189, page 280 and Figure 185B, page 276). This point should lie over the sciatic nerve as it makes its exit from the pelvis through the greater sciatic notch of the iliac bone (Figure 185 A and B, page 276).

Precautions

Aspirate.—Aspiration tests should be made before injection. With the exception of an intravascular injection, little danger is incurred in performing this block.

Do Not Allow Patient to Move.—Once the landmarks are drawn, do not allow the patient to move. In heavy patients the buttocks may distort the landmarks if the patient moves a slight amount.

Procedure

1. The sterilizer control is checked to be sure the equipment has been sterilized. The area is aseptically prepared and draped.

2. The anesthetist stands facing the buttocks of the patient.

3. The patient is instructed to say *"Now"* and not to move as soon as he feels a "tingle" or an "electric shock" go down his leg. *Paresthesias of the sciatic nerve are characterized by sharp, spraying, electric shock-like sensations which radiate down the leg to the toes, the heel, or the foot.*

4. An intradermal wheal is raised at the determined point with the ¾-inch (2 cm.) 25-gauge Huber point security Lok-needle.

5. Deep infiltration is then carried out with a 1½-inch (3.8 cm.), 22-gauge security Lok-needle.

6. A 3-inch (7.5 cm.) or 4-inch (10 cm.), 22-gauge security Lok-needle, depending on the size of the patient, without a syringe attached, is inserted at the wheal perpendicular to the skin in all planes and advanced until paresthesias of the sciatic nerve are elicited or bone is encountered.

7. When paresthesias are elicited, the needle is fixed and 15 to 25 cc. of the anesthetic solution is injected (Figure 190, page 281 and Figure 191, page 282). Depending on the size of the buttocks, the depth to which the needle must be inserted may vary from 2 inches (5 cm.) to 4 inches (10 cm.).

8. When the bone, usually the rim around the greater sciatic notch, i.e., the spine of the ischium and the bone in its immediate vicinity, has been encountered, the needle depth should be noted. The needle never need be inserted in any direction more than ¾ inch (2 cm.) past this depth. The nerve usually lies above this part of the iliac bone in this region, and paresthesias are often encountered before or just as the bone is contacted.

9. If paresthesias are not encountered, the needle point is withdrawn slightly and re-inserted in various directions, i.e., a little more upward or downward in the plane of the body marked by the line perpendicular to the line between the posterior superior iliac spine and the greater trochanter (Figure 192, page 283), until paresthesias occur. Should this maneuver fail to produce paresthesias and if bone has been encountered on each try, an attempt should be made to slip into the sciatic notch by directing the point of the needle slightly sacrally in an effort to obtain paresthesias of the sciatic nerve as it courses through the notch.

10. If after numerous endeavors no paresthesias are obtained, 15 to 20 cc. of the local anesthetic solution should be injected as the needle point is moved along the bony rim around the greater sciatic notch, in hopes of anesthetizing the nerve by diffusion of the local anesthetic agent. The diffusion technique of blocking the sciatic nerve is usually unsatisfactory and the percentage of failures or partial failures is high.

TECHNIQUE OF FEMORAL NERVE BLOCK

If a barbiturate has not been given or if the patient is apprehensive at the completion of

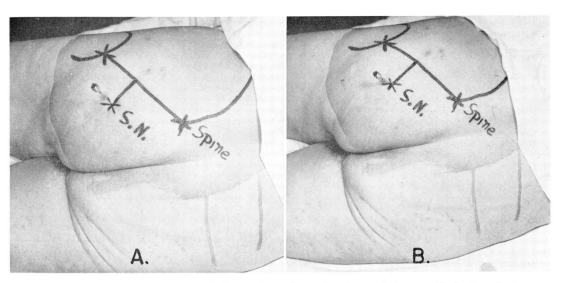

Figure 190. S. N. Sciatic Nerve. A. 4-inch (10 cm.) needle in place for a sciatic nerve block. Paresthesias were just elicited. Note the perpendicular position of the needle. B. Needle walked upward and another paresthesia was elicited. As the sciatic nerve crosses the rim of bone of the greater sciatic foramen it is approximately ¾ inch (2 cm.) to 1 inch (2.5 cm.) in width. Therefore, more than one paresthesia may be elicited.

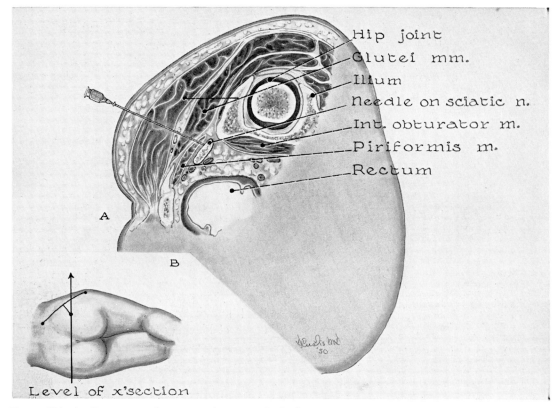

Figure 191. A. Cross-sectional anatomy of area in which the sciatic nerve is injected with the needle in the sciatic nerve. B. Level of cross section.

the sciatic nerve block, 100 mg. (1½ gr.) to 200 mg. (3 gr.) of pentobarbital is given prior to the femoral nerve block. Paresthesias of the femoral nerve are not sought and if added sedatives are given *slowly intravenously* at this point the patient seldom remembers the femoral nerve block or is discomforted by it.

Position and Landmarks

1. The patient lies supine with hands clasped behind his head.

2. The inguinal ligament and the femoral artery are located by palpation. An X is made on the skin 1 inch (2.5 cm.) below the inguinal ligament and just lateral to the femoral artery (Figure 193, page 283). This X marks the femoral nerve.

Precaution

Aspirate.—Aspiration tests should be made

before injection. With the exception of an intravascular injection, little danger is incurred in performing this block.

Procedure

1. The area is aseptically prepared and draped.

2. The anesthetist stands facing the side of the patient to be blocked.

3. An intradermal wheal is raised at the determined point with the 25-gauge Huber point security Lok-needle.

4. If the anesthetist is right-handed, the index finger of the left hand palpates and retracts the artery medially (Figure 194A, page 284). If the anesthetist is left-handed the right hand is used.

5. A 1½-inch (3.8 cm.) security Lok-needle without the syringe attached is inserted per-

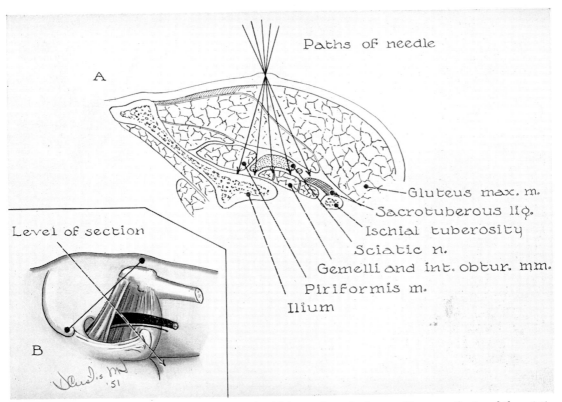

Figure 192. A. Direction in which the needle should be readjusted when seeking paresthesias of the sciatic nerve. B. Level of oblique section A.

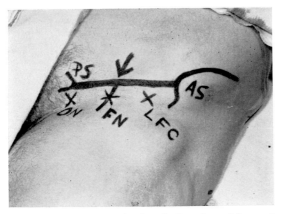

Figure 193. Shows the landmarks for a lateral femoral cutaneous nerve block, femoral nerve block, and obturator block. AS, anterior superior spine of the iliac bone; LFC, lateral femoral cutaneous nerve; FN, femoral nerve; PS, pubic tubercle (spine); ON, obturator nerve. Line between anterior superior spine and pubic tubercle represents the ilioinguinal (Poupart's) ligament. Arrow points to femoral artery which is represented by line extending below ilioinguinal ligament. Note landmarks for femoral nerve, lateral femoral cutaneous nerve, and obturator nerve all lie on a straight line which is approximately 1 inch (2.5 cm.) below and parallel to the ilioinguinal ligament.

pendicular to the skin and advanced until its point lies in close approximation to the lateral side of the artery (Figure 194A, B, and C, page 284 and Figure 195, page 285). The artery is usually ½ inch (1.3 cm.) to 1 inch (2.5 cm.) below the skin. Piercing the vessel need cause little concern. The needle is merely withdrawn from the lumen of the vessel and redirected slightly laterally. When the operator removes his hand from the needle, it should pulsate with each heart beat.

6. 20 cc. of the local anesthetic solution is now injected in a fan-wise direction lateral to the artery (Figure 194D, page 284 and Figure 196, page 285). The anesthetic solution is injected as the needle moves in and out. Care should be taken to see that a wall of anesthetic solution extends from the skin to a depth of 1¼ inches (3.2 cm.) and from the artery laterally at least 1 inch (2.5 cm.). It is best to err on the deep and lateral sides since in those areas there are no structures

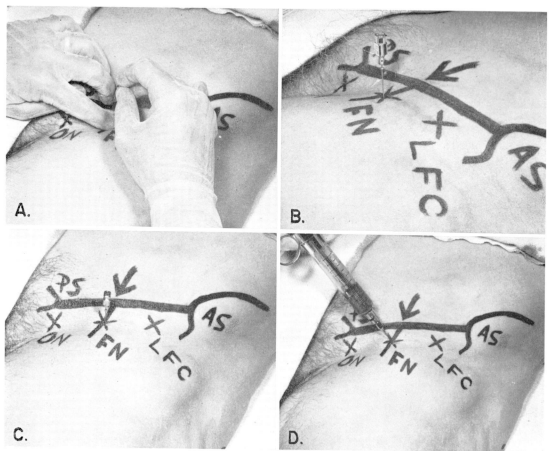

Figure 194. Technique of femoral nerve block. AS, anterior superior spine of the iliac bone; LFC, lateral femoral cutaneous nerve; FN, femoral nerve; PS, pubic tubercle (spine); ON, obturator nerve. A. Index finger of the left hand palpates pulsations of femoral artery. Right hand places 1½-inch (3.8 cm.) needle immediately lateral to artery and slightly deeper than the artery. B. Lateral view of position of needle following placement. C. Anterior view of needle following placement. D. Infiltration in fan-wise direction for 1 inch lateral to the femoral artery, maintaining depth of original insertion.

that can be harmed. This fan-wise injection should be made along an imaginary line projected through the cross-sectional plane of the body (Figure 196, page 285).

7. No attempt at eliciting paresthesias is made, since the diffusion technique of blocking the femoral nerve gives close to 100 percent results. If paresthesias should occur, the needle is fixed and after aspiration 5 cc. of the anesthetic solution injected. *Paresthesias of the femoral nerve are characterized by "electric shocks" in the knee or over the medial side of the leg.*

DISTRIBUTION OF ANESTHESIA

Sciatic Nerve: This nerve supplies the mus-
cles of the back of the thigh and those of the leg and foot. It supplies the skin of the back of the thigh, the back and lateral aspect of the leg and the lateral side, bottom and all the toes of the foot with the occasional exception of the dorsal surface of the big toe (Figure 197, page 286). It sends articular branches to the hip joint, knee joint, and ankle joint.

Femoral Nerve: In the lower extremities this nerve supplies the muscles of the quadriceps femoris group and the skin over the medial aspect of the thigh, leg, foot, and occasionally the dorsal surface of the big toe (Figure 197, page 286). It sends articular branches to the hip and knee joints.

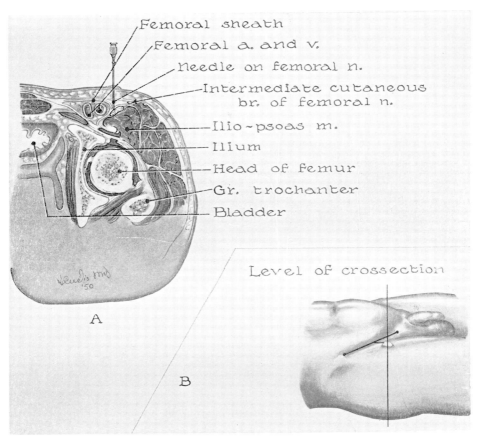

Femoral sheath
Femoral a. and v.
needle on femoral n.
Intermediate cutaneous
br. of femoral n.
Ilio-psoas m.
Ilium
Head of femur
Gr. trochanter
Bladder

A

Level of crossection

B

Figure 195. A. Anatomy of the femoral nerve at the level of the injection. B. Shows the level of the cross section.

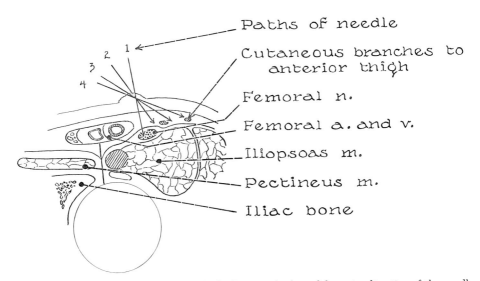

Paths of needle
Cutaneous branches to anterior thigh
Femoral n.
Femoral a. and v.
Iliopsoas m.
Pectineus m.
Iliac bone

Figure 196. Cross section through the thigh showing the lateral fan-wise direction of the needle as the femoral nerve is injected. This cross section is through the same area as shown in Figure 195.

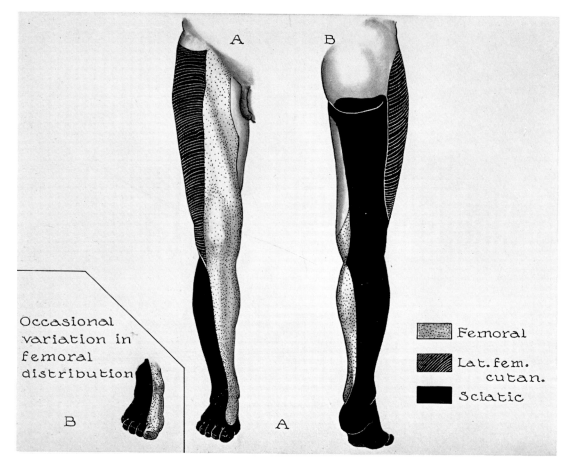

Figure 197. A. Area of skin anesthesia resulting from a sciatic nerve, femoral nerve, or lateral femoral cuta-neous nerve block. B. Variation in distribution of the femoral nerve in the foot.

COMPLICATIONS

Toxic Reactions (intravascular injections, etc.): See Chapter 3, page 19.

REMARKS

Femoral Nerve Innervates Quadriceps Femoris Muscle: If the femoral nerve has been adequately anesthetized, the patient will be unable to extend the leg at the knee. This movement is dependent upon the quadriceps femoris muscle which is innervated by the posterior division of the femoral nerve.

Sciatic Nerve Eliminates Motion of Toes: If the sciatic nerve has been adequately anesthetized, the patient will in most instances be unable to move the toes on the blocked foot.

Elicit Paresthesias of Sciatic Nerves: Par-esthesias of the sciatic nerve should be elicited to assure an adequate block. *Do not be misled!* In the lightly premedicated patient be sure the paresthesias radiate to the *foot.* Sensations radiating to the thigh and calf may have been referred by the periosteum. Remember the dictum, *"No paresthesias, no anesthesia,"* and failures will be minimal.

When performing a sciatic nerve block on a child under basal narcosis, a heavily medicated adult, or on a stoic patient, the anesthetist should pay particular attention to the leg and foot being blocked. When the sciatic nerve in these patients is stimulated, often the leg or foot will suddenly twitch or move.

If Needle Is Constantly Moving, Aspiration Is Not Necessary: When injecting fan-wise, as in the femoral nerve block, aspiration is not necessary, providing the needle is constantly moving back and forth while the anesthetic solution is being deposited. As long as the needle is constantly moving, there is little chance of depositing a large amount of anesthetic solution in a blood vessel.

Spinal Block Indicated for Open Operations On or Above Knee: Open operations on or above the knee cannot be carried out under the combination of sciatic and femoral nerve blocks unless the lateral femoral cutaneous and obturator nerves are also blocked. Even in the most experienced hands, blocking of the obturator nerve is often unsatisfactory. Therefore, if the patient's physical status dictates that regional analgesia should be employed in these cases it seems best to resort to a more certain method, e.g., spinal block.

Infection Below Knee No Contraindication to Block: Infections in the lower extremity below the knee, particularly if the patient is on chemotherapy or an antibiotic drug, are not a contraindication to the use of a sciatic and femoral nerve blocks as described. The increased circulation of the extremity following the block may actually be beneficial in shortening the course of the infection.

Paresthesias of Femoral Nerve Not Sought: Paresthesias of the femoral nerve are not always easy to obtain, and no effort to elicit them is necessary. Paresthesias of the sciatic nerve are usually easily stimulated and every effort to find them should be made. When the combination of these two blocks is not adequate for a surgical procedure on the ankle or foot, the femoral nerve is usually the one that has been missed. It cannot be emphasized too strongly that when the fan-wise injection of the femoral nerve is executed, it must be done carefully so that an adequate block of the femoral nerve is accomplished.

Sciatic Nerve Block May Be Used to Produce Sympathetic Block: If the patient cannot be positioned for a block of the lumbar sympathetic ganglia or the physician does not wish to attempt a block of the lumbar sympathetic ganglia, sciatic nerve block may be used as a means of blocking most of the sympathetic nerves to the leg. When the sciatic nerve is blocked to alleviate vasoconstriction, it should be remembered that a somatic nerve block with loss of motor and sensory function also occurs. Therefore, a block of the sciatic nerve may be used as a therapeutic measure, but not as a diagnostic test to prognosticate the results of a lumbar sympathectomy.

Sciatic and Femoral Nerve Blocks Are the Peripheral Nerve Blocks of Choice for Operations Below the Knee: The combination of sciatic nerve block at the greater sciatic notch and femoral nerve block just below the inguinal ligament is favored for the following reasons.

First, it produces complete analgesia for either surgical procedures or closed manipulations of the lower extremity from 2 inches (5 cm.) below the inferior border of the patellar tendon on down. The larger percentage of injuries to the lower extremity occur in this region.

Second, closed reductions and manipulations of fractures of the middle or lower third of the femur may in most cases be performed.

Third, either block by itself will usually provide inadequate analgesia because of the variations in the terminal distribution of the two nerves. The anesthetist should not overlook the wide and varied distribution of the saphenous branch of the femoral nerve over the dorsum of the foot, the medial malleolus, and the big toe (Figure 197, page 286).

Fourth, only if the two nerves are blocked can the pneumatic tourniquet be applied to the thigh without marked discomfort. If the sciatic and femoral nerves are blocked at or below the knee, a tourniquet placed on the thigh will cause pain. Since the advent of the pneumatic tourniquet, most surgeons prefer a bloodless field; this should always be present in the anesthetist's mind when blocking the nerves of the lower extremity.

Fifth, this block is very applicable to the diabetic since many complications peculiar to diabetes occur in the lower leg and foot. Most diabetics have arteriosclerosis but if this associated disease has not progressed too far, the block may actually increase the circulation of the extremity and promote healing. Thus it has served a double purpose.

Sixth, in crushing injuries of the foot or leg with associated shock and vascular spasm, this combination is the anesthesia of choice; it will release the spasm, correct the shock, if not due to hemorrhage, and provide anesthesia.

Seventh, the execution of sciatic and femoral nerve block is easy to master.

Eighth, this block produces quicker, more constant, and more satisfactory operating analgesia of the leg and foot with less technical difficulty than blocking of the branches of these nerves below the knee.

Ninth, complications other than toxic reactions from blocks performed as advocated in this chapter are negligible.

Tenth, following individual blocks of the peroneal nerve just below the knee and anterior or posterior tibial nerves at the ankle, it is not uncommon for the patient to complain of painful paresthesias of these nerves when wearing shoes, particularly high shoes or boots, tight riding pants, or when he bumps his leg in the region of the nerve.

Lastly, digital block is avoided because gangrene of a toe following it is not uncommon.

Because of the circumstances listed above, sciatic and femoral nerve block is the only procedure other than local infiltration and spinal block which the author recommends for operations below the knee. When operations of minor significance are to be accomplished under regional analgesia and the surgeon agrees not to use a tourniquet, local infiltration as described in Chapter 10, page 62, is usually performed by the surgeon. An example is surgery of ingrown toenail, which perhaps does not warrant sciatic and femoral nerve blocks.

Tourniquet Pain Not Completely Eliminated by Sciatic and Femoral Nerve Blocks: If a tourniquet is placed on the thigh and inflated following a block of the sciatic and femoral nerves, the patient may complain of some discomfort in the thigh. The pain may be eliminated by: (1) sedation, *e.g.*, 100 mg. (1½ gr.) to 200 mg. (3 gr.) of pentobarbital or 8 mg. (⅛ gr.) to 10 mg. (⅙ gr.) of morphine; or (2) blocking of the lateral femoral cutaneous nerve.

Recover Broken Needle(s): All needles should be tested before use. If a needle breaks, every effort to recover it, including surgery, should be made. Unremoved needles have a tendency to migrate and may cause permanent injuries as well as medicolegal complications.

Repeat Block When Analgesia Is Inadequate: If the desired results from the first block attempt are unsatisfactory, do not hesitate to reblock the patient if time permits. Most patients will think nothing about being reblocked if the second attempt is prefaced by a statement such as: "Well, I guess we will have to inject a little more medicine if we are going to freeze this area."

However, do not exceed the maximum safe dosage of the local anesthetic solution for both blocks. If to reblock the patient the maximum safe dose of the local anesthetic solution must be exceeded, 45 minutes should elapse between blocks.

CHAPTER 34

Obturator Nerve Block

INDICATIONS

Surgical: Combined with sciatic, femoral, and lateral femoral cutaneous nerve blocks for surgical procedures on or above the knee.

Diagnostic: Localization of hip joint pain.

Therapeutic: Relief of hip joint pain and spasm of the adductor group of muscles.

ANATOMY

The obturator nerve arises from the ventral division of the second, third, and fourth lumbar nerves (Figure 187, page 277). It leaves the pelvis through the upper part of the obturator foramen (Figure 198A and B, page 289). It enters the thigh and divides into anterior and posterior branches. The anterior

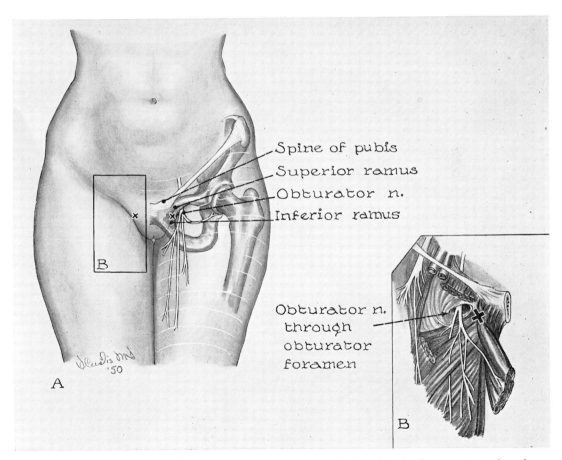

Spine of pubis
Superior ramus
Obturator n.
Inferior ramus

Obturator n. through obturator foramen

Figure 198. A. Anatomy of the obturator nerve as it passes through the obturator foramen. B. Enlarged area of A. with detailed anatomy. X marks the spot of entrance of the needle for an obturator nerve block.

branch supplies an articular branch to the hip joint, muscular branches to the adductor longus muscle, gracilis muscle, adductor brevis muscle, and occasionally the pectineus muscle. It also occasionally supplies cutaneous branches to the knee region and upper third of the tibial side of the leg. The posterior branch supplies muscular branches to the obturator externus muscle, adductor magnus muscle, adductor brevis muscle, and an articular branch to the knee joint.

PREMEDICATION

When the block is performed for a diagnostic or therapeutic procedure, no premedication is necessary because no attempts to elicit paresthesias are made and the block is not painful if adequate infiltration is performed as the needle is advanced.

When the block is performed in conjunction with sciatic, femoral, and lateral femoral cutaneous nerve blocks for operation on the leg, the same medications as given for sciatic and femoral block are sufficient. See Chapter 33, page 276.

DRUGS

Tetracaine (Pontocaine)

Dosage.—20 cc. to 25 cc. of 0.15 to 0.25 per-cent solution with or without 0.1 cc. of epinephrine (Adrenalin) 1:1000 in each 20 cc. of solution.* 150 TRU of hyaluronidase may be of aid in this block (see page 43).

Onset.—Operating analgesia is established in 15 to 30 minutes.

Duration.—Operating analgesia lasts 3½ to 6 hours, with stronger concentrations and solutions containing epinephrine giving the upper limits.

Procaine (Novocain)

Dosage.—20 to 25 cc. of a 1.0 to 2.0 percent solution with or without 0.1 cc. of epinephrine (Adrenalin) 1:1000 in each 20 cc. of solution.* 150 TRU of hyaluronidase may be of aid in this block (see page 43).

Onset.—Operating analgesia is established in 10 to 20 minutes.

Duration.—Operating analgesia lasts 1 to 1½ hours, with stronger concentration and solutions containing epinephrine giving the upper limits.

Lidocaine (Xylocaine) or Mepivacaine (Carbocaine)

Dosage.—20 cc. to 25 cc. of 1.0 to 1.5 per-cent solution with or without 0.1 cc. of epinephrine (Adrenalin) 1:1000 in each 20 cc. of solution.* 150 TRU of hyaluronidase may be of aid in this block (see page 43).

Onset.—Operating analgesia is established in 5 to 20 minutes.

Duration.—Operating analgesia lasts 1¼ to 3 hours, with stronger concentrations and solutions containing epinephrine giving the upper limits.

MATERIALS

Regional tray (see Chapter 9, page 51) or:

1. One ¾-inch (2 cm.), 25-gauge Huber point security Lok-needle.

2. One 1½-inch (3.8 cm.), 22-gauge security Lok-needle, preferably with short bevel.

3. One 3-inch (7.5 cm.), 22-gauge security Lok-needle, preferably with short bevel.

4. One tuberculin Lok-syringe for measuring epinephrine.

5. One 10 cc. Lok-syringe, preferably with finger rings.

6. One graduated measuring cup, preferably stainless steel, for mixing solution.

7. One prep cup, preferably stainless steel.

8. Four sterile towels.

9. Six sterile sponges.

10. One sterilizer control.

---

*Optimal concentration of epinephrine is 1:200,000, that is, 0.1 cc. of epinephrine 1:1000 in 20 cc. of the local anesthetic solution (see page 39).

TECHNIQUE

Position and Landmarks

1. The patient lies in the dorsal recumbent position with his hands behind his head and his legs slightly abducted (Figure 199, page 291).

2. The spine of the pubic bone is palpated and an X marked on the skin ½ inch (1.3 cm.) below and ½ inch (1.3 cm.) lateral to it (Figure 198, page 289 and Figure 199, page 291).

Precautions

*Avoid Burning Patient with Antiseptic Solu-*tion.—Care should be taken so that the antiseptic solution does not burn the patient's genitalia. This may be avoided by using an aqueous preparation or careful placement of a sponge in the groin.

Aspirate.—Careful aspiration for blood should be performed.

Procedure

1. The sterilizer control is checked to be sure the equipment has been sterilized.

2. The area is aseptically prepared and draped.

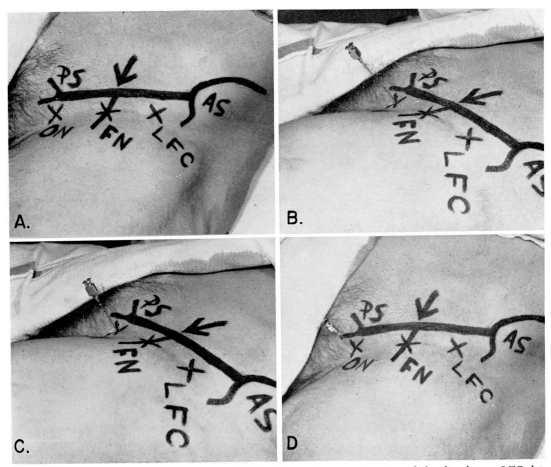

Figure 199. A. Landmark for obturator nerve block. AS. anterior superior spine of the iliac bone; LFC, lateral femoral cutaneous nerve; FN, femoral nerve; PS, pubic tubercle (spine); ON, obturator nerve. B. Three-inch needle rests on inferior ramus of pubic bone. Note it is perpendicular in all planes to the skin. C. Lateral view of 3-inch (7.5 cm.) needle in place in obturator foramen for an obturator nerve block. The *hub* of the needle has been moved slightly cephalad from its position in B. and slightly lateral so that it slides off the lateral edge of the inferior ramus and caudad to the superior ramus of the pubic bone. Paresthesias to the hip joint and knee joint were elicited, but these are not a necessity to establish adequate analgesia. D. View of needle from foot of table to show lateral slope.

3. A skin wheal is made at the X with a ¾-inch (2 cm.), 25-gauge Huber point security Lok needle (Figure 200, page 292).

4. Local infiltration is then performed with the 1½-inch (3.8 cm.), 22-gauge security Lok-needle from the skin to the inferior ramus of the pubic bone.

5. The 3-inch (7.5 cm.), 22-gauge security Lok-needle is then inserted through the wheal perpendicular to the skin and slowly advanced, maintaining this relationship until the inferior ramus of the pubic bone is contacted at a depth of ½ inch (1.3 cm.) to 1½ inches (3.8 cm.) (Figure 199B, page 291 and Figure 200, page 292). This depth is noted.

6. Now, withdraw the needle from the inferior ramus of the pubic bone and change its direction so that it points ½ inch (1.3 cm.) laterally and ⅛ inch (0.3 cm.) caudally from its position in step 5. Then, reinsert it to a depth slightly greater than when the inferior ramus was initially contacted. The inferior

ramus should not be felt and the needle's point should lie lateral to it and caudad to the superior ramus of the pubic bone (Figure 199C and D, page 291 and Figure 200, page 292). If the inferior ramus is still felt, move the needle laterally another ¼ inch (0.6 cm.).

7. When the needle's point no longer contacts bone, it should lie at the upper inner portion of the obturator foramen—this is the area through which the obturator nerve passes (Figure 198, page 289). Now, the needle is advanced inward ¾-inch (2 cm.) to 1 inch (2.5 cm.) (Figure 199C and D, page 291 and Figure 200, page 292).

While executing steps 6 and 7, the most common mistake is the directing of the point of the needle cephalad, i.e., decreasing the angle of the shaft of the needle to less than 90 degrees with the skin. If this is done, the needle passes above the superior ramus of the pubic bone and under the ilioinguinal (Poupart's) ligament toward the abdominal cavity—not caudad to the superior ramus and into the obturator foramen.

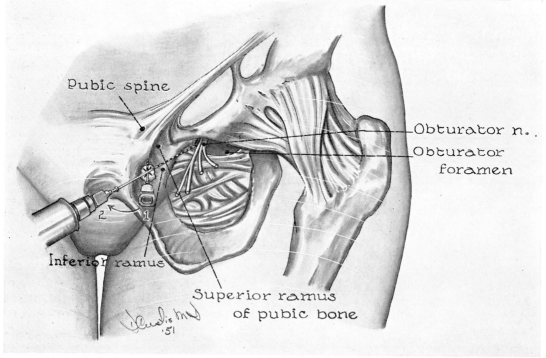

Figure 200. Method of injecting the obturator nerve. The needle point at position 1 rests against the inferior ramus of the pubic bone. At position 2 the needle slides into the upper inner portion of the obturator foramen.

8. 15 cc. of local anesthetic solution is injected as the needle is moved forward and backward ½ inch (1.3 cm.) in the obturator foramen.

9. 10 cc. of the local anesthetic solution is injected as the needle is *slowly* withdrawn.

EXTENT OF ANALGESIA

Anesthesia of the obturator nerve is difficult to determine from the skin area anesthetized. No skin may be anesthetized or the anesthetized area in the inner upper thigh may be very small. If an adequate obturator block has been performed, the patient will be unable to adduct his leg strongly.

COMPLICATIONS

Toxic Reactions (intravascular injections, etc.): See Chapter 3, page 19.

REMARKS

Paresthesias of the Obturator Nerve Are Seldom Obtained: It is rare to obtain paresthesias of the obturator nerve and anesthesia of the nerve depends on adequately flooding the upper part of the obturator foramen where the nerve usually lies.

Do Not Exceed Maximum Dosage of Drugs When Obturator Nerve Block Is Combined with Block of Other Nerves of Lower Extremity: When an obturator block is performed in conjunction with sciatic, femoral, and lateral femoral cutaneous nerve blocks, the total amount of local anesthetic solution employed for all the individual blocks should not exceed the maximum advocated dosage of the local anesthetic agent in question; for example, a total of 90 to 100 cc. of a 0.15 percent solution of tetracaine should not be exceeded for all four blocks (see page 17).

Obturator Nerve Block May Be Used to Prognosticate Result of Obturator Neurectomy: One of the surgical procedures which has been used to relieve hip pain is obturator neurectomy. The outcome of the operation may often be prognosticated from the results of a diagnostic block. The anesthetist should remember that the hip joint is also innervated by branches of the sciatic and femoral nerves, and that in 20 percent of the cases there is an accessory obturator nerve which also sends a branch to the hip joint. Therefore, if pain persists or is only partially relieved following an obturator nerve block, one of the other nerves may be the offender, and unless these nerves are also evulsed, the patient's pain will usually continue after neurectomy.

To Assure Regional Block of Lower Extremity Use Spinal Block: Even in the most expert hands an obturator block is often missed. Therefore, when it is imperative that the patient receive no supplementary anesthesia, be it inhalation or intravenous, during an operation on the extremity, it is best to employ a spinal block rather than to try to block the obturator, sciatic, femoral, and lateral femoral cutaneous nerves.

Recover Broken Needle(s): All needles should be tested before use. If a needle breaks, every effort to recover it, including surgery, should be made. Unremoved needles have a tendency to migrate and may cause permanent injuries as well as medicolegal complications.

Repeat Block When Analgesia Is Inadequate: If the desired results from the first block attempt are unsatisfactory, do not hesitate to reblock the patient if time permits. Most patients will think nothing about being reblocked if the second attempt is prefaced by a statement such as: "Well, I guess we will have to inject a little more medicine if we are going to freeze this area."

However, do not exceed the maximum safe dosage of the local anesthetic solution for both blocks. If to reblock the patient the maximum safe dose of the local anesthetic solution must be exceeded, 45 minutes should elapse between blocks.

CHAPTER 35

Block of the Lateral Femoral Cutaneous Nerve

INDICATIONS

Surgical: Operations confined to the skin and subcutaneous tissue overlying the lateral aspect of the thigh. It is often combined with sciatic, femoral, and obturator nerve blocks for operations on or above the knee.

Diagnostic: Differentiation of neuralgias in the thigh.

Therapeutic: Relief of pain limited to the distribution of the nerve, *e.g.*, meralgia paraesthetica.

ANATOMY

The lateral femoral cutaneous nerve is formed by branches of the second and third lumbar nerves (Figure 187, page 277). It emerges from the deep tissues beneath the inguinal ligament to become subfascial (below the fascia lata) 1 inch (2.5 cm.) medial to the anterior superior spine (Figure 201, page 295). It pierces the fascia lata a little further caudad to lie in the subcutaneous tissue (Figure 201, page 295).

PREMEDICATION

When the block is performed for a diagnostic or a therapeutic procedure no premedication is necessary because no attempts to elicit paresthesias are made and the block is not painful if adequate infiltration is performed as the needle is advanced.

When the block is performed in conjunction with other blocks of the leg for a surgical procedure, the same medications as given for sciatic and femoral nerve blocks are sufficient (see Chapter 33, page 276).

DRUGS

Tetracaine (Pontocaine)

Dosage.—10 cc. to 25 cc. of 0.15 to 0.25 percent solution with or without 0.1 cc. of epinephrine (Adrenalin) 1:1000 in each 20 cc. of solution.*

Onset.—Operating analgesia is established in 15 to 30 minutes.

Duration.—Operating analgesia lasts 3½ to 6 hours, with stronger concentrations and solutions containing epinephrine giving the upper limits.

Procaine (Novocain)

Dosage.—10 cc. to 25 cc. of 1.0 to 2.0 percent solution with or without 0.1 cc. of epinephrine (Adrenalin) 1:1000 in each 20 cc. of solution.*

Onset.—Operating analgesia is established in 10 to 20 minutes.

Duration.—Operating analgesia lasts 1 to 1½ hours, with stronger concentrations and solutions containing epinephrine giving the upper limits.

Lidocaine (Xylocaine) or Mepivacaine (Carbocaine)

Dosage.—10 cc. to 25 cc. of 1.0 to 1.5 percent solution with or without 0.1 cc. of epinephrine (Adrenalin) 1:1000 in each 20 cc. of solution.*

Onset.—Operating analgesia is established in 10 to 20 minutes.

*Optimal concentration of epinephrine is 1:200,000, that is, 0.1 cc. of epinephrine 1:1000 in 20 cc. of the local anesthetic solution (see page 39).

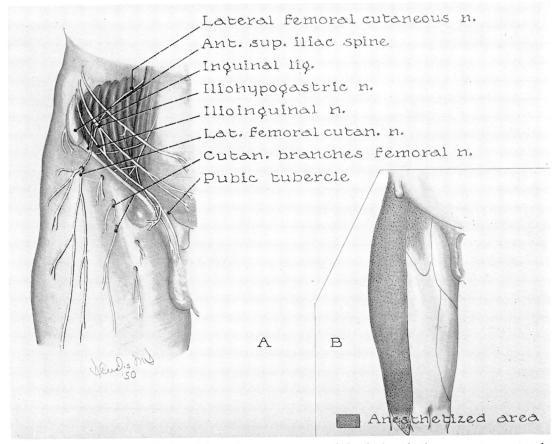

Figure 201. A. Anatomy of the lateral femoral cutaneous nerve of the thigh and other nerves innervating the thigh just below the inguinal (Poupart's) ligament. B. Skin area anesthetized by a block of the lateral femoral cutaneous nerve.

Duration.—Operating analgesia lasts 1¼ to 3 hours, with stronger concentrations containing epinephrine giving the upper limits.

MATERIALS

Regional tray (Chapter 9, page 51) or:

1. One ¾-inch (2 cm.), 25-gauge Huber point security Lok-needle.

2. One 1½-inch (3.8 cm.), 22-gauge security Lok-needle.

3. One 2-inch (5 cm.), 22-gauge security Lok-needle.

4. One tuberculin Lok-syringe for measuring epinephrine.

5. One 10 cc. Lok-syringe, preferably with finger rings.

6. One stainless steel ruler.

7. One graduated measuring cup, preferably stainless steel, for mixing solution.

8. One prep cup, preferably stainless steel.

9. Four sterile towels.

10. Six sterile sponges.

11. One sterilizer control.

TECHNIQUE

Position and Landmarks

1. The patient lies in the supine position with or without a pillow, and his hands are clasped behind his head.

2. The anterior superior spine of the iliac bone is determined and an X marked 1 inch (2.5 cm.) medial and 1 inch (2.5 cm.) caudad to it (Figure 202A, page 296 and Figure 203A,

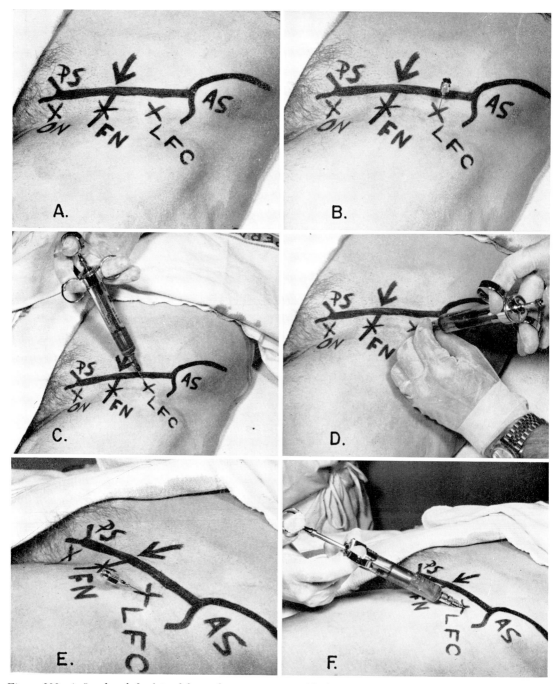

Figure 202. A. Landmark for lateral femoral cutaneous nerve block. AS, anterior superior spine of the iliac bone; LFC, lateral femoral cutaneous nerve; FN, femoral nerve; PS, pubic tubercle; ON, obturator nerve. B. 1½-inch (3.8 cm.) needle has just contacted fascia lata. (Syringe has been removed from needle for photographic clarity.) C. Injection 1 inch (2.5 cm.) lateral to initial insertion. D. Injection 1 inch (2.5 cm.) medial to initial injection. E. Needle has contacted iliac bone between anterior superior spine and anterior inferior spine. F. Needle redirected to slide to inside of iliac bone.

page 297). The X must be located below the ilioinguinal (Poupart's) ligament.

Precaution

Aspirate.—Aspiration for blood should be carefully performed.

Procedure

Paresthesias are not sought. This technique is a field block of the lateral femoral cutaneous nerve.

1. The sterilizer control is checked to be sure the equipment has been sterilized.

2. The area is aseptically prepared and draped.

3. The anesthetist stands at the side to be blocked.

4. An intradermal wheal is raised at the X with the 25-gauge Huber point security Lok-needle.

5. At the X, the lateral femoral cutaneous nerve lies immediately under the fascia lata. The fascia lata is tough, dense, and fibrous. The 1½-inch (3.8 cm.) or 2-inch (5 cm.) needle with the full 10 cc. syringe attached is introduced perpendicular through the skin wheal (Figure 202B, page 296 and Figure 203A and B, page 297).

6. The needle is advanced downward *very slowly* until it meets the resistance of the fascia lata (Figure 203B, page 297).

7. Then, if the anesthetist again exerts *gentle* pressure downwards, he will feel the point of the needle "pop" through the fascia lata.

8. One cc. of the local anesthetic solution is injected with the point of the needle lying just below the fascia lata.

9. As the point of the needle is withdrawn from the fascia lata, another 1 cc. of solution is injected.

10. Steps 6, 7, 8, and 9 are repeated in a fan-like direction both medially and laterally in a cross-sectional plane of the body for 1 inch (2.5 cm.) on each side of the X (Figure 202 C and D, page 296 and Figure 203B, page

297). A total of 10 to 15 cc. of solution is injected. As noted previously, the lateral femoral cutaneous nerve usually lies immediately under the fascia lata at the X (Figure 201A,

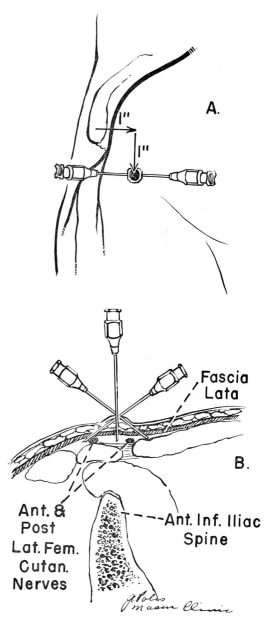

Figure 203. Landmarks for the injection of the lateral femoral cutaneous nerve at the thigh. A. Fan-wise injection along the imaginary line representing the cross section in Figure B. B. Cross section just below anterior superior iliac spine and just above anterior inferior iliac spine. Needles have pierced fascia lata—the anesthetic solution is injected just above and below fascia lata.

page 295). However, 1 cc. of solution is injected as the needle is withdrawn from the fascia lata to block the nerve should it have pierced the fascia lata above the X.

11. Now, the point of the needle is directed so as to contact the iliac bone just below the anterior superior spine (Figure 202E, page 296 and Figure 204A and B, needle position 1, page 298).

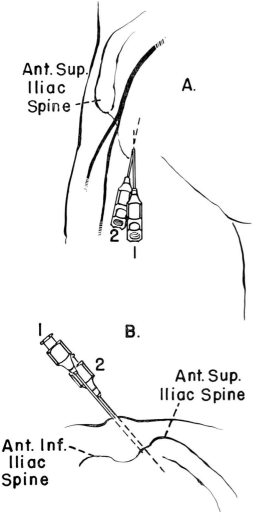

Figure 204. Method of depositing the local anesthetic solution in area coursed by the lateral femoral cutaneous nerve as it exits from the pelvis. Needle 1 rests on iliac bone between anterior superior and anterior inferior spines. Needle 2 lies on medial side of shelving surface of iliac bone ½ (1.3 cm.) to 1 inch (2.5 cm.) deeper than the bone contacted by needle in position 1. A. Anterior view. B. Lateral inside view.

12. After the bone is contacted, the needle is slightly withdrawn, redirected medially, and reinserted for a distance of 1 inch (2.5 cm.) immediately adjacent to the medial side of shelving edge of that bone (Figure 202F, page 296 and Figure 204A and B, needle position 2, page 298). This is the area through which the lateral femoral cutaneous nerve courses as it makes its exit from the pelvis (see Figure 201, page 295).

13. As the needle is moved forward and backward ¼ inch (0.6 cm.) to ½ inch (1.3 cm.), 10 cc. of the local anesthetic solution is injected and the needle removed.

14. *For a successful block, the local anesthetic solution should be placed both along the shelving (inside) edge of the iliac bone and below and above the fascia lata.*

EXTENT OF ANALGESIA

Dermal and subcutaneous analgesia results over the distribution of the nerve (Figure 197, page 286 and Figure 201B, page 295).

COMPLICATIONS

Toxic Reactions (intravascular injections, etc.): See Chapter 3, page 19.

REMARKS

To Relieve Pain a Series of Blocks Must Be Performed: When the block is performed to relieve pain over the distribution of the nerve, a series of injections are often necessary.

Do Not Exceed Maximum Dose of Drugs When Lateral Femoral Cutaneous Nerve Block Is Combined with Block of Other Nerves of Lower Extremity: When a lateral femoral cutaneous block is performed in conjunction with sciatic, femoral, and obturator nerve blocks, the total amount of solution employed for all the individual blocks should not exceed the maximum advocated dosage of the local anesthetic agent in question; for example, a total of 90 to 100 cc. of a 0.15 percent solution of tetracaine should not be exceeded for all four blocks (see page 17).

Recover Broken Needle(s): All needles should be tested before use. If a needle breaks, every effort, including surgery, should be made to recover it. Unremoved needles have a tendency to migrate and may cause permanent injuries as well as medicolegal complications.

Repeat Block When Analgesia Is Inadequate: If the results from the first block attempt are unsatisfactory, do not hesitate to reblock the patient if time permits. Most patients will think nothing about being reblocked if the second attempt is prefaced with a statement such as: "Well, I guess we will have to inject a little more medicine if we are going to freeze this area."

However, do not exceed the maximum safe dosage of the local anesthetic solution for both blocks. If to reblock the patient the maximum safe dose of the local anesthetic solution must be exceeded, 45 minutes should elapse between blocks.

CHAPTER 36

Block of the Suprascapular Nerve

INDICATIONS

Surgical: None.

Diagnostic: Localization of pain of the shoulder girdle.

Therapeutic: Relief of painful shoulder disorders such as acute bursitis, chronic bursitis with or without calcium deposits, partial capsular tear, and pain in the shoulder for which no diagnosis can be established .

ANATOMY

The suprascapular nerve arises from a trunk formed by the union of the fourth, fifth, and sixth cervical nerves (Figure 134, page 222). It enters the supraspinatus fossa via the suprascapular notch and then divides (Figure 205, page 300). It is important to note that the nerve does not branch until it has passed through the suprascapular notch (Figure 205, page 300). Its branches supply the supraspi-

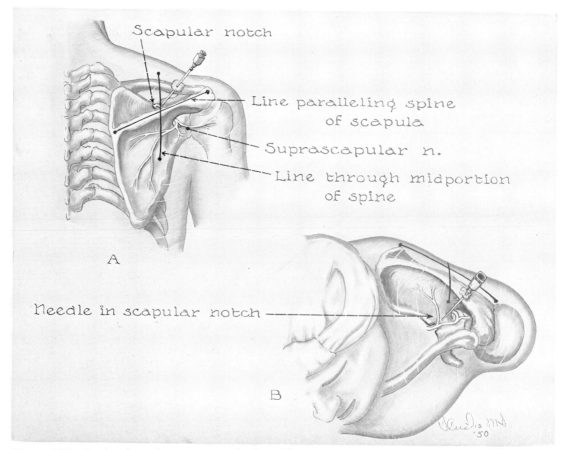

Figure 205. Landmarks and anatomy involved in blocking the suprascapular nerve. A. Posterior view. B. Superior view.

natus and infraspinatus muscles and the shoulder joint.

PREMEDICATION

No premedication is necessary for the following reasons. First, the block is not painful if local infiltration of anesthetic solution is carefully carried out before placing the needle. Second, no attempts to elicit paresthesias are made. However, occasionally paresthesias characterized by a "electric shock-like" sensation radiating to the shoulder may occur. Third, most patients are treated on an outpatient basis. Lastly, the patient is placed in the sitting position for the block.

DRUGS

Tetracaine (Pontocaine)

Dosage.—10 cc. to 20 cc. of 0.10 to 0.25 percent solution with or without 0.1 cc. of epinephrine (Adrenalin) 1:1000 in 20 cc. of solution.*

Onset.—Analgesia is established in 10 to 20 minutes.

Duration.—Analgesia from the anesthetic agent lasts 3½ to 6 hours, with stronger concentrations and solutions containing epinephrine giving the upper limits. However, relief of the patient's pain may be permanent.

Procaine (Novocain)

Dosage.—10 cc. to 20 cc. of 1.0 to 2.0 percent solution with or without 0.1 cc. of epinephrine (Adrenalin) 1:1000 in 20 cc. of solution.*

Onset.—Analgesia is established in 5 to 15 minutes.

Duration.—Analgesia from the anesthetic agent lasts 1 to 1¾ hours, with stronger concentrations and solutions containing epinephrine giving the upper limits. However, relief of the patient's pain may be permanent.

Lidocaine (Xylocaine) or Mepivacaine (Carbocaine)

Dosage.—10 cc. to 20 cc. of 1.0 to 1.5 percent solution with or without 0.1 cc. of epinephrine (Adrenalin) 1:1000 in 20 cc. of solution.*

Onset.—Analgesia is established in 5 to 15 minutes.

Duration.—Analgesia lasts 1¼ to 3 hours, with stronger concentrations and solutions containing epinephrine giving the upper limits.

MATERIALS

Regional tray (see Chapter 9, page 51) or:

1. One ¾-inch (2 cm.), 25-gauge Huber point security Lok-needle.

2. One 3-inch (7.5 cm.), 22-gauge security Lok-needle, preferably with a short bevel.

3. One tuberculin Lok-syringe for measuring epinephrine.

4. One 10 cc. Lok-syringe, preferably with finger rings.

5. One graduated measuring cup, preferably stainless steel, for mixing solution.

6. One prep cup, preferably stainless steel.

7. Four sterile towels.

8. Six sterile sponges.

9. One sterilizer control.

TECHNIQUE

Position and Landmarks

1. The patient sits on the edge of the operating room cart or table with his arms folded across his abdomen.

2. The spine of the scapula is located and a line drawn along it from the tip of the acromion to the scapular border (Figure 205, page 300 and Figure 206, page 302).

3. The midpoint of this line is determined and a vertical line parallel to the spines of the

*Optimal concentration of epinephrine is 1:200,000, that is, 0.1 cc. of epinephrine 1:1000 in 20 cc. of the local anesthetic solution (see page 39).

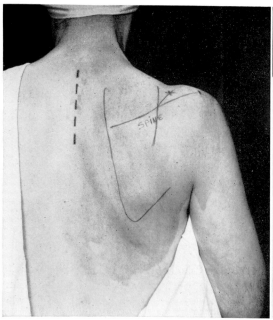

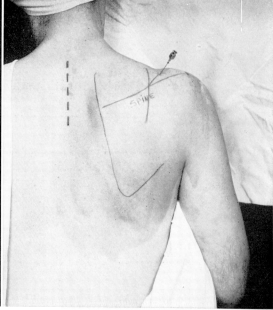

Figure 206. Shows the position of the patient for a suprascapular nerve block with the landmarks drawn on the skin. Note that the vertical line through the spine of the scapula is parallel to the spines of the vertebrae.

Figure 207. The 3-inch (7.5 cm.) needle rests in the suprascapular notch. Note its direction. This patient was blocked for an acute bursitis with marked relief on an outpatient basis. Note the downward, inward, and slightly forward direction of the needle. The shaft of the needle is practically at a 90 degree angle in all planes in relationship to the natural slope of the shoulder. Paresthesias were elicited.

vertebral column is drawn through it, forming four quadrants (Figure 205, page 300 and Figure 206, page 302).

4. The angle of the upper outer quadrant is then bisected with a line and an X marked on this line 1 inch (2.5 cm.) from the apex of the angle (Figure 205, page 300 and Figure 206, page 302).

Precautions

Aspirate.—The suprascapular artery and vein are separated from the suprascapular nerve by the superior transverse ligament of the scapula. Nevertheless, they may be punctured and careful aspiration tests should always be performed before injecting any solution.

Procedure

1. The sterilizer control is checked to be sure the equipment has been sterilized.

2. The area is aseptically prepared and draped.

3. A skin wheal is made at the X with a ¾-inch (2 cm.), 25-gauge Huber point security Lok-needle.

4. The subcutaneous tissue and suprascapular muscle are infiltrated with the local anesthetic solution.

5. The 3-inch (7.5 cm.), 22-gauge short beveled security Lok-needle is introduced perpendicular to the skin in all planes and then advanced slowly downward, maintaining its perpendicular position in relationship to the skin until bone is contacted (Figure 207, page 302). This depth varies from 2 inches (5 cm.) to 2½ inches (6.3 cm.), depending on the build of the patient. It is of utmost importance that the relationship of the needle to the skin be 90 degrees in all planes to give the inward, downward, and forward

direction which is necessary to locate the notch (Figure 207, page 302).

6. When bone is contacted, the needle usually lies on the bone surrounding the suprascapular notch. The needle is then slightly withdrawn and redirected laterally, medially, or superiorly until it is felt to slide into the notch. 10 cc. of anesthetic solution is injected. The position is checked by withdrawing the needle slightly and re-inserting it medially and laterally to see if the walls of the notch can be contacted. The needle is then replaced in the notch and an additional 5 cc. of anesthetic solution is deposited.

7. If bone is not contacted and the needle has been advanced deeper than 2½ inches (6.3 cm.), it is possible that the needle lies in the notch or has passed over the superior edge of the scapula. Its position should be checked as in step 6 above and 10 cc. of anesthetic solution deposited if the position is correct.

EXTENT OF ANALGESIA

No skin analgesia exists so that all indications of a successful block rest with the relief of the subjective signs and symptoms.

COMPLICATIONS

Toxic Reactions (intravascular injections, etc.): See Chapter 3, page 19.

Pneumothorax: This complication is rare and occurs in less than 1 percent of the cases. It is usually caused by advancing the needle deeper than recommended. See Chapter 30, page 237.

REMARKS

A Series of Blocks May Be Necessary to Relieve Pain: If only temporary relief occurs after the first block, the doctor should not consider the procedure a failure. It is often necessary to repeat the block three to five times, once or twice a week, and this point must be impressed on the patient as well as the doctor.

This technique does not give good results when the shoulder pain is caused by arthritis, metastatic cancer, myositis, and dislocations.

Use Block Early in Treatment of Pain—Not as Last Resort: This type of block has been extremely useful when all other treatment for chronic bursitis fails. Therefore, it should be used early in the treatment of this disease in conjunction with other therapy, *e.g.,* physiotherapy and x-ray, and not as a last resort when this other therapy fails.

Recover Broken Needle(s): All needles should be tested before use. If a needle breaks, every effort, including surgery, should be made to recover it. Unremoved needles have a tendency to migrate and may cause permanent injuries as well as medicolegal complications.

Repeat Block When Analgesia Is Inadequate: If the results from the first block attempt are unsatisfactory, do not hesitate to reblock the patient if time permits. Most patients will think nothing about being reblocked if the second attempt is prefaced by a statement such as: "Well, I guess we will have to inject a little more medicine if we are going to freeze this area."

CHAPTER 37

Digital Nerve Block

INDICATIONS

Surgical: Operations on the fingers and toes.

Diagnostic: None.

Therapeutic: None.

ANATOMY

The dorsal nerves which supply the back of the fingers are the terminal branches of the radial and ulnar nerves (Figure 152, page 236). The volar nerves which supply the palmar surface of the fingers are the terminal branches of the median and ulnar nerves (Figure 152, page 236). The nerves which supply the plantar surface and dorsum of the toes are the terminal branches of the sciatic nerves via the tibial and peroneal nerves (Figure 197A, page 286). Occasionally, however, the dorsal surface of the big toe receives part of its innervation from the terminal portion of the femoral nerve via the saphenous nerve (Figure 197 B, page 286).

PREMEDICATION

None is necessary because: (1) no attempts to elicit paresthesias are made; (2) the block is not painful; and (3) this block is frequently performed on outpatients.

DRUGS

Tetracaine (Pontocaine)

Dosage.—10 cc. to 50 cc. of 0.15 to 0.25 percent solution *without* a vasoconstrictor agent, depending on the number of digits to be anesthetized. 10 cc. per finger or toe should not be exceeded.

Onset.—Operating analgesia is established in 10 to 15 minutes.

Duration.—Operating analgesia lasts 3½ to 6 hours, with stronger solutions giving the upper limits.

Procaine (Novocain)

Dosage.—10 cc. to 50 cc. of 1.0 to 2.0 percent solution *without* a vasoconstrictor agent, depending on the number of digits to be anesthetized. 10 cc. per finger or toe should not be exceeded.

Onset.—Operating analgesia is established in 5 to 10 minutes.

Duration.—Operating analgesia lasts 1 to 1½ hours, with stronger solutions giving the upper limits.

Lidocaine (Xylocaine) or Mepivacaine (Carbocaine)

Dosage.—10 cc. to 50 cc. of 0.5 to 1.0 percent solution *without* a vasoconstrictor agent, depending on the number of digits to be anesthetized. 10 cc. per finger or toe should not be exceeded.

Onset.—Operating analgesia is established in 5 to 10 minutes.

Duration.—Operating analgesia lasts 1¼ to 3 hours, with stronger solutions giving the upper limits.

MATERIALS

Regional tray (see Chapter 9, page 51) or:

1. One ¾-inch (2 cm.), 25-gauge Huber point seurity Lok-needle.

2. One 1½-inch (3.8 cm.), 22-gauge, security Lok-needle, preferably with short bevel.

3. One 10 cc. Lok-syringe, preferably with finger rings.

4. One graduated measuring cup, preferably stainless steel, for mixing solution.

5. One prep cup, preferably stainless steel.

6. Four sterile towels.

7. Six sterile sponges.

8. One sterilizer control.

TECHNIQUE

Position and Landmarks

On the dorsolateral aspect of the finger or toe at the interdigital folds, two X's are made (Figure 208B, page 305).

Precaution

Restrict Volume of Local Anesthetic Solution.—Do not exceed 10 cc. of anesthetic solution for each finger or toe.

Procedure

1. The finger or toe to be blocked is aseptically prepared and draped.

2. The anesthetist stands at the side to be blocked.

3. Skin wheals are raised at the X's at the interdigital folds with the ¾-inch (2 cm.), 25-gauge Huber point security Lok-needle (Figure 208, page 305).

4. A ring of local anesthetic solution is then placed around the finger or toe from the bone to the skin by a fan-wise placement of the needle through the points at the interdigital folds (Figure 208A, page 305).

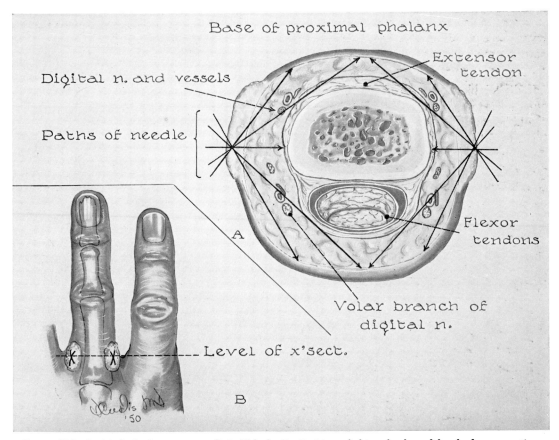

Figure 208. A. Method of executing a digital block. B. Position of skin wheals and level of cross section.

DISTRIBUTION OF ANALGESIA

Anesthesia of the finger or toe blocked distal to the ring of anesthesia.

COMPLICATIONS

Toxic Reactions (intravascular injections, etc.): See Chapter 3, page 19.

REMARKS

Digital Block Is Frequently Used: The author realizes that many men in a general practice utilize this block for minor lesions of the fingers and toes, ruptured tendons, paronychia, and ingrown nails without having any serious complications. For this reason, as well as to point out its danger and limitations, it was included in the book.

Digital Block Is Seldom Used by Author: It is still the author's opinion that digital blocks should be avoided, since gangrene of the finger or toe following the block is not uncommon. In addition, this block alone does not permit the pneumatic tourniquet to be applied to the arm or thigh without pain to the patient.

If digital blocks are to be performed and gangrene is to be avoided, the following points should be carefully observed. First, more than 8 cc. to 10 cc. of local anesthetic solution should never be injected around any one finger or toe. Second, vasoconstrictor agents should never be added to the local anesthetic solution. Lastly, massage of the tissue where the anesthetic solution was deposited should be adequately vigorous in order to facilitate spread of the solution and increase its absorption. 150 TRU of hyaluronidase may be useful to accomplish the spread of the local anesthetic solution if the operating time is to be quite brief. Without a vasoconstrictor in the solution in which hyaluronidase is used, the duration of operating analgesia is greatly reduced (see Chapter 6, page 43).

Recover Broken Needle(s): All needles should be tested before use. If a needle breaks, every effort to recover it, including surgery, should be made. Unremoved needles have a tendency to migrate and may cause permanent injuries as well as medicolegal complications.

Repeat Block When Analgesia Is Inadequate: If the results from the first block attempt are unsatisfactory, do not hesitate to reblock the patient if time permits. Most patients will think nothing about being reblocked if the second attempt is prefaced by a statement such as: "Well, I guess we will have to inject a little more medicine if we are going to freeze this area."

CHAPTER 38

Regional Block of the Upper or Lower Extremity by the Intravenous Injection of a Local Anesthetic Solution

INDICATIONS

Surgical: Operations and manipulations of one and three-quarters hours or less on the upper and lower extremities from the lower pneumatic tourniquet peripherally. This procedure is most suited for soft tissue operations, *e.g.,* ganglionectomy, Dupuytren's contractures, etc. Fractures may be reduced, but the application of the Esmarch bandage will cause discomfort. Also, manipulations of the ulnar, median, or radial nerves will cause paresthesias that may not be tolerated by the patient.

Diagnostic: None.

Therapeutic: None.

ANATOMY

The only pertinent anatomy is the distribution and location of the veins of the hand, the cubital fossa, the foot, ankle, and leg (Figure 209, page 308; Figure 210, page 309; and Figure 211, page 309).

PREMEDICATION

Use Heavy Medication: Paresthesias are not sought and the initial application of the upper pneumatic tourniquet and the Esmarch bandage may cause marked discomfort for 10 to 20 minutes. The average patient (age 20 to 50, weight 150 pounds or over, approximate height 5 feet, 5 inches or over, and good physical status) receives:

1. 200 mg. (3 gr.) of pentobarbital (Nembutal) by mouth at hour of sleep the night before surgery.

2. 200 mg. (3 gr.) of pentobarbital by mouth 1½ to 2 hours before the estimated *block* time.

3. 15 mg. (¼ gr.) of morphine and 0.6 mg. (¹⁄₁₀₀ gr.) of scopolamine intramuscularly ¾ to 1 hour before the estimated *block* time.

Reduction of Premedication: It is seldom necessary to increase this premedication irrespective of the over-all size of the patient until the patient arrives in either the anesthesia or operating room. However, it is very common to reduce this medication under various circumstances; for example, for the geriatric patient, the adolescent patient, the debilitated or cachectic patient, and for patients whose surgery is complicated by other disease, *e.g.,* myxedema, diabetes, heart disease, etc. In the patient over 60 years of age, barbiturates and especially scopolamine may often cause disorientation. Therefore, in these patients atropine is usually substituted for scopolamine and the dosage of the barbiturate omitted or greatly reduced, *i.e.,* to 50 mg. (¾ gr.) or less. *Always err on the light side.*

Inadequate Premedication: If medication is inadequate either for the block or for the surgical procedure, intravenous pentobarbital 50 mg. (¾ gr.) to 100 mg. (1½ gr.) or intravenous morphine 8 mg. (⅛ gr.) to 15 mg. (¼ gr.) may be given slowly. Judicious use of added sedation is extremely important. Often small supplementary doses of morphine or pentobarbital will make a block successful, especially when a patient interprets touch and motion as pain.

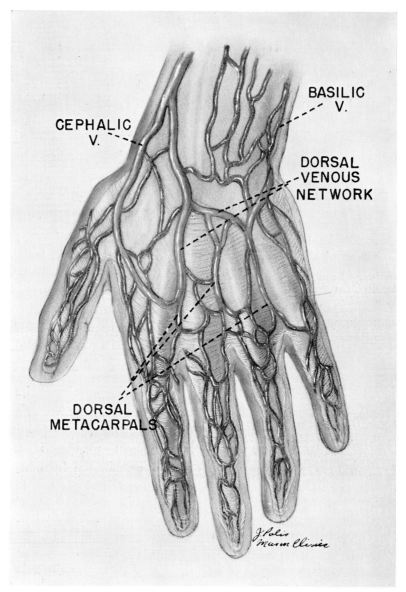

Figure 209. Anatomy of veins of dorsum of hand and wrist. Either cephalic or large veins on the dorsum of the hand are preferred to the dorsal metacarpal or basilic veins.

DRUGS

Lidocaine (Xylocaine): This is the drug most frequently injected to produce intravenous regional block and it should not contain either a preservative or a drug to prevent oxidation (see Remarks, page 317).

Dosage.—To anesthetize the upper and lower extremity, 50 cc. and 100 cc., respectively,

of 0.5 percent solution without epinephrine (Adrenalin) are necessary.

Onset.—Operating analgesia is established in 5 to 15 minutes.

Duration.—Operating analgesia lasts one and one-half to one and three-quarter hours. Occasionally analgesia may last two hours. When the surgery is completed and pneumatic

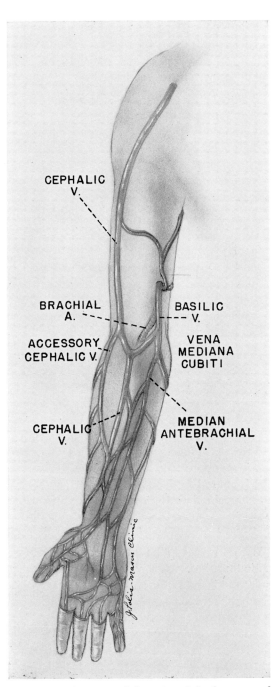

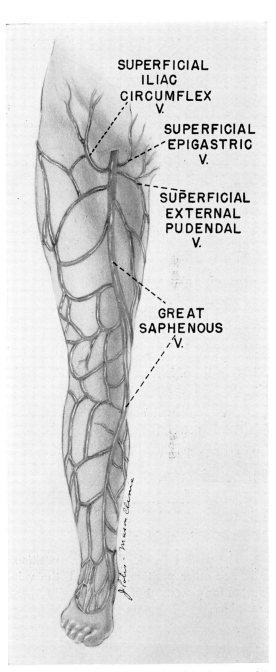

Figure 210. Anatomy of the veins of the forearm and cubital fossa. If the basilic vein in the cubital fossa is selected, be sure it—not the brachial artery—is cannulated.

Figure 211. Anatomy of the veins of the leg. For this technique a vein on the dorsum of the foot or the saphenous vein at the ankle is preferred. Veins above the middle of the leg, i.e., those in the popliteal fossa or thigh, should be avoided.

tourniquet deflated, sensory and motor function return within 5 to 10 minutes.

MATERIALS

1. One rubber tourniquet, *i.e.,* 12 to 18 inches (30 to 45 cm.) of ⅞ inch (2.3 cm.) Penrose drain.

2. One 16, 17, or 18-gauge plastic needle with stylet (Figure 2, page 8).

3. One 500 cc. or 1000 cc. bottle of intravenous fluid and one intravenous infusion set for placing the needle and maintaining its patency until the plastic stylet is placed in the needle. The remaining amount of solution and the infusion set may be used to start an intravenous infusion in another extremity.

4. Two pneumatic tourniquets.

5. One Esmarch bandage.

6. One ¾-inch (2 cm.), 25-gauge Huber point security Lok-needle.

7. One 10 cc. Lok-syringe, preferably with finger rings.

8. One graduated measuring cup, preferably stainless steel, for mixing the solution.

9. One sterilizer control.

10. Adhesive tape.

TECHNIQUE

Position and Landmarks

1. The patient lies in the supine position, or in any other position, provided, the vein selected for placement of the needle is readily accessible.

2. For surgery on the elbow, the needle is placed in the forearm or cubital fossa. For surgery of the forearm and hand, a vein on the dorsum (back) of the hand is used. And, for surgery of the lower extremity, a vein in the foot, ankle, or lower leg is selected.

Precautions

Maintain Needle Position in Vein.—Care must be taken to keep the needle in the vein during: (1) elevation of the arm; (2) application and removal of the Esmarch bandage; (3) inflation of the pneumatic tourniquet; and (4) injection of the local anesthetic solution. For this reason, we prefer the plastic needle rather than a steel needle.

Test and Constantly Check Pneumatic Tourniquet Pressure.—The pressure in the pneumatic tourniquets must be constantly checked. If the pneumatic tourniquet pressure fails and the local anesthetic agent rapidly reaches the general circulation, a systemic toxic reaction may ensue.

Warn Patient of Pain from Esmarch Bandage and Inflated Pneumatic Tourniquet.—This pain will last until: (1) anesthesia is established; (2) the lower pneumatic tourniquet is inflated; and (3) the upper pneumatic tourniquet released, *i.e.,* 15 to 20 minutes. During this time some patients may require additional sedation or light anesthesia.

Completely Exsanguinate Extremity.—Failure to completely remove the blood from the extremity will result in: (1) poor anesthesia; (2) blood in the operative field; (3) hematoma formation at the injection site; (4) increased incidence of systemic toxic reactions; and (5) a blotchy appearance of the skin (cutis marmorata) which is of no significance and is caused by blood being forced from the deeper veins into the subcuticular capillaries.

Procedure

With the exception of placing the pneumatic tourniquets, the procedure is performed under sterile conditions. Figure 212, page 311, through Figure 216, page 316, depict the steps in the procedure for the upper extremity. No illustrations are included to depict the procedure for the lower extremity, but the steps are comparable except 100 cc. rather than 50 cc. of the local anesthetic solution is used.

1. One of the two pneumatic tourniquets is applied as high as possible on the extremity to be anesthetized (Figure 212A, page 311).

2. The skin is aseptically prepared and the sterile Penrose rubber tourniquet is applied 3

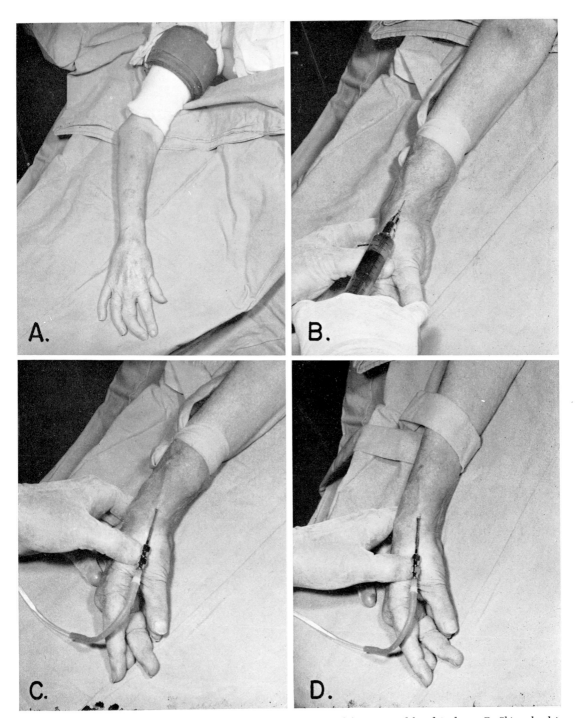

Figure 212. A. Upper tourniquet applied to arm. Sterile prep of forearm and hand is done. B. Skin wheal is raised 3 inches below ⅞-inch sterile Penrose tourniquet at cephalic vein preparatory to placing plastic needle. C. Plastic needle partially inserted into vein. D. Penrose tourniquet released.

inches (7.5 cm.) above the point at which the plastic needle (Rochester needle, Figure 2, page 8) is to be inserted (Figure 212B, page 311).

3. A skin wheal is raised with the ¾-inch (2 cm.), 25-gauge Huber point security Lok-needle at the site selected for insertion of the needle (Figure 212B, page 311).

4. The plastic needle is connected to the infusion set and fluids are run through the needle to assure its patency. Then the fluids are shut off.

5. The needle is inserted through the skin wheal and into the vein (Figure 212C, page 311).

6. The rubber tourniquet used to place the plastic needle is removed (Figure 212D, page 311).

7. The intravenous fluids are turned on and the introducing steel needle is withdrawn ¾ inch (2 cm.) (Figure 213A, page 313). The plastic needle is cannulated up the vein (Figure 213B, page 313).

8. The intravenous infusion is turned off and disconnected from the hub of the steel introducing needle (Figure 213 C, page 313).

9. The introducing steel needle is completely withdrawn, leaving the plastic needle in the vein (Figure 213D, page 313).

10. The intravenous solution is now connected to the hub of the plastic needle and the solution is permitted to run through the plastic needle to ascertain that the lumen of the needle is in the vein and that the shaft of the plastic needle does not leak (Figure 214A, page 314). Leakage is most likely to occur where the plastic tube is swedged on to the metal hub. If leakage from the plastic needle occurs or if the intravenous fluids extravasate into the tissues, another plastic needle must be inserted.

11. When neither leakage nor extravasation results, the intravenous fluids are disconnected from the hub of the needle and the plastic stylet (Figure 2, page 8) is inserted into the plastic needle to prevent blood entering the needle with subsequent clotting and blocking of the lumen of the needle (Figure 214 B and C, page 314).

12. The extremity is raised above the level of the body for 2 to 3 minutes (Figure 214D, page 314).

13. The patient is warned to expect discomfort and the entire extremity is tightly wrapped with an Esmarch bandage to effect exsanguination (Figure 215A, page 315).

14. The patient is again warned to expect discomfort.

15. The pneumatic tourniquet is inflated—for the upper extremity 260 mm. of mercury pressure (5 pounds of air pressure) and for the lower extremity 520 mm. of mercury pressure (10.5 pounds of air pressure).

16. The Esmarch bandage is removed (Figure 215 B, page 315). The plastic stylet is removed from the plastic needle and no blood should appear at the hub of the needle if exsanguination by the Esmarch bandage has been effective (Figure 215 C, page 315).

17. The local anesthetic solution is injected—upper extremity 50 cc. and lower extremity 100 cc. (Figure 215D, page 315). When refilling the syringe, the local anesthetic solution may drip from the hub of the plastic needle. To shorten the time the hub of the needle is opened, two syringes instead of one may be employed. We use only one syringe, but when doing the procedure, asepsis, including the use of sterile gloves, is maintained. Therefore, when refilling the syringe, a gloved finger is placed over the hub of the needle to prevent fluid from refluxing (Figure 216 A, page 316).

18. The plastic needle is removed (Figure 216 B, page 316). Pressure is applied at the site of puncture of the vein for 2 to 3 minutes by an assistant or nurse (Figure 216 C, page 316). A small amount of the local anesthetic solution may leak from the vein but no blood should extravasate if the exsanguination of the arm was effectively performed and if the pneumatic tourniquet was effective.

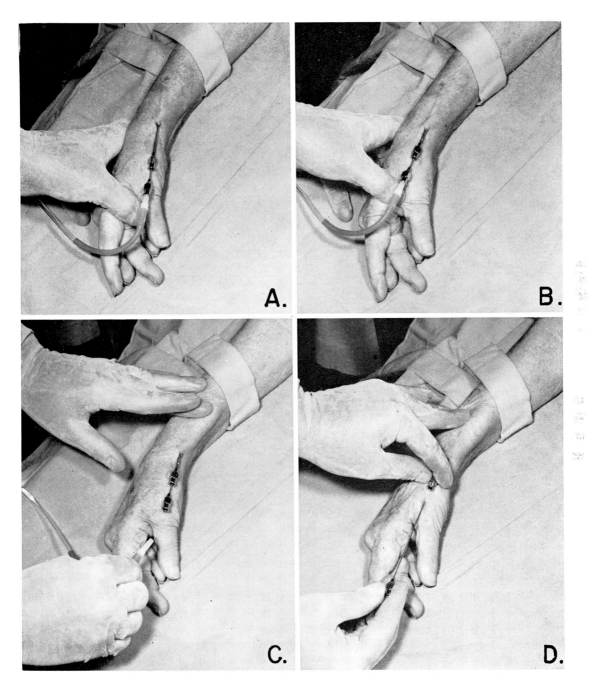

Figure 213. A. Introducing needle partially removed. B. Plastic needle cannulated up vein with intravenous fluids running. C. Intravenous fluids removed from introducing needle while middle finger of left hand compresses vein to prevent bleeding into needle. Also, at this point, it may be necessary to hold hub of plastic needle with thumb and index finger as shown in D. D. Introducing needle removed.

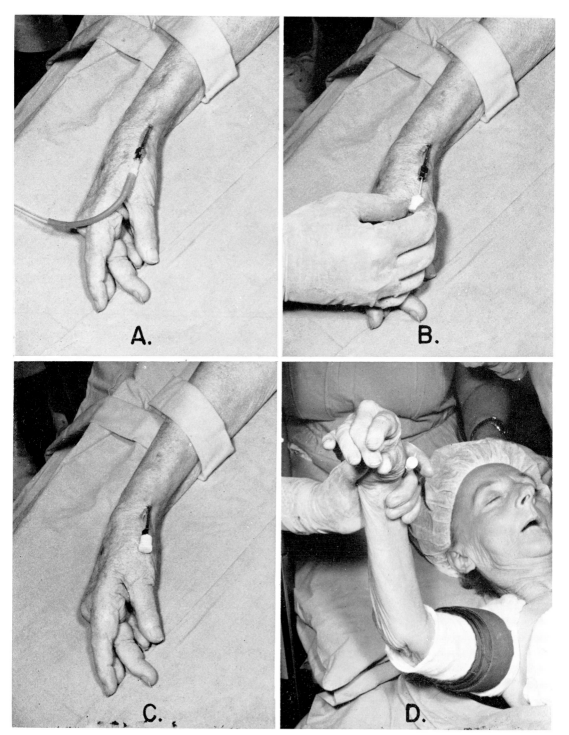

Figure 214. A. Intravenous fluids connected to plastic needle to test for leak. B. Intravenous fluid removed and plastic stylet introduced into plastic needle. C. Plastic stylet locked on plastic needle. D. Arm held above level of body for 2 to 3 minutes—note that patient is heavily sedated for next step is painful.

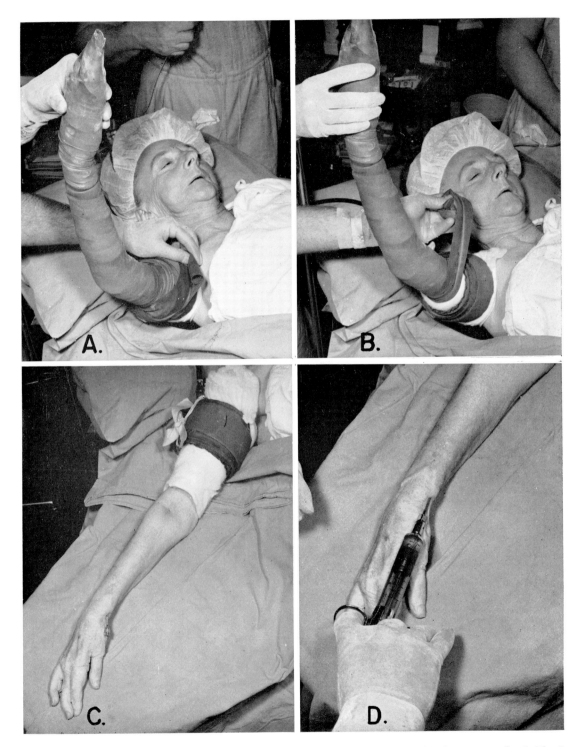

Figure 215. A. Esmarch bandage applied and tourniquet inflated. B. Esmarch bandage removed. C. Plastic stylet removed from plastic needle. No blood appears at hub of needle indicating exsanguination of arm is complete. D. Local anesthetic solution injected into vein.

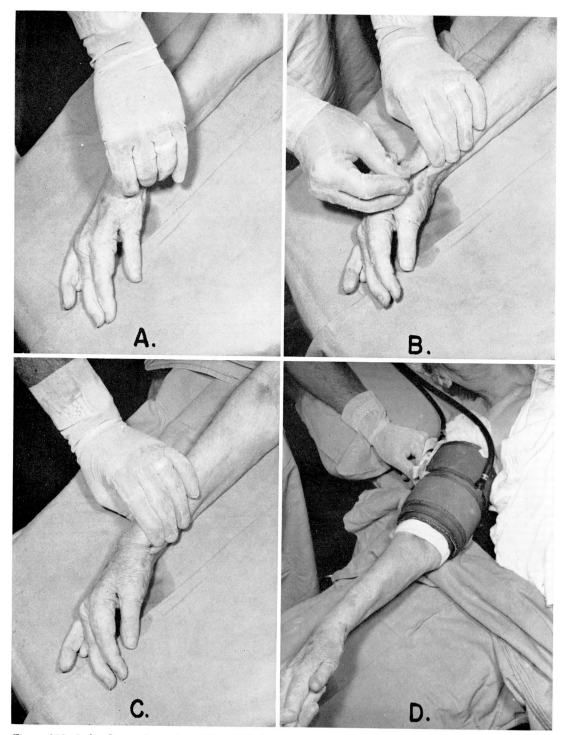

Figure 216. Index finger of anesthetist's hand blocking needle hub to prevent reflux of local anesthetic solution between doses. B. Plastic needle being withdrawn. C. Pressure being applied over vein from which plastic needle was withdrawn. D. Second tourniquet applied below first tourniquet, second tourniquet inflated, and upper tourniquet (first tourniquet) released.

19. The second pneumatic tourniquet is applied immediately below the inflated first pneumatic tourniquet (Figure 216 D, page 316).

20. After anesthesia of the extremity has established (5 to 15 minutes), the lower pneumatic tourniquet is inflated to the pressures noted in step 15 and the pressure in the upper pneumatic tourniquet is released. This maneuver usually eliminates all pneumatic tourniquet pain because the lower pneumatic tourniquet exerts pressure in an anesthetized area.

21. When the operation is complete, the pressure in the lower pneumatic tourniquet is released and after 15 seconds reinflated for 2 minutes. This is repeated 2 to 4 times to prevent all of the local anesthetic agent being "dumped" rapidly into the general circulation and a subsequent systemic toxic reaction resulting.

EXTENT OF ANALGESIA

Anesthesia of both sensory and motor function of the extremity ensues from the lower border of the upper pneumatic tourniquet peripherally. Usually sensory anesthesia is more profound than motor. Following removal of the pneumatic tourniquet, both motor and sensory function return within 5 to 10 minutes.

COMPLICATIONS

Toxic Reactions (intramuscular injections, etc.): See Chapter 3, page 19. Such reactions will occur with greater frequency if the deflation-reinflation technique for removing the pneumatic tourniquet is not observed (step 21 under Procedure, page 317). If any evidence of a systemic toxic reaction occurs, usually only minor signs of cortical stimulation appear, e.g., dizziness, feeling of impending loss of consciousness, etc.

Pneumatic Tourniquet Pain: This may on occasion cause discomfort and may require additional sedation

REMARKS

Avoid Solutions Containing Methylparaben and Metabisulfite: These drugs are often added to commercially prepared local anesthetic solutions to prevent oxidation and as a preservative. Solutions containing them are not recommended for intravenous regional anesthesia, for they may be responsible for the inflammation of the vein and the thrombophlebitis which has occurred following intravenous anesthesia in a few cases.

Methylparaben.—Methylparaben is a preservative and fungistatic agent.

Metabisulfite.—Metabisulfite is an antioxidizing agent.

Peripheral Vascular Disease and Infection Are Contraindications: In peripheral vascular diseases where a pneumatic tourniquet is contraindicated, this technique should not be used. Also, this method is not indicated when squeezing of the extremity with the Esmarch bandage may spread infection.

Explain Procedure to Patient: This should be done with any regional block method, but with this technique the discomfort of the Esmarch bandage and the upper pneumatic tourniquet must be emphasized.

Use of Plastic Needle with Hub or Scalp Infusion Metal Needle without Hub: Some physicians prefer to use the scalp infusion metal needle for the injection of the local anesthetic solution because it has no hub and, therefore, does not cause pressure when the Esmarch bandage is applied. The plastic needle with hub and a stylet is preferred by us because: (1) there is less chance of it being dislodged from the vein; (2) wrapping of the hub of the needle and the cap of the stylet under a tightly applied Esmarch bandage for 2 to 3 minutes does not cause either pain or tissue damage; (3) the plastic needle has a larger lumen and this speeds injection of the local anesthetic solution; and (4) with a stylet in place, blood cannot enter the needle, coagulate, and plug it.

Avoid Placement of Intravenous Needle in Artery: When the needle is placed in the hand, wrist, foot, ankle, or lower leg, such placement is most unlikely. But, when the cubital fossa is used, inadvertent placement in the brachial artery or its branches (radial and ulnar arteries) is not a rarity. Since the solution injected is a local anesthetic drug, the consequences may not be serious but intraarterial injections should be avoided.

Omit Esmarch Bandage in Fractures: In fractures the application of the Esmarch bandage is painful. In these cases the elevation of the extremity for 5 minutes to drain the blood from it *may* remove enough of the blood to permit adequate anesthesia without the use of the Esmarch bandage.

Release of Pneumatic Tourniquet Prior to Completion of Operation: Often near the completion of an operation where a pneumatic tourniquet was used the surgeon will request its release so that bleeding may be detected and stopped prior to closing the wound and applying the dressing. If this is done, the duration of operating time which will remain (5 to 10 minutes) may be inadequate.

Is Inflation and Deflation Technique for Removing Pneumatic Tourniquet at End of Operation a Necessity? This precaution is mandatory if the operative procedure is of short duration, *i.e.,* less than 45 minutes. If the operation lasts more than 45 minutes, some authors feel that this intermittent deflation and inflation of the pneumatic tourniquet is unnecessary for in their experiences systemic toxic reactions do not occur and the technique predisposes to bleeding into the operative site.

Operating Time Limited: The duration of operating analgesia is limited by: (1) the duration of action of the local anesthetic agent, and (2) the length of time the pneumatic tourniquet can be inflated without tissue damage resulting. While the operating time could be prolonged by releasing the pressure in the pneumatic tourniquet allowing circulation to be re-established in the extremity, and repeating the anesthetic procedure, this poses certain hazards, *e.g.,* infection of the operative site, etc., and is seldom done.

No Postoperative Analgesia: With other forms of regional block, postoperative analgesia is usually present for varying periods of time. With this technique, sensation returns within 10 minutes.

PART II

PERIPHERAL NERVE BLOCK
ANESTHESIA

SECTION IV

MISCELLANEOUS

CHAPTER 39

Transtracheal Injection

INDICATIONS

A NY PROCEDURE requiring topical analgesia of the lower pharynx, larynx, and trachea. These include: (1) bronchoscopy and esophagoscopy; (2) endotracheal intubation; (3) prophylactic prevention of laryngospasm when an anesthetic agent which may irritate the larynx must be given rapidly (for example, ether); and (4) releasing of severe laryngospasms. The most severe laryngospasms occur when the patient is in the light planes of anesthesia, *i.e.*, induction and emergence. In these stages of anesthesia, the cough reflexes are still very active, particularly those initiated by irritation of the upper tracheal mucosa. If a topical anesthetic agent is placed directly into the trachea during a severe laryngospasm, the patient will in most instances cough, spray the cords, and automatically release the spasm.

ANATOMY

The cricoid cartilage is the only complete ring of cartilage in the neck. The membrane which usually lies between the thyroid and cricoid cartilages is the cricothyroid membrane (Figure 217, page 322).

PREMEDICATION

No special medication is given for this block as it is practically painless. Whatever premedication is administered for the subsequent anesthetic technique is adequate.

DRUGS

Tetracaine (Pontocaine)

Dosage.—2 to 4 cc. of a 0.5 percent solution (10 to 20 mg.).

Onset.—Analgesia is established in 2 to 5 minutes.

Duration.—Variable.

Lidocaine (Xylocaine)

Dosage.—2 to 4 cc. of a 2.0 percent solution (40 to 80 mg.).

Onset.—Analgesia is established in 1 to 5 minutes.

Duration.—Variable.

Cocaine

Dosage.—3 cc. of a 4.0 percent solution (120 mg.).

Onset.—Analgesia is established in 2 to 5 minutes.

Duration.—Variable.

MATERIALS

1. One 1½-inch (3.8 cm.), 22-gauge Huber point Lok-needle.

2. One 5 cc. Lok-syringe.

3. One sterilizer control.

TECHNIQUE

Position and Landmarks

1. The patient lies in the dorsal recumbent position with or without a "donut" under his head, and his arms at his sides (Figure 218, page 322).

2. The head is placed in maximum extension (Figure 218, page 322).

3. The thyroid and cricoid cartilages are palpated and an X marked on the skin over-

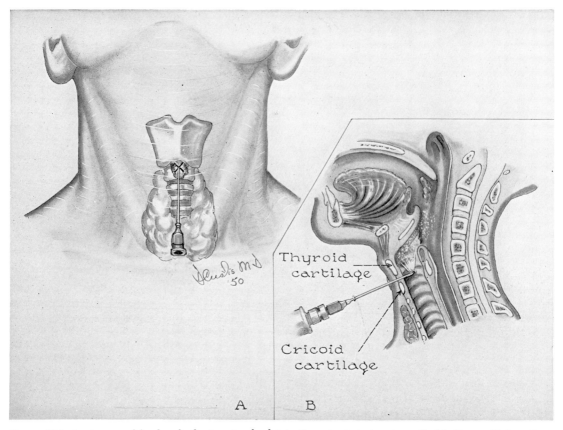

Figure 217. Anatomy and landmarks for transtracheal injection. A. Anterior view. B. Median sagittal section.

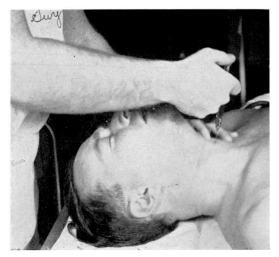

Figure 218. Position of patient and anesthetist during execution of the transtracheal injection.

lying the membrane between the two. This mark locates the cricothyroid membrane (Figure 217, page 322).

Precaution

Use Sterile Technique.—Be sure the equipment has been sterilized.

Procedure

1. The procedure is explained carefully to the patient and he is cautioned not to cough, swallow, or talk until told to do so.

2. The area is aseptically prepared with an alcohol sponge.

3. The anesthetist stands at the head of the operating table facing the patient's feet (Figure 218, page 322). If the anesthetist is right-handed, the index finger of the left hand palpates the cricothyroid membrane where the X is marked on the skin (Figure 218, page 322). The patient is cautioned that he will feel a "stick" in the neck.

4. With a quick thrust the 1½-inch (3.8 cm.), 22-gauge Huber point Lok-needle attached to the Lok-syringe, containing the exact amount of the local anesthetic solution, is pushed perpendicularly through the X on the skin and the cricothyroid membrane into the lumen of the trachea (Figure 217, page 322).

5. The plunger of the syringe is withdrawn to be sure air is aspirated and the needle is correctly placed.

6. The contents of the syringe are rapidly discharged and the needle withdrawn.

7. The patient will usually cough automatically and he should be encouraged to repeat these coughs three or four times.

EXTENT OF ANALGESIA

The upper portion of the trachea, larynx, and the lower portion of the pharynx.

COMPLICATIONS

Toxic Reactions: (See Chapter 3, page 19). This type of reaction is usually due to rapid absorption of the local anesthetic solution. Reactions of this type, which occur from absorption from the mucous membrane of the trachea or the alveoli of the lungs, have a rapid onset and are severe. Rapid *correct* treatment is essential.

Puncture of the Esophagus or Soft Tissues: Either of these may occur, but we have seen no complications from them. Just withdraw the needle and replace it in the trachea.

REMARKS

Spray Nose, Mouth, and Pharynx: If the patient is to be intubated or bronchoscoped while awake or in light planes of anesthesia, the nose, mouth, and pharynx are sprayed with a nebulizer to assure topical analgesia above the glottis.

Use Huber Point Needle: The use of the Huber point needle is encouraged so that the anesthetic agent may be placed with some degree of accuracy. If the patient is to be in-

tubated, the bevel is directed upward since anesthesia of the lower trachea is not so important (Figure 217, page 322). If the injection is used for bronchoscopy, the bevel should be pointed downward so as to spray the solution as far down the trachea as possible. This precaution may be superfluous since before an expulsive cough can be produced, the patient must take a deep breath, which aids in drawing the anesthetic solution down the trachea.

Choking or Gagging Is Normal: If the conscious patient seems to choke or gag immediately after the injection, the anesthetist should not become alarmed. The patient will clear his own airway and will not suffocate.

Bleeding or Fistula From Technique No Problem: The danger of producing severe bleeding or creating a fistula from this injection is minimal.

Technique 96 Percent Effective: This method of laryngeal and tracheal analgesia is effective in over 96 percent of the cases and is an excellent method of controlling the autonomic reflexes during intubation. The 4 percent failures are treated by spraying the laryngeal cords under direct vision as they are exposed. Presumably such failures occur because the local anesthetic agent passed the cords at a rapid rate when the patient gave the explosive cough, and thus the pharyngeal side of the cords may have been only partially anesthetized.

Do Not Exceed Maximum Dose: The maximum dose of anesthetic solution advocated must not be exceeded since this dosage rarely incites a reaction after this procedure, but a greater dosage may do so. When a systemic toxic reaction occurs, an overdose of the drug, *i.e.*, a high blood level type reaction, not an allergic type, usually is the reason (see page 19).

Use Transtracheal Injection for Esophagoscopy: While in esophagoscopy the larynx is not entered, transtracheal injection is advocated since the esophagoscopist often produces severe laryngospasm by inadvertent stimulation of the larynx. This is singularly true if thiopental (Pentothal) anesthesia is being administered.

Thiopental (Pentothal) Analgesia May Be Used With Transtracheal Injection: This procedure usually is performed with the patient awake. It may be performed under thiopental *analgesia* with good results if the anesthetist does not wish the patient to remember the "stick" in the neck. However, the patient must not have lost his lid reflex; transtracheal injec-tion cannot be performed if the cough mechanism has been suppressed by previous anesthesia.

Succinylcholine (Anectine) is Method of Choice to Correct Severe Laryngospasm: Succinylcholine (Anectine) 40 to 60 mg. given intravenously or intramuscularly is usually the preferred method of correcting a severe laryngospasm, but, if the drug is not available, transtracheal injection may be lifesaving.

CHAPTER 40

Intracapsular Blocks of the Shoulder Joint and Knee Joint

INDICATIONS

Surgical: Closed reduction of a dislocated shoulder or a "locked" or dislocated knee.

Diagnostic: Differentiation of intracapsular pain from extracapsular pain.

Therapeutic: Occasionally pain caused by trauma or an acute bursitis may be relieved by a lavage.

ANATOMY

The joint capsules are innervated by nerve endings in the synovial membranes. The shoulder joint is innervated by the axillary and supracapsular nerves. The knee joint is innervated by the obturator, femoral, tibial, and common peroneal nerves. The joints normally contain clear synovial fluid. When injury has occurred, this fluid is usually bloody.

PREMEDICATION

No attempts to elicit paresthesias are made, and the procedure is not painful. However, the injury is often quite painful, and since cooperation and relaxation of the patient are highly important to the success of the technique, heavy premedication is advised.

Heavy Premedication: The average patient (age 20 to 50, weight 150 pounds or over, height 5 feet, 5 inches or over, and good physical status) receives:

1. 200 mg. (3 gr.) of pentobarbital (Nembutal) by mouth at hour of sleep on night previous to surgery.

2. 200 mg. (3 gr.) of pentobarbital 1½ to 2 hours before the estimated *block* time. However, since most of these injuries are treated

immediately as emergencies, this medication (1 and 2) is often omitted until the opiate and belladonna drug have been given by the intravenous route. Then, if they are not adequate, 100 mg. (1½ gr.) to 200 mg. (3 gr.) of pentobarbital is administered intravenously. At least 15 minutes should elapse between the intravenous injection of the opiates and the barbiturates so that maximum effect of the morphine will be realized.

3. 15 mg. (¼ gr.) of morphine and 0.6 mg. (¹⁄₁₀₀ gr.) of scopolamine are given intramuscularly ¾ to 1 hour before the estimated *block* time. If, however, the patient is to be treated immediately, the above dosage is given slowly, intravenously. *Be sure, if the patient has been referred, whether or not a previous injection of an opiate has been administered.*

Reduction of Premedication: It is seldom necessary to increase this premedication irrespective of the over-all size of the patient until the patient arrives in either the anesthesia or operating room. However, it is very common to reduce this medication under various circumstances; for example, in the case of the geriatric patient, the adolescent patient or child, the debilitated or cachectic patient, and for those whose surgery is complicated by other disease, *e.g.,* myxedema, diabetes, heart diseases, etc. In the patient over 60 years of age, barbiturates and especially scopolamine often cause disorientation. Therefore, in these patients atropine is usually substituted for scopolamine and the dosage of the barbiturate omitted or greatly reduced, *i.e.,* to 50 mg. (¾ gr.) or less. *Always err on the light side.*

Inadequate Premedication: If medication is inadequate either for the block or for the surgical procedure, intravenous pentobarbital 50 mg. (¾ gr.) to 100 mg. (1½ gr.) or intravenous morphine 8 mg. (⅛ gr.) to 15 mg. (¼ gr.) may be given slowly. Judicious use of added sedation is extremely important. Often small supplementary doses of morphine or pentobarbital will make a block successful, especially when a patient interprets touch and motion as pain.

DRUGS

Tetracaine (Pontocaine)

Dosage.—20 cc. to 50 cc. of 0.15 to 0.25 percent solution with or without 0.25 cc. of epinephrine (Adrenalin) 1:1000 in 50 cc. of solution.*

Onset.—Analgesia is established in 10 to 30 minutes.

Duration.—3½ to 6 hours, with stronger concentrations and solutions containing epinephrine giving the upper limits.

Procaine (Novocain)

Dosage.—20 cc. to 50 cc. of 1.0 to 2.0 percent solution with or without 0.25 cc. of epinephrine (Adrenalin) 1:1000 in 50 cc. of solution.*

Onset.—Analgesia is established in 5 to 20 minutes.

Duration.—1 to 1½ hours, with stronger concentrations and solutions containing epinephrine giving the upper limits.

Lidocaine (Xylocaine) or Mepivacaine (Carbocaine)

Dosage.—20 cc. to 50 cc. of 1.0 percent solution with or without 0.25 cc. of epinephrine (Adrenalin) 1:1000 in 50 cc. of solution.*

Onset.—Analgesia is established in 5 to 20 minutes.

Duration.—1 to 3 hours, with solutions containing epinephrine giving the upper limits.

---

*Optimal concentration of epinephrine is 1:200,000, that is, 0.1 cc. of epinephrine 1:1000 in 20 cc. of the local anesthetic solution (see page 39).

MATERIALS

Regional tray (see Chapter 9, page 51) or:

1. One ¾-inch (2 cm.), 25-gauge Huber point security Lok-needle.

2. One 2-inch (5 cm.), 22- or 20-gauge security Lok-needle.

3. One tuberculin Lok-syringe for measuring epinephrine.

4. One 10 cc. Lok-syringe, preferably with finger rings.

5. One stainless steel graduated measuring cup, for mixing solutions.

6. One stainless steel prep cup.

7. Four towels.

8. Six sponges.

9. One sterilizer control.

TECHNIQUE

Position and Landmarks

1. The position is that in which the patient is most comfortable.

2. A definite landmark through which to insert the needle through synovial membrane cannot be indicated emphatically, since much depends on the type of dislocation and more than one approach may be necessary before the synovia is entered.

Precautions: None.

Procedure

1. The sterilizer control is checked to be sure the equipment has been sterilized.

2. The area over the shoulder joint or knee joint is aseptically prepared and draped.

3. An intradermal wheal with the ¾-inch (2.0 cm.), 25-gauge Huber point is made over the joint, avoiding bone obstructions such as the acromial process and the patella (Figure 219, page 327 and Figure 220, page 327).

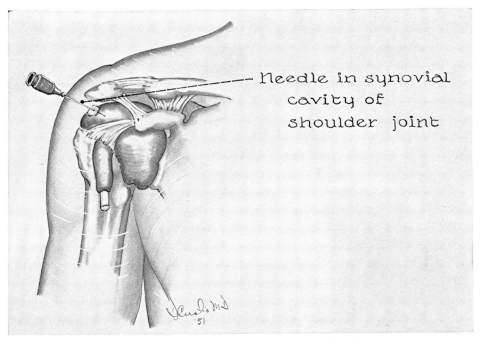

Figure 219. Injection of the synovial cavity of the shoulder joint.

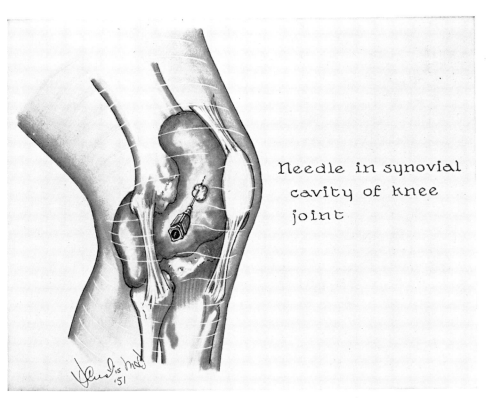

Figure 220. Injection of the synovial cavity of the knee.

4. The 2-inch (5 cm.), 22 or 20-gauge Lok-needle with the half-full Lok-syringe attached is then advanced through the skin wheal, through the synovial membrane, into the joint space, injecting small amounts of anesthetic solution as the needle advances (Figure 219, page 327 and Figure 220, page 327).

5. Frequent attempts at aspiration are made so that as soon as the joint space is entered, synovial fluid will be aspirated, showing that this space has been entered.

6. As much as possible of synovial fluid, which may be blood-tinged, if the injury is severe, is withdrawn, discarded, and replaced with local anesthetic solution. No less than 20 cc. and, if possible, 30 to 40 cc. of the local anesthetic solution should be placed inside the joint capsule.

7. Adequate time is allowed for the anesthetic to take effect.

EXTENT OF ANALGESIA

The synovia of the joint injected.

COMPLICATIONS

Toxic Reactions (intravascular injections, etc.): See Chapter 3, page 19. These occur extremely infrequently.

REMARKS

Incidence of Satisfactory Analgesia Less Than With Other Block Techniques: This type of analgesia is not as satisfactory as brachial plexus block, or sciatic and femoral nerve block, or spinal analgesia; however, it is satisfactory in over 90 percent of the cases and avoids a more complicated anesthetic procedure. If it fails, the above mentioned anesthetic techniques or general anesthesia may be employed.

Allow Adequate Time for Analgesia to Establish: It must be stressed that adequate time must be allowed for the local anesthetic agent to anesthetize the synovial membrane.

Bloody Synovial Fluid Is No Contraindication: Withdrawal of bloody synovial fluid is no contraindication to the injection of the local anesthetic solution.

Recover Broken Needle(s): All needles should be tested before use. If a needle breaks, every effort to recover it, including surgery, should be made. Unremoved needles have a tendency to migrate and may cause permanent injuries as well as medicolegal complications.

Repeat Block When Analgesia Is Inadequate: If the results from the first block attempt are unsatisfactory, do not hesitate to reblock the patient if time permits. Most patients will think nothing about being reblocked if the second attempt is prefaced by a statement such as: "Well, I guess we will have to inject a little more medicine if we are going to freeze this area."

However, do not exceed the maximum safe dosage of the local anesthetic solution for both blocks. If to reblock the patient the maximum safe dose of the local anesthetic solution must be exceeded, 45 minutes should elapse between blocks.

CHAPTER 41

The Therapeutic Use of Absolute Alcohol in Peripheral Nerve Block

A LCOHOL BLOCK of the peripheral nerves is not without serious complications. Often the complication, in particular the neuritis which is commonly produced by alcohol, is as severe or more severe than the original pain problem for which it was employed. Therefore, it behooves the beginner in regional analgesia, or the physician who does the occasional block, to avoid it. Its use should be limited to larger institutions or specialists whose reputation in this work can compensate for poor results.

When one or two nerves are to be injected, such as in tic douloureux, treatment on an outpatient basis is satisfactory; however, arrangements should be made so that the patient may rest for one to two hours following the injection, because about 10 percent of the patients become nauseated and vomit following the injection of the alcohol. For extensive alcohol injections, *e.g.*, celiac plexus block, the patient should be hospitalized.

INDICATIONS

Surgical: None.

Diagnostic: Occasionally an alcohol block of the branches of the trigeminal nerve or of the lumbar sympathetic ganglia is performed to prognosticate the advisability of a surgical procedure. However, alcohol is usually not employed in diagnostic procedures.

Therapeutic: Relief of intractable disabling pain, *i.e.*, trigeminal neuralgias, carcinoma, etc., and alleviation of vascular deficiencies where operations are not indicated.

PREMEDICATION

We do not administer premedication prior to performing peripheral nerve blocks with alcohol because: (1) often accurate paresthesias are essential to correctly place the needle; (2) pain during injection of the alcohol confirms correct placement of the needle; and (3) medicolegal involvement is avoided (see page 334). After a successful block, the average patient who had severe pain prior to the block will seldom complain of pain or of the paresthesias caused by either the placement of the needle or the injection of the alcohol, provided the technique is carefully explained beforehand. The pain from the injection of the alcohol will prevail for a short time, 5 to 10 seconds. The patient can tolerate this and the relief that will follow is so marked that it is unusual for a patient to object to a repeat block if it is necessary at a later date.

PROPERTIES OF ABSOLUTE ALCOHOL

Mode of Action on the Nerve Tissue: Alcohol scleroses the nerve tissue by its dehydrating action. Typical wallerian degeneration occurs. The myelinated nerves regenerate, but the time required for this varies with each individual and with the region of the body. Often the small unmyelinated nerve fibers may be permanently destroyed if an adequate amount of alcohol has been employed.

Dosage: 0.5 to 50 cc. depending on the concentration of alcohol, the nerve(s) injected, and the location of the nerve(s).

Onset: Immediate if the needle is in the correct location.

Duration: Area of analgesia over the distribution of the nerve involved lasts six weeks to six months. However, the patient may be free from pain from a few weeks to years, and occasionally the pain never recurs. In most instances, the average period of pain relief is six to fifteen months.

Toxicity: Alcohol, *itself*, injected in the stated quantities is not systemically toxic. Superficial injections may cause blistering and sloughing.

MATERIALS

Regional block tray or the equipment listed under each block. A 2 or 3 cc. Lok-syringe or a tuberculin syringe should always be included so that small amounts of the alcohol may be accurately measured. The syringe which is to be used for the injection of alcohol should not be used to measure any other solution—it should be used only to measure and inject the alcohol.

TECHNIQUE

1. Explain in detail to the patient the reasons why an alcohol block is being performed and the technique step by step. Warn the patient of the severe discomfort and the fact that it will disappear in a matter of seconds or minutes. Stress that his cooperation is essential for a successful result.

2. The local anesthetic agent is employed in making the skin wheal and for superficial infiltration only. *Under no circumstances should the nerve tissue in question be blocked with the local anesthetic agent to decrease the pain of the alcohol injection.* This dilutes the alcohol and may cause poor results.

3. The needles are placed according to the directions given for the block in question and all the precautions must be carefully observed. When using alcohol, paresthesias of the peripheral somatic nerve to be injected *must* be elicited.

4. The quantity of alcohol is carefully measured and injected.

5. 2 cc. of air is then blown through the needle to evacuate the alcohol and the needle is removed. This maneuver is advocated to

prevent: (1) sinus tracts from forming between the alcohol deposit and the site of injection of the needle and (2) drops of alcohol from being deposited on other nerves, particularly motor divisions, as the needle is withdrawn.

SOME OF THE COMMON CONDITIONS WHICH MAY BE TREATED BY ABSOLUTE ALCOHOL NERVE BLOCK

It is obvious that all conditions may not and should not be covered in this book, but the following are those which occur most frequently and which may be treated with relative safety, although the complications which occur may be permanent.

Trigeminal Neuralgia (Tic Douloureux)

General Considerations

1. Trigeminal neuralgias are usually excited by trigger points in one of the three divisions of the fifth cranial nerve. The trigger area most frequently lies in the maxillary division, occasionally in the mandibular division, and rarely in the ophthalmic division; however, it is not uncommon to have the trigger point in one division cause referred pain in another division. This is particularly true of the maxillary division, which often causes referred pain over or around the eye. Blocking of the division containing the trigger area usually alleviates the referred pain.

2. Gasserian (semilunar) ganglion block should not be done with alcohol because of the following reasons. First, it eliminates the normal corneal reflex of the eye on the blocked side and as a result corneal ulcers occur in a high percentage of cases. These ulcers may cause loss of sight in the affected eye if not carefully treated by an ophthalmologist. Second, the dangers of placing alcohol solutions within the cranial cavity and in close proximity to the brain are numerous, *e.g.*, paralysis of other nerves, etc. Third, the sclerosing action of alcohol on the gasserian ganglion makes future surgical section of it an arduous task because adhesions and fibrous tissue forma-

tions make the identification of its components difficult. Fourth, blocking of either the mandibular or maxillary divisions or their terminal branches as they leave their respective foramina is just as satisfactory and does not carry the above complications. The area of anesthesia produced is limited to the one division blocked and does not affect the whole face. And, fifth, twenty-five to thirty percent of gasserian ganglion blocks are unsuccessful.

3. Only the terminal branches, supraorbital and supratrochlear, of the ophthalmic nerve should be blocked. Attempts to block the ophthalmic nerve, *per se,* may lead to damage of the eyeball or oculomotor nerve or its branches.

4. More than 1.5 cc. of alcohol should not be injected at any one time in any of the divisions of the trigeminal nerve. It is seldom necessary to use more than ½ cc. of absolute alcohol when blocking the terminal branches (supraorbital, supratrochlear, infraorbital, and mental) of the divisions of the fifth cranial nerve.

5. Blocking of more than one division or reblock of the same division should not be done unless at least 24 hours and preferably 72 hours have been allowed to elapse. Often, in spite of an adequate block, the patient may experience sensations which resemble the old tic pain for this period of time before complete relief of pain is experienced.

6. It is not uncommon for the patient to have a peculiar feeling in his face following an alcohol block, which he describes as "woody" with "the feeling of worms crawling over the face." When this occurs, the patient should be assured that this is a normal reaction and that it will gradually disappear. The patient should also be impressed with the fact that the tic pain is not returning.

7. If after three days the typical tic pain is still present, reblock of the same division, if anesthesia does not exist over its distribution or block of one of the other divisions of the trigeminal nerves, is indicated.

8. If an elderly patient with trigeminal neuralgia receives relief from an alcohol block, and pain should return at a later date, at least one or two more alcohol blocks should be administered before resorting to surgery, since they may allow him to live his life span without undergoing a surgical procedure. However, if a young patient with trigeminal neuralgia receives relief from an alcohol block and the pain returns, section of the nerve is preferred to repeated blocks.

9. It is not uncommon for a trigeminal neuralgia patient to come to the office following a successful block merely to be assured that the block will not disappear and the tic type pain return. At this time, with careful choice of words, the patient can be prepared for a reblock or surgery should the effect of the alcohol block be dissipated after a year or so.

Alcohol Block of the Mandibular Maxillary Divisions and Their Terminal Branches or the Terminal Branches of the Ophthalmic Compared to Immediate Surgical Resection or Alcohol Block of the Gasserian (Semilunar) Ganglion

1. The advantages of alcohol block before surgical resection may be summarized as follows. First, the outcome of surgical resection can be prognosticated with virtual certainty, *i.e.,* if an injection affords relief, the operation should afford the same relief, and if the injection affords no relief, the operation may not be successful. Some physicians may challenge this statement but in most instances it applies. Second, the prolonged numbness of the face with gradual recovery gives the patient ample time to consider whether he prefers a permanent numbness of his face to his original pain. Third, if the trigeminal neuralgia has been long-standing, most patients are debilitated, as pain is initiated by the process of eating. In these patients, temporary relief of six to fifteen months allows them to restore their general nutrition and health, making them a better surgical risk. Fourth, this block may allow the very old patients to complete their life span without operation. Fifth, there is the occasional patient who may receive permanent relief. Cases of relief of over thirty years have been recorded. Lastly, alcohol has not been

placed on the gasserian (semilunar) ganglion and thus the surgical resection of the ganglion is not complicated by adhesions if it is elected to perform such surgery at a future date.

2. The disadvantages are those listed as complications under maxillary nerve block (page 108) and mandibular nerve block (page 99). Since alcohol is the blocking agent, these complications may be permanent.

Ulceration, Slough, and Gangrene of the Area Innervated by the Terminal Branches of the Maxillary Division of the Fifth Nerve: Following alcohol block of the maxillary nerve at the foramen rotundum or the infraorbital nerve in its canal, ulceration and severe slough of the skin of the ala of the nose, the upper alveolar ridge, the soft or hard palate, or a combination of these can occur. This is not the result of the alcohol alone, for it occurs following surgical section of the maxillary nerve at the gasserian ganglion.

Two such cases resulted following blocks by us. The first case followed a block of the maxillary nerve after it had emerged from the foramen rotundum and was passing through the pterygopalatine fossa. In this instance, the posterior portion of the superior alveolar ridge of the maxillary bone and its surrounding tissue sloughed. The second case followed block of the infraorbital nerve in a patient who previously had three such alcohol blocks at one-year intervals without any complications. In this patient, the skin around the ala of the nose sloughed, as did a portion of the hard palate.

The cause of this infrequent complication is difficult to determine. Faulty technique, vascular changes, reflex, or involvement of the sympathetic nervous system have all been considered as possible causes, but none accepted as fact.

This complication, in relation to the number of times the branches of the fifth nerve are sectioned either surgically or chemically, occurs too infrequently to condemn such treatment of trigeminal neuralgia on its account. However, the seriousness of the complication should make the physician cognizant that he must explain its possible occurrence to the patient prior to the block.

The treatment of these cases is often difficult but includes antibiotic drugs; hot, wet packs; incision and drainage; debridement of the sloughed ulcer and gangrenous area; and skin grafting. In instances where the ulcerated area remains infected in spite of the above treatment and/or cannot be prepared for grafting, temporary sympathetic denervation by blocking the stellate ganglion may be indicated to improve circulation to the involved area. A plastic surgeon should treat this complication.

Intractable Disabling Pain and Inoperable Carcinomas

General Considerations.—Alcohol blocks other than spinal (subarachnoid) injections are usually limited to the cranial nerves, the autonomic nervous system, and occasionally the cervical nerves. When good results are to be accomplished with alcohol blocks in a patient with pain, they should be performed before the patient becomes addicted to narcotics; otherwise, in spite of an adequate block, he will still complain of pain in hopes of receiving a narcotic.

Peripheral Somatic Nerves.—If the nerves of the thoracic region, lumbar region, and sacral region are blocked extradurally with alcohol rather than by the spinal route, the neuralgias from the block may be as disabling as the original pain. Also, the possible involvement of motor function from overflow or direct injection of a combined sensory and motor nerve is an important consideration and may present a serious complication, particularly if the extremities are involved.

Chronic Pancreatitis and Cancer of Pancreas, Stomach, Liver, or Gallbladder.—The pain of chronic pancreatitis or the pain of cancer of the pancreas, stomach, liver, or gallbladder can be alleviated for 3 to 5 months or longer—occasionally 1 year—by blocking the celiac (splanchnic) plexus with alcohol. The needles are placed as described under celiac plexus block, page 156. A total of 50 cc. of 50 percent alcohol is injected, *i.e., 25 cc. through each needle.* The physician prepares the 50 percent alcohol by mixing 25 cc. of absolute alcohol with 25 cc. of normal saline.

The patient receives no premedication for this block because the unmedicated patient can significantly aid the physician performing the block. When the needles are in place, and the aspiration tests are negative, the anesthetist injects 1 cc. of the alcohol solution. If the patient reports a somatic nerve paresthesia, the needle should be repositioned. If, however, he reports feeling pressure like "a kick in the solar plexus" and not being able to breathe, the needle is properly placed and the alcohol is injected. Following the injection of the alcohol, patients report that it "burns like fire" for a period of thirty seconds to one minute, and then this pain subsides. The needle is cleared by injecting 2 cc. of air before it is withdrawn in order to prevent spilling some of the solution on the first lumbar somatic nerve. Neuritis of this nerve has been reported, but has not been seen by us.

The progressive degeneration of the nerve fibers caused by the alcohol takes place gradually over a period of days. Hence, the immediate anesthetic effects of the alcohol are usually not as pronounced as those which will appear several days after the block. Thus, 2 to 4 days should pass to allow the block to exert its maximum effects before it is evaluated or repeated.

During celiac plexus block, accidental intravascular, subarachnoid, or intraperitoneal injection may occur. These are easily avoided by frequent aspirations and by careful control of the needle as the solution is being injected. None of these have been seen by us. The only two complications which have occurred are: (1) pain in the back that lasted approximately 24 to 48 hours, and (2) hypotension similar to that which accompanies a splanchnicectomy. Presumably, the tissue irritation from the alcohol causes the pain in the back at the site of the injection. This pain for control sometimes requires small amounts of an analgesic compound (Empirin) containing phenacetin, 150 mg. (2½ gr.); acetylsalicylic acid, 200 mg. (3 gr.); caffeine, 30 mg. (½ gr.); and 30 mg. (½ gr.) of codeine.

Hypotension, which results from interrupting the vasoconstrictor fibers to a wide area, is no problem in the young subjects who can compensate by vasoconstriction in the unaffected vessels. However, the older, arteriosclerotic patients frequently feel faint when they are ambulated. These patients are treated with a tight abdominal binder and elastic stockings. In three to five days, they apparently compensate for this splanchnic vascular dilatation and no longer need the stockings and binder. Oral administration of ephedrine is effective to combat this type of hypotension, but is not used by us. Because of the possibility of hypotension and feeling of faintness or dizziness following the block, the patient is warned about fainting or feeling faint when in an upright position, and the following orders are written on the patient's chart: (1) wrap both legs to midthigh with a six-inch elastic bandage; (2) apply a tight abdominal binder before ambulation; (3) ambulate only with an assistant on each side; (4) check blood pressure and pulse every fifteen minutes for two hours; and (5) if systolic pressure falls below ____, notify Dr. _____, telephone number _____.

Vascular Insufficiencies

Upper Extremities.—Alcohol block of the thoracic sympathetic ganglia (1 through 4) for anginal pain should be left to the expert because: (1) pneumothorax with deposit of alcohol in the pleural cavity is not uncommon; (2) alcohol injections in severe cases may carry a mortality rate of more than 10 percent; and (3) intercostal neuritis, particularly below the third thoracic nerve, may be as disabling as the anginal pain.

Alcohol block of the stellate ganglion by any of the neck approaches is to be avoided because: (1) a persistent Horner's syndrome with diplopia often results; (2) involvement of the brachial plexus with prolonged weakness and neuritis of the arm may result; and (3) involvement of the recurrent laryngeal nerve with prolonged hoarseness and difficult swallowing frequently follows.

Lower Extremities.—Alcohol injection of the lumbar sympathetic chain may be performed without complications other than an associated neuritis or temporary paralysis of the lumbar somatic nerves. If this injection is performed, up to 4 cc. of alcohol may be placed on each ganglion, *i.e.*, if the second, third, and fourth lumbar sympathetic ganglia are injected, a total of 12 cc. of absolute alcohol may be employed.

Since occasionally it may be difficult to prognosticate the outcome of a lumbar sympathectomy from a single injection or repeated injections of the ganglia with a local anesthetic blocking agent, it is at times helpful to produce a prolonged block with alcohol. If after one to three months of an effective chemical sympathectomy no beneficial results are obtained, it may be safe to assume that little could be gained from an operation. Thus, the patient is spared the expense and discomforts of an operation which would not have alleviated his difficulties.

Comment.—With the present advances in anesthetic and surgical techniques, it is only the exceptional case that warrants an alcohol block for a vascular insufficiency. The results from surgery are far more satisfactory both to the patient and the anesthetist.

If alcohol is injected prior to surgery as a diagnostic or therapeutic procedure its sclerosing action may make identification of the anatomy difficult. This may cause a poor surgical result.

REMARKS

Do Not Use Alcohol Until Block Technique Is Mastered: Alcohol should not be employed by an anesthetist until he has mastered the block procedure with which it is to be administered. When complications occur from the spread of local anesthetic agents to the surrounding tissues, they will be automatically corrected within a few hours. On the other hand, complications resulting from the use of alcohol may be semipermanent or permanent.

Take Precautions Which May Avoid Medicolegal Action: While it is permissible to premedicate a patient who is to have a neurolytic drug injected into a peripheral nerve, the gasserian ganglion, or a sympathetic ganglion, it is preferable not to do so since a complication may result. If the patient is not medicated or anesthetized he is clearly consenting to the treatment and is not undergoing any type of therapy which might be objectionable to him. The one patient who was blinded by me (Figure 55, page 109, and Figure 56, page 109) is a typical example of the efficacy of this precaution—although the patient consulted a lawyer who contacted our insurance company, no suit developed and no settlement was made. The lawyer for our insurance company was of the opinion the case could be successfully fought on the basis that the plaintiff had willingly submitted to the treatment knowing the possible complications. Certainly a block procedure, particularly one in which neurolytic drugs are to be used, should never be performed against the will of the patient, for he may seek retribution on the basis of "technical assault."

The patient should be made to understand the risks involved in an alcohol block and a signed permit for execution of the block is a necessity (see page 10). Under no circumstances should a nerve containing motor fibers be injected with absolute or dilute alcohol unless the patient understands and is willing to accept the associated motor disability, whether it be partial or complete.

Perform Diagnostic Block With Local Anesthetic Solution Before Using Alcohol: A day or two before performing most alcohol blocks, a block with a long-acting local anesthetic agent such as tetracaine (Pontocaine) should be employed because it allows: (1) the patient to experience for a short time the results that may be expected for a prolonged period when alcohol is injected; (2) the anesthetist to find out what complications may result from his technique before they are incurred for a period of three weeks to a year by the use of alcohol; and (3) the anesthetist to determine the exact amount of alcohol necessary to accomplish the desired results and thus evaluate the feasibility of the procedure, *i.e.*, small measured amounts of local anesthetic solutions comparable to the amount of alcohol advocated should be used first as a test dose.

Do Not Anesthetize the Nerve(s) With a Local Anesthetic Solution Immediately Prior to the Injection of Alcohol: If a local anesthetic solution is injected into or onto a nerve to anesthetize it prior to the injection of alcohol in an effort to eliminate the pain caused by the alcohol, the volume of the local anesthetic solution will dilute the alcohol and the block may not be as effective.

Should Roentgenograms be Taken? The taking of roentgenograms during a block procedure is time-consuming, inconvenient, and the information obtained is not always accurate. Therefore, even when alcohol is injected, x-ray seldom is employed for the routine therapeutic or diagnostic blocks described herein.

When a block is being learned, when paresthesias are difficult to elicit, or if there is any question as to whether or not the needle is correctly placed, x-rays of the needles in place and a competent radiologist to interpret the needle's position may be extremely valuable.

As an added precaution, 35 percent iodopyracet (Diodrast) solution may be employed as the solvent for the crystals of the local anesthetic agent. In this manner, if x-rays are taken within five to ten minutes following the injection of the solution, the exact spread of the solution may be ascertained. The only drawback to the injection of an iodopyracet solution is the fact that in 10 to 15 percent of the cases it may intensify the pain, cause a new type of pain, or create a new distribution of the pain after the anesthesia from the local anesthetic drug has been dissipated.

Roentgenograms do have the following advantage: (1) when taken during the block with a short-acting local anesthetic agent, they serve as a means of comparison with the films taken when the needle or needles are placed for the alcohol block; and (2) they will establish a permanent, visible record of the position of the needle or needles if the alcohol block is repeated at a later date.

Record Amount of Alcohol Used: The exact amount of alcohol injected should always be recorded on the patient's chart.

Use Small Sterile Ampules of Alcohol: Absolute alcohol for block procedures should come in small sterile ampules (2 cc. size) which should be opened at the time of the injection. Highly concentrated alcohol will absorb moisture from the air and may contain spores if it has been allowed to stand open or loosely stoppered.

Inadvertent Intravenous Injection of Alcohol Causes No Problems: Injection of absolute alcohol intravenously involves few complications other than an occasional thrombosis of the vessel in question.

Surgery May Be Preferable to Alcohol Block: At the present time we do not have a good permanent solution to destroy nerve tissue. Alcohol is satisfactory for blocking the cranial nerves and for spinal (subarachnoid) injections, but when employed in other regions it causes severe neuritis in a large percentage of cases.

With the exception of alcohol injection of the cranial nerves and the celiac (splanchnic) plexus, it is probably best that surgery, *i.e.*, sensory root sections, sympathectomies, cordotomies, and lobotomies, should be carried out wherever feasible in preference to alcohol blocking. Alcohol blocking of the peripheral nerves other than the cranial nerves and the celiac plexus for intractable pain of carcinoma and vascular deficiencies is in general unsatisfactory and causes both the anesthetist and the patient unwarranted trouble.

Long-Acting Agents Other Than Alcohol or Phenol Must Be Used With Care: When alcohol or phenol (see page 336) is contraindicated for therapeutic block of pain problems of the peripheral nerves, preparations of local anesthetic agents which are credited with prolonged duration of analgesia such as Intracaine in oil, Zylcaine, Protocaine, Dolamin, Eucupine, and Efocaine have been employed.

When contemplating the injection of one of these preparations the following comments should be evaluated:

1. Preparations in oil, if placed too superficially in the body tissues, often cause severe slough.

2. Many physicians feel that any results which are obtained from these preparations, most of which contain benzyl alcohol as a preservative, can be attributed to the benzyl alcohol.

3. Intravenous injections of oily substances may be fatal.

4. When employing these substances the toxic dose of the local anesthetic drug incorporated in the preparation should not be exceeded. If a toxic reaction to the local anesthetic agent occurs it should be treated as described in Chapter 3, page 19.

5. Eucupine is a very toxic drug and has been known to cause visual disturbances as well as blindness when used internally. Its injection is also quite painful. For these two reasons many hesitate to use the drug.

6. Alleviating painful problems usually requires repeated injections. This is true whether the above preparations or a local anesthetic agent by itself is injected. Therefore, it may not be wise to run the added risk which an oily preparation involves.

7. Dolamin is not an oily substance and is nontoxic to the body tissues. The occasional dramatic result which follows the use of this ammonium sulfate preparation may warrant its trial.

8. When local anesthetic agents are incorporated in an oil, propylene glycol or polyethylene glycol base, a severe neuritis of 3 to 4 weeks duration may occur following injection into peripheral nerves. Also, varying degrees of paralysis and death have resulted from them entering the subarachnoid space or spinal cord following their placement paravertebrally.

Solutions injected paravertebrally and intraneurally may reach the subarachnoid space or the spinal cord via the perineural spaces of peripheral nerves. The perineural spaces of the peripheral nerves are actual, not just theoretical, avenues to the spinal cords when solutions are injected intraneurally.

9. *The duration of analgesia from the above-mentioned preparations is unpredictable.* A poor result from the use of these preparations is the rule rather than the exception.

Phenol May Be Substituted for Alcohol: 5 to 7 percent phenol may be used for peripheral nerve block in the same fashion as absolute alcohol. However, to date its use has not been as extensive as alcohol in blocking the peripheral nerves. Complications from its use are those which occur with alcohol.

CHAPTER 42

Intra-abdominal Anesthesia by Peritoneal Lavage

GENERAL CONSIDERATIONS

A SHORT chapter on this type of regional anesthesia is included because of the safety and simplicity of this procedure. This procedure may answer difficult problems occurring during surgery or peritoneoscopy. Often during either regional anesthesia or general anesthesia the peritoneum and its contents are not adequately anesthetized. This may be caused by inadequate anesthesia, or in a prolonged operation, the effective duration of the local anesthetic agent may have elapsed. Peritoneal lavage will in most cases help correct this condition.

DRUGS

A large volume of a relatively dilute solution of the local anesthetic agent gives the best results.

Tetracaine (Pontocaine)

Dosage.—200 cc. of 0.1 percent solution.

Onset.—Analgesia is established in 5 to 8 minutes.

Duration.—Operating analgesia lasts approximately 1 to 1¼ hours.

Procaine (Novocain)

Dosage.—200 cc. of 0.5 to 1.0 percent solution.

Onset.—Operating analgesia is established in 3 to 8 minutes.

Duration.—Operating analgesia lasts 30 to 40 minutes.

Lidocaine (Xylocaine)

Dosage.—200 cc. of 0.5 percent solution.

Onset.—Operating analgesia is established in 3 to 8 minutes.

Duration.—Operating analgesia lasts ½ to 1 hour.

TECHNIQUE

1. The local anesthetic solution is poured into the peritoneal cavity either through a nick in the peritoneum or into the open peritoneum.

2. The peritoneum is closed either by a pack or by pulling its edges together.

3. The solution is allowed to remain in the abdomen 5 to 8 minutes.

4. Then the solution is withdrawn by suction.

REMARKS

Systemic Toxic Reactions Seldom Result: The fact that toxic reactions are neglible seems to indicate that rapid absorption of the local anesthetic solution or agent by the peritoneum does not occur. However, if the doses listed are exceeded, reactions to the local anesthetic drug may ensue.

Intestine Shrinks Markedly: The relaxation which follows the maneuver is quite astounding. The intestine shrinks until it is the size of a large grapefruit, and the peritoneum may be picked up and pulled together without difficulty. However, this characteristic response may not be seen under the following circumstances: (1) peritoneal soilage from infection or hemorrhage; (2) dilated bowel caused by pathological conditions of the contents of the peritoneal cavity; for example, intestinal obstruction, volvulus, emboli of mesenteric vessels, etc.; and (3) the use of local anesthetic solutions whose concentration is greater than those advocated.

Agent of Choice Is Procaine (Novocain) or

Lidocaine (Xylocaine): Procaine is usually more adaptable to this type of procedure than tetracaine. The onset of its action is more rapid and the anesthesia somewhat better. Lidocaine has been employed with results reported to be more satisfactory than those with procaine.

PART III

SPINAL (SUBARACHNOID),

EPIDURAL (PERIDURAL), AND

CAUDAL ANESTHESIA

CHAPTER 43

Single-Dose Spinal (Subarachnoid) Anesthesia

INDICATIONS

Surgical: Operations below the innervation of the third intercostal nerve.

Diagnostic: Differentiation of autonomic nervous system diseases from organic diseases; for example, arteriosclerotic vascular insufficiencies from vasospastic diseases.

Therapeutic: Treatment of vascular occlusions and spasms of the lower extremity (see Chapter 29, page 211). Emboli usually are not in themselves aided, but the associated spasm is relieved, which may give a more advantageous amputation site.

Spinal block may relieve pain such as that caused by acute pancreatitis or mesenteric thrombosis, which is difficult to control with opiates.

Reversal of anuria caused by chemotherapy and blood transfusions may be aided by spinal block provided hypotension from the block does not ensue or, if it does, steps to correct it are taken.

ANATOMY

In the lumbar region, the spinous processes of the vertebrae have very little slope as compared to those in the thoracic region (Figure 221, page 342 and Figure 222, page 343). They are covered by the supraspinous ligament and connected by the interspinal ligaments (Figure 222, page 343). The ligamenta flava connect the lamina of the arches of the vertebrae and are tough fibrous bands (Figure 222, page 343). Between the ligamenta flava and the dura is a space which is filled with very loose areolar tissues, fat, and blood vessels. This is known as the epidural space (Figure 222, page 343 and Figure 270, page 409). The dura with its contents lies supported in the vertebral canal. Cephalad, the dura fuses with the skull at the foramen magnum. Caudad, the dura ends at the level of the second sacral foramen, but the spinal cord, *itself*, ends at the level of the first lumbar vertebra (Figure 223, page 343). The spinal cord is sparsely supplied with blood vessels (Figure 318, page 482).

PREMEDICATION

Paresthesias are not sought. Heavy medication, particularly for the surgical patient, is advised except in the geriatric patient, the pregnant patient, and the patient with a poor physical status.

Heavy Premedication: The average patient (age 20 to 50, weight 150 pounds or over, approximate height 5 feet, 5 inches or over, and good physical status) receives:

1. 200 mg. (3 gr.) of pentobarbital (Nembutal) by mouth at hour of sleep the night before surgery.

2. 100 mg. (1½ gr.) to 200 mg. (3 gr.) of pentobarbital with one ounce of water by mouth 1½ to 2 hours before estimated *block* time.

3. 15 mg. (¼ gr.) of morphine and 0.6 mg. (1/100 gr.) of scopolamine intramuscularly ¾ to 1 hour before estimated *block* time.

Reduction of Premedication: It is seldom necessary to increase this premedication irrespective of the over-all size of the patient until the patient arrives in either the anesthesia or operating room. However, it is very common to reduce this medication under various circumstances; for example, in the case of the geriatric patient, the adolescent patient or

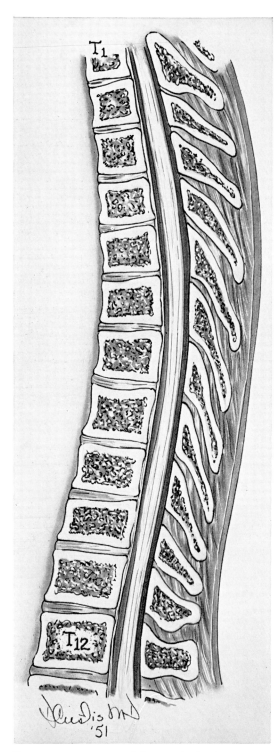

Figure 221. Anatomy of the vertebral column in the thoracic region (T1 - T12) showing the marked slant of the spinous processes of the thoracic vertebrae.

child, the debilitated or cachectic patient, the pregnant patient, and for those whose surgery is complicated by other disease, e.g., myxedema, diabetes, heart disease, etc. In the patient over 60 years of age, barbiturates and especially scopolamine often cause disorientation. Therefore, in these patients atropine is usually substituted for scopolamine and the dosages of the barbiturate omitted or greatly reduced, i.e., 50 mg. (¾ gr.) or less. *Always err on the light side.*

Inadequate Premedication: If medication is inadequate for surgery or the block procedure, pentobarbital 50 mg. (¾ gr.) to 100 mg. (1½ gr.), morphine 10 mg. (⅙ gr.), or preferably small amounts of 0.6 percent thiopental (Pentothal) or 0.2 percent methohexital (Brevital) may be given slowly intravenously until the desired effect results. Judicious use of added sedation is extremely important. Often small supplementary doses of thiopental or methohexital, will make a block successful when a patient interprets touch and motion as pain. When either of these two drugs is employed, a slow intravenous drip may be needed throughout the entire block and surgical procedure.

Premedication of the Patient in Labor: All barbiturates, narcotics, belladonna derivatives, tranquilizers, and combinations of these drugs will pass the placenta and equilibrate in the fetus in the same period of time as they do in the mother. Therefore, little or no premedication is advised—the spinal block will relieve the pain.

If premedication is to be given to allay the parturient's fears and apprehensions, a reasonable dosage of drugs which will not significantly depress the fetus should be used, e.g., meperidine (Demerol) 50 mg. and promethazine (Phenergan) 25 mg.

DRUGS

Anesthetic Agents: The agents used by us include: (1) tetracaine (Pontocaine); (2) procaine (Novocain); and (3) dibucaine (Nupercaine). For methods and dosages, refer to Chapter 44, page 370.

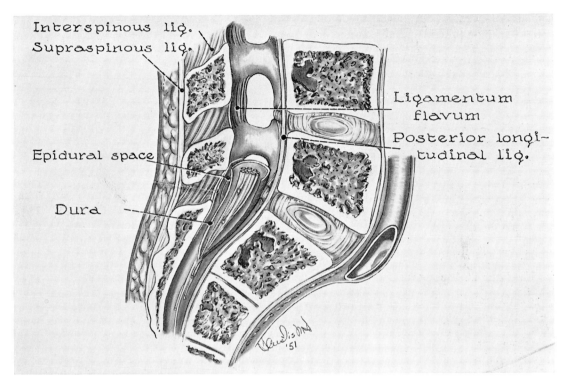

Figure 222. Anatomy of the vertebral column and its contents in the lower lumbar and upper sacral regions.

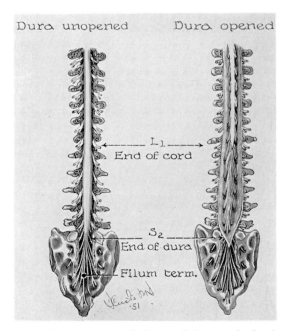

Figure 223. Anatomical sketch of the vertebral column and its contents showing the levels at which the spinal cord and the dura end.

Lidocaine (Xylocaine) and mepivacaine (Carbocaine) are not used by us (see page 15).

Vasoconstrictor Agents: The agents used subarachnoidally to prolong duration of operating analgesia are epinephrine (Adrenalin) 1:1000 and phenylephrine (Neo-Synephrine) 1 percent (see Chapter 51, page 481).

Local Anesthetic Solution for Skin Wheal: 2 cc. ampules of 1 percent procaine (Novocain) solution.*

MATERIALS

Regional tray (see Chapter 9, page 51) or:

1. One ¾-inch (2 cm.), 25-gauge Huber point security Lok-needle.

2. One 1½-inch (3.8 cm.), 22-gauge security Lok-needle.

*This size ampule is obtained from Vitarine Company, Queens, New York.

3. One 21 or 22-gauge, 3½-inch (9 cm.) spinal Lok-needle (Greene type) or one 26-gauge, 3½-inch (9 cm.) spinal Lok-needle.*

4. One 3 cc. Lok-syringe.

5. One 5 cc. Lok-syringe.

6. One 10 cc. Lok-syringe.

7. One prep cup, preferably stainless steel.

8. One Allis forceps.

9. One sponge forceps.

10. One Pitkin or thin-walled needle guide for 21- or 22-gauge spinal needle or a 21-gauge needle introducer for the 26-gauge needle.*

11. Four towels.

12. Four 4 x 4 sponges.

13. One sterilizer control.

TECHNIQUE

Landmarks

A line is drawn between the iliac crests (Figure 224, page 344). This line crosses either the spinous process of the fourth lumbar ver-

---

*These items may be obtained from Becton, Dickinson and Company, Rutherford, N. J. Order numbers are: 21- or 22-gauge Greene point spinal needle, G462LNR and specify 3½ inch; 26-gauge, 3½-inch spinal needle and 21-gauge, 2-inch introducer come as a combination, C462LNRB; Pitkin needle guide, PNG; and thin-walled needle guide, 01-0027 (state size of needle which will be placed through guide).

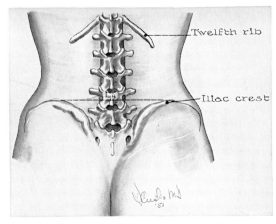

Figure 224. Landmarks for determining the site of the spinal (lumbar) puncture. Dotted line crosses the spine of the fourth lumbar vertebra.

tebra or the interspace between the spinous processes of the fourth and fifth lumbar vertebrae, *i.e.*, fourth lumbar interspace (Figure 224, page 344). Counting cephalad the third or second lumbar interspace may be easily determined.

Position

Lateral Decubitus (Side).—This position is the most frequently employed position as it requires the least effort on the part of the patient and assistants are not necessary. The patient is placed on his right or left side with his knees drawn up to his stomach, his upper arm lying across his chest, his lower arm at right angles to his body, and his head flexed, resting on a small pillow (Figure 225 A and B,

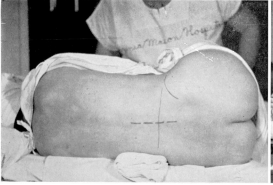
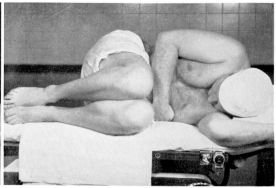

Figure 225. A. and B. Lateral decubitus (side) position for a spinal (lumbar) puncture. The straight line passes through the spinous process of the fourth lumbar vertebra. A. (*Left*) Posterior view. Head is supported on small pillow, upper arm is folded across chest, and knees flexed on abdomen. B. (*Right*) Anterior view.

page 344). Every effort is made to keep the spinous processes of the vertebral column parallel to the table and the patient well flexed so as to open the interspaces.

If an assistant is not available to hold the patient in the above position, it may be simulated by the patient clasping his hands either around his knees and pulling up his knees toward his stomach (Figure 226 A and B,

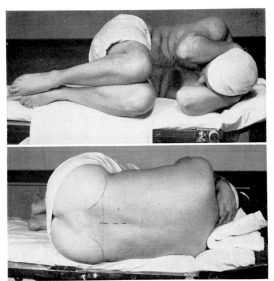

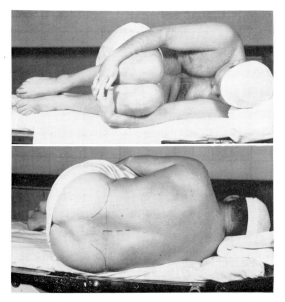

Figure 226. Method of obtaining a good spinal (lumbar) puncture position by having the patient pull his knees up to his stomach when an assistant is not available. A. *(Bottom)* Posterior view. B. *(Top)* Anterior view.

page 345), or behind his head and trying to make his elbows and knees touch (Figure 227 A and B, page 345).

With the patient in this position, the anesthetist should be cognizant of the following: (1) in an obese patient the skin line marking the middle of the back may be pulled by the weight of the fat so that it lies 1 inch (2.5 cm.) to 1½ inches (3.8 cm.) below the spinous processes; and (2) if the spinal fluid pressure is low, and this often goes hand in hand with a low blood pressure, except in pathological conditions of the central nervous system, it may be necessary to use aspiration to obtain spinal fluid. If either of these conditions

Figure 227. Method of obtaining a good spinal (lumbar) puncture position by folding the patient's hands behind his head and trying to touch the knees with the elbows. A. *(Top)* Anterior view. B. *(Bottom)* Posterior view.

make it difficult to obtain spinal fluid, use the sitting position.

Sitting.—The patient sits on the edge of the table with his legs over the side of the table, his feet on a stool, his head flexed on the chest, and his arms folded across his upper abdomen (Figure 228A, page 346). An assistant should at all times steady the patient so that he does not fall off the table (Figure 228B, page 346). Often a patient, after heavy sedation, will feel faint when placed in this position. This is probably due to the fact that the barbiturates and opiates cause peripheral vasodilatation and with the patient in the upright position there is a tendency for the blood to pool in the lower extremities, thus compromising the blood supply to the brain.

Furthermore, the vasodilatation caused by the premedication will be accentuated by the vasodilatation which the anesthesia will bring about. And, if the patient is required to sit up for a period of time following the administration of the spinal block to assure a low level of analgesia, he may lose consciousness. When this occurs, the patient should be *immediately*

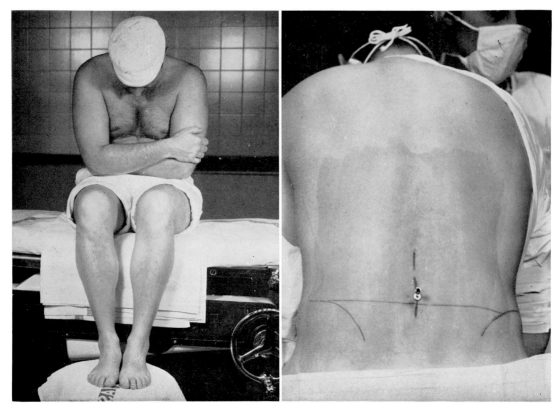

Figure 228. A. and B. Sitting position for spinal (lumbar) puncture. A. *(Left)* Anterior view. Feet rest on a stool, the arms are folded across the chest, and the head is flexed for the best results. B. *(Right)* Posterior view with spinal (lumbar) needle in place. The straight line between the iliac crests crosses the cephalad portion of the spinous process of the fourth lumbar vertebra. Note drop of spinal fluid at hub of needle.

placed in the supine position and given oxygen.

The sitting position is advised for the following patients: (1) those who have a low spinal fluid pressure—in a sitting position, the weight of the column of spinal fluid increases the pressure of the spinal fluid; (2) the patient who is obese—the sitting position does not let the subcutaneous fat droop and distort the relationship of the topographical landmarks to the vertebral column; (3) the obstetrical patient who is to have a vaginal delivery —under this circumstance, the solutions usually employed are hyperbaric (heavier than the specific gravity of spinal fluid) and a low spinal block is usually desired; and (4) the patient with an intratrochanteric fracture—it is easier for such patient to sit up than turn on his side.

Prone.—The patient lies on his abdomen with the middle of the iliac bones resting over the flexion point of the operating table (Figure 229 A and B, page 347). The table is flexed so as to drop the legs and head and thus open the distance between the spines of the lumbar vertebrae. In this position aspiration often is necessary to obtain spinal fluid. The prone position usually is used only in orthopedic problems, and rectal and sacral procedures where a hypobaric (lighter than the specific gravity of spinal fluid) solution is employed.

Precautions

Prior to Performing a Spinal Block Take the Blood Pressure.—A preanesthetic check of the blood pressure is mandatory.

Bloody Tap Is Contraindication to Spinal Block.—Check carefully for a bloody spinal

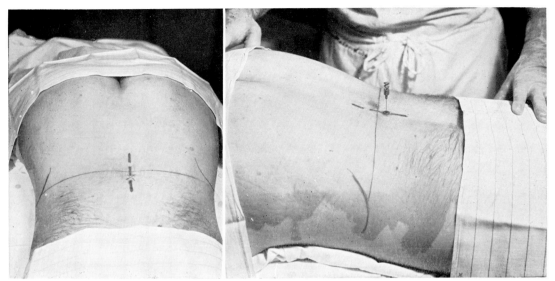

Figure 229. A. and B. A. *(Left)* Posterior view. Prone position for spinal subarachnoid tap. The straight line joining the iliac crests crosses the spine of the fourth lumbar vertebra. Note that the patient is in the jack-knife (Buie) position which tends to increase the intravertebral space. B. *(Right)* Lateral view. Spinal needle in place for injection of the local anesthetic agent.

tap. A bloody spinal fluid is a contraindication to a spinal block. It is not uncommon, when performing a spinal tap, for the first few drops of the spinal fluid to contain blood. Usually after five to six drops of spinal fluid the blood will disappear and the fluid will be clear. If, however, after ten or fifteen drops the spinal fluid still contains blood, the spinal puncture should be repeated at another interspace. Then if the spinal fluid still contains blood, another anesthetic technique should be substituted for spinal block.

Start Intravenous Fluids.—Prior to executing a spinal block, intravenous fluids should be running, preferably with a plastic needle (Figure 2, page 8). Hypotension is the most frequent complication of spinal block and its treatment is the intravenous administration of a vasoconstrictor drug.

Procedure

The author recognizes that there are many excellent ways to do a spinal puncture. The one described below is the one which is employed by the author. Other techniques may give equally satisfactory results.

1. The sterilizer control is checked to be sure the equipment has been sterilized.

2. The anesthetist puts on sterile gloves, aseptically prepares the skin, and places a sterile towel over the "up" side.

3. A skin wheal is raised over the selected interspace with the ¾-inch (2 cm.), 25-gauge Huber point security Lok-needle using 0.2 cc. to 0.3 cc. of a 1.0 percent procaine (Novocain) solution (Figure 230, page 347).

4. 0.8 cc. to 1.5 cc. of the procaine solution is infiltrated into the interspinous ligament.

5. The introducer is placed through the wheal into the interspinous ligament (Figure

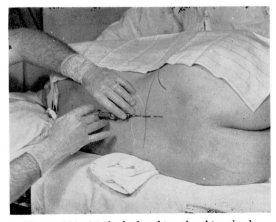

Figure 230. Method of making the skin wheal.

231 A and B, page 348 and Figure 232, page 348). The index and middle (long) fingers of the free hand should straddle the interspace into which the introducer is to be placed (Figure 231 A and B, page 348). Great care should be taken that this introducer lies in the same plane as the spinous processes and perpendicular to the transverse processes. If it points upward or downward, or if the patient's back is not at a 90-degree angle in the vertical plane

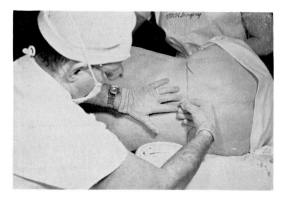

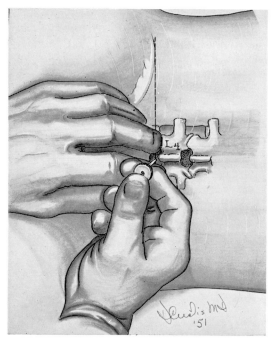

Figure 231. Placing the introducer. The index and middle (long) fingers of the left hand straddle the third lumbar interspace, thereby marking it as the introducer is inserted. A. *(Top)* Placement in a patient. B. *(Bottom)* Schematic drawing of A. with the underlying landmarks (position of the patient reversed).

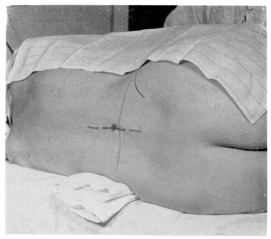

Figure 232. Introducer in place.

with the table, the spinal needle will not travel a true course (Figure 233, page 349).

With the Pitkin or thin-walled introducer, which is 1⅛ inch (2.8 cm.) and 1 inch (2.5 cm.) in length, respectively, puncture of the dura is unlikely. On the other hand, if the 2-inch (5 cm.), 21-gauge needle is used as an introducer for placement of the 26-gauge spinal needle, the dura may be tapped in a thin or medium sized person when the introducing needle is inserted to its hub.

6. The spinal needle is carefully checked for weaknesses and to be sure that it has an easily removable stylet. The relationship of the markings on the hub of the needle to the bevel of the needle are always noted—usually, the opening in the bevel is on the same side as the notch in the hub of the needle (Figure 252, page 389).

7. The spinal needle is held by the anesthetist so that the thumb rests on the head of the stylet and the shaft of the needle rests between the index and middle fingers (Figure 234, page 349.) This prevents displacement of the stylet and allows the anesthetist to steady his hand by resting the ring and little fingers on the patient's back (Figure 234, page 349).

8. The spinal needle is then inserted through the introducer. If carefully and *slowly* advanced through the interspinous ligament, it

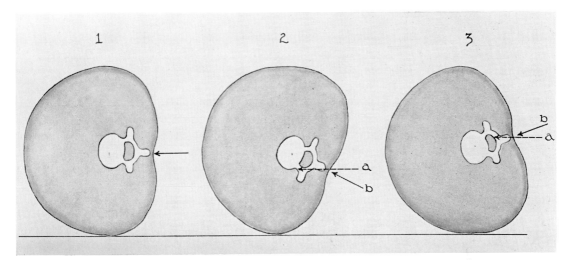

Figure 233. Schematic drawing showing that the physician, when performing a spinal (subarachnoid) puncture, must at all times be cognizant of the patient's position. As shown in 2 and 3, when the patient is tilted, the needle must not be inserted parallel to the table but must be inserted in the same plane as the spinous processes and perpendicular to the transverse processes if a satisfactory tap is to be performed. In drawings 2 and 3 "a" represents the incorrect plane of insertion and "b" the correct plane of insertion.

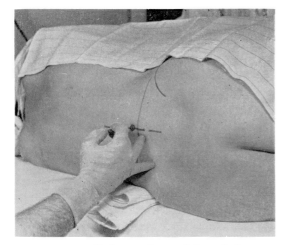

Figure 234. Needle being advanced through the introducer into the subarachnoid space. Note how little and ring fingers support the hand so that slow advancement of the needle is easily performed.

will be felt to pierce the ligamentum flavum, pass through the epidural space where less resistance is felt, and "pop" through the dura as slight resistance is met (Figure 222, page 343). The anesthetist should note that if the needle is advanced slowly, he will feel the first decrease in resistance as the needle passes through the ligamentum flavum and the point of the needle rests in the epidural space. It

then must be advanced through the dura (Figure 222, page 343).

9. The stylet is withdrawn and spinal fluid allowed to appear at the hub of the needle. If no fluid is obtained, the needle should be rotated 180 degrees without the stylet. The dura or nerve root may be blocking the lumen of the needle (Figure 235 A and B, page 350 and Figure 236 A and B, page 350). Then if no fluid appears, it should be slowly advanced, since the point of the needle may still lie in the epidural space (see step 8). If the needle has been advanced too rapidly, it will pass through the dura, impinge on the body of the vertebra or rest in the nucleus pulposus, and spinal fluid will not be obtained (Figure 237 A, page 351). If this occurs, the needle should be slowly withdrawn ⅛ inch (0.3 cm.) or so (Figure 237 B, page 351).

If at any point in this step the anesthetist thinks the bevel of the spinal needle should be inside the dura but obtains no spinal fluid, the 3 cc. Lok-syringe with 1.0 to 1.5 cc. of air in it should be attached to the needle and the 1.0 to 1.5 cc. of air should be discharged through the needle. If no air returns into the syringe, an attempt to withdraw spinal fluid is made. This maneuver is done for four reasons. First,

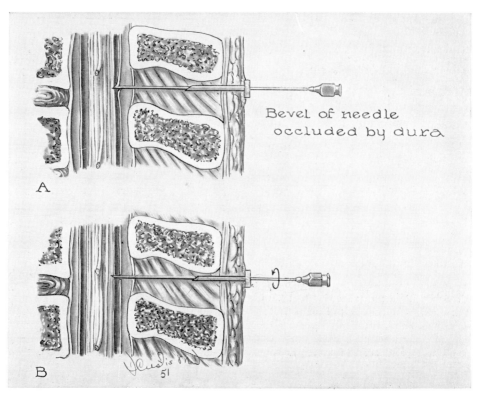

Figure 235. A. The needle has pierced the dura and the dura rests against the bevel of the needle preventing or hindering the flow of spinal fluid. B. Rotation of the spinal needle 180 degrees will free the bevel and allow the spinal fluid to flow freely.

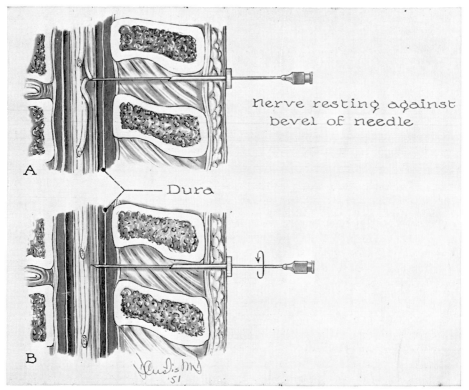

Figure 236. A. The needle is inside the dura but its bevel is resting against a nerve. B. Rotation of needle 180 degrees frees the bevel, allowing a free flow of spinal fluid.

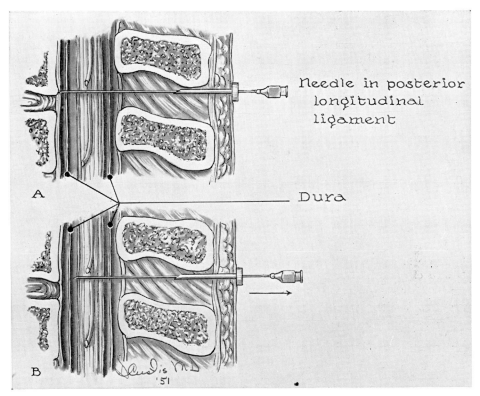

Figure 237. A. The spinal needle has been advanced too far into the spinal canal. B. Slight withdrawal of the needle allows its bevel to rest in the subarachnoid space.

it is not uncommon for a small particle of tissue to plug the needle, especially if the stylet is slightly displaced during the insertion of the spinal needle—the pushing of air through the needle will usually clear a tissue plug from the needle. Depositing of a minute sterile tissue plug into the subarachnoid space does not cause complications. Second, if after pushing the air from the syringe, the air returns into the syringe, the point of the needle probably lies in the anterior portion of the interspinous ligament or the ligamentum flavum and must be advanced. Third, if air is easily pushed from the syringe, if no air returns, and if spinal fluid cannot be aspirated, then the bevel of the needle probably lies in the epidural space and must be advanced. Lastly, occasionally during the use of the lateral decubitus position and often during the use of the prone position, the spinal fluid pressure will be too low to cause the spinal fluid to drip from the needle—aspiration allows the anesthetist to obtain spinal fluid.

With the 26-gauge spinal needle, 5 to 10 seconds should be allowed to pass before the above maneuver is executed. The small lumen of the needle allows the spinal fluid to pass through it very slowly.

10. When a free drip of spinal fluid is obtained, the syringe containing the anesthetic solution is attached (Figure 238, page 352 and Figure 239, page 352). During this maneuver, if the anesthetist is right-handed, he should firmly grip the hub of the spinal needle between the index finger and thumb of his left hand as the back of the left hand rests against the patient's back (Figure 239, page 352; Figure 240, page 352 and Figure 241, page 353). This steadies and prevents displacement of the needle. When attaching the Lok-syringe to the spinal Lok-needle, the syringe should be held firmly in the right hand with the ring finger or little finger resting against the plunger to prevent its moving, and wrist motion used to lock the syringe on the needle (Figure

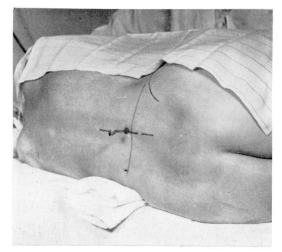

Figure 238. Needle in position in the subarachnoid space. Note drop of spinal fluid at the hub of the needle.

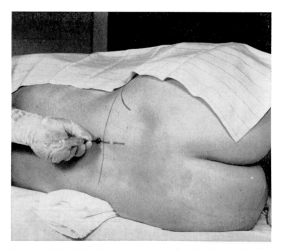

Figure 239. Hand rests against the back and holds the needle and syringe firmly so that the needle will not be moved during the aspiration or injection.

240 A and B, page 352 and Figure 241 A and B, page 353). The syringe should not be rolled in the fingers. A counterclockwise twist of the wrist allows the lock mechanism of the syringe and needle to engage and then a clockwise twist of the wrist locks the syringe on the needle (Figure 240 A and B, page 352 and Figure 241, page 353).

11. A small amount of spinal fluid is then withdrawn into the syringe and the subarachnoid injection is made at the rate of 1 cc. per second. *If a free flow of spinal fluid into the*

syringe is not obtained, the needle should be adjusted or reinserted; otherwise, unsatisfactory analgesia can be expected.

12. When the injection is completed, the anesthetist withdraws 0.3 to 0.5 cc. from the spinal canal and reinjects it to be sure that the needle has remained in the subarachnoid space during the initial injection.

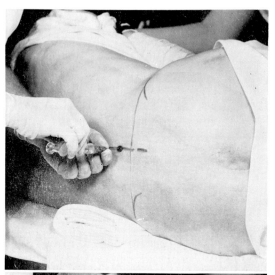

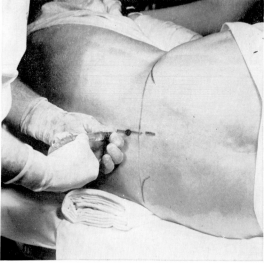

Figure 240. Connecting the Lok-syringe to the spinal needle. The needle is held firm at all times by the left hand. A. (*Top*) The syringe, with the ring finger of the right hand resting against the plunger to prevent its moving, is fitted to the hub of the needle. B. (*Bottom*) With a turn of the wrist of the hand holding the syringe, the syringe is locked on the needle.

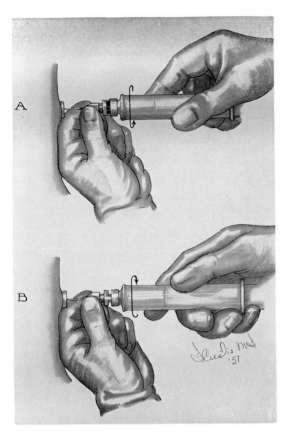

Figure 241. Correct method of holding the syringe as it is connected to the spinal needle. Either the ring finger or the little finger should rest against the barrel of the syringe to prevent loss of the measured local anesthetic solution in the syringe. A. Counterclockwise rotation of the syringe as it is placed on the needle. B. Clockwise rotation of the syringe to lock it on the spinal needle.

13. The needle and introducer are withdrawn and the patient immediately placed in the position necessary to obtain the desired analgesia. See Chapter 44, page 370, for positions.

14. The blood pressure and the level of anesthesia should be checked immediately and at frequent intervals. The rate at which the agent is ascending or descending in the spinal canal is as important to know as the blood pressure. An Allis forceps is used to pinch the skin since its use will usually determine the level of analgesia more accurately than pricking the skin with a pin.

EXTENT OF ANALGESIA

This depends on the technique employed (Chapter 44, page 370). It is possible to produce anesthesia of part or all of the dermatomes of the body (Figure 242, page 354).

COMPLICATIONS

High or Total Spinal Block: This, *itself*, is not considered individually since its signs, symptoms, and treatment are those discussed below: hypotension, nausea and vomiting, respiratory arrest and, if these go untreated, cardiac arrest. To avoid deaths, early recognition of these complications is essential.

When total spinal block occurs, the question often arises: Should spinal fluid be withdrawn and should the subarachnoid space be lavaged? In most instances, when a total spinal block occurs, the anesthetist is too busy resuscitating the patient to withdraw spinal fluid and lavage the subarachnoid space—the correction of hypotension, respiratory arrest, and cardiac arrest must come first. By the time the patient's vital signs are stable, withdrawal of spinal fluid and lavage may not be indicated.

Withdrawal of Spinal Fluid.— A total of 50 to 60 cc. of spinal fluid may be withdrawn, provided: (1) it can be done slowly without herniating the medulla; and (2) it can be done immediately—most local anesthetic drugs "fix" in 15 to 30 minutes.

Lavage of Subarachnoid Space.—Lavage with normal saline or distilled water is not indicated, since both are unphysiologic solutions and could cause irreparable damage to the cord. If lavage is to be done, a physiologic solution, *e.g.*, Ringer's, must be used.

Hypotension

Signs and Symptoms.—Usually occur within ten minutes after the subarachnoid injection. Cardiac output is decreased, resulting in lowered systolic pressure, lowered pulse pressure, and increased circulatory time. Diastolic pressure falls very little. Bradycardia may occur.

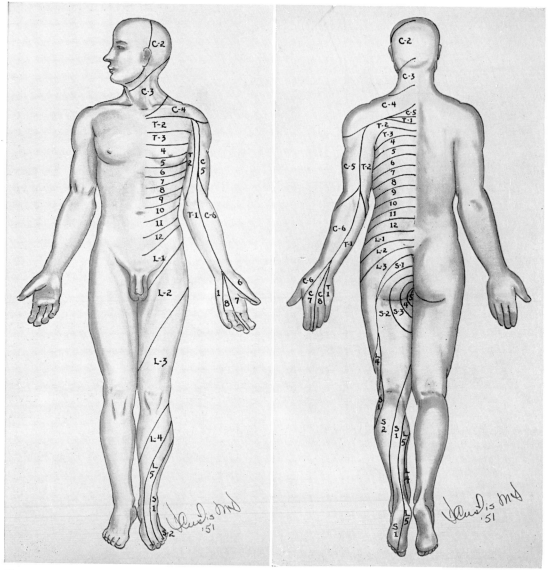

Figure 242. Schematic drawing of the sensory dermatome sections of the human body. A. *(Left)* Anterior view. B. *(Right)* Posterior view.

Etiology.—Hypotension is a result of: (1) a sudden relaxation of the vascular and muscular systems in the areas anesthetized and (2) decreased rate of blood flow returning to the heart. The latter is probably caused by decreased intercostal muscle function and consequent decrease in the respiratory pumping action which normally facilitates the return of the blood to the heart.

Treatment.—First, give oxygen by mask. Many of the minor falls in blood pressure may be corrected by this type of therapy. It should always be the first step in the treatment of hypotension following the execution of spinal anesthesia. Oxygen should be given while the vasoconstrictor drug is being prepared for administration.

If the lithotomy position is to be used for the operation, *e.g.,* vaginal hysterectomy, vaginal delivery, hemorrhoidectomy, etc., put the patient's legs in the stirrups. The autotransfusion from the legs may be adequate to correct a relative hypovolemia resulting from vascular dilatation produced by blockade of the sympathetic nervous system (see Remarks, page 366). However, remember that when the lithotomy position is resolved at the completion of surgery the opposite effect may result.

Then, if the hypotension is not corrected, ephedrine sulfate 25 mg. (⅜ gr.), or phenylephrine (Neo-Synephrine) 1 mg. to 2 mg., or any of the other vasoconstrictor drugs which may be preferred, is administered intravenously. If a low pressure persists, add 1 cc. of phenylephrine 1 percent (10 mg. per cc.) to 500 cc. or 1000 cc. of intravenous fluids and maintain blood pressure at preanesthetic level by varying the drip. Phenylephrine is a powerful vasoconstrictor and should be used in very dilute solutions. The phenylephrine drip may be continued into the postoperative period to maintain the patient's blood pressure until the local anesthetic agent has been dissipated (see page 36).

If the anesthetist makes it a routine procedure to start an intravenous infusion before performing the spinal puncture, a severe or persistent hypotension may usually be treated easily. Blood pressure should always be checked just before injecting a vasoconstrictor drug as oxygen therapy or the compensatory mechanisms of the body may have corrected a transient blood pressure fall.

Remember that hypotension during spinal analgesia may occur from hemorrhage, and this type of hypotension should be treated by blood replacement therapy. In an emergency, plasma, osmotic volume expanders, vasoconstrictor drugs, or all three may be administered until whole blood is obtained.

Nausea and Vomiting

Signs and Symptoms.—If caused by hypotension, the patient becomes pale, lips blanch, and the patient becomes nauseated and then vomits. Blood pressure is low. This type of reaction may occur at any time during the anesthetic procedure or operation, but is most common immediately after the injection of the local anesthetic agent into the subarachnoid space.

If caused by hypertension, there is increased blood pressure, flushed face, nausea, and vomiting. This type may occur at any time during the anesthetic or surgical procedure, but usually follows the intramuscular or intravenous injection of a vasoconstrictor agent.

If caused by traction reflexes, pulse and respirations do not vary, but the patient often complains of chest pain and nausea, which is followed by vomiting. The blood pressure may or may not fall. This type of reaction occurs during surgery.

Etiology.—Nausea and vomiting are a result of: (1) hypotension with a stagnant type of anoxia; (2) hypertension from vasoconstrictor drugs given prophylactically or for correction of hypotension; (3) traction reflexes which usually are transmitted by the autonomic nervous system; and (4) miscellaneous reasons, *e.g.*, premedication, motion during change of positions, and apprehension.

Treatment.—Always check blood pressure before treating nausea and vomiting. If caused by hypotension, give oxygen by mask and elevate blood pressure (see Table V, page 26).

If caused by hypertension, give oxygen by mask and if blood pressure becomes dangerously high, give chlorpromazine (Thorazine) intravenously (see page 41).

If nausea and vomiting are caused by traction reflexes, they may be treated by light inhalation or intravenous anesthesia—0.6 percent thiopental (Pentothal) by the intravenous drip method and N_2O (2 L.) plus O_2 (2 L.) via the anesthetic machine is extremely satisfactory.

If this complication is caused by any of the miscellaneous conditions (see Etiology, item 4), 50 mg. of dimenhydrinate (Dramamine) intravenously will usually correct the condition immediately.

Respiratory Arrest

Signs and Symptoms.—Patient complains of inability to breathe, becomes restless, and stops breathing. Signs of hypoxia ensue, such as tachycardia and later bradycardia, restlessness, air hunger, cyanosis, and convulsions.

Etiology.—High spinal anesthesia with paralysis of the intercostal and phrenic nerves, central depression from cerebral anemia caused by hypotension, or both.

Treatment.—If caused by high spinal, give artificial respiration by bag and mask until spinal anesthesia is dissipated. Be sure airway is established and patent. If necessary, do not hesitate to use an oral airway or endotracheal tube. *Watch for vomiting and aspiration of emesis* (see page 30).

If caused by central depression, administer oxygen by bag and mask and vasoconstrictor drugs intravenously (see Table V, page 26).

Cardiac Failure: This complication is rare.

Signs and Symptoms.—These include: (1) peripheral vascular collapse; (2) cessation of normal cardiac action and absence of peripheral pulse; (3) cessation of respiration; and (4) if an ophthalmoscope is available, cessation of blood flow in ocular vessels may be seen.

Etiology.—Usually unknown, but may be caused by an overactive vagus in the presence of anesthetized sympathetic fibers. This situation may occur when spinal anesthesia extends to T5 or above. Even though sensory analgesia exists only to T5, it is possible that the small sympathetic fibers above this level may be anesthetized by minute quantities of the local anesthetic agent which have migrated higher but are not sufficiently strong to produce sensory analgesia. Also, hypoxia of a stagnant type may be a potent inciting factor.

Treatment.—See page 28.

Pulmonary Collapse: This complication is extremely rare.

Signs and Symptoms.—Fever with generalized toxic manifestations is often present before administration of anesthesia. The signs of pulmonary collapse are cessation of respiration and cessation of cardiac action.

Etiology.—It is thought to be caused by an unbalanced autonomic nervous system with a predominance of the parasympathetic division, namely, the vagus, causing reflex contraction of the lung. It usually occurs in the presence of: (1) high spinal; (2) intraperitoneal manipulation; and (3) severe apprehension or fear.

Treatment.—Prophylactic treatment consists of avoiding spinal analgesia where a strongly unbalanced autonomic nervous system is suspected and giving large doses of atropine if a spinal block is administered. The atropine should be repeated during long surgical procedures, especially in patients showing severe emotional distress, high basal metabolic demands or oxygen intake, and toxemia, or who are to have their lower thoracic and lumbar sympathetic nerves sectioned.

Active treatment consists of: (1) administering intravenous atropine 0.6 mg. ($\frac{1}{100}$ gr.); (2) giving oxygen under pressure by mask and bag—if a closed system cannot be obtained, a cuffed endotracheal tube should be used; and (3) treatment of cardiac failure if it should occur (see Table V, page 26).

Toxic Reactions (intravascular injections, etc.): Seldom occur (see Chapter 3, page 19).

Headache: Occurs in 2 to 9 percent of cases.

Signs and Symptoms.—Headache appears usually 24 hours after the spinal puncture. It is usually absent when the patient is lying flat and is accentuated by the upright position. And, it is characterized by a severe throbbing, usually in the occipital region, and may persist from several days to weeks.

Etiology.—Headache may be the result of leakage of spinal fluid through the hole in the dura after the spinal needle has been withdrawn, irritation of the dura or the nerves by the local anesthetic agent, infection, or all three (see Table VII, page 357).

Treatment.—See Table VIII, page 357. When a spinal headache from leakage of spinal fluid occurs, treatment should be vigorous, for headache often precedes an abducens nerve paralysis.

TABLE VII

PROBABLE MECHANISM OF HEADACHE FROM LEAKAGE OF SPINAL FLUID OR MENINGITIS

Etiology	Area of Head to which Pain is Referred
LEAKAGE OF SPINAL FLUID (Hypotension of Spinal Fluid)	
I. Traction on:	
A. Veins passing to sagittal and transverse sinus	Front, top, and side of head
B. Middle meningeal arteries	From eyes posterior to ears
C. Intracranial portion of internal carotid arteries and main component of circle of Willis or pia arachnoid	Region of eyes, or front, top, or sides of the head
D. Basilar and vertebral arteries and branches	Back of head and neck
II. Displacement of entire intracranial arterial system from left to right or vice versa.	Generalized headache from eyes to neck
INFLAMMATION OF STRUCTURES AT BASE AND CONVEXITY OF BRAIN (Hypertension of Spinal Fluid)	
I. Posterior fossa	Chiefly, back of head
II. Supratentorial fossa	Chiefly, frontal or vertical

TABLE VIII

TREATMENT OF POSTSPINAL HEADACHES FROM LOWERED SPINAL FLUID PRESSURES

I. When diagnosis is made one or more of the following orders are written, usually A; B; and C will correct the headache.

A. **Apply abdominal binder** snugly over 2 bath towels before patient sits up or is ambulatory.
Rationale: Pressure on vena cava slows emptying of epidural venous plexus which in turn decreases epidural space and increases spinal fluid pressure.

B. **Codeine 30 mg. (½ gr.) and acetylsalicylic acid (Aspirin) 600 mg. (10 gr.)** p.r.n. for headache.
Rationale: Symptomatic relief of headache.

C. **Measured oral intake** of at least 3,000 cc. of water for 4 days. If this is not met, supplement with 5% dextrose in distilled water intravenously.
Rationale: Hydration to assure ample body fluids for production of cerebrospinal fluid.

D. **Nicotinamide 100 mg. (1½ gr.)** intramuscularly 3 times a day for 2 days.
Rationale: Dilatation of choroid plexus to increase the production of cerebrospinal fluid.

E. **Surgical pituitrin (1:2000) 1 cc.** intramuscularly 3 times a day.
Rationale: Antidiuretic action.
N. B. Watch for "pituitrin shock;" if it occurs, stop pituitrin. Do not give drug to patient with heart disease, hypertension, toxemia, pre-eclampsia, or eclampsia.

II. If severe headache persists after this treatment, a **lumbar epidural block** or **caudal block** with the injection of 30 to 40 cc. of normal saline should be evaluated. It usually is definitive treatment.
Rationale: Decrease epidural space, increase spinal fluid pressure.

NOTE: Treatment as described takes 3 days—the length of time a mild or moderate postspinal headache of this nature lasts—and therefore its efficacy may be questioned. Nevertheless, the patient feels an attempt to help his problem is being made.

Prophylaxis.—Many headaches from leakage of spinal fluid may be avoided by: (1) hydration; (2) using 22-gauge or smaller needles, *e.g.*, 26; (3) using spinal needles without cutting bevels; (4) placing the spinal needle with cutting bevel correctly; and (5) a combination of these.

HYDRATION: A positive water balance on which the choroid plexus may draw to produce spinal fluid is essential. It has been shown that adequate hydration favors regeneration of spinal fluid at a rate sufficient to replace that lost via a large dural leak, while inadequate fluid intake or hypertonic dextrose solutions may aggravate the effect of even a small dural leak. An intake of 3000 cc. a day prior to surgery and following surgery should be maintained even if it requires intravenous administration of fluids.

22-GAUGE OR SMALLER GAUGE NEEDLE: The incidence of spinal headache is markedly reduced by the use of 22- to 26-gauge needles when compared with 21- or larger gauge needles.

SPINAL NEEDLES WITHOUT CUTTING BEVELS: The bevels of most spinal needles are ground in such a fashion that they have cutting edges—the Greene point needle and the Whitacre "pencil point" needles do not (Figure 243, page 358). Even when inserted correctly, a spinal needle with cutting edges on the bevel cuts the longitudinal fibers of the dura while either the Greene point needle or the Whitacre point needle separates them. When the longitudinal fibers of the dura are separated rather than cut, they approximate following removal of the needle and the hole in the dura is smaller (compare Figure 244 B, page 359 with Figure 245 B, page 359).

PLACEMENT OF NEEDLE: Most of the fibers of the dura run longitudinally, *i.e.*, parallel to the spinal cord. When a needle whose bevel has a cutting edge is used, the bevel should be inserted parallel to the fibers of the dura so that the needle will tend to split or spread them rather than cut them (Figure 245, page 359). This type of placement will result in a slit-shaped, small wound, while cutting across the fibers will result in a crescent-shaped hole which will tend to gape as the fibers retract (com-

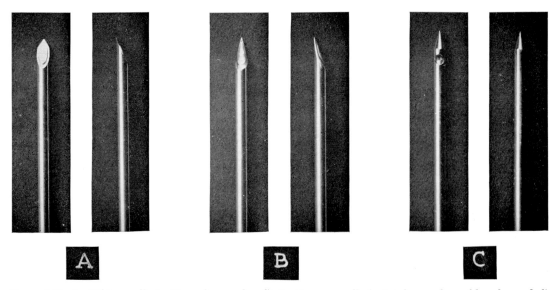

Figure 243. A. Pitkin needle (cutting edges on bevel). B. Greene needle (point sharp, edges of bevel rounded). C. Whitacre pencil point needle (point sharp, bevel completely rounded). The Greene and Whitacre needles are obtained from Becton, Dickinson and Company, Rutherford, N. J., and the order numbers are G462LNR and W462LNR, respectively.

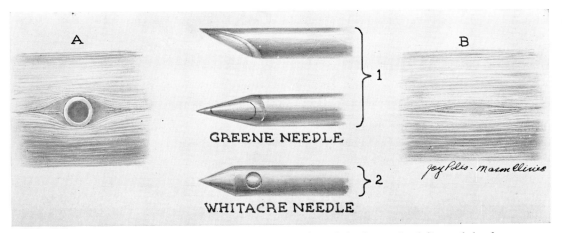

Figure 244. A. Greene or Whitacre needle in place. Only a few of the longitudinal fibers of the dura are severed; most are spread—not cut. B. When the needle is removed, fibers tend to approximate.

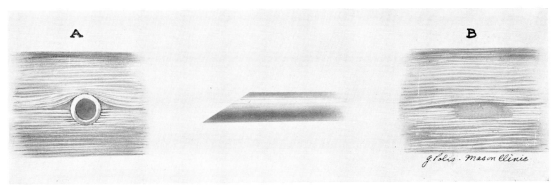

Figure 245. A. Pitkin needle in place in the subarachnoid space after being *correctly* inserted with the sharp cutting edges of its bevel parallel to the longitudinal fibers of the dura. When a needle with sharp cutting edges on the bevel is inserted in this manner, it cuts fewer fibers of the dura (about one-half as many) than when it is inserted at right angles to the fibers. B. The hole in the dura is smaller than that produced in Figure 246 because fewer dural fibers have been severed.

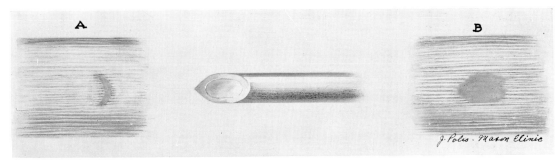

Figure 246. A. Crescent-shaped cut in dura made by the sharp cutting edges of the bevel of the Pitkin needle which has been introduced into the dura with the bevel of the needle at right angles to the longitudinal fibers of the dura. A maximum number of fibers are severed when a needle with this type of bevel is *incorrectly* inserted in this position into the subarachnoid space. B. Needle removed. The hole in the dura gaps widely.

pare Figure 245, page 359 with Figure 246, page 359).

Pain at the Site of Spinal Puncture

Signs and Symptoms.—Patient complains of pain in lumbar area.

Etiology.—Backache is the result of: (1) trauma to the periosteum of the vertebra with or without a hematoma; (2) straightening of the normal lumbar curve of the back—this may occur under any anesthesia which relaxes the sacrospinalis group of muscles (Figure 247, page 360); (3) lying in bed; (4) infection; or (5) a combination of these. *Most backaches following a spinal anesthesia are not the fault of the anesthetic technique but of faulty position, etc.*

Treatment.—Treatment consists of: (1) ambulation; (2) heat and physiotherapy; (3) psychotherapy; (4) chemotherapy or antibiotic therapy; or (5) a combination of these.

Meningitis or Meningismus

Signs and Symptoms.—These range from a slightly stiff neck and headache to a typical meningitis.

Etiology.—Meningitis or meningismus is a result of: (1) faulty aseptic technique; (2) irritation from the local anesthetic agent; (3) bloody tap; (4) lumbar puncture in presence of a septicemia or local infection; or (5) a combination of these.

Treatment.—If symptoms are minor, none is necessary. If a typical meningitis occurs, it should be treated with the antibiotics, etc., and a neurologist should be called to treat the patient.

Palsies and Paralysis

Signs and Symptoms.—Palsies and paralysis occur postoperatively and are usually peripheral in type. The cranial nerves, particularly the sixth, are most often involved.

Etiology.—They are the result of: (1) hypotension of spinal fluid, contaminated equipment, detergents, cold sterilization, unknown factors; (2) pre-existing diseases—pre-existing central nervous system diseases such as

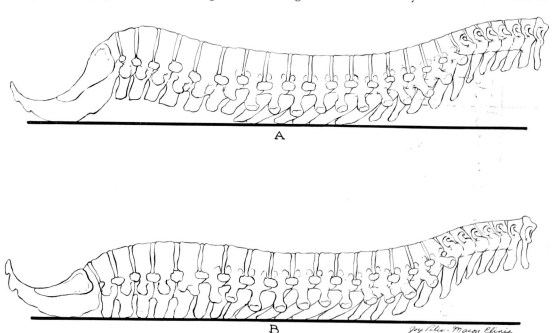

Figure 247. A. Normal lumbar curve. B. Lumbar curve "flattened or straightened" as a result of the paralysis of the sensory and motor nerves of the dermatomes and consequent relaxation of the muscles of the vertebral column.

cord degeneration from pernicious anemia, amyotrophic lateral sclerosis, etc., may be accentuated by spinal anesthesia; (3) bleeding following a spinal puncture in a patient with a blood dyscrasia or one who is receiving anticoagulant therapy; (4) too concentrated a local anesthetic agent or a high alkalinity of the spinal fluid; and (5) spinal puncture above the second lumbar interspace with injury to the cord.

Treatment.—Treatment consists of: (1) large doses of thiamine (B_1), *i.e.*, 100 mg. (1½ gr.) t.i.d.; (2) physiotherapy; (3) psychotherapy; (4) myelogram or spinal tap for diagnostic value; (5) exploratory laminectomy to ascertain whether or not a spinal cord tumor is present; and (6) a combination of these. Electromyography should be done to establish type of lesion and approximate time of onset. A neurologist should be called and he should treat the patient.

Urinary Retention

Signs and Symptoms.—The bladder becomes distended and although the urgency to urinate is present, the patient cannot void. Pain is severe until the patient successfully voids or is catheterized.

Etiology.—Usually, urinary retention is attributed to pre-existing urinary infection or difficulty, the anesthesia, the horizontal position of the patient, the pain of injured tissues, the surgical procedure, and drugs, such as opiates. The incidence of urinary retention is about the same whether regional block or general anesthesia is employed. The primary factor in urinary retention is trauma to the bladder during surgery or obstetrical deliveries.

Treatment.—If the bladder has not been traumatized during surgery, treatment consists of one or two catheterizations, after which the patient usually voids voluntarily. Voluntary urination may be encouraged by hot packs to the perineum, standing or sitting the patient in the upright position and suggesting another catheterization in the patient's presence. Neostigmine (Prostigmin), 1 ampule, *i.e.*, (1:2000), every four hours until the patient urinates seems to be of value in some cases. If the bladder has been traumatized, the treatment is twofold; first, further damage to the bladder must be prevented and, second, residual urine should be avoided. An indwelling catheter for 4 to 6 days will accomplish this.

REMARKS

Factors Influencing the Level of Spinal Analgesia Which May Be Controlled by the Anesthetist

Volume of the Solution Employed.—The greater the volume the higher the level of analgesia.

Site of Lumbar Puncture.—The highest point in the lumbar curve of the vertebral column of a supine patient is usually the fourth lumbar vertebra (Figure 248, page 361). Therefore, if solutions heavier than spinal fluid are injected at the fourth interspace, they tend to

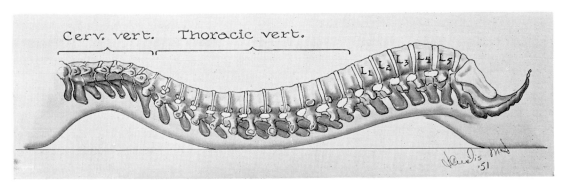

Figure 248. Anatomical normal curve of the spinal column.

gravitate caudad, and if injected at the second or third lumbar interspace, they tend to gravitate cephalad.

Rate of Injection.—The more rapid the rate of injection, the higher the level of analgesia.

Specific Gravity.—The normal specific gravity of spinal fluid varies between 1.003 and 1.009. If the anesthetic solution has a specific gravity less than 1.003, then it is *hypobaric* and tends to gravitate to the highest point in the spinal canal; for example, if the buttocks are higher than the head, then this solution will gravitate toward the buttocks (Figure 249, page 362).

If the anesthetic solution has a specific gravity of more than 1.009, it is *hyperbaric* and tends to gravitate to the lowest point in the spinal canal; for example, if the buttocks are higher than the head, then this solution will gravitate toward the head (Figure 249, page 362).

If the anesthetic solution has a specific gravity of 1.003 to 1.009, it is *isobaric* and its diffusion is unpredictable.

Position of the Patient Following Injection.—The anesthetic solution may go upward or downward, depending on the specific gravity of the local anesthetic solution in relationship to the specific gravity of the spinal fluid.

Dosage of the Drugs.—The greater the concentration, the higher the level of analgesia in most instances.

Factors Influencing the Level of Spinal Analgesia Which Cannot Be Controlled by the Anesthetist: These include: (1) variations in spinal fluid pressures—the greater the

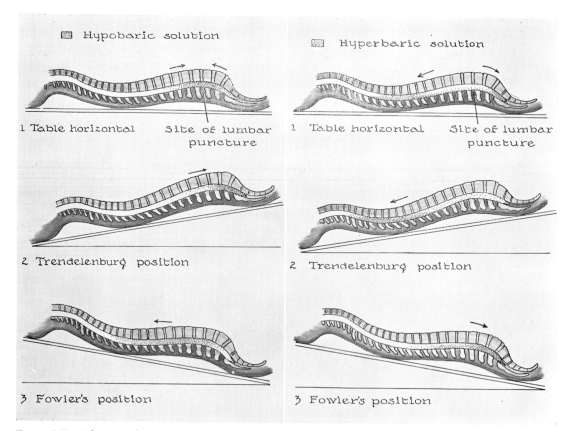

Figure 249. Schematic drawing showing the effects of Trendelenburg's and Fowler's positions on the gravitation of hyperbaric and hypobaric solutions.

pressure, the higher the anesthetic level; (2) length of the spinal cord; (3) diameter of the spinal cord; and (4) curve of the vertebral column.

Factors Influencing the Duration of Spinal Analgesia

Drug Employed.—The duration of analgesia varies with the drug, *e.g.*, procaine (Novocain) ¾ to 1 hours, tetracaine (Pontocaine) 1½ hours, etc.

Use of Vasoconstrictors Subarachnoidally.— See Chapter 51, page 481.

Dosage of the Drug.—Relatively little influence.

Contraindications to Spinal Analgesia: With the exception of severe hemorrhage, hemorrhagic blood dyscrasias and infections, whether systemic or localized, contraindications to spinal analgesia are relative and depend on the doctor's ability to cope with the complications which may occur. In general, the patient who is in poor physical condition is not a good risk for spinal analgesia. The following conditions are relative rather than absolute contraindications, and as the technique of spinal analgesia is mastered, it may be the anesthesia of choice in many of these cases.

Diseases of the Cardiovascular System, e.g., Myocardial Diseases, Arrhythmias, Decompensation, and Hypertension.—When spinal blocks are given in these cases, they should usually be confined to procedures below the umbilicus.

Pre-existing Neurological Diseases, e.g., Paralysis from Nerve Injuries, Poliomyelitis, etc., as well as Degenerative Nervous System Diseases, e.g., Pernicious Anemia, Amyotrophic Lateral Sclerosis, etc.—In the presence of these complications, if spinal analgesia must be used, consultation with another doctor and the entering of a note on the patient's chart listing the pre-existing disabilities may prevent many medicolegal complications (see page 10). In such a patient, the vasoconstrictor drugs probably should be omitted from the anesthetic solution as they may constrict the blood vessels of the dura and the cord. This may add to the cord damage by causing anoxia of the spinal cord.

Disturbances in Blood Morphology, i.e., Anemias Other Than Pernicious Anemia.— When during placement of a spinal needle trauma to a blood vessel occurs in a patient with a blood dyscrasia, uncontrollable hemorrhage into the epidural or subarachnoid space may result and this can cause paralysis. Also, the possibility of profuse hemorrhage into the soft tissue must not be disregarded in such a patient.

Increased Abdominal Pressure.—If the anesthetist remembers that increased intra-abdominal pressure, *e.g.*, pregnancy, intestinal obstruction, obesity, etc., usually results in a high level of anesthesia and he reduces the volume and dosages of drugs to be injected by one-third to one-half of the ordinary dose, serious difficulties do not arise.

Psychotic Patients.—If these patients are correctly medicated or if light intravenous thiopental (Pentothal) analgesia is given previous to the anesthetic procedure and during surgery, there will be no difficulty.

Extremes of Age.—While these are usually considered to be contraindications to spinal block, the following considerations are relevant: (1) spinal block may be administered to children if the dosage is greatly reduced and if the patient is correctly sedated with rectal thiopental (see page 246) and (2) the geriatric patients, in spite of their arteriosclerosis and labile blood pressures, tolerate carefully administered spinal analgesia extremely well.

Chronic Backache and Preoperative Headache.—These complaints speak for themselves and if a spinal block is administered in these cases the anesthetist is courting trouble.

Moribund Conditions.—These patients are poor risks under any anesthesia, but in most instances general anesthesia carefully administered or bilateral intercostal nerve block supplemented with light general anesthesia is preferable for abdominal work and blocking of the peripheral nerves is preferable for operations on the extremities.

Proven Allergy to Local Anesthetic Drugs.— See Chapter 4, page 32.

Arthritis or Spondylitis.—These often make the spinal tap mechanically difficult or impossible.

Hypotension.—Further lowering of the blood pressure with a high spinal anesthesia in a patient who is hemorrhaging or who is moribund may result in a hypotension that will not respond to treatment. However, patients who normally have a low blood pressure tolerate most spinal anesthetic procedures without difficulty.

Anticoagulant Therapy.—If spinal block is used during this type of therapy and a blood vessel is punctured, bleeding into the epidural space or subarachnoid space may result in neurological complications. The possibility of profuse hemorrhage into the soft tissues must also not be overlooked.

Term "Subarachnoid Block" May Be Preferable to Term "Spinal Block": Perhaps, anesthesia and operating personnel, as well as the house staff, should get into the habit of using the terms "local," "subarachnoid block" (S.A.B.), or "lumbar block" in preference to "spinal block." This is psychologically desirable since the term "spinal" in general causes a certain amount of fear and trepidation in the general public.

However, such terms should not be used to delude the patient into thinking he is not having spinal anesthesia.

Administer Oxygen During Block: Every anesthetist should remember that spinal blocks produce a stagnation type of anemia and either intermittent (every five or ten minutes) or continuous oxygen by mask or nasal catheter should be administered during surgery and postoperatively until the effects of the anesthesia are dissipated. This is particularly true in the older arteriosclerotic patient or in one who has suffered with mild or severe hemorrhage at any time.

Should Vasoconstrictor Drugs Be Administered Prophylactically? There is a difference of opinion as to when to give a vasoconstrictor drug. Some anesthetists feel it should be given intravenously only when a fall in blood pressure occurs—I agree with this view (see page 42). Others believe in administering a vasoconstrictor drug intramuscularly before the lumbar puncture to prevent severe falls in blood pressure, *i.e.*, "prophylactically."

If a spinal block is employed for a cesarean section, a vaginal delivery, or any other surgery where an oxytocic drug may be given, a long-acting vasoconstrictor drug should not be administered either to prevent or correct hypotension. A severe, persistent, dangerous hypertension and even rupture of a cerebral blood vessel which may cause brain damage and hemiplegia can result from the combined effect of a long-acting vasoconstrictor, *e.g.*, methoxamine (Vasoxyl) and an oxytocic drug which have been administered to a patient within three to six hours of one another (see page 41).

This does not preclude the addition of 0.2 cc. of 1:1000 epinephrine (Adrenalin) or 5 mg. of phenylephrine (Neo-Synephrine) to the solution to be injected subarachnoidally. The vascular supply of the subarachnoid space and the spinal cord is sparse (page 482). Therefore, these drugs, when administered subarachnoidally, are not absorbed into the general circulation in an appreciable quantity.

Position of Anesthetist When Performing Block: While placing the spinal needle the anesthetist should sit on a stool which is adjusted to a comfortable height. After the needle is correctly located, the anesthetist stands.

Explain Procedure to Patient: The patient should be notified of every step in the procedure before it is done so that he will not jump or become tense.

When Tap Cannot Be Done at One Interspace Try Another: When a spinal puncture cannot be successfully executed at one lumbar interspace, another may be tried.

Monitor Patient: Blood pressure, pulse, and respiration should be checked at least every five minutes, and if complications arise, much more frequently.

The patient with a spinal block should never be unattended, and constant contact by conversation with the patient should be maintained for the first twenty minutes following the injection of the local anesthetic agent into the subarachnoid space. Many of the common complications of spinal block occur in these first twenty minutes and complaint of the patient as well as changes in his sensorium are valuable aids in detecting some of the earliest signs of complications.

Make Patient Amnesic: When a spinal block is inadequate and the patient is restless, or if the surgeon wishes to teach and discuss the case with a consulting physician or visit, 0.6 percent thiopental (Pentothal) or 0.2 percent methohexital (Brevital) by the intravenous drip technique should be administered until the patient is amnesic. These are ideal solutions to employ in conjunction with spinal blocks. *However, it is often best not to start them, especially in intra-abdominal procedures, until the level of anesthesia is established.*

When amnesia or unconsciousness is produced by these drugs, the blood pressure may fall 10 to 20 millimeters of mercury. This blood pressure fall is a normal occurrence whenever a patient is no longer conscious of his surroundings. Also, it may result from the too rapid administration of either drug.

Vasoconstrictor Drugs and Oxygen Must Be Available: Vasoconstrictor drugs and a means of administering oxygen should always be readily available.

Raise Head on Pillow: When solutions heavier than spinal fluid, *i.e.*, tetracaine (Pontocaine) with glucose (dextrose) or 5 percent procaine (Novocain), are employed, the head should be flexed on a pillow so that the anesthetic solution will not rise above the cervical region (Figure 261 C, page 397). In spite of this precaution, total spinal blocks occasionally result.

Spinal Block Is Not Contraindication for Early Ambulation: A spinal block is not a contraindication to early ambulation. It has been shown that the percentage of headaches is approximately the same whether the patient is placed in a flat position for twenty-four hours or allowed to sit up or be ambulatory.

Do Not Attempt to Block Vagus Nerves or Phrenic Nerves When Performing a Spinal Block: Abolition of intrapleural and intra-abdominal traction reflexes and noxious stimuli from the diaphragm require blocking of the vagus nerves and phrenic nerves, respectively. No attempt to block such reflexes with a spinal block should be made, *i.e.*, levels of analgesia higher than the third or fourth thoracic dermatomes (Figure 242, page 354) seldom should be sought. Heavy premedication, light general anesthesia, or both should be used when necessary to abolish these reflexes.

Is Spinal Block Indicated for Hysterectomy, Oophorectomy, or Both? Women who are passing through menopause or who are castrated at surgery often have symptoms postoperatively which resemble a spinal headache but which are actually not due to the spinal block. These menopausal symptoms often are very prolonged and difficult to treat. If the patient has had a spinal block for surgery at this time, she will be very prone to blame the anesthetic technique. Therefore, in these patients, if other anesthetic techniques are available and safe, spinal blocks may best be avoided.

Spinal Block May Be Used to Treat Vascular Emergencies of Lower Extremity: When acute vascular emergencies of the lower extremities arise (see Chapter 29, page 211) and proficiency at blocking the lumbar sympathetic ganglia has not been acquired, spinal block should be considered in preference to the lumbar sympathetic ganglia block.

Elevation of Legs May Be Used to Raise Blood Pressure: Spinal block causes a profound relaxation of the muscles and blood vessels of the legs. This relaxation makes it possible for a large volume of blood to pool in the lower extremities. If the legs have not been wrapped as previously described (Chapter 1, page 7), a severe hypotension may ensue.

The reservoir of blood in the lower extremities may be useful in correcting a persistent hypotension (Figure 250, page 366). If the legs are raised above the body level, the blood may be emptied from the legs, the effective circulating blood increased, and the hypotension corrected. This method is only a temporary expedient to correct a hypotension—the underlying cause must be treated to correct the situation permanently.

Conversely, when the legs are lowered, pooling of the blood in them occurs with a subsequent decrease in the effective circulating blood volume and a decrease in the blood pressure. Therefore, whenever the patient's legs are lowered, the blood pressure should be carefully monitored.

Rapid Changes in Position Are Not Tolerated: Under no circumstances should a patient under the effects of a spinal block be moved from one position to another position rapidly. If this rule is not carefully observed deaths will occur, since the rapid shunting of blood is not well tolerated. This dictum holds true under any form of anesthesia or analgesia but is especially true of spinal analgesia.

Spinal Block Will "Fix" in 20 Minutes: In most instances, when tetracaine (Pontocaine),

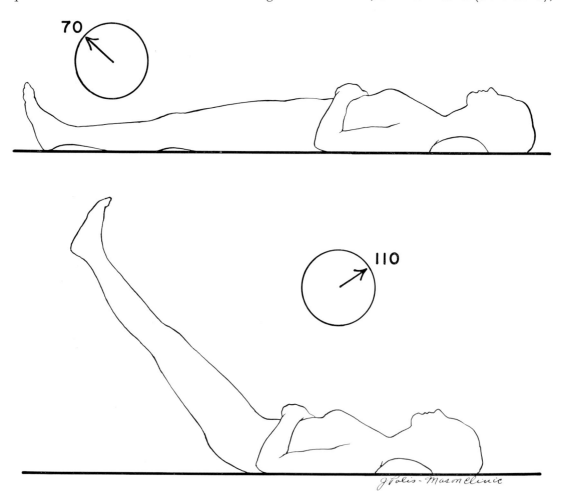

Figure 250. Autotransfusion with a subsequent rise in blood pressure can be accomplished by elevating the patient's legs. Approximately 500 cc. of blood may be pooled in the lower extremity. The lowering of the legs may have the opposite effect.

procaine (Novocain), or dibucaine (Nupercaine) are administered, a spinal block will "fix," *i.e.*, height of anesthesia will not vary after 15 to 20 minutes. However, in rare instances the level may vary with positional changes until the anesthesia has dissipated itself. Often, lidocaine (Xylocaine) and mepivacaine (Carbocaine) do not "fix" in this period of time (see page 15).

Peripheral Nerve Block Is Preferable to Spinal Block: Physicians after reading this and the next chapter may justly ask: "Why master other regional blocks of the lower extremities and trunk when one block, *i.e.*, spinal block, which may be used to produce analgesia at least to the nipple line with relative safety, is much simpler to perform and the percentage of satisfactory results usually higher?" As a matter of fact, when regional procedures are indicated, peripheral nerve block techniques are preferable whenever possible to spinal block, epidural block, or caudal block.

Literature and medical talks containing unfavorable remarks about spinal, epidural, and caudal blocks have been made available for public consumption. As a result, many patients are opposed to having such a block if it can be avoided but will take a peripheral nerve block without hesitation. Furthermore, the annoying complications of spinal, epidural, and caudal blocks, *i.e.*, hypotension, nausea and vomiting, bladder or bowel dysfunction, total anesthesia, backaches, headaches, and major neurological complications, are avoided to a large degree.

Is Caudal or Epidural Block Safer Than Spinal Block? With epidural or caudal block, the minor complications of spinal block, *e.g.*, headache, usually are avoided. However, the incidence of major complications, such as, total spinal block, hypotension, systemic toxic reactions, and neurologic complications, is as great or greater with caudal and epidural blocks when compared with spinal block.

This should be expected because: (1) larger volumes and higher concentrations of the local anesthetic solution must be used for epidural or caudal block; (2) often, the site of the epi-

dural tap is made at or above the second lumbar interspace—the site where the spinal cord usually ends; (3) an inadvertent subarachnoid placement of the needle thought to be in the epidural space may go unrecognized; (4) often, a concentration of epinephrine (Adrenalin) greater than 1:200,000 is employed in the local anesthetic solution injected into the epidural space; (5) with a continuous caudal or epidural technique, total subarachnoid block may result after a *reinforcing* dose (page 467); and (6) the experience of most physicians is not as great with epidural or caudal block as with spinal block.

Insert Introducer or Spinal Needle at Caudad Edge of Spinous Process: When placing the introducer or using the spinal needle without an introducer, the insertion should be made just caudad to the spinous process and the shaft advanced so that the point is inclined slightly cephalad (Figure 251, page 367). This position usually allows the spinal needle to pass through the interspinous space where it is the widest.

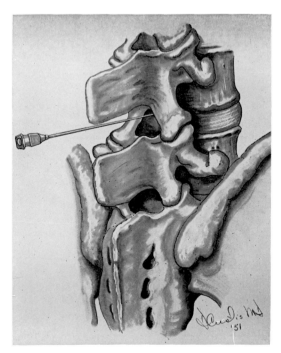

Figure 251. Shows the spinal needle being inserted just caudad to the inferior edge of the spinous process with a slight slant of the needle cephalad.

Use Introducer: The introducer is used to avoid the introduction of skin plugs or skin bacteria into the subarachnoid space.

Chlorpromazine (Thorazine) Plus Spinal Block Results in Severe Hypotension: If chlorpromazine is given before or during a spinal, caudal, epidural, or celiac plexus block, a severe hypotension may develop. In this case the low blood pressure is of such a nature that it seldom *adequately* responds to the usual dosage of the common vasoconstrictor drugs, *e.g.*, ephedrine sulfate, phenylephrine (Neo-Synephrine), methoxamine (Vasoxyl), or levarterenol (Levophed). Levarterenol or phenylephrine, if run rapidly, will usually elevate the pressure. But stopping them before either the regional block or the dosage of chlorpromazine has been dissipated may again lower the blood pressure to a precarious level. Therefore, chlorpromazine is not used by us for sedation when one of the above-mentioned procedures is to be or has been used. Likewise, the corollary to this should be noted, *i.e.*, if the patient received chlorpromazine therapy within a 24-hour period prior to surgery, general anesthesia or a peripheral nerve block is indicated—not a spinal, epidural, caudal, or celiac plexus block.

Subdural Cavity: What normally is referred to as the dura is anatomically two membranes composed of the dura mater and the arachnoid (Figure 270, page 409). Between these two membranes is a *potential* cavity known as the *subdural cavity*. The dura mater and arachnoid are, in fact, in contact with each other except where they are separated by a minute quantity of fluid which serves to moisten the apposed surfaces. If the dura mater and arachnoid are entered with a needle, the subdural cavity theoretically could contain a significant amount of spinal fluid as a result of leakage from the subarachnoid space through the hole in the arachnoid into the subdural cavity.

Such a situation is more likely to occur in a patient who had a diagnostic spinal tap, *e.g.*, myelogram; who the next day is brought to surgery; and in whom spinal anesthesia is administered for the surgical procedure. If leakage of spinal fluid into the subdural cavity occurred following the myelogram, then the anesthetist could: (1) place the spinal needle in the subdural cavity, (2) obtain a free flow of spinal fluid, (3) think the needle was in the subarachnoid space, (4) inject the local anesthetic solution, and (5) obtain little or no anesthesia because the solution has not entered the subarachnoid space. While this can occur, and could be the explanation of unsatisfactory spinal anesthesia, it is the author's opinion that its actual occurrence is extremely rare—over 500 intervertebral discs have been removed under spinal block which were preceded by myelograms and our incidence of unsatisfactory anesthesia in this procedure is less than 1 percent.

Avoid Solutions Containing Methylparaben and Metabisulfite: These drugs are often added to commercially prepared local anesthetic solutions to prevent oxidation and as a preservative. Usually, they are not added to solutions specifically prepared for spinal block and other local anesthetic solutions containing them are not recommended for spinal blocks.

Methylparaben.—Methylparaben is a preservative and fungistatic agent.

Metabisulfite.—Metabisulfite is an antioxidizing agent.

Recover Broken Needle(s): All needles should be tested before use. If a needle breaks, every effort to remove it, including surgery, should be made. Unremoved needles have a tendency to migrate and may cause permanent injuries as well as medicolegal complications.

When a spinal needle breaks, there is little doubt in the anesthetist's mind of what has happened. A distinct click is felt. This usually happens when the needle is being inserted and the stylet is still in the needle. If the anesthetist suspects that the needle has broken, he should not remove the stylet. If the needle breaks after the stylet was removed, the portion containing the hub of the needle should not be moved. The stylet and hub end of the needle are valuable guides to locating the broken end of the needle. When the anesthetist suspects that the needle has been broken, he should release his hold on it and have an x-ray taken immediately.

Repeat Block When Analgesia Is Inadequate: Most failures to establish spinal blocks are due to the fact that the local anesthetic solution is not placed subarachnoidally. If after fifteen to thirty minutes there is *no* analgesia from a spinal block, it may be repeated with relative safety, using the same drug mixture. However, if there is an inadequate level of analgesia present, one must never overlook the fact that it is not uncommon for a high spinal block to ensue when a spinal block is repeated under this circumstance. Therefore, when some analgesia is present the supplementary dosage is reduced by about ⅓ to ½ of the original dosage.

It may often take at least fifteen minutes to realize the full extent of a spinal block. This is mentioned so that in case of a slow onset, the spinal is not repeated before adequate time has been allowed for the first block to take effect. To be safe, it is best to allow one-half hour before repeating spinal anesthesia. Even then, it may be better to use another technique, *i.e.*, inhalation, etc., if available.

CHAPTER 44

Method of Administration of Single-Dose Spinal (Subarachnoid) Anesthesia for Some of the Common Surgical Procedures

I⊤ ɪs ᴏʙᴠɪᴏᴜs to the reader that all methods of administration, as well as the techniques involving all local anesthetic agents, cannot be included here. The ones given below have a relatively wide margin of safety, and are likely to keep the anesthetist out of difficulty and yet produce adequate analgesia in better than 95 percent of the cases. The dosage and drugs advocated for the following operations are those employed by the author in *adult* patients, *i.e.*, patients over 14 years of age, irrespective of complicating diseases, *i.e.*, cardiac, respiratory, etc., unless noted under *Remarks*. Children in general are poor subjects for spinal analgesia unless it is administered by a physician anesthetist who has been trained to meet their idiosyncrasies; then, with correct medication, it may be the anesthesia of choice. No one drug is advocated for every procedure, but each agent is chosen for its relative safety and adaptability to the operation and the surgical position in which the patient is to be placed. Before any attempt to use these techniques is undertaken, Chapter 43, page 341, Single-Dose Spinal (Subarachnoid) Anesthesia, should be read so that the technique and the common complications of spinal anesthesia, which are not dealt with individually here, may be understood. Also, Chapter 51, page 481, The Use of Vasoconstrictor Drugs in the Subarachnoid Space to Prolong Spinal Block, should be reviewed.

CESAREAN SECTION

Drugs and Techniques

Tetracaine (Pontocaine) with Dextrose (Glucose)

1. The following drugs are mixed together in a 5 cc. Lok-syringe:

   0.2 cc. epinephrine (Adrenalin) solution 1:1000.

   0.8 cc. (8 mg.) of a 1 percent tetracaine solution.

   1.0 cc. of a 10 percent dextrose solution.
   _____

   2.0 cc. Total. This is a hyperbaric mixture, *i.e.*, the specific gravity is greater than the specific gravity of the spinal fluid.

2. The spinal puncture is performed with the patient in the lateral decubitus or sitting position. The second or third lumbar interspace, preferably the second, is employed if the patient is over 5 feet, 3 inches and the third or the fourth lumbar interspace, preferably the third, when the patient is 5 feet, 3 inches or shorter.

3. The syringe containing the above mixture is connected to the spinal needle and 0.5 cc. of spinal fluid is aspirated into the syringe, making a total of 2.5 cc. in the syringe.

4. The content of the syringe is discharged subarachnoidally at the rate of 1 cc. per second.

5. A small amount of spinal fluid, not to exceed 0.3 cc. to 0.5 cc., is then withdrawn into the syringe and reinjected. This maneuver assures the anesthetist that the needle point rests subarachnoidally at the completion of the injection.

6. The needle and introducer are withdrawn and the patient is turned into the supine position with her head and shoulders elevated by a pillow.

7. The table remains level. *NO TRENDELENBURG* or other positional changes should be made for at least 20 minutes. In most instances the anesthetic level will be "fixed," *i.e.*, will not vary, after this period of time has elapsed.

8. Operating analgesia is established in five to ten minutes and lasts 2 to 2¼ hours.

Procaine (Novocain)

1. The following drugs are mixed together in a 5 cc. Lok-syringe:

   0.2 cc. of epinephrine (Adrenalin) solution 1:1000.

   1.8 cc. of distilled water, normal saline, or spinal fluid.

   100 mg. of procaine crystals is dissolved in the above solutions.

   ───────

   2.0 cc. Total. This is a hyperbaric mixture, *i.e.*, the specific gravity is greater than the specific gravity of the spinal fluid.

2. The spinal puncture is performed with the patient in the lateral decubitus or sitting position. The second or the third lumbar interspace, preferably the second, is employed if the patient is over 5 feet, 3 inches and the third or the fourth lumbar interspace, preferably the third, when the patient is 5 feet, 3 inches or shorter.

3. The syringe containing the above mix-

ture is connected to the spinal needle and 0.5 cc. of spinal fluid is aspirated into the syringe, making a total amount of 2.5 cc. in the syringe.

4. The content of the syringe is discharged subarachnoidally at the rate of 1 cc. per second.

5. A small amount of spinal fluid, not to exceed 0.3 cc. to 0.5 cc., is then withdrawn into the syringe and reinjected. This maneuver assures the anesthetist that the needle point rests subarachnoidally at the completion of the injection.

6. The needle and introducer are withdrawn and the patient is turned into the supine position with her head and shoulders elevated by a pillow.

7. The table remains level. *NO TRENDELENBURG* or other positional changes should be made for 20 minutes. In most instances the anesthetic level will be "fixed," *i.e.*, will not vary, after this period of time has elapsed.

8. Operating analgesia is established in five minutes and lasts 1 to 1½ hours.

Extent of Analgesia: Analgesia usually rises to the fifth or sixth thoracic dermatomes with the above techniques. This is adequate for cesarean section. The rise of analgesia should be checked with an Allis forceps at frequent intervals, although with the recommended dosages it will seldom rise above T6. If the level of anesthesia rises above T6, place the patient in Fowler's (head-up) position immediately.

Following the operation, if a tetracaine solution with a vasoconstrictor drug is employed, the patient may be unable to move her legs for two to eight hours. The anesthetist should not become alarmed by such a duration and he should explain to the patient that feeling will return in approximately this period of time (see page 484).

Remarks

Administer Oxygen.—Oxygen by bag and mask is given through the entire process. It usually prevents nausea and vomiting even if the blood pressure should fall.

Use Additional Sedation.—*After the baby is delivered,* 0.6 percent thiopental (Pentothal) by the intravenous drip method is often administered until the eyelid reflex but not the corneal reflex is lost, *i.e.,* 200 mg. to 400 mg., for the following reasons: (1) the patient desires to go to sleep; (2) it is necessary to explore the upper abdomen; and (3) oxytocic drugs are given intravenously. Pitocin or ergotrate given intravenously often causes nausea and vomiting if the patient is conscious. This is disconcerting to the patient, obstetrician and anesthetist, and should, if possible, be avoided. If these two drugs are to be given and thiopental is contraindicated, 50 mg. of dimenhydrinate (Dramamine) intravenously 10 minutes before their injection will usually prevent nausea and vomiting.

Monitor Patient Carefully.—Blood pressure readings should be taken at frequent intervals so that a sudden fall will not be overlooked. *A sudden fall in blood pressure is the most common complication associated with the use of spinal anesthesia in cesarean section, and it must be remedied immediately.* To combat sudden falls in blood pressure, which primarily endanger fetal oxygenation, the anesthetist should do the following. First, start an intravenous infusion prior to the execution of the spinal block, so that a means of giving drugs intravenously is available. Avoid salt solutions in eclampsia and pre-eclampsia and dextrose solutions in the diabetic. If dextrose solutions are administered to the diabetic, be sure the amount to be given is covered by insulin. Second, start the administration of 100 percent oxygen by mask and bag as soon as the spinal block has been given. And, third, treat hypotension immediately with: (1) a rapid drip of the infusion fluid, (2) vasoconstrictor drugs, or (3) both (see page 36).

When a cesarean section is being performed, increasing the drip of the intravenous fluids and administering 500 cc. to 700 cc. of the solution rapidly may be the method of choice because: (1) normally this amount of fluid corrects the relative hypovolemia which is a result of vascular dilatation from the spinal block; (2) usually the patient's blood pressure returns to a normal level and profusion of the uterus is maintained; (3) no vasoconstrictor drug is used—thus, if an oxytocic drug is necessary, a severe hypertension is less likely to occur (see page 41); and (4) if the hypotension was a result of the supine hypotensive syndrome or a combination of it and the spinal block, emptying of the uterus may correct the hypotension. The elevation of blood pressure obtained from the administration of 500 cc. to 700 cc. of intravenous fluids is maintained *only* for approximately 15 to 20 minutes—usually this is sufficient time to deliver the fetus. Once the fetus is delivered, a blood pressure of 80 to 100 millimeters of mercury in an obstetrical patient of good physical status causes little concern.

The advocates of a rapid infusion of fluids emphasize that vasoconstrictor drugs constrict uterine vessels with a subsequent decrease in perfusion of the placenta and that this may be detrimental to the fetus. Whether the fetus is compromised is debatable—vasoconstrictor drugs have been used to correct hypotension from spinal anesthesia in many thousands of obstetrical patients with no apparent untoward effects on the fetus.

Do Not Over Medicate Patient Prior to Birth of the Infant.—Meperidine (Demerol) 50 mg. and promethazine (Phenergan) 25 mg. are the preanesthetic medications of choice as such amounts do not significantly depress the baby's respiration. Scopolamine or atropine, 0.4 mg. (¹⁄₁₅₀ gr.) to 0.6 mg. (¹⁄₁₀₀ gr.), may be substituted for the promethazine. Pentobarbital (Nembutal) or another barbiturate preoperatively is to be avoided, but may be given the night before the operation to assure the patient a good night's sleep.

Hemorrhage Is Contraindication for Spinal Block.—In cases of severe hemorrhage, such as abruptio placentae, etc., spinal analgesia should be avoided.

Reduce Dosage in Short and/or Obese Patient.—In the extremely obese or short patient (under five feet tall), the quantities of drugs and spinal fluid should be reduced by one-third so that the total volume injected is one-third less than that advocated in the average patient. The third, or preferably the fourth, lumbar interspace is chosen as the site for the lumbar puncture. This is very important if complications are to be avoided.

Vasoconstrictor Drug Plus Oxytocic Drug May Cause Severe Hypertension.—Long-acting vasoconstrictor drugs, *e.g.*, methoxamine (Vasoxyl), must not be used either to prevent or correct a hypotension in the obstetrical patient or any other patient who may receive an oxytocic drug (see page 41).

Do Not Mistreat Psychogenic Reactions.—Obstetrical patients, particularly those who are to have cesarean section and to whom a spinal has been administered, are often under great strain and may present various complaints, which are purely psychogenic. These include inability to breathe, feeling of faintness, crying, nausea, interpretation of touch as pain, hysteria, and a host of others. Reassurance that everything is as it should be is often the only treatment necessary. Should symptomatic treatment be indicated, it consists of the administration of oxygen and, if no premedication was given, meperidine (Demerol) 50 mg. and promethazine (Phenergan) 25 mg. intravenously. *Do not exceed this amount, otherwise depression of the baby may occur.* These cases are called to the anesthetist's attention so that before he automatically treats any symptoms, he checks blood pressure, pulse, respirations, and the anesthetic level to ascertain the causes. Many of these psychogenic responses simulate the complications of spinal analgesia.

Omission of Vasoconstrictor Drug from Local Anesthetic Solution Shortens Duration of Analgesia.—The vasoconstrictor agent may be omitted at any time from the local anesthetic mixture, but the operating time will be noticeably shortened, *i.e.*, to ¾ to 1 hour with procaine, and 1 to 1½ hours with tetracaine.

To Markedly Prolong Duration of Analgesia Substitute Phenylephrine (Neo-Synephrine) for Epinephrine (Adrenalin).—See page 482.

ANORECTAL SURGERY

Hemorrhoidectomy, fistulectomy, pilonidal cystectomy, coccygectomy, rectal biopsy, etc.

Drugs and Techniques

Tetracaine (Pontocaine) with Dextrose (Glucose)

1. The following drugs are mixed together in a 5 cc. Lok-syringe:

> 0.2 cc. epinephrine (Adrenalin) solution 1:1000.
>
> 0.6 cc. (6 mg.) of a 1 percent tetracaine solution.
>
> 0.8 cc. of a 10 percent dextrose solution.
> ———
> 1.6 cc. Total. This is a hyperbaric mixture, *i.e.*, the specific gravity is greater than that of the spinal fluid.

2. The spinal puncture is performed at the third or fourth lumbar interspace with the patient in the sitting position. The relationship of the bevel of the needle to the markings on the hub of the needle should be noted before puncture, and the bevel should point caudad in the subarachnoid space.

3. The syringe containing the above mixture is connected to the spinal needle with the bevel pointing downward, and 0.4 cc. of spinal fluid is aspirated into the syringe, making a total amount of 2.0 cc. in the syringe.

4. The content of the syringe is *slowly* discharged into the subarachnoid space at the rate of 0.1 cc. per second.

5. A small amount of spinal fluid, not to exceed 0.3 cc. to 0.5 cc., is then withdrawn into the syringe and reinjected. This maneuver assures the anesthetist that the needle point rests subarachnoidally at the completion of the injection.

6. The needle and introducer are withdrawn and the patient is allowed to remain in the sitting position for two to three minutes because the anesthetic solution is heavier than spinal fluid. Then he may be placed in the lithotomy position with his head on a pillow. Trendelenburg position or other positional changes are to be avoided until they are requested by the surgeon to facilitate his work.

7. If the Buie (jackknife) or prone position is desired, the patient remains in the sitting position for five minutes and then is lowered in the supine position, in which he remains another 15 minutes before being positioned. Even with this precaution, a high anesthesia may result. In most cases the anesthetic level will be "fixed," *i.e.*, it will not vary, after 20 minutes have elapsed.

8. Operating analgesia is established in five to ten minutes and lasts 2¼ to 3¾ hours.

Procaine (Novocain)

1. The following drugs are mixed together in a 5 cc. Lok-syringe:

> 0.2 cc. of epinephrine (Adrenalin) solution 1:1000.
>
> 1.0 cc. of distilled water, normal saline, or spinal fluid.
>
> 50 mg. of procaine crystals are dissolved in the above solution.
>
> ————
>
> 1.2 cc. Total. This is a hyperbaric mixture, *i.e.*, the specific gravity is greater than the specific gravity of the spinal fluid.

2. The spinal puncture is performed at the third or fourth lumbar interspace with the patient in the sitting position. The relationship of the bevel of the needle to the markings on the hub of the needle should be noted before puncture, and the bevel should point caudad in the subarachnoid space.

3. The syringe containing the above mixture is connected to the spinal needle, the bevel of which points downward, and 0.4 cc. of

spinal fluid is aspirated into the syringe, making a total amount of 1.6 cc. in the syringe.

4. The content of the syringe is discharged subarachnoidally at the rate of 0.1 cc. per second.

5. A small amount of spinal fluid, not to exceed 0.3 cc. to 0.5 cc., is then withdrawn into the syringe and reinjected. This maneuver assures the anesthetist that the needle point rests subarachnoidally at the completion of the injection.

6. The needle and introducer are withdrawn and the patient is allowed to remain in the sitting position for two to three minutes as the anesthetic solution is heavier than spinal fluid. Then he may be placed in the lithotomy position with his head on a pillow. Trendelenburg position or other positional changes are to be avoided until requested by the surgeon to facilitate his work.

7. If the Buie (jackknife) or prone position is desired, the patient remains in the sitting position for five minutes and then is lowered to the supine position, in which he remains another 15 mintues before being positioned. Even with this precaution, a high anesthesia may result. In most cases the anesthetic level will be "fixed," *i.e.*, it will not vary, after twenty minutes have elapsed.

8. Operating analgesia is established in five minutes and lasts 1½ to 2 hours.

Light Dibucaine (Nupercaine), i.e., 1:1500, or Light Tetracaine (Pontocaine), i.e., 0.1 Percent, Without a Vasoconstrictor Agent.—These are hypobaric solutions, *i.e.*, the specific gravity is less than the specific gravity of spinal fluid.

1. 6 cc. or 7 cc. of a 1:1500 dibucaine solution or 6 cc. to 7 cc. of a 0.1 percent tetracaine solution are drawn into a 10 cc. Lok-syringe. Vasoconstrictor agents are usually not added.

2. The spinal puncture is performed with the patient in the sitting, lateral decubitus (side), or prone position, using the third or fourth lumbar interspace.

3. The syringe containing the above mixture is attached to the spinal needle and enough spinal fluid, not to exceed 0.5 cc., is withdrawn to assure a free flow through the needle.

4. The content of the syringe is discharged subarachnoidally at the rate of 1 cc. per second.

5. A small amount of spinal fluid, not to exceed 0.3 to 0.5 cc., is then withdrawn into the syringe and reinjected to assure the anesthetist that the needle point rests subarachnoidally at the completion of the injection.

6. The needle and introducer are withdrawn and if the sitting or lateral decubitus position was employed, the patient is *immediately* placed in the prone position.

7. The table is *immediately* flexed into a jackknife position (Buie position) and tilted into a 10 to 20 degree Trendelenburg position. The dibucaine or tetracaine solutions are lighter than spinal fluid (hypobaric) and can only move caudally in the spinal canal if this position is assumed (see Figure 224, page 344).

8. Operating analgesia is established in five to ten minutes and lasts 3 to 4 hours with dibucaine and 1½ to 2 hours with tetracaine.

Extent of Analgesia: The area of analgesia is confined mostly to the perineum and sacral regions.

Following the operation, if a light dibucaine solution without epinephrine or a heavy tetracaine solution with a vasoconstrictor drug is employed, the patient may be unable to move his legs for two to eight hours. The anesthetist should not become alarmed by such a duration and he should explain to the patient that feeling will return in approximately this period of time (see page 484).

Remarks

Light Anesthetic Solutions Advocated for Prone Position.—When the prone position (Buie position, *i.e.*, jackknife position) is advocated, the technique using light dibucaine or light tetracaine is the one of choice. The

local hypobaric anesthetic solution cannot gravitate cephalad since it is lighter than the spinal fluid.

Do Not Alter Dose for Obese and/or Short Patient.—These dosages need not be changed for height or weight of patient.

To Markedly Prolong Duration of Analgesia When Hyperbaric Solutions Are Used, Substitute Phenylephrine (Neo-Synephrine) for Epinephrine (Adrenalin).—See page 482.

Omission of Vasoconstrictor Drug from Hyperbaric Local Anesthetic Solution Shortens Duration of Analgesia.—The vasoconstrictor agent may be omitted at any time from the mixture but the operating time will be noticeably shortened, *i.e.*, to 1 to 1½ hour with procaine, and 1½ to 2 hours with tetracaine.

GENITAL SURGERY

Circumcision, orchiectomy, perineorrhaphy, transurethral resection, and vasectomy, and

LOWER EXTREMITY SURGERY

Vein ligations, open and/or closed manipulation, and operations of the hip, thigh, leg, and foot, etc.

Drugs and Techniques

Tetracaine (Pontocaine) with Dextrose (Glucose)

1. The following drugs are mixed together in a 5 cc. Lok-syringe:

> 0.2 cc. epinephrine (Adrenalin) solution 1:1000.

> 0.6 cc. (6 mg.) of a 1 percent tetracaine solution.

> 0.8 cc. of a 10 percent dextrose solution.

> ―――

> 1.6 cc. Total. This is a hyperbaric mixture, *i.e.*, the specific gravity is greater than the specific gravity of the spinal fluid.

2. Spinal puncture is performed at the second or third lumbar interspace with the patient

in the sitting or lateral decubitus (side) position. The lateral decubitus (side) position and the second lumbar interspace usually are preferable. However when the patient has a fractured hip, the sitting position is preferred (see page 346).

3. The syringe containing the above mixture is connected to the spinal needle and 0.4 cc. of spinal fluid is aspirated into the syringe, making a total amount of 2.0 cc. in the syringe.

4. The content of the syringe is discharged subarachnoidally at the rate of 1 cc. per second.

5. A small amount of spinal fluid, not to exceed 0.3 cc. to 0.5 cc., is then withdrawn into the syringe and reinjected. This maneuver assures the anesthetist that the needle point rests subarachnoidally at the completion of the injection.

6. The needle and introducer are withdrawn, and the patient is then immediately put in the supine position with his head and shoulders elevated on a pillow. The table remains level. *NO TRENDELENBURG* or other positional changes should be made for at least twenty minutes as the anesthetic solution is heavier than spinal fluid and will gravitate in the direction of dependency. In most instances the anesthetic level will be "fixed," *i.e.*, will not vary, after this period of time has elapsed.

7. Operating analgesia is established in five to 10 minutes and lasts 2¼ to 3¾ hours.

Procaine (Novocain)

1. The following drugs are mixed together in a 5 cc. Lok-syringe:

0.2 cc.   epinephrine (Adrenalin) solution 1:1000.

1.4 cc.   of distilled water or normal saline.

100 mg. of procaine crystals are dissolved in the above solution.

_____

1.6 cc.   Total. This is a hyperbaric mix-

ture, *i.e.*, the specific gravity is greater than the specific gravity of the spinal fluid.

2. The spinal puncture is performed, with the patient in the sitting or lateral decubitus (side) position, at the second or third lumbar interspace. The lateral decubitus (side) position and the second lumbar interspace are preferred. However when the patient has a fractured hip, the sitting position is preferred (see page 346).

3. The syringe containing the above mixture is connected to the spinal needle and 0.4 cc. of spinal fluid is aspirated, making a total amount of 2.0 cc. in the syringe.

4. The content of the syringe is discharged subarachnoidally at the rate of 1 cc. per second.

5. A small amount of spinal fluid, not to exceed 0.3 cc. to 0.5 cc., is then withdrawn into the syringe and reinjected to assure the anesthetist that the needle point rests subarachnoidally at the completion of the injection.

6. The needle and the introducer are withdrawn and the patient is immediately placed in the supine position with his head and shoulders elevated on a pillow. The table remains level. *NO TRENDELENBURG* or other positional changes should be made for at least twenty minutes as the anesthetic solution is heavier than spinal fluid and will gravitate in the direction of dependency. In most instances the anesthetic level will be "fixed," *i.e.*, will not vary, after this period of time has elapsed.

7. Operating analgesia is established in five minutes and lasts 1½ to 2 hours.

Extent of Analgesia: Anesthesia is usually established somewhere between the pubic bone and the umbilicus in most cases. This height is adequate for transurethral resections, and bladder distention with distilled water is not painful. The rise of analgesia should be checked with an Allis forceps at frequent intervals, although with the recommended dosages it will seldom rise to or above T10 (the umbilicus). If the level of anesthesia rises above T10, place the patient in Fowler's (head-up) position immediately.

Following the operation, if a tetracaine solution with a vasoconstrictor drug is employed, the patient may be unable to move his legs for two to eight hours. The anesthetist should not become alarmed by such a duration and he should explain to the patient that feeling will return in approximately this period of time (see page 484).

Remarks

Reduce Dosage in Short and/or Obese Patient.—For extremely obese patients or short patients (under five feet tall), the quantities of drugs and spinal fluid should be reduced by one-third so that the total volume injected is one-third less than that advocated for the average patient. The third lumbar interspace is usually preferred in these patients as the site for the lumbar puncture. This is very important if complications are to be avoided.

To Markedly Prolong Duration of Analgesia Substitute Phenylephrine (Neo-Synephrine) for Epinephrine (Adrenalin).—See page 482.

Omission of Vasoconstrictor Drug from Anesthetic Solution Shortens Duration of Analgesia.—The vasoconstrictor agent may be omitted at any time from the mixture, but the operating time will be noticeably shortened, *i.e.,* to 1 to 1½ hours with procaine, and 2 to 3 hours with tetracaine.

Abdominal Pain May Indicate Rupture of Bladder.—If a patient who is having a transurethral resection under spinal block and whose anesthesia has been satisfactory suddenly complains of severe abdominal pain, the anesthetist should not supplement the block until the surgeon has checked to be sure the bladder has not ruptured. An alert anesthetist may in these cases often aid in the diagnosis of a ruptured bladder.

Sitting Position More Comfortable Than Side Position When Hip is Fractured.—Often patients who have fractures of the lower extremity are more comfortable in the sitting position than the lateral decubitus position while the spinal tap is being performed. Such a patient may be placed in the sitting position without placing his legs over the side of the table.

HERNIA SURGERY

Inguinal, direct and indirect; femoral; incisional hernias below the umbilicus if no intraabdominal manipulation is to be performed; and

EXTRAPERITONEAL BLADDER SURGERY

Suprapubic prostatectomy; extraperitoneal bladder exploration; and

VAGINAL HYSTERECTOMY

Drugs and Techniques

Tetracaine (Pontocaine) with Dextrose (Glucose)

1. The following drugs are mixed together in a 5 cc. Lok-syringe:

  0.2 cc. epinephrine (Adrenalin) solution 1:1000.

  1.0 cc. (10 mg.) of a 1 percent tetracaine solution.

  1.2 cc. of a 10 percent dextrose solution.

  ___

  2.4 cc. Total. This is a hyperbaric mixture, *i.e.,* the specific gravity is greater than the specific gravity of the spinal fluid.

2. The spinal puncture is performed at the second or third lumbar interspace with the patient in the sitting or lateral decubitus position.

3. The syringe containing the above mixture is connected to the spinal needle and 0.6 cc. of spinal fluid is aspirated into the syringe, making a total amount of 3.0 cc. in the syringe.

4. The content of the syringe is discharged subarachnoidally at the rate of 1 cc. per second.

5. A small amount of spinal fluid, not to exceed 0.3 cc. to 0.5 cc., is then withdrawn into the syringe and reinjected. This maneuver assures the anesthetist that the needle point rests subarachnoidally at the completion of the injection.

6. The needle and introducer are withdrawn. The patient is immediately put in the supine position with his head and shoulders elevated on a pillow. The table remains level. NO TRENDELENBURG or other positional changes should be made for at least 20 minutes as the anesthetic solution is heavier than spinal fluid and will gravitate in the direction of dependency. In most instances the anesthetic level will be "fixed," i.e. will not vary, after this period of time has elapsed.

7. Operating analgesia is established in five to ten minutes and lasts 2 to 2½ hours.

Procaine (Novocain)

1. The following drugs are mixed together in a 5 cc. Lok-syringe.

> 0.2 cc.   of epinephrine (Adrenalin) solution 1:1000.
>
> 2.0 cc.   of distilled water, normal saline, or spinal fluid.
>
> 100 mg. of procaine crystals are dissolved in the above solution.
>
> ———
>
> 2.2 cc.   This is a hyperbaric mixture, *i.e.*, the specific gravity is greater than the specific gravity of the spinal fluid.

2. The spinal puncture is performed at the second or third lumbar interspace with the patient in the sitting or lateral decubitus position.

3. The syringe containing the above mixture is connected to the spinal needle and 0.8 cc. of spinal fluid is aspirated into the syringe, making a total amount of 3.0 cc. in the syringe.

4. The content of the syringe is discharged subarachnoidally at the rate of 1 cc. per second

5. A small amount of spinal fluid, not to exceed 0.3 cc. to 0.5 cc., is then withdrawn into the syringe and reinjected. This maneuver assures the anesthetist that the needle point rests subarachnoidally at the completion of the injection. The needle and introducer are withdrawn.

6. The patient is immediately put in the supine position with his head and shoulders elevated on a pillow. NO TRENDELENBURG or other positional changes should be made for at least 20 minutes as the anesthetic solution is heavier than spinal fluid and will gravitate in the direction of dependency. In most instances the anesthetic level will be "fixed," i.e., will not vary, after this period of time has elapsed.

7. Operating analgesia is established in five minutes and lasts 1 to 1½ hours.

Extent of Analgesia: Analgesia extends between the xiphoid process and umbilicus in most cases, *i.e.*, T8. The rise of analgesia should be checked with an Allis forceps at frequent intervals, although with the recommended dosages it will seldom rise above T8. If the level of anesthesia rises above T8, place the patient in Fowler's (head-up) position immediately.

For vaginal hysterectomies, analgesia must extend above the umbilicus; otherwise, traction reflexes on the peritoneum which result from manipulating the uterus cause the patient discomfort.

Following the operation, if a tetracaine solution with a vasoconstrictor drug is employed, the patient may be unable to move his legs for two to eight hours. The anesthetist should not become alarmed by such a duration and he should explain to the patient that feeling will return in approximately this period of time (see page 484).

Remarks

Reduce Dosage in Short and/or Obese Patient.—In the extremely obese or short patient (under 5 feet tall), the quantities of drugs and spinal fluid should be reduced by one-third so that the total volume injected is one-third less than that advocated for the average patient. The third lumbar interspace is usually preferred in these patients as the site for the lumbar puncture. This is very important if complications are to be avoided.

Examine Bowel When It Is Incarcerated.— When a spinal block is given for an incarcerated hernia, the incarcerated bowel should always be inspected to see if it is viable, whether strangulation is or is not suspected. Occasionally in this type of case a spinal block will give sufficient relaxation for the involved bowel to slip back into the abdomen. This is no indication to postpone surgery as the bowel may be gangrenous.

Omission of Vasoconstrictor Drug from Local Anesthetic Solution Shortens Duration.— The vasoconstrictor agent may be omitted at any time from the mixture but the operating time will be noticeably shortened, *i.e.*, to ¾ to 1 hour with procaine and 1¼ to 1¾ hours with tetracaine.

To Markedly Prolong Duration of Analgesia Substitute Phenylephrine (Neo-Synephrine) for Epinephrine (Adrenalin).—See page 482.

INTRA-ABDOMINAL SURGERY

Appendectomy, cholecystectomy, gastric resection, bowel resection, hysterectomy, ventral hernia with intraperitoneal manipulation, bladder resections, splenectomy, and intestinal obstruction, and

RETROPERITONEAL SURGERY

Nephrectomy, ureteral lithotomy, and lumbar sympathectomy.

Drugs and Techniques

Tetracaine (Pontocaine) with Dextrose (Glucose)

1. Depending on the height of the patient, one of the following combinations of drugs is mixed together in a 5 cc. Lok-syringe:

	Height of Patient		
Drugs	5' - 5'5"	5'6" - 6'	Over 6'
Epinephrine (Adrenalin) solution 1:1000	0.2 cc.	0.2 cc.	0.2 cc.
1% tetracaine solution	1.2 cc. (12 mg.)	1.5 cc. (15 mg.)	1.8 cc. (18 mg.)
10% dextrose solution	1.4 cc.	1.7 cc.	2.0 cc.
Total	2.8 cc.	3.4 cc.	4.0 cc.

These are hyperbaric mixtures, *i.e.*, the specific gravity is greater than the specific gravity of spinal fluid.

2. The spinal puncture is performed with the patient in the lateral decubitus or sitting position. The second, third, or fourth lumbar interspace may be used in any patient, but as a "rule of thumb" the third or fourth lumbar interspace is employed in the short patient, and the second or third lumbar interspace in the tall patient.

3. The syringe containing one of the above mixtures is connected to the spinal needle and 0.3 cc. of spinal fluid is aspirated into the syringe.

4. The content of the syringe is discharged subarachnoidally at the rate of 1 cc. per second.

5. A small amount of spinal fluid, not to exceed 0.3 cc. to 0.5 cc., is then withdrawn into the syringe and reinjected. This maneuver assures the anesthetist that the needle point rests subarachnoidally at the completion of the injection.

6. The spinal needle and the introducer are withdrawn and the patient is turned into the supine position with his head and shoulders elevated by a pillow.

7. The table is tilted to a 10-degree Trendelenburg position and the abdomen tested at frequent intervals with an Allis forceps.

8. When skin analgesia exists to the fifth thoracic dermatome (between the nipple line and the xiphoid process), and skin hypesthesia (decrease in normal sensations) to the

fourth thoracic dermatome (Figure 242, page 354), the table should be leveled or put in a 5-degree Fowler's position. This will usually assure complete analgesia to the third or fourth thoracic dermatome.

9. The table now should remain in the level or Fowler's position for twenty minutes before Trendelenburg position is instituted or any other positional changes are made.

10. Operating analgesia is established in 5 to 15 minutes and lasts 2 to 2¼ hours. If the operative procedure requires a period of 2¼ to 3½ hours, phenylephrine (Neo-Synephrine) 5 mg. should be substituted for the epinephrine (see page 482).

Procaine (Novocain)

1. Depending on the height of the patient, one of the following combinations is mixed together in a 5 cc. Lok-syringe:

Drugs	Height of Patient		
	5' - 5'5"	5'6" - 6'	Over 6'
Epinephrine (Adrenalin) solution 1:1000	0.2 cc.	0.2 cc.	0.2 cc.
Distilled water, normal saline, or spinal fluid	2.5 cc.	3.0 cc.	3.5 cc.
Procaine crystals (dissolved in the above solutions)	120 mg.	150 mg.	180 mg.
Total	2.7 cc.	3.2 cc.	3.7 cc.

These are hyperbaric mixtures, *i.e.*, the specific gravity is greater than the specific gravity of spinal fluid.

2. The spinal puncture is performed with the patient in the lateral decubitus or sitting position. The second, third, or fourth lumbar interspace may be employed, but as a "rule of thumb" the third or fourth lumbar interspace is used in the short patient and the second or third lumbar interspace in the tall patient.

3. The syringe containing one of the above mixtures is connected to the spinal needle and 0.3 cc. of spinal fluid is aspirated into the syringe.

4. The content of the syringe is discharged subarachnoidally at the rate of 1 cc. per second.

5. A small amount of spinal fluid, not to exceed 0.3 cc. to 0.5 cc., is then withdrawn into the syringe and reinjected. This assures the anesthetist that the needle point rests subarachnoidally at the completion of the injection.

6. The spinal needle and introducer are withdrawn and the patient is turned into the supine position with his head and shoulders elevated by a pillow.

7. The table is tilted to a 10-degree Trendelenburg position and the abdomen tested at frequent intervals with an Allis forceps.

8. When skin analgesia exists to the fifth thoracic dermatome (between the nipple line and the xiphoid process), and skin hypesthesia (decrease in normal sensations) to the fourth thoracic dermatome, the table should be leveled or put in a 5-degree Fowler's position. This will usually assure complete analgesia to the third or fourth thoracic dermatome.

9. The table now should remain in the level or Fowler's position for twenty minutes before Trendelenburg position is instituted or any other positional changes are made.

10. Operating analgesia is established in 5 to 10 minutes and 1 to 1½ hours of analgesia may be expected with this technique. If the operative procedure requires long periods, *i.e.*, 1¾ to 2 hours, phenylephrine (Neo-Synephrine) 5 mg. should be substituted for the epinephrine (see page 482).

Remarks

Monitor Patient.—When a high spinal block is given, a constant check of the blood pressure and the height of analgesia is necessary, especially during the immediate post-administration period.

For Intra-abdominal Surgery Analgesia to T4 Must Exist.—Whenever the peritoneum is invaded, analgesia must extend to the fourth thoracic dermatome even if the surgery is below the umbilicus. Even then, in many cases, traction on the peritoneum and mesentery will cause the patient discomfort, which usually manifests itself in chest pain, nausea and vomiting.

Use Thiopental (Pentothal) to Supplement Spinal Block.—0.6 percent thiopental analgesia and oxygen by nasal catheter or mask are used in conjunction with most intraperitoneal and retroperitoneal procedures, especially if they are above the umbilicus. Traction and manipulation in these regions may cause the patient to feel pain, become nauseated, or hiccup. These reflexes often occur in spite of somatic analgesia to the fourth dermatome and are mediated via the vagus nerve, which a spinal block does not anesthetize unless total spinal anesthesia occurs. Likewise, if the surgeon palpates the dome of the liver, the patient may feel severe pain in the shoulders. This pain is transmitted by the phrenic nerve, which is also not anesthetized by spinal anesthesia unless the level reaches the fourth cervical vertebra. It is best for the surgeon who is giving spinal anesthesia himself not to push the anesthetic level too high. He should not try to abolish traction reflexes, etc., by allowing the anesthetic level to rise to the first or second thoracic dermatomes—such a level will probably not abolish them anyway. The spinal block should be used for relaxation of the abdominal wall and its contents, which usually means anesthesia between the xiphoid process and the nipple line. Then, if the patient is uncomfortable, thiopental and oxygen as advocated above should be given by the person attending the case.

Reduce Dosage in Short and/or Obese Patient, Patients with Distention, and Those with Large Tumors.—In obese patients, in patients with large abdominal tumors that cause the abdomen to protrude, and in patients with abdominal distention such as that seen in intestinal obstruction, the quantities of drugs and the spinal fluid should be reduced by one-third so that the total volume injected is one-third less than that advocated for the average

patient of that height. The lumbar puncture should be made in the third or fourth lumbar interspace. *In the extremely obese, one-half the listed amounts should be employed.* This is extremely important if complications are to be avoided.

In patients who are under 5 feet tall, the quantities of drugs and spinal fluid advocated for the 5 foot to 5 foot, 5 inch patient should be reduced by one-third so that the total volume injected is one-third less.

Use Spinal Block with Care in the Debilitated Patient.—In general, the old, debilitated patient is not a good candidate for intra-abdominal procedures under *high* spinal anesthesia, *i.e.*, analgesia to the third or fourth thoracic dermatome. *High* is emphasized because *low* spinal anesthesia, *i.e.*, analgesia to or below the tenth thoracic dermatome (the level of the umbilicus), may be a suitable anesthesia for many procedures, *e.g.*, transurethral resection, reduction of a fractured hip, anorectal surgery, etc., in the elderly patient.

When Abdominal Relaxation Is Inadequate to Close Peritoneum, Use d-Tubocurarine or Peritoneal Lavage.—If the surgery is longer than contemplated and the patient's abdomen is difficult to close because motor function of the abdominal muscles has returned, the following two points should be remembered. First, a small amount of intravenous *d*-tubocurarine (curare), *i.e.*, 1 to 2 cc., may be added as a supplement to relax the muscles which are only partially relaxed by the dissipating spinal anesthesia. Larger doses of *d*-tubocurarine are to be avoided since severe respiratory depression or arrest may occur. However, the 1 cc. dose may be repeated in five to ten minutes if necessary. Second, peritoneal reflexes are usually responsible for the tightening of the abdominal muscles and these may be abolished by peritoneal lavage with a local anesthetic agent (see Chapter 42, page 337).

Is Spinal Block Indicated When Patient Has Intestinal Obstruction? Opinion differs as to whether spinal anesthesia or general anesthesia should be used for operation for intestinal obstruction, particularly acute intestinal obstructions. The arguments for and against usually center on the following points.

When spinal anesthesia exists to the fourth thoracic dermatome, the sympathetic portion of the autonomic system innervating the abdomen is blocked and the predominance of the parasympathetic portion via the vagus nerve causes the bowel to contract. Although this improves the surgical conditions, it may, on the rare occasion, cause a gangrenous bowel to rupture. Since antibiotic therapy is successful in treating a fecal peritonitis, provided the rent in the bowel is immediately corrected, this rare complication may not be as serious a problem as it once was.

With spinal analgesia the pharyngeal and laryngeal reflexes are not abolished, and the conscious patient may protect his own airway from vomitus. On the other hand, if a patient under spinal anesthesia does vomit and is uncooperative or cannot expel the vomitus because a forceful expiration is not possible with the thoracic and abdominal muscles blocked, aspiration may occur and present a serious problem. It should be remembered that the diaphragm, even though it still functions during spinal anesthesia, may not be effective in producing a forceful expiration strong enough to eject vomitus, since the abdominal muscles are relaxed and the diaphragm has nothing to push against.

Spinal anesthesia usually gives ideal relaxation, while even expert hands may have difficulty in managing a general anesthesia for such cases. If general anesthesia is used, either an awake intubation or a rapid induction of anesthesia as well as rapid placement of an endotracheal tube with an inflatable cuff is necessary to prevent vomitus from contaminating the tracheobronchial tree. Both of these techniques require an extremely well-trained anesthetist, usually a specialist.

Regardless of Type of Anesthesia Selected for Intestinal Obstruction, Empty Stomach and Be Prepared to Treat Vomiting.—As with any anesthetic situation, the method to be employed depends on what type of anesthesia is available and which type can be best administered; however, irrespective of which anes-

thetic method is employed, the potential possibility of vomiting with aspiration is perhaps the most serious complication. A chemical pneumonia caused by aspiration of gastric contents is extremely difficult to treat.

Therefore, the following points are pertinent, whichever method of anesthesia is employed. First, aspiration of the stomach contents with a Levin tube, or preferably an Ewald tube, just prior to the administration of anesthesia, is essential. Second, if the patient's condition and severity of the obstruction permit, decompression with a Miller-Abbott tube of the distended bowel, correction of the fluid imbalance, and the postponement of surgery for a day or two may greatly reduce the anesthetic risk. Remember that the Miller-Abbott tube does not empty the stomach, and that before anesthesia is administered, the stomach should be emptied by "sinking" a Levin or Ewald tube. And, third, suction apparatus and instruments for clearing the airway and maintaining a clear airway should be immediately available (see page 52 to page 55).

Omission of Vasoconstrictor Drugs from Local Anesthetic Solution Shortens the Duration.—The vasoconstrictor agent may be omitted at any time from the mixture but the operating time will be noticeably shortened, e.g., ¾ to 1 hour with procaine and 1¼ to 1¾ hours with tetracaine.

Prolonged Anesthesia of Legs May Follow Use of Vasoconstrictor Drug in Subarachnoid Space.—Following the operation, especially if a tetracaine solution with a vasoconstrictor drug is employed, the patient may be unable to move his legs for two to eight hours or longer. The anesthetist should not become alarmed and he should explain to the patient that feeling will return in approximately this period of time (see page 484).

BACK AND SPINE OPERATIONS

Laminectomy below the seventh thoracic dermatome and spinal fusion.

Drugs and Techniques

Tetracaine (Pontocaine) and Dextrose (Glucose)

1. The following drugs are mixed together in a 5 cc. Lok-syringe:

> 0.2 cc. of epinephrine (Adrenalin) solution 1:1000.
>
> 1.0 cc. (10 mg.) of a 1 percent tetracaine solution.
>
> 1.2 cc. of a 10 percent dextrose solution.
>
> ————
>
> 2.4 cc. Total. This is a hyperbaric mixture, *i.e.*, the specific gravity is greater than the specific gravity of spinal fluid.

2. The spinal puncture is performed at the second or third lumbar interspace with the patient in the sitting or lateral decubitus position.

3. The syringe containing the above mixture is connected to the spinal needle and 0.6 cc. of spinal fluid is aspirated into the syringe, making a total amount of 3.0 cc. in the syringe.

4. The content of the syringe is discharged subarachnoidally at the rate of 1 cc. per second.

5. A small amount of spinal fluid, not to exceed 0.3 cc. to 0.5 cc., is then withdrawn into the syringe and reinjected. This maneuver assures the anesthetist that the needle point rests subarachnoidally at the completion of the injection.

6. The needle and introducer are withdrawn. The patient is immediately placed in the supine position with his head and shoulders elevated on a pillow. The table should remain level and *NO TRENDELENBURG* or other positional changes made.

7. After twenty minutes, the patient may be turned *slowly* into the prone position for surgery. In most instances the anesthetic level will be "fixed," *i.e.*, will not vary, after this period of time has elapsed.

8. Operating analgesia is established in 5 to 10 minutes and lasts 2 to 3 hours. If the operation is in the lower lumbar or sacral area, analgesia may be even more prolonged.

Procaine (Novocain)

1. The following drugs are mixed together in a 5 cc. Lok-syringe:

> 0.2 cc. of epinephrine (Adrenalin) solution 1:1000.
>
> 2.0 cc. of distilled water, normal saline, or spinal fluid.
>
> 100 mg. of procaine crystals are dissolved in the above solution.
>
> ————
>
> 2.2 cc. Total. This is a hyperbaric mixture, *i.e.*, the specific gravity is greater than the specific gravity of the spinal fluid.

2. The spinal puncture is performed at the second or third lumbar interspace with the patient in the sitting or lateral decubitus position.

3. The syringe containing the above mixture is connected to the spinal needle and 0.8 cc. of spinal fluid is aspirated into the syringe, making a total amount of 3.0 cc. in the syringe.

4. The content of the syringe is discharged subarachnoidally at the rate of 1 cc. per second.

5. A small amount of spinal fluid, not to exceed 0.3 cc. to 0.5 cc., is then withdrawn into the syringe and reinjected. This maneuver assures the anesthetist that the needle point rests subarachnoidally at the completion of the injection.

6. The needle and introducer are withdrawn. The patient is immediately put in the supine position with his head and shoulders elevated on a pillow. *NO TRENDELENBURG* or other positional changes are made.

7. After twenty minutes, the patient may be turned *slowly* into the prone position for surgery. In most instances the anesthetic level

will be "fixed," *i.e.*, will not vary, after this period of time has elapsed.

8. Operating analgesia is established in five minutes and lasts 1 to 2 hours.

Extent of Analgesia: Analgesia with this technique usually extends to the eighth thoracic dermatome. The rise of analgesia should be checked with an Allis forceps at frequent intervals, although with the recommended dosages it will seldom rise above T8. If the level of anesthesia rises above T8, place the patient in Fowler's (head-up) position immediately.

Following the operation, if a tetracaine solution with a vasoconstrictor drug was employed, the patient may be unable to move his legs for two to eight hours. The anesthetist should not become alarmed by such a duration and he should explain to the patient that feeling will return in approximately this period of time (see page 484).

Remarks

Turn Patient Slowly.—When the patient is shifted from the supine to the prone position, he should be moved slowly. Rapid motion may cause rapid shunting of the blood with loss of consciousness and, occasionally, death.

Additional Sedation Usually Is Required.—The prone position is a difficult position for the patient to maintain for a prolonged period. Therefore additional sedation is often indicated.

Reduce Dosage in Short or Obese Patient.—In obese patient or patients under five feet tall, the quantity of drugs and spinal fluid used should be reduced by one-third so that the total volume injected is one-third less than that advocated for the average patient.

Omission of Vasoconstrictor from Local Anesthetic Solution Shortens Duration.—The vasoconstrictor agent may be omitted at any time from the mixture but the operating time will be noticeably shortened, *i.e.*, ¾ to 1 hour with procaine and 1¼ to 1¾ hours with tetracaine.

To Markedly Prolong Duration of Analgesia Substitute Phenylephrine (Neo-Synephrine) for Epinephrine (Adrenalin).—See page 482.

Following Myelography, It May Be Difficult to Obtain Spinal Fluid or If It Is Obtained No Anesthesia May Occur.—If a myelogram has been performed a day or two before surgery, leakage of spinal fluid may be sufficient to preclude the obtaining of spinal fluid when performing the lumbar tap for anesthesia purposes even if the patient is placed in the sitting position for the tap. If this should occur, general anesthesia should be contemplated, or the local anesthetic solution may be injected if the anesthetist is quite certain that the needle point rests subarachnoidally. If no anesthesia results after the injection of the local anesthetic solution, it is best to change to general anesthesia without further attempts at spinal anesthesia.

If spinal fluid is obtained but no anesthesia results when the local anesthetic solution is injected, it may be due to a separation of the dura mater and the arachnoid with pooling of spinal fluid between them (see Subdural Cavity, page 368).

VAGINAL OBSTETRICAL DELIVERIES

Drugs and Techniques

Tetracaine (Pontocaine) with Dextrose (Glucose)

1. The following drugs are mixed together in a 3 cc. Lok-syringe:

   0.2 cc. of epinephrine (Adrenalin) solution 1:1000.

   0.5 cc. (5 mg.) of a 1 percent tetracaine solution.

   0.5 cc. of 10 percent dextrose solution.

   1.2 cc. Total. This is a hyperbaric mixture, *i.e.*, the specific gravity is greater than the specific gravity of spinal fluid.

2. The spinal puncture at the third or

fourth lumbar interspace is performed with the patient in the sitting position.

3. The syringe containing the above mixture is connected to the spinal needle and 0.2 cc. of spinal fluid is aspirated to assure a free flow through the needle.

4. Between labor pains the content of the syringe is discharged at the rate of 0.33 cc. per second.

5. A small amount of spinal fluid, not to exceed 0.3 cc. to 0.5 cc., is withdrawn into the syringe and reinjected. This assures the anesthetist that the needle point rests subarachnoidally at the completion of the injection.

6. The spinal needle and introducer are withdrawn and the patient is allowed to remain in the sitting position for 30 seconds. She is then placed in the supine position with her head on a pillow. *NO TRENDELENBURG* or other positional changes should be made for at least twenty minutes. In most instances the anesthetic level will be "fixed," *i.e.*, it will not vary, after this period of time has elapsed.

7. Operating analgesia is established in 5 to 10 minutes and lasts 2 to 2¼ hours.

Procaine (Novocain)

1. The following drugs are mixed together in a 3 cc. Lok-syringe:

0.2 cc. of epinephrine (Adrenalin) solution 1:1000.

1.0 cc. of distilled water, normal saline, or spinal fluid.

50 mg. of procaine crystals are dissolved in the above solution.

1.2 cc. Total. This is a hyperbaric mixture, *i.e.*, the specific gravity is greater than the specific gravity of spinal fluid.

2. The spinal puncture at the third or fourth lumbar interspace is performed with the patient in the sitting position.

3. The syringe containing the above solution is connected to the spinal needle and 0.2 cc. of spinal fluid is aspirated to assure a free flow through the needle.

4. Between labor pains the content of the syringe is discharged at the rate of 0.33 cc. per second.

5. A small amount of spinal fluid, not to exceed 0.3 cc. to 0.5 cc., is withdrawn into the syringe and reinjected. This assures the anesthetist that the needle point rests subarachnoidally when the injection is completed.

6. The spinal needle and introducer are withdrawn and the patient is allowed to remain in the sitting position for 30 seconds. She is then placed in the supine position with her head on a pillow. *NO TRENDELENBURG* or other positional changes should be made for at least twenty minutes. In most instances the anesthetic level will be "fixed," *i.e.*, it will not vary after this period of time has elapsed.

7. Operating analgesia is established in five to fifteen minutes and lasts 1 to 1½ hours.

Heavy Dibucaine (Nupercaine).—This solution contains 2.5 mg. of dibucaine per cubic centimeter of 5 percent dextrose and it is a hyperbaric mixture, *i.e.*, the specific gravity is greater than the specific gravity of spinal fluid.

1. 1 cc. of heavy dibucaine is drawn into a 2 or 3 cc. Lok-syringe. *No vasoconstrictor is employed.*

2. The spinal puncture at the third or fourth lumbar interspace is performed with the patient in the sitting position.

3. The syringe containing the above mixture is connected to the spinal needle and 0.2 cc. of spinal fluid is aspirated to assure a free flow through the needle.

4. Between labor pains the content of the syringe is discharged at the rate of 0.33 cc. per second.

5. A small amount of spinal fluid, not to exceed 0.3 cc. to 0.5 cc., is withdrawn into the syringe and reinjected. This assures the anesthetist that the needle point rests subarachnoidally when the injection is completed.

6. The spinal needle and introducer are withdrawn and the patient allowed to remain in the sitting position for 30 seconds. She is then placed in the supine position with her head on a pillow. *NO TRENDELENBURG* or other positional changes should be made for at least 20 minutes. In most instances the anesthetic level will be "fixed," *i.e.*, it will not vary, after this period of time has elapsed.

7. Operating analgesia is established in 5 to 15 minutes and lasts 1¾ to 3 hours.

Extent of Analgesia: Analgesia with these techniques usually extends to the tenth thoracic dermatome (umbilicus). The rise of analgesia should be checked with an Allis forceps at frequent intervals, although with the recommended dosages it will seldom rise above T10. If the level of anesthesia rises above T10, place the patient in Fowler's (head-up) position immediately. The technique as described herein produces a "low spinal block." If a true "saddle block" is desired, the patient is allowed to remain in the sitting position for a minimum of three minutes. A saddle block is defined as anesthesia of that area of the female perineum that would touch a saddle if the patient were riding a horse.

Following the delivery, if a dibucaine solution without a vasoconstrictor drug or a tetracaine solution with a vasoconstrictor drug is employed, the patient may be unable to move her legs for two to eight hours. The anesthetist should not become alarmed by such a duration and he should explain to the patient that feeling will return in approximately this period of time (see page 484).

Remarks: When spinal block is used for vaginal delivery, some of the remarks found under Continuous (Intermittent) Caudal Block, page 465 to 472, are applicable and review of them is advised.

Hypotension.—Hypotension following low spinal or saddle block for vaginal delivery does not occur with as great a frequency as following spinal block for cesarean section. If it occurs, the patient's legs are placed immediately in stirrups to effect an autotransfusion (see page 365), and oxygen is administered by bag and mask. If these two measures do not correct the hypotension, use: (1) a rapid drip of intravenous fluids (see page 372); (2) vasoconstrictor drugs (see page 36); or (3) both. If a vasoconstrictor drug is used, one with a short action, *e.g.*, ephedrine sulfate or a phenylephrine drip, is advocated. If an oxytocic drug must then be used, severe persistent hypertension is less likely to result (see page 41).

Do Not Alter Dosage for Short and/or Obese Patient.—These methods are adaptable without varying dosages for patients of all types and builds.

For Version and Extraction, Relaxation May Be Inadequate.—Analgesia is adequate by these techniques for midforceps, low forceps, episiotomy, and repair. If an obstetrical procedure requiring profound relaxation of the uterus and cervix, such as version and extraction or a breech delivery, is necessary, the technique to be used must be carefully selected. Uterine contractility during labor is considered to be autonomous and not affected by regional block techniques. Therefore, even though the sensory fibers from the uterus, vagina, and vulva may be anesthetized, a constriction ring may prevent delivery of the head of the fetus. A constriction ring may present no problem to the skilled obstetrician. Nonetheless, in breech deliveries or versions and extractions general anesthesia is considered by many physicians to be a safer procedure than spinal anesthesia.

If Block Slows Labor, the Uterus Will Respond to Oxytocic Drugs.—Spinal block may slow labor, but the exact underlying etiology is not clearly established. While regional block can abolish the pain of labor, it does not interfere with the contractility of the uterus—uterine contractility is autonomous. Regardless of the regional block procedure employed, the uterus will respond to oxytocic drugs.

Increase in Forceps Delivery.—The incidence of forceps deliveries with spinal block is increased because the involuntary urge to bear down, which is necessary during the second stage of labor, is absent—Fergusson's reflex is blocked by this block. However, when the analgesic level is not above the tenth thoracic dermatome with this block and when the parturient is cooperative, she can bear down and often she can deliver the fetus. She should be coached to do so during her contractions by either the anesthetist or the obstetrician, and moderate pressure should be exerted on the fundus of the uterus to prevent the uterus being pushed anteriorly as the diaphragm moves caudad.

To Markedly Prolong Duration of Analgesia with Tetracaine or Procaine, Substitute Phenylephrine (Neo-Synephrine) for Epinephrine (Adrenalin).—See page 482.

Omission of Vasoconstrictor Drug from Local Anesthetic Solution Shortens Duration of Analgesia.—The vasoconstrictor agent may be omitted at any time from the procaine or the tetracaine mixture but the operating time will be noticeably shortened, *i.e.*, to ¾ to 1 hour with procaine and 1¼ to 1¾ hours with tetracaine.

Vasoconstrictor Drug Plus Oxytocic Drug May Cause Severe Hypertension.—If a spinal block is employed for a vaginal delivery, a long-acting vasoconstrictor drug should not be administered either to prevent or correct a hypotension when an oxytocic drug is to be given. A severe, persistent, dangerous hypertension and even rupture of a cerebral blood vessel which may cause brain damage and hemiplegia can result from the combined effect of a vasoconstrictor drug, *e.g.*, methoxamine (Vasoxyl) and an oxytocic drug which have been administered to a patient within three to six hours of one another (see page 41).

This does not preclude the addition of either epinephrine or phenylephrine to the solution to be injected subarachnoidally. The vascular supply of the subarachnoid space and the spinal cord is sparse (see page 484). Therefore, these drugs are not absorbed into the general circulation in an appreciable quantity when they are injected into the subarachnoid space.

Inject Local Anesthetic Solution Between Labor Pains.—Early studies indicated that cerebrospinal fluid pressure during uterine contractions, with the patient not bearing down, is slightly to moderately increased. However, recent studies show that uterine contraction itself does not have an effect on the cerebrospinal fluid pressure but that changes in intra-abdominal and intrathoracic pressures from bearing down and rapid deep breathing do elevate the cerebrospinal fluid pressure. For these reasons, it is probably best not to inject solutions into the subarachnoid space during uterine contractions.

A True Saddle Block May Not Relieve Pain Caused by Contraction of the Uterus.—With saddle block analgesia, the pains caused by the contractions of the uterus are not relieved. Only the perineum is anesthetized.

Analgesia of the Perineum May be Prolonged.—When a low spinal block is administered, analgesia of the perineum may last from 3 to 5 hours, although the pain from uterine contractions may return within a 2½-hour period.

CHAPTER 45

Continuous (Intermittent) Spinal (Subarachnoid) Anesthesia

INDICATIONS

WHENEVER spinal (subarachnoid) anesthesia is indicated and single-dose spinal block will not produce sufficient analgesia time, this method may be used.

Surgical: See page 341.

Diagnostic: See page 341.

Therapeutic: See page 341.

ANATOMY

Same as for single-dose spinal anesthesia. See page 341.

PREMEDICATION

Same as for single-dose spinal anesthesia. See page 341.

DRUGS

Local Anesthetic Agents: The two agents usually used are tetracaine (Pontocaine) and procaine (Novocain). The author prefers tetracaine. A solution of one of these drugs is prepared in a 10 cc. Lok-type syringe as follows, depending on the agent selected.

Tetracaine (Pontocaine) and Dextrose (Glucose)

> 4.0 cc. (40 mg.) of a 1 percent tetracaine solution.

> 6.0 cc. of a 10 percent dextrose solution.

> _____

> 10 cc. Total. This is a hyperbaric mixture, *i.e.*, the specific gravity is greater than the specific gravity of spinal fluid.

Procaine (Novocain)

> 10 cc. of distilled water, normal saline or, preferably, spinal fluid.

> 300 mg. of procaine are dissolved in the solution.

> _____

> 10 cc. Total. This is a hyperbaric mixture, *i.e.*, the specific gravity is greater than the specific gravity of spinal fluid.

Vasoconstrictor Drugs: With a continuous spinal block, the addition of a vasoconstrictor drug to the local anesthetic solution to prolong its duration is of no advantage.

Local Anesthetic Agent for Skin Wheal: 2 cc. ampules of 1 percent procaine (Novocain) solution.*

MATERIALS

Regional tray (see Chapter 9, page 51) or:

1. One ¾-inch (2 cm.), 25-gauge Huber point security Lok-needle.

2. One 1½-inch (3.8 cm.), 22-gauge security Lok-needle.

3. One 3 cc. Lok-syringe.

4. One 10 cc. Lok-syringe, preferably with finger rings.

5. One prep cup, preferably stainless steel.

6. One Allis forceps.

7. One sponge forceps.

_____

*This size ampule may be obtained from the Vitarine Company, Queens, New York.

8. One Pitkin needle guide or thin-walled needle guide.*

9. Four towels.

10. Four 4 x 4 sponges.

11. One sterilizer control.

To this basic equipment must be added the following special items.

1. One 3-inch (7.5 cm.), 18-gauge thin-walled spinal needle with a Tuohy (directional) bevel (Figure 252, page 389 and Figure 264, page 402).*

2. One vinyl plastic tubing (Figure 253, (page 390 and Figure 263, page 401).* The tubing is marked with a felt marking pen or ball point pen 5¾ inches (14.5 cm.) from the end to be placed in the subarachnoid space.

3. One wire stylet for the vinyl tubing (Figure 253, page 390).*

4. One ¾-inch (2 cm.), 23-gauge Lok-needle, preferably with a short bevel, or a Tuohy-Borst catheter-syringe adapter (Figure 253, page 390; Figure 264, page 402 and Figure 265, page 402).* Either the needle or the Tuohy-Borst adapter is employed as a connector so that the syringe containing the local anesthetic solution as well as the one-way stopcock may be attached to the plastic tubing.

5. One spring clip female to male Lok one-way stopcock (Figure 253, page 390 and Figure 264, page 402).*

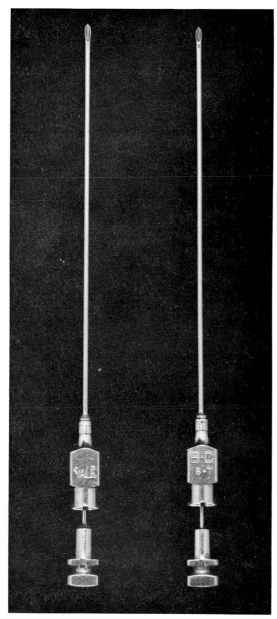

Figure 252. 3-inch (7.5 cm.), 18-gauge thin-walled Tuohy (directional) needles for inserting plastic tubing into either the subarachnoid space or epidural space. The notch in the hub of the needle and the opening in the bevel of the Tuohy needle are on the same side. The engraving on the hub of the needle, i.e., Yale or B-D, 18-T, varies from one needle to the next.

*This equipment may be obtained from Becton, Dickinson and Company, Rutherford, New Jersey. Order numbers are: Pitkin needle guide, PNG; thin-walled needle guide, 01-0027; Tuohy needle, T466LNRH; plastic tubing regular, VX020 and radiopaque, RVX020 or CRVX020; wire stylet for plastic tubing, 01-0041; Tuohy-Borst adapter, 610A; female to male Lok one-way stopcock, MS09; and plug for female Lok outlet, 417A.

Two types of radiopaque tubing are available—the RVX020 which does not permit observation of the lumen and the CRVX020, which does permit observation of the lumen. The CRVX020 allows detection of blood or spinal fluid more easily when the aspiration tests are performed. It also permits observation of the wire stylet. For illustrations, the RVX020 was employed because photographs of it are better.

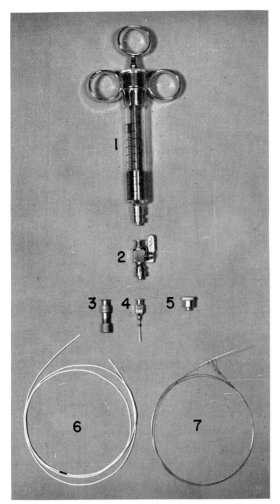

Figure 253. Continuous equipment: (1) 10 cc. Lok-syringe with finger rings; (2) female to male Lok one-way stopcock; (3) Tuohy-Borst adapter; (4) ¾-inch (2 cm.), 23-gauge Lok needle; (5) plug for female Lok outlet; (6) plastic tubing marked with felt marking pen 5¾ inches from end to be placed into the subarachnoid or epidural space; and (7) wire stylet.

6. One plug for female Lok outlet (Figure 253, page 390 and Figure 264, page 402).

TECHNIQUE

Landmarks: Same as for single dose spinal anesthesia. See page 344.

Position: Same as for single dose spinal anesthesia although the lateral decubitus (side) position is most frequently employed (Figure 254A, page 391). See page 344.

Precautions: Same as for single dose spinal anesthesia. See page 346.

Procedure: Since the introduction of plastic tubing, the technique using the ureteral catheter or the technique using the malleable needle and special mattress (the Lemmon method) is seldom employed. The following description is the plastic tubing technique.

1. The sterilizer control is always checked to see that the equipment is sterile.

2. The anesthetist puts on sterile gloves, prepares the skin, and sterile towels are placed over the up side and under the down side.

3. A skin wheal is raised over the third or fourth lumbar interspace with the ¾-inch (2 cm.), 25-gauge Huber point security Lok-needle using 0.2 cc. to 0.3 cc. of a 1.0 percent procaine (Novocain) solution (Figure 254A, page 391).

4. 0.8 cc. to 1.5 cc. of the procaine solution is infiltrated into the interspinous ligament.

5. A hole is made in the skin wheal with either the Pitkin or the thin-walled needle guide (Figure 254B, page 391) and the guide withdrawn. Usually, this prevents the spinal needle carrying with it a skin plug and skin bacteria into the subarachnoid space.

6. The relationship of the opening in the bevel of the Tuohy spinal needle to the markings on the hub are noted. The notch in the hub of the needle into which the projection in the top of the stylet fits is on the same side as the opening in the bevel of the Tuohy needle (Figure 252, page 389).

7. The 18-gauge, thin-walled Tuohy needle is held by the anesthetist so that the thumb exerts pressure on the stylet's top and the shaft is supported between the index and middle fingers (Figure 254C, page 391). This prevents displacement of the stylet and allows the anesthetist to steady his hand by resting the ring and little fingers on the patient's back (Figure 254C, page 391).

The index and middle (long) fingers of the free hand should straddle the interspace into

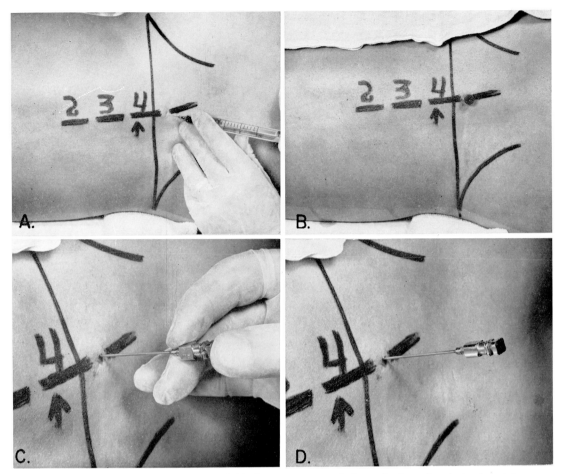

Figure 254. Technique of continuous spinal block. A. Raising of skin wheal at fourth lumbar interspace. B. Hole being made in skin wheal with introducer. C. Tuohy needle inserted through hole into interspinous ligament with opening in bevel facing cephalad. D. Prior to inserting the needle into subarachnoid space the bevel of needle is turned toward the ceiling.

which the needle is to be placed. Great care should be taken that the needle lies in the same plane as the spinous processes and perpendicular to the transverse processes. If it points upward or downward, or if the patient's back is not at a 90-degree angle in the vertical plane with the table, the spinal needle may not travel a true course (Figure 233, page 349).

The Tuohy needle is inserted through the hole in the wheal with the opening in the bevel pointed cephalad (Figure 254C, page 391). It is carefully advanced into the interspinous ligament for approximately 1 inch (5 cm.) to 1¼ inches (3.2 cm.). If the needle is not inserted through the skin and the ligament with its bevel in this direction, the nee-

dle will tend to deviate to one side or the other.

8. When the point of the needle rests in the anterior portion of the interspinous ligament or ligamentum flavum, the opening in the bevel of the needle is pointed toward the ceiling (Figure 254D, page 391). Now the bevel of the needle is parallel to the fibers of the dura and will not cut a large hole in the dura (Figure 245, page 359).

9. The needle is slowly advanced through the epidural space and into the subarachnoid space. When the stylet is withdrawn, the spinal fluid should run out *rapidly,* and this should not alarm the anesthetist (Figure 255A, page 392).

The stylet is replaced in the needle (Figure 255B, page 392). A slow drip of spinal fluid may be obtained when only part of the opening in the bevel of the Tuohy needle, e.g., ⅟₁₆ inch (0.15cm.), lies in the subarachnoid space. If a slow drip rather than a rapid drip results, slowly advance the needle ⅟₁₆ inch (0.15 cm.) to ⅛ inch (0.3 cm.) deeper. *Be sure the entire opening in the bevel, which is ⅛ inch (0.3 cm.) in length, lies in the subarachnoid space* (Figure 256, page 393). Unless the entire opening in the bevel is in the subarachnoid space, the plastic tubing will not pass through it.

10. Now, the opening in the bevel of the Tuohy needle is pointed cephalad. Thus, the plastic tubing is directed toward the patient's head (Figure 255B, page 392).

11. The wire stylet in the plastic tubing is withdrawn slightly so that it is ½ inch (1.3 cm.) from the end to be inserted into the Tuohy spinal needle. If the anesthetist is right-handed, the thumb and index finger of the left hand grasp the hub of the Tuohy needle while the remaining fingers hold the plastic tubing. The back of the left hand rests against the pa-

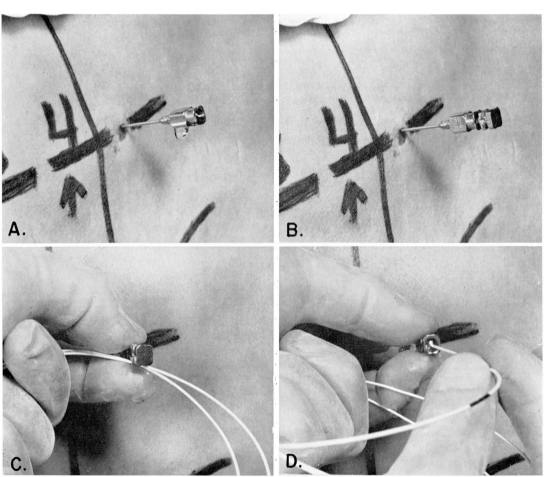

Figure 255. Technique of continuous spinal block (con't.). A. Spinal fluid rapidly drips from hub of needle. B. Stylet replaced in needle to keep spinal fluid loss to minimum, the needle is advanced ⅛ inch (0.3 cm.) to be sure the entire bevel rests in subarachnoid space. The Tuohy needle is rotated slowly so that the bevel's opening again points cephalad. C. Method of holding the needle for the initial ½ inch (1.3 cm.) insertion of the tubing into the subarachnoid space by the right-handed anesthetist. The left hand rests firmly against the back, holding the hub of the needle securely with the thumb and index finger and the tubing with the middle, ring, and little fingers. D. Stylet removed by right hand and tubing is "fed" slowly through the needle by the right hand.

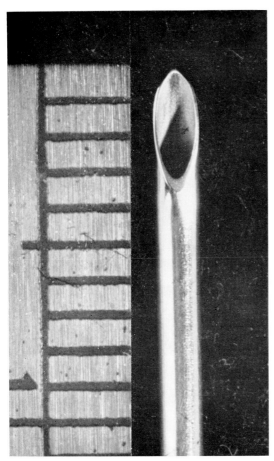

Figure 256. The opening in bevel of Tuohy needle is ⅛ inch (0.3 cm.).

tient's back (Figure 255C, page 392). The right hand withdraws the stylet from the needle and puts it in the regional block tray. Now, the right hand feeds the plastic tubing through the needle (Figure 255D, page 392). The plastic tubing will stop when its end hits the curve of the point of the needle. Then, the plastic tubing is pushed ½ inch (1.3 cm.) beyond the bevel of the needle. Moderate pressure on the plastic tubing may be required for this to be accomplished and, *therefore, the needle must be held securely* (Figure 255C and D, page 392).

12. Once the first ½ inch (1.3 cm.) of the plastic tubing passes beyond the point of the Tuohy needle it is no longer necessary to hold the hub of the needle with the left hand. The index finger and thumb of the left hand release

their hold on the hub of the needle (Figure 257 A, page 394). The tubing is carefully removed from the middle, ring, and little fingers. The tubing is straightened and the stylet is withdrawn 2 inches (5 cm.). Now the tubing is advanced this distance through the needle until the mark on the plastic tubing is at the hub of the needle (Figure 257A and B, page 394). If the bevel of the needle rests in the subarachnoid space, the tubing should advance easily with *light* and *delicate* pressure —no resistance should be encountered and there should be no need to hold the needle (Figure 257A, page 394). If the tubing is difficult to thread, the bevel of the needle probably does not lie in the subarachnoid space.

If the stylet is not withdrawn prior to the insertion of the tubing beyond the point of the Tuohy needle, the physician probably will not be able to remove the stylet from the tubing, although he may be able to withdraw the 18-gauge needle over the tubing and the stylet. Even in a situation where the Tuohy needle can be removed, the stylet may not be dislodged from the tubing. Thus, the procedure to this point will have to be repeated. This difficulty occurs because the Tuohy needle has a curved point and the tubing and the stylet are bent at an acute angle where they enter the subarachnoid space.

Once the plastic tubing has passed the point of the needle, do not try to withdraw it, as the needle may cut it off or shred it. If a readjustment is necessary, the needle and the plastic tubing must be removed as one, and the procedure repeated to this point.

13. The Tuohy needle is now withdrawn from the patient's back over the plastic tubing and stylet. This is a critical maneuver. Again, the thumb and index finger of the left hand hold the hub of the needle (Figure 257C, page 394). The plastic tubing with stylet in it is grasped firmly 1 inch (2.5 cm.) distal to the hub of the needle by the thumb and index finger of the right hand (Figure 257C, page 394). Then, the thumb and index finger of the left hand pull the needle out of the patient until the hub touches the thumb and index finger

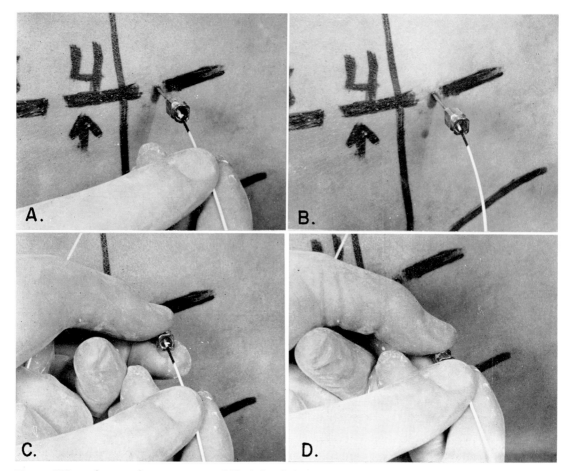

Figure 257. Technique of continuous spinal block (con't.). A. Tubing being threaded through needle with gentle pressure—the left hand need not hold needle. B. The mark, 5¾ inches (14.5 cm.) from tip of tubing, rests at hub of needle. C. In preparation to remove the needle, the tubing is gripped firmly with thumb and index finger of right hand 1 inch (2.5 cm.) from needle hub to prevent it being either inserted further into the subarachnoid space or withdrawn as the needle is removed. The needle is gripped with the thumb and index finger of the *left* hand. D. The left hand pulls the needle back over the tubing and stylet until the hub contacts the index finger and thumb of the *right* hand—*do not move right hand.* The maneuver detailed in C. and D. is repeated two or three times until the needle's tip emerges from the skin.

of the right hand—do not move the right hand (Figure 257D, page 394). This maneuver is repeated two or three times until the point of the needle emerges from the skin. If this maneuver is executed carefully, the plastic tubing will not be dislodged from its position in the subarachnoid space.

14. As soon as the point of the needle emerges from the skin, the plastic tubing is fixed by the thumb and index finger of the left hand at its point of entrance into the skin (Figure 258A, page 395). The needle is slipped to the end of the plastic tubing (Fig-

ure 258B, page 395). The stylet is withdrawn (Figure 258C, page 395), and the needle removed (Figure 258D, page 395). The distance of the mark on the plastic tubing from the skin should be checked—by doing this, it can be determined whether the plastic tubing was dislodged from the subarachnoid space when the spinal needle was withdrawn (Figure 259A, page 396).

15. The Tuohy-Borst tubing adapter or the 23-gauge short-beveled ¾-inch (2 cm.) Lok-needle is affixed to the plastic tubing (Figure

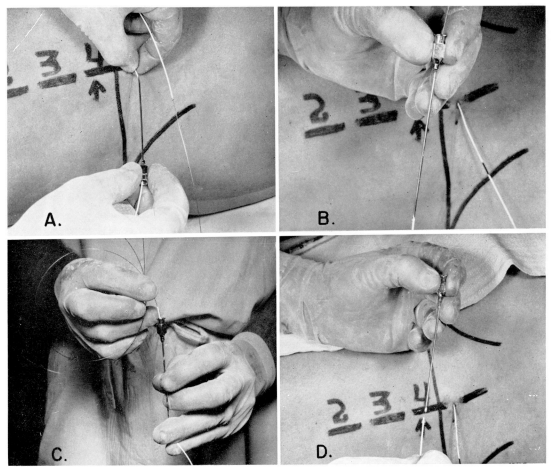

Figure 258. Technique of continuous spinal block (con't.). A. Plastic tubing is gripped by index finger and thumb of left hand at its entrance into skin. B. The needle is slipped to the end of the plastic tubing with the right hand. C. The thumb and index finger of the left hand hold the needle and the ring and little fingers hold the tubing. Now, the stylet is *slowly* withdrawn from the plastic tubing by the right hand. D. The stylet is placed on the table with the anesthetic equipment. The right hand holds the tubing and the needle is removed from it.

259 B and C, page 396). We prefer the 23-gauge needle.

16. The one-way stopcock is connected to either the Tuohy-Borst adapter or the 23-gauge needle (Figure 259 D, page 396 and Figure 260 A, page 396).

17. Spinal fluid is allowed to appear at the open end of the stopcock—for this to occur, the plastic tubing may have to be held below the top of the table (Figure 260 A, page 396).

If no spinal fluid appears and if the anesthetist thinks he has placed the tubing correctly, he should place the table in 10 to 15 degree Fowler's position. This increases the spinal fluid pressure, and if the tubing is placed subarachnoidally, spinal fluid should appear. If it does not, gentle aspiration with an empty syringe should be attempted. Then, if no spinal fluid appears, the plastic tubing is withdrawn 1 inch (2.5 cm.) from the patient—if the tubing was kinked in soft tissues during withdrawal of the Tuohy needle, this maneuver will straighten the tubing. Now if spinal fluid still is not obtained, the tubing should be withdrawn and another attempt with sterile equipment should be made to insert the tubing.

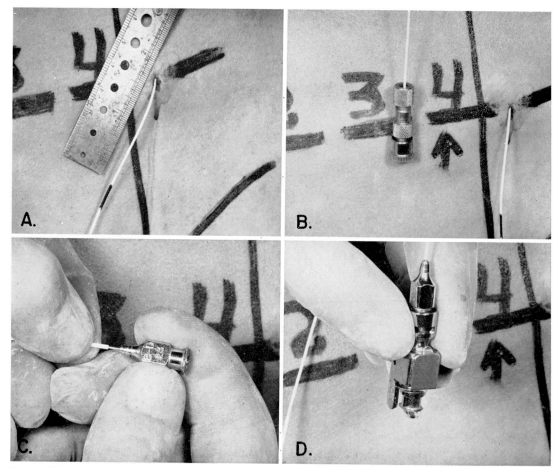

Figure 259. Technique of continuous spinal block (con't.). A. The distance from the skin to the mark on the plastic tubing is examined. B. Tuohy-Borst adapter affixed to tubing. C. ¾-inch (2 cm.), 23-gauge needle affixed to tubing—we prefer to use the needle. As the 23-gauge needle is inserted into the tubing it is rotated back and forth between the thumb and index finger of the right hand to facilitate it sliding into the tubing. D. One-way stopcock attached to 23-gauge needle.

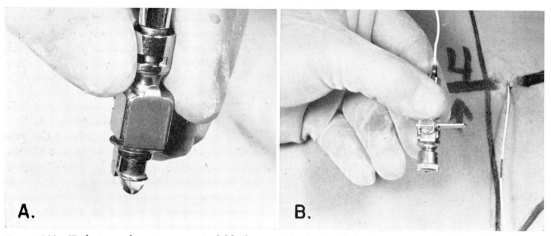

Figure 260. Technique of continuous spinal block (con't.). A. Spinal fluid is permitted to fill needle and one-way stopcock. B. Stopcock closed and plug placed in stopcock.

18. When spinal fluid is obtained, the stopcock is turned off, and the stopcock is sealed with the plug for the female outlet (Figure 260 B, page 396).

19. A piece of gauze is taped under the plastic tubing as it emerges from the skin (Figure 285 D, page 433), and the plastic tubing taped to the back, either to the right or left of the spinous processes (Figure 261 A, page 397).

20. The patient is instructed to turn on his back. He may do this himself, providing the anesthetist prevents pull on the tubing by placing his hand over the entrance of the plastic tubing through the skin (Figure 261 B, page 397).

21. The knee restraint straps, shoulder braces, and wrist cuffs are snugly adjusted so that the patient will not move when tilted. His head and shoulders are elevated on pillows (Figure 261 C, page 397).

22. The plug is removed from the stopcock, the syringe containing the hyperbaric local anesthetic solution is attached to the stopcock, and the syringe is fastened at the head of the table with adhesive tape (Figure 261 D, page 397). The table is placed in a 10-degree Trendelenburg (Figure 261 D, page 397).

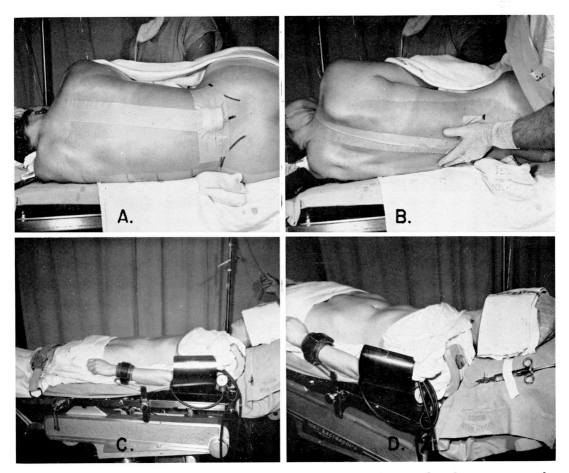

Figure 261. Technique of continuous spinal block (con't.). A. Plastic tubing taped in place—sponge is under tubing. B. Patient is turned supine—hand of anesthetist holds tubing in place at its entrance into skin. C. Patient correctly positioned on table—head elevated, shoulder brace in place, wrist cuffs fastened, knee strap secured, and arm protector in place. D. Syringe attached to stopcock, fastened to head of table, and table in 10 degrees Trendelenburg.

23. The stopcock is opened and 0.2 cc. of the anesthetic solution is slowly injected to fill the plastic tubing, needle, and stopcock (Figure 262, syringe 1 and 2, page 399).

24. The calculated dose is then very slowly injected—1 cc. every 8 to 10 seconds. The initial dose should be one-fourth less than that of tetracaine or procaine given for single-dose spinal blocks (see page 370 to page 387). *It cannot be too strongly stressed that the injection must be slow so that the local anesthetic solution just drips out of the tubing. If a rapid injection is made, the local anesthetic solution will come out of the tubing in a jet-like stream because of the small diameter of the tubing, and increase the danger of high or total analgesia!*

25. After the initial dose is injected, the stopcock is shut (Figure 262, syringe 3, page 399).

26. At the end of each 45 minutes after a procaine injection and at the end of each 1¼ to 1½ hours after a tetracaine injection, a reinforcing dose is given. The milligram dosage of the first reinforcing dose usually is reduced to three-fourths of the initial dose.

27. To reduce the number of milligrams in the reinforcing doses, but maintain the volume, the stopcock is opened and the local anesthetic solution remaining in the syringe, tubing, needle, and stopcock, is diluted with spinal fluid by aspirating until the syringe again contains 10 cc. The withdrawal of spinal fluid into the syringe may be very slow and tedious due to the small inner diameter of the plastic tubing. The anesthetist must have patience at this point and *"tease"* the spinal fluid into the syringe by either gentle traction on the plunger of the syringe or opening the stopcock 10 to 15 minutes prior to the first reinforcing dose and allowing the spinal fluid pressure to slowly fill the syringe to the 10 cc. mark. The amount of solution necessary to fill the plastic tubing, needle, and stopcock (0.2 cc.) is reinjected and then the calculated reinforcing dose is injected *very slowly.* For example, using tetracaine:

The plastic tubing, needle, and stopcock hold approximately 0.2 cc. (Figure 262, syringe 2, page 399).

If the initial dose was 10 mg. or 2.5 cc. of the tetracaine solution, the contents of the plastic tubing, needle, and stopcock (0.2 cc.) plus the contents of the syringe (7.3 cc.) will amount to 30 mg. (4 mg. per cc.) or 7.5 cc. of tetracaine solution (Figure 262, syringe 3, page 399).

The first reinforcing dose should be approximately three-fourths of the initial 10 mg. dose or 7.5 mg. of tetracaine. To assure an adequate volume, the tetracaine solution in the plastic tubing, needle, and stopcock, i.e., 0.2 cc., *plus 2.5 cc. of spinal fluid,* is aspirated until there is 10 cc. in the syringe. Now each cubic centimeter of the tetracaine solution in the syringe contains 3 mg. (Figure 262, syringe 4, page 399).

0.2 cc. is reinjected to fill the tubing, needle, and stopcock (Figure 262, syringe 5, page 399) and then the reinforcing dose of 7.5 mg. of tetracaine in 2.5 cc. of solution is injected (Figure 262, syringe 6, page 399). The stopcock is shut. *After the first reinforcing dose, successive reinforcing doses are given without further dilution of the anesthetic solution remaining in the syringe and tubing. Such doses are usually slightly smaller than the first reinforcing dose, i.e., 6 mg. of tetracaine (2 cc. of solution) in the above example.*

The operating table is usually placed in a 5- to 10-degree Trendelenburg position for the reinforcing injection. The reinforcing dose should be carefully watched to see that it does not rise too high. Should the operating table be in steep Trendelenburg, *i.e.,* more than 10 degrees, all the reinforcing doses may have to be reduced to ½ of the initial dose to avoid high levels of anesthesia.

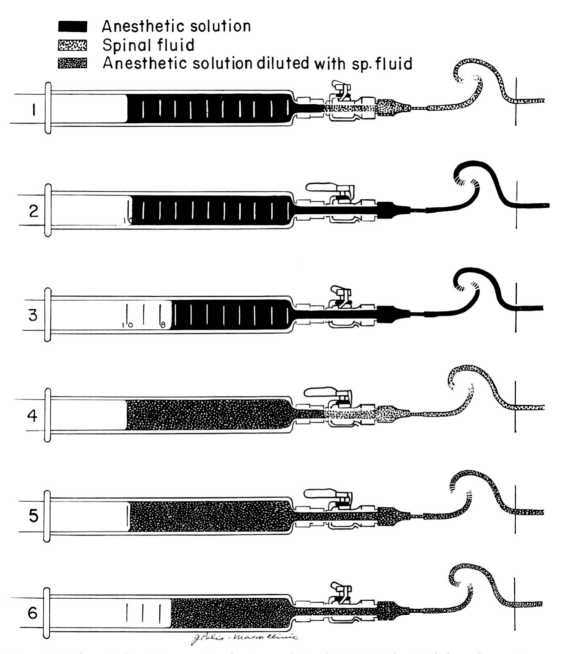

Figure 262. Schematic drawing representing the steps used in administering the initial dose of a continuous spinal anesthetic as well as the reinforcing dose. 1. Syringe filled with the local anesthetic agent. 2. Tubing filled with the local anesthetic solution. 3. Initial dose given. 4. Local anesthetic solution diluted with spinal fluid in preparation for the first reinforcing dose. 5. Tubing filled with the local anesthetic solution which has been diluted with spinal fluid. 6. Administration of the first reinforcing dose.

28. If the 40 mg. of tetracaine is not adequate for the entire surgical procedure, the syringe is disconnected and 2.0 cc. of a 1 percent solution of tetracaine (20 mg.) and 3 cc. of a 10 percent dextrose solution are drawn into it through a sterile needle. The syringe is reconnected to the stopcock, the stopcock opened, and 2 cc. of spinal fluid added to the

solution in the syringe. Each 1.0 cc. of solution in the syringe now contains approximately 3 mg. of tetracaine and further reinforcing doses can be injected.

Actually, each cubic centimeter of solution will contain slightly less than 3 mg. of tetracaine because a very small amount of local anesthetic agent from the previous dose is in the tubing, needle, and stopcock. This small amount less can be disregarded.

29. When the operation is completed, either the tubing may be slowly withdrawn or it may be left in the subarachnoid space for a 12- to 24-hour period.

At our institution, most resections of the abdominal aorta are performed with continuous spinal block and at the end of the operation the tubing is not removed for at least two reasons. First, temporary vascular insufficiency of a lower extremity may develop which is relieved by sympathetic block—this is effected by the injection of 3 mg. of tetracaine in 1.0 cc. of 10 percent dextrose into the subarachnoid space through the plastic tubing. Second, if a serious vascular insufficiency of the lower extremity develops which requires emergency surgery, the means of immediately establishing anesthesia is available. Plastic tubing which is left in the subarachnoid space for 12 to 24 hours does not cause serious complications, provided reasonable antiseptic precautions are taken. If signs of meningeal irritation, i.e., stiff neck or headache, develop; the tubing is removed immediately and the signs of meningeal irritation disappear in 6 to 12 hours.

30. When the tubing is withdrawn, it should be examined to be sure that it is the same length as it was when it was introduced into the subarachnoid space.

EXTENT OF ANALGESIA

Any number of dermatomes can be anesthetized with this block. The surgical procedure determines the number of dermatomes which must be paralyzed (see pages 370 to 387).

COMPLICATIONS

Same as single-dose spinal block. See page 353.

REMARKS

The remarks found under Single-Dose Spinal (Subarachnoid) Block, page 361 to 369, also apply here and should be reviewed.

Use of Vasoconstrictor Drugs in Subarachnoid Space Has Reduced Need of Continuous Technique: The use of vasoconstrictor drugs subarachnoidally has greatly reduced the necessity of employing continuous spinal analgesia. Even in upper abdominal operations single dose spinal analgesia with tetracaine will last 3 to 4 hours when phenylephrine (Neo-Synephrine) is incorporated in the local anesthetic solution and 2 to 2¼ hours when epinephrine (Adrenalin) is used (see Table XI, page 482).

Whenever Possible, Continuous Techniques Are Avoided: Most anesthetists avoid continuous spinal analgesia whenever possible because of the technical difficulties and the length of time necessary to place the tubing and establish analgesia.

Sterilization of Tuohy Needle, Plastic Tubing, Tuohy-Borst Adapter, One-way Stopcock, and Plug for Stopcock: All of these items are heat sterilized in separate containers—for method of heat sterilization (see page 50). When a continuous technique is to be used, the additional items needed are opened and emptied onto the regional block tray.

Plastic Tubing.—Heat will kill bacteria but steam is necessary to eliminate spores. Steam will neither pass through the wall of the plastic tubing nor will it enter the lumen of a small tube—an air lock is formed in its lumen. Therefore, the lumen of the plastic tubing can not be sterilized by heat unless it contains water which becomes steam when the temperature in the autoclave rises above 250 degrees Fahrenheit. Furthermore, steam will not penetrate the sealed plastic bag in which the tubing with its stylet is placed for sterilization—

some means of assuring steam entering the bag or forming in the bag must be provided.

For these reasons the following steps are performed when the plastic tubing is heat sterilized. First, it is marked with a felt marking pen 5¾ inches (14.5 cm.) from the end to be inserted into the subarachnoid space. Second, the tubing is filled with 0.2 cc. of water. Third, the stylet is inserted into the tubing. Fourth, the tubing and stylet are placed in a plastic bag. Fifth, 1 cc. of water is placed in the plastic bag and the bag sealed or the bag is sealed and holes are punched in the bag so that the steam can enter it. Sixth, the bag is wrapped in a towel with a sterilizer control (Diack). Seventh, sterilizer control tape is used to keep the towel from opening. Eighth, the package is dated and signed by the person

preparing the package. And, then the package is autoclaved immediately (Figure 263, page 401).

Tuohy Needle, 23-Gauge Needle, Stopcock, and Plug for Stopcock.—These are placed in a large test tube and sterilized together. They are the items most frequently used by the author for a continuous technique (Figure 264, page 402).

Tuohy-Borst Adapter.—The adapter should be disassembled and the parts should be sterilized in a large test tube. The adapter is reassembled at the time it is to be used. This adapter relies on the compression of a rubber gasket to form a tight seal around the tubing. If the gasket is brittle, etc., a complete seal will not be effected. Since the adapter must be

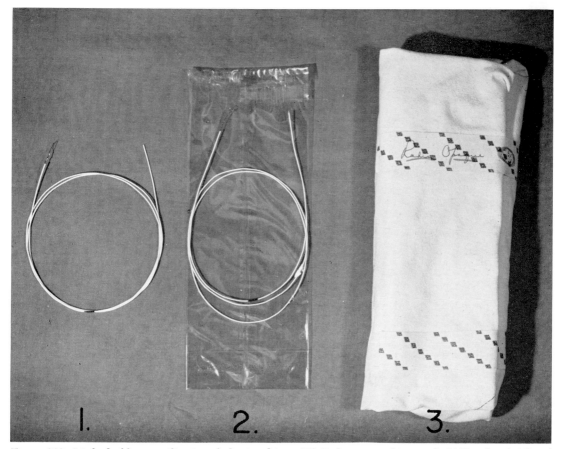

Figure 263. Method of heat sterilization of plastic tubing. (1) Radiopaque tubing marked 5¾ inches (14.5 cm.) from the end to be inserted. 0.2 cc. of water is placed in lumen of tube and stylet inserted. (2) Tubing placed in plastic bag. 1 cc. of water placed in plastic bag. Bag sealed. (3) Bag wrapped in wrapper with sterilizer control (Diack). Wrapper sealed with sterilizer tape. Package then autoclaved.

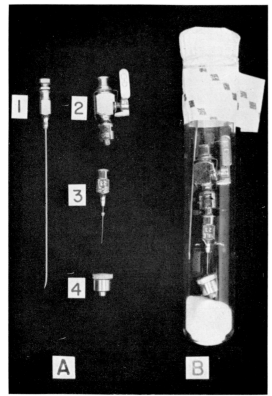

Figure 264. A. 1. Tuohy needle. 2. One-way stop-cock. 3. 23-gauge needle. 4. Plug for adapter. B. The items in A are all placed in a test tube and heat sterilized. When a continuous technique is to be used, they are dumped onto the open regional block tray.

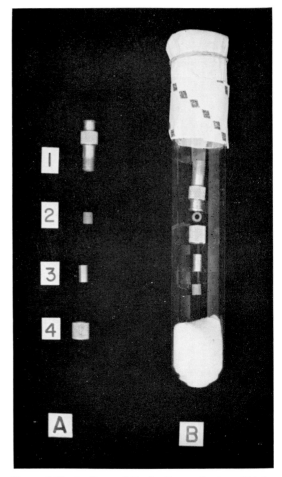

Figure 265. A. Parts of Tuohy-Borst adapter: (1) female end; (2) rubber gasket; (3) metal compressor collar; and (4) screw nut. B. The adapter parts should be heat sterilized together in a large test tube and assembled at time the adapter is to be used. This adapter relies on compression of the rubber gasket around the tubing. If the gasket is brittle—this can occur from repeated heat sterilizations—a complete seal will not be effected. The adapter must be tightened securely on the tubing, otherwise it will leak. Usually two rubber gaskets are sterilized as a precautionary measure.

tightened securely on the tubing to prevent leakage, the gasket must be examined prior to assembly to be sure it is in good condition. The 23-gauge needle is preferred to the Tuohy-Borst adapter by us because of the mechanical difficulties that can arise with the adapter (Figure 265, page 402).

Monitor Patient Carefully: The patient should be carefully watched through the entire procedure but, in particular, after the injection of each dose whether it be the initial or reinforcing dose. Blood pressure falls and complications, which are more likely to occur after an injection, should not go untreated.

Establishment of Surgical Analgesia May Be Slow: Surgical analgesia may not be established for as long as 10 minutes with procaine solutions and 15 minutes with tetracaine solutions.

Give Reinforcing Dose Before Patient Has Pain: The analgesia must not be allowed to wear off. Once it has and the patient feels pain, it may be difficult to re-establish satisfactory analgesia.

Number of Reinforcing Doses Are Not Limited: There is no limit to the number of reinforcing doses which may be given for an operation.

Incidence of Spinal Headache Is Increased: With the use of a large needle and the insertion of the plastic tubing, there is some increase in the incidence of headaches over that of single dose spinal.

Use Stylet in Plastic Tubing: The stylet remains in the plastic tubing while threading it through the needle to facilitate its introduction. The plastic tubing for continuous spinal blocks does not come with a stylet and the manufacturer states that none is necessary for its insertion. However, it has been found through unfortunate experiences that this is not true. Stylets may be purchased (see footnote, page 389), obtained from a number 5 ureteral catheter, or a stylet may be made from 28- or 26-gauge stainless steel surgical wire available in the supply room of most operating suites. *The stylet should be partially removed with each advancement of the tubing beyond the point of the needle.* If this is not done, withdrawal of the stylet may be extremely difficult.

Continuous Spinal Block May Be Used To Produce Prolonged Sympathetic Block: When prolonged lumbar sympathetic block is indicated in the treatment of a vascular insufficiency of the extremity in a hospitalized patient and repeated lumbar sympathetic blocks are contraindicated, a continuous spinal block may be helpful. If this procedure is instituted, care of the bladder and rectum are of prime importance and the need for such care should be anticipated. Tachyphylaxis to repeated doses of tetracaine or procaine in the subarachnoid space has not been observed.

Mark Distance Plastic Tubing Is To Be Inserted: The distance the plastic tubing is to be inserted should be marked with a felt marking pen or a ball point pen prior to sterilization. Marking of the plastic tubing serves two purposes: (1) it permits placement of the tubing the correct distance into the subarachnoid space, and (2) it allows the physician to recognize whether the tubing was dislodged from the subarachnoid space when the 18-gauge needle and stylet are withdrawn. This mark should be approximately 5¾ inches (14.5

cm.) from the end which is to be placed subarachnoidally—3 inches (7.5 cm.) for the length of the shaft of the needle; ¾ inch (2.0 cm.) for the length of the hub of the needle; and 2 inches (5 cm.) for beyond the point of the needle.

Can the Position of the Plastic Tubing in the Subarachnoid Space Consistently Be Predicted? The spinal fluid offers little or no resistance to the passage of the tubing, nor does it fix the tubing in place in the subarachnoid space. Therefore, when the plastic tubing is placed in the subarachnoid space for a distance greater than 2 inches (5 cm.), the answer to this question is "No." *Only by inserting radiopaque tubing and checking its placement by x-ray can its direction in the subarachnoid space be ascertained with any certainty (Figure 266, page 404 and Figure 267, page 405).* For this reason, we seldom insert the tubing more than 2 inches (5 cm.) in the subarachnoid space. When the tubing is inserted for only 2 inches (5 cm.) the tip's approximate position is usually known and the dose can be determined more accurately.

Difficulties May Be Encountered When Plastic Tubing Is Inserted More Than 2 Inches (5 cm.) Into the Subarachnoid Space: If the plastic tubing is inserted more than 2 inches (5 cm.) into the subarachnoid space, the following may occur: (1) it may kink; (2) turn 180 degrees and go in the opposite direction to that in which it was inserted; (3) wrap around a nerve and be difficult to remove; (4) elicit severe paresthesias; and (5) a combination of these. Also, when the tubing is inserted purposely or inadvertently for more than 2 inches (5 cm.) in a cephalad direction a high or total spinal may result, unless the doses are markedly reduced.

Should Regular or Radiopaque Plastic Tubing be Used? The principal disadvantage of the non-radiopaque tubing is that its location cannot be determined if the block is inadequate or if the tubing breaks. The principal disadvantage of the radiopaque tubing is the ability to locate it if it does break.

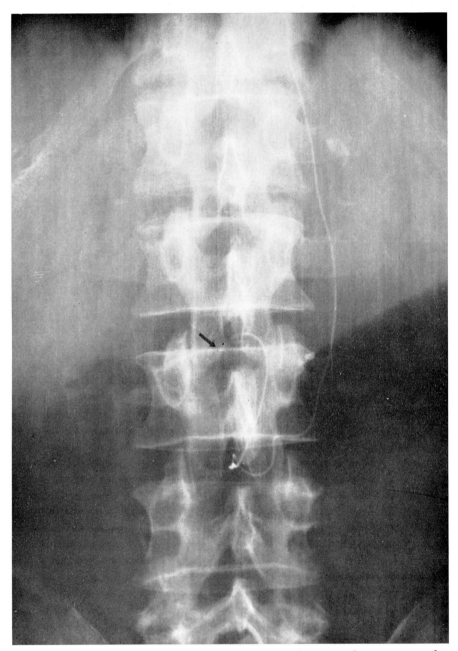

Figure 266. X-ray of the plastic tubing in the subarachnoid space. Tubing was inserted at the interspace between the second and third lumbar vertebrae, using a Tuohy needle with the opening in the bevel pointing cephalad. It was threaded 2 inches into the subarachnoid space, and after moving cephalad to the interspace between the second and third lumbar vertebrae, it turned to point caudad (arrow). This patient had a repair of a hiatus hernia. She is 5 feet, 3 inches tall; weighs 235 pounds; and is 48 years old. The initial dose of hyperbaric tetracaine (Pontocaine) was 8 mg. The table was in 10-degree Trendelenburg. Anesthesia level was to the third thoracic dermatome.

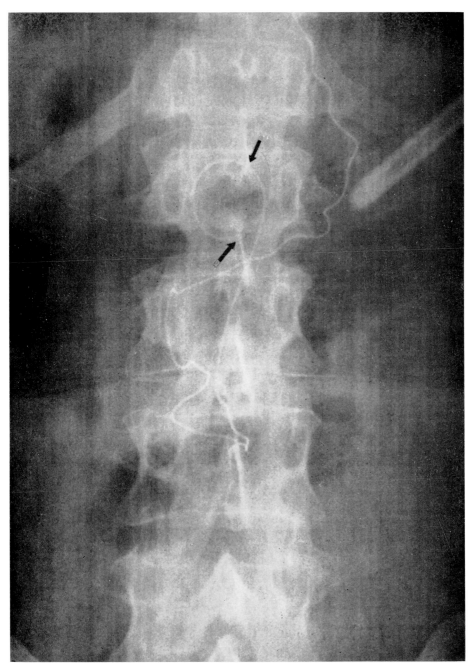

Figure 267. X-ray of plastic tubing in the subarachnoid space. Tubing was inserted at the interspace between the second and third lumbar vertebrae with the opening in the bevel of the Tuohy needle pointing cephalad. It was inserted for 4 inches (10 cm.) into the subarachnoid space. It went cephalad to the first lumbar vertebra, turned 180 degrees and its tip lies at the interspace between the first and second lumbar vertbrae (arrows). This 61 year old patient had a cystotomy and bladder tumor removed. He is 5 feet, 7 inches tall and weighs 122 pounds. The initial dose of hyperbaric tetracaine (Pontocaine) was 10 mg. The table was level. Anesthesia level was to the sixth thoracic dermatome.

Vinyl plastic tubing is inert and when left in the body, seldom, if ever, causes any difficulty. But if it can be located in the subarachnoid space, the question arises: Should it be removed? To remove it may subject the patient to an unnecessary, hazardous operation. To not remove it may provoke a medicolegal situation—the ramifications of which are too numerous to list.

Therefore, the type of tubing a physician selects is one of personal choice. Regardless of which type is selected, a broken piece of tubing in a patient presents a difficult problem. Whether an attempt to retrieve the tubing is made depends on the circumstances and should involve consultation with other specialists and the anesthetist's insurance company. Nonetheless, the patient must be informed of such a mishap and should participate in the decision as to whether the tubing should be removed.

Inject Anesthesia Solution Slowly: *With the catheter technique, very slow injection of the local anesthetic solution is mandatory, i.e., no faster than 1.0 cc. every 8-10 seconds. The solution should not be instilled subarachnoidally in a jet-like stream.*

Close One-way Stopcock Between Doses: If this is not done, too great a dilution of the local anesthetic solution may result.

Recover Broken Needle(s): See page 369.

CHAPTER 46

Single-Dose Epidural (Peridural) Block

M ANY ANESTHETISTS are electing to perform epidural blocks rather than spinal blocks. Probably several reasons account for this: (1) publicity in medical publications, newspapers, and lay magazines has emphasized the theory that neurological complications developing after spinal anesthesia are necessarily a result of the anesthetic technique itself; (2) the courts have awarded large sums of money to patients paralyzed after spinal anesthesia, without demanding proof that the anesthetic technique or negligence was involved; that is, simply on the basis of "res ipsa loquitur" (meaning, "the condition speaks for itself"); (3) many malpractice policies will not cover the administration of spinal anesthesia; and (4) epidural blocks usually circumvent the minor complications of spinal anesthesia such as headache and backache and the objection of some patients to spinal anesthesia (see page 424).

DEFINITION

An epidural block results from the injection of the local anesthetic solution into the epidural space in the cervical, thoracic, or lumbar area of the vertebral column.

INDICATIONS

Surgical: It may be used for operations of the retroperitoneal area, back, chest, abdominal wall, abdominal cavity, perineum, and lower extremities. It can be employed for cesarean sections and vaginal deliveries.

Diagnostic: Differentiation of autonomic nervous system diseases from organic diseases; for example, arteriosclerotic vascular insufficiencies from vasospastic diseases.

Therapeutic: Treatment of vascular occlusions and spasms of the lower extremity (see page 211). Emboli usually are not in themselves aided, but the associated spasm is relieved, which may give a more advantageous amputation site.

Relief of pain such as that caused by acute pancreatitis or mesenteric thrombosis, which is difficult to control with opiates.

Treatment of anuria caused by chemotherapy and blood transfusions.

ANATOMY

The epidural space lies between the dura mater on the one side and, on the other side, the ligaments and periosteum lining the vertebral canal (Figure 268, page 408 and Figure 269, page 408). It extends from the foramen magnum, where the periosteum of the skull and the dura fuse, to the sacrococcygeal membrane.

The epidural space is filled with loose areolar tissue, blood vessels, and lymphatics, but solutions injected into it can pass up and down between these anatomical structures (Figure 270, page 409). The arterial supply is meager, but the plexuses of veins are numerous and they are found principally in the lateral aspect of the epidural space (Figure 270, page 409).

PREMEDICATION

Paresthesias are not sought. Heavy medication is advised except in the geriatric patient, the pregnant patient, and patient of poor physical status.

Heavy Premedication: The average patient (age 20 to 50, weight 150 pounds or over,

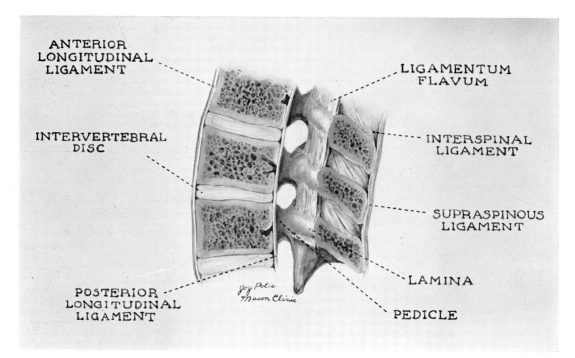

ANTERIOR
LONGITUDINAL
LIGAMENT

INTERVERTEBRAL
DISC

POSTERIOR
LONGITUDINAL
LIGAMENT

LIGAMENTUM
FLAVUM

INTERSPINAL
LIGAMENT

SUPRASPINOUS
LIGAMENT

LAMINA

PEDICLE

Figure 268. Sagittal section of ligaments and bones of the vertebrae which form the outside wall of the epidural space.

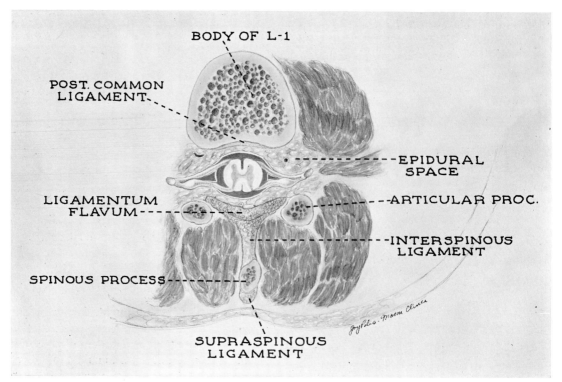

BODY OF L-1

POST. COMMON
LIGAMENT

LIGAMENTUM
FLAVUM

SPINOUS PROCESS

SUPRASPINOUS
LIGAMENT

EPIDURAL
SPACE

ARTICULAR PROC.

INTERSPINOUS
LIGAMENT

Figure 269. Cross section at level of the first lumbar vertebra showing structures of epidural space and the surrounding anatomy.

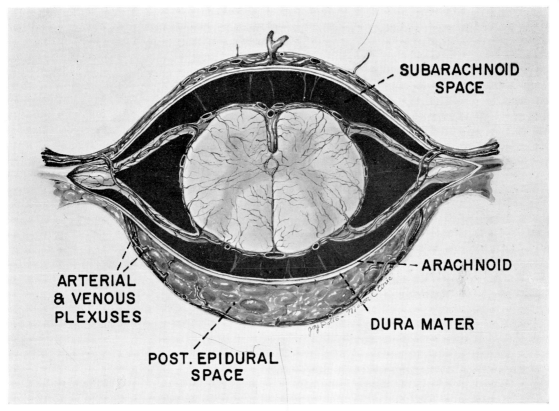

Figure 270. Cross section of epidural space and its contents.

height 5 feet, 5 inches or over, and good physical status) receives:

1. 200 mg. (3 gr.) of pentobarbital (Nembutal) by mouth at hour of sleep the night before surgery.

2. 100 mg. (1½ gr.) to 200 mg. (3 gr.) of pentobarbital with one ounce of water by mouth 1½ to 2 hours before estimated *block* time.

3. 15 mg. (¼ gr.) of morphine and 0.6 mg. (¹⁄₁₀₀ gr.) of scopolamine intramuscularly ¾ to 1 hour before estimated *block* time.

Reduction of Premedication: It is seldom necessary to increase this premedication irrespective of the over-all size of the patient until the patient arrives in either the anesthesia or operating room. However, it is very common to reduce this medication under various circumstances; for example, in the case of the geriatric patient, the adolescent patient or

child, the debilitated or cachectic patient, the pregnant patient (see page 410), and for those whose surgery is complicated by other disease, *e.g.*, myxedema, diabetes, heart disease, etc. In the patient over 60 years of age, barbiturates and especially scopolamine often cause disorientation. Therefore, in these patients atropine is usually substituted for scopolamine and the dosage of the barbiturate omitted or greatly reduced, *i.e.*, to 50 mg. (¾ gr.) or less. *Always err on the light side.*

Inadequate Premedication: If medication is inadequate for surgery or the block procedure, pentobarbital 50 mg. (¾ gr.) to 100 mg. (1½ gr.), morphine 10 mg. (¹⁄₆ gr.), or preferably small amounts of 0.6 percent thiopental (Pentothal) or 0.2 percent methohexital (Brevital) may be given slowly intravenously until the desired effect results. Judicious use of added sedation is extremely important. Often small supplementary doses of thiopental or methohexital, will make a block successful when a patient interprets touch and motion as pain.

Premedication of the Patient in Labor: All barbiturates, narcotics, belladonna derivatives, tranquilizers, and combinations of these drugs will pass the placenta and equilibrate in the fetus in the same period of time as they do in the mother. Therefore, little or no premedication is advised—the epidural block will relieve the pain.

If premedication is to be given to allay the parturient's fears and apprehensions, a reasonable dosage of drugs which will not significantly depress the fetus should be used, e.g., meperidine (Demerol) 50 mg. and promethazine (Phenergan) 25 mg.

DRUGS

Tetracaine (Pontocaine) or procaine (Novocain) alone is seldom selected for epidural block. The rapid onset and constant results of lidocaine (Xylocaine), mepivacaine (Carbocaine), and chloroprocaine (Nesacaine) make them the agents of choice for this block.

Solutions containing methylparaben and metabisulfite should not be used (see Remarks, page 425).

Lidocaine (Xylocaine) or Mepivacaine (Carbocaine)

Dosage.—10 cc. to 20 cc. of 1.0 to 1.5 percent solution with or without 0.1 cc. of epinephrine (Adrenalin) 1:1000 in 20 cc. of the local anesthetic solution.*

Onset.—Operating analgesia is established in 10 to 20 minutes.

Duration.—Operating analgesia lasts 1¼ to 2 hours, with stronger concentrations containing epinephrine giving the upper limits.

Lidocaine (Xylocaine) or Mepivacaine (Carbocaine) with Tetracaine (Pontocaine): Tetracaine may be incorporated in either a lidocaine or mepivacaine solution to prolong the duration of action of these two solutions. Either of these mixtures is the author's choice for executing an epidural block.

Dosage.—10 to 20 cc. of the following solution is injected. *More than 20 cc. of this solution should not be used for any one dose, and in many surgical procedures a smaller volume is adequate, particularly when the segmental type of analgesia is sought.*

> 25 cc. of a 1.5 percent solution of lidocaine or mepivacaine.
>
> 50 mg. of tetracaine crystals.
>
> 0.1 cc. of epinephrine (Adrenalin) 1:1000.*
>
> ———
>
> 25.1 cc.

Onset.—Operating analgesia is established in 10 to 20 minutes.

Duration.—Operating analgesia lasts 2½ to 3 hours.

Chloroprocaine (Nesacaine): See Remarks, page 425.

Dosage.—10 to 20 cc. of a 2.0 percent solution with or without 0.1 cc. of epinephrine (Adrenalin) 1:1000 in 20 cc. of the local anesthetic solution.*

Onset.—Operating analgesia is established in 10 to 20 minutes.

Duration.—Operating analgeisa lasts ¾ to 1¼ hours, with solutions containing epinephrine giving the upper limits.

MATERIALS

Regional tray (see Chapter 9, page 51) or:

1. One ¾-inch (2 cm.), 25-gauge Huber point security Lok-needle.

2. One 1½-inch (3.8 cm.), 22-gauge security Lok-needle.

3. One 19-gauge, 3-inch (7.5 cm.) spinal Lok-needle, preferably with a short bevel.

———

*Optimal concentration of epinephrine is 1:200,000, that is, 0.1 cc. of epinephrine 1:1000 in 20 cc. of the local anesthetic solution (see page 426).

4. One tuberculin Lok-syringe for measuring epinephrine.

5. One 3 cc. Lok-syringe.

6. One 5 cc. Lok-syringe.

7. One 10 cc. Lok-syringe.

8. One prep cup.

9. One graduated measuring cup, preferably stainless steel, for mixing solution.

10. One Allis forceps.

11. One sponge forceps.

12. One Pitkin or thin-walled needle guide.*

13. Four towels.

14. Four 4 x 4 sponges.

15. One sterilizer control.

TECHNIQUE

Landmarks

A line is drawn between the iliac crests (Figure 224, page 344 and Figure 271 A, page 412).

2. This line crosses either the spinous process of the fourth lumbar vertebra or the interspace between the spinous processes of the fourth and fifth lumbar vertebrae, i.e., fourth lumbar interspace (Figure 224, page 344).

3. Counting cephalad, the desired lumbar interspace may be easily determined.

4. Theoretically, at least, the epidural space may be entered through C1 through L5. It may also be entered via the caudal canal (see Chapter 48, page 439). While the epidural space may be entered via the interspaces of the vertebrae from C1 through L5, the site of choice for the physician who is learning epidural block is in the midline in the lumbar region, i.e., the interspaces between T12 to L5

*These items may be obtained from Becton, Dickinson and Company. Order number for Pitkin needle guide is PNG and for thin-walled needle guide is 01-0027.

because of the following anatomical reasons: (1) the interspinous ligaments and ligamenta flava are thickest in the midline; (2) the epidural space is widest in the midline (Figure 270, page 409); (3) the venous sinuses and the arterial supply are less dense in the midline than they are laterally; and (4) the angle of the slopes of the spinous processes of the lumbar vertebrae are less acute (compare Figure 221, page 342 with Figure 222, page 343).

Position

Lateral Decubitus (Side).—This position is the most frequently employed position since it requires the least effort on the part of the patient and assistants are not a necessity. The patient is placed on his right or left side with his knees drawn up to his stomach, his upper arm lying across his chest, his lower arm at a right angle to his body, and his head flexed, resting on a small pillow (Figure 225, page 344 and Figure 271 A, page 412). Every effort is made to keep the spinous processes of the vertebral column parallel to the table and the patient well-flexed so as to open the interspaces.

If an assistant is not available to hold the patient in the above position, it may be simulated by the patient clasping his hands either behind his head and trying to make his elbows and knees touch (see Figure 227, page 345) or under his knees and pulling up his knees toward his stomach (see Figure 226, page 345).

Regarding this position, the anesthetist should recognize that in an obese patient the skin line marking the middle of the back may be pulled by the weight of the fat so that it lies 1 inch (2.5 cm.) to 1½ inches (3.8 cm.) below the spinous process.

Sitting.—The patient sits on the edge of the table with his legs over the side of the table, his feet on a stool, his head flexed on the chest, and his arms folded across his upper abdomen (Figure 228 A and B, page 346). An assistant should at all times steady the patient so that he does not fall off the table (Figure

228, page 346). See comment on page 345 under *Sitting*.

Precautions

Monitor Blood Pressure.—A preanesthetic check of the blood pressure is mandatory.

Aspirate for Spinal Fluid and Blood.—Check carefully by aspiration in four planes, *i.e.,* 90 degree rotation of the needle each time, for spinal fluid or blood. *The large amounts of anesthetic solution required by the block (15 times the dosage for spinal block) make either an inadvertent dural puncture or an intravascular injection a very serious complication. Therefore, this procedure must not be undertaken unless the physician is prepared to han-*

dle a serious systemic toxic reaction or a long lasting total spinal anesthesia.

Procedure

1. The sterilizer control is checked to be sure the equipment is sterile.

2. The anesthetist aseptically prepares the skin, and places a sterile towel over the side.

3. A skin wheal is raised over the selected interspace with the ¾-inch (2 cm.), 25-gauge Huber point security Lok-needle, using 0.2 cc. to 0.3 cc. of the local anesthetic solution (Figure 271 B, page 412).

4. 0.8 cc. to 1.5 cc. of the local anesthetic solution is infiltrated into the interspinous ligament.

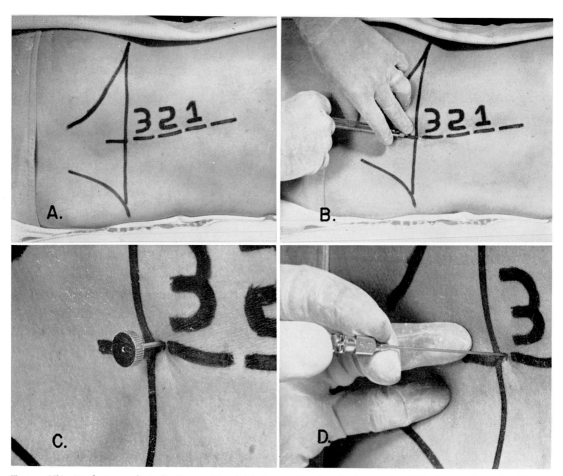

Figure 271. Technique of single dose epidural block. A. Landmarks for epidural block. B. Skin wheal being made at second lumbar interspace. C. Hole made in skin wheal with needle introducer. D. 19-gauge spinal needle placed in interspinous ligament.

5. The Pitkin or thin-walled needle guide is placed through the skin wheal to make a hole in the skin which will accommodate the 19-gauge spinal needle (Figure 271C, page 412). The needle guide is removed. Usually, this prevents the 19-gauge needle carrying with it a skin plug and skin bacteria into the epidural space.

6. The 19-gauge spinal needle with a short bevel is held by the anesthetist so that the thumb exerts pressure on the stylet's top and the shaft is supported between the index and middle fingers (Figure 271 D, page 412). This prevents displacement of the stylet and allows the anesthetist to steady his hand by resting the ring and little fingers on the patient's back (Figure 271 D, page 412).

7. The needle is then inserted through the hole in the skin wheal and carefully and slowly advanced 1 inch (2.5 cm.) to 1¼ inches (3.2 cms.) until its point lies in the substance of the interspinous ligament (Figure 271 D, page 412).

The index and middle (long) fingers of the free hand should straddle the interspace into which the needle is to be placed. Great care should be taken that the needle lies in the same plane as the spinous processes and perpendicular to the transverse processes. If it points upward or downward, or if the patient's back is not at a 90-degree angle in the vertical plane with the table, the spinal needle may not travel a true course (Figure 233, page 349).

8. One of two principal methods is generally used to ascertain when the epidural space has been entered by the needle. We prefer the "loss of resistance" method.

NEGATIVE PRESSURE METHOD.— The stylet is removed from the 19-gauge needle and a drop of the local anesthetic solution is placed in the hub of the needle—this is commonly referred to as the "hanging drop method" (Figure 272A, page 413 and Figure 273A, page 414).*

*A variation of the negative pressure method is the use of the glass adapter (Figure 274, page 414 and Figure 275, page 415).

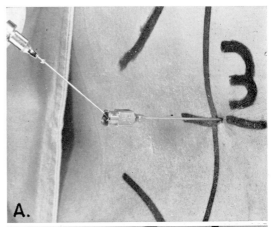

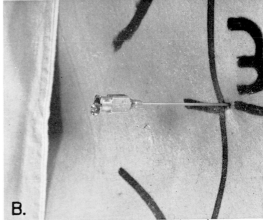

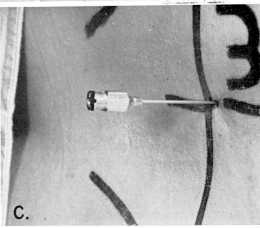

Figure 272. Hanging drop method of entering epidural space. A. Drop of fluid is placed in hub of needle whose point rests in ligamentum flavum or anterior portion of interspinous ligament. B. Large drop of fluid at opening in hub. C. As needle is slowly advanced into epidural space and drop of fluid is sucked into needle.

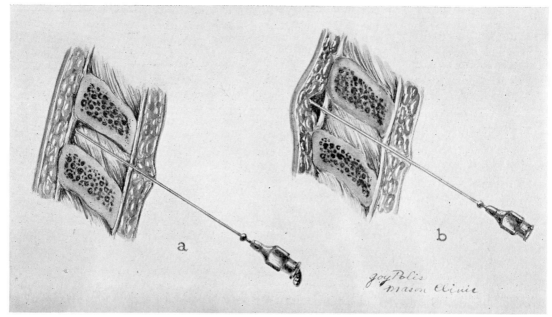

Figure 273. Sagittal section demonstrating hanging drop. A. Drop of fluid is placed in hub of needle whose point rests in ligamentum flavum or anterior portion of interspinous ligament. B. As needle is slowly advanced into epidural space the drop of fluid is sucked into needle.

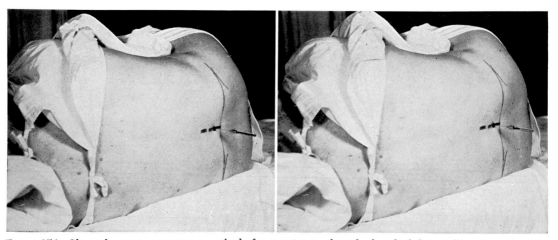

Figure 274. Glass adapter or manometer method of ascertaining when the bevel of the needle rests in the epidural space. A. *(Left)* Needle rests in the interspinous ligament. The glass adapter is filled. N.B. Indigo carmine was used in the glass adapter for photographic illustration. B. *(Right)* Needle rests in epidural space. The fluid in the glass adapter has been sucked in.

The needle is now *slowly* advanced until it is felt to pierce the ligamentum flavum and the drop of fluid in the hub of the needle is sucked inward by the apparent negative pressure in the epidural space (Figure 272 C, page 413 and Figure 273 B, page 414). *Remember that if the needle is advanced slowly it will pass* *through the tough ligamentum flavum with somewhat of a snap.*

When the point of the needle first enters the epidural space in the cervical, thoracic, or lumbar area, air or fluid is sucked from the needle into the epidural space. Yet it is highly unlikely that a

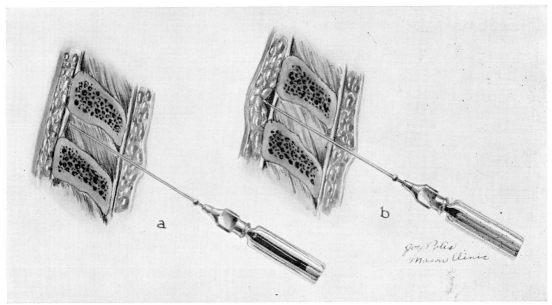

Figure 275. Sagittal section demonstrating glass tubing or manometer method of ascertaining when the bevel of the needle rests in the epidural space. A. Needle rests in the interspinous ligament. The glass adapter is filled. B. Needle rests in epidural space. The fluid in the glass adapter has been sucked in.

pre-existing negative pressure in the epidural space is responsible for this phenomenon. It has been fairly conclusively shown that the apparent negative pressure is created by tenting of the dura. This is a result of the needle pushing ahead of it the anatomical structures of the epidural space and the dura (Figure 276, page 416).

LOSS OF RESISTANCE (PRESSURE) METHOD.*—The stylet is removed from the 19-gauge needle and a Lok-syringe, preferably a 3 cc. size, filled with sterile normal saline is attached to the needle (Figure 277, page 416 and Figure 278 A, page 417).

If the anesthetist is right-handed, the index finger and thumb of the right hand grasp the hub of the needle while the other fingers and back of the hand rest firmly against the patient's back (Figure 277, page 416 and Figure 278 A, page 417).

Pressure is exerted against the plunger

---

*A variation of the "loss of resistance" method is the Macintosh balloon (Figure 280, page 419 and Figure 281, page 420).

The "loss of resistance" method, used for locating the epidural space, is based on the principle that if the needle lies in the posterior part of the interspinous ligament or the epidural space and pressure is applied to the plunger of the syringe, fluid will escape. If, on the other hand, the bevel of the needle lies in the anterior portion of the interspinous ligament or the ligamentum flavum, constant hard pressure on the plunger of the syringe will not force fluid from the syringe. Therefore, when performing an epidural puncture with this method the following may be observed. As the needle is placed through the skin and slowly advanced into the posterior portion of the interspinous ligament, fluid may be forced from the syringe. This continues to be possible until the bevel of the needle enters the anterior portion of the interspinous ligament or the ligamentum flavum. At this point no fluid can be forced from the syringe when pressure is exerted on its plunger. This is the cue for the physician administering the anesthesia to proceed carefully. *Constant, unremitting* pressure is now exerted on the plunger of the syringe by one hand as the other slowly advances the needle. As soon as the bevel of the needle or a portion of the bevel enters the epidural space, there is a sudden release of the fluid from the syringe which signals that the epidural space has been entered.

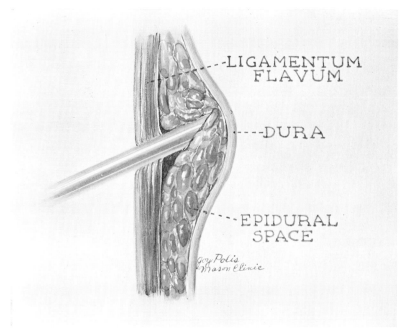

Figure 276. Tenting of dura. Needle pushing contents of epidural space and dura anteriorly—probably this creates negative pressure phenomenon.

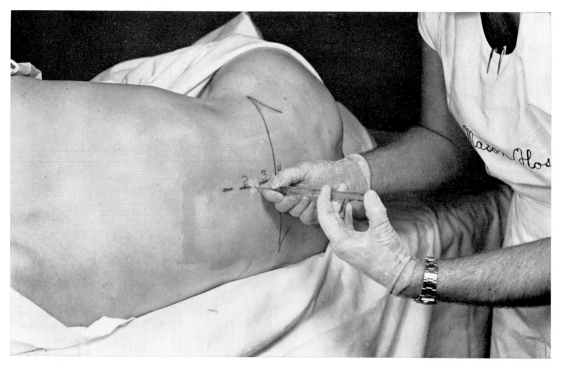

Figure 277. Pressure method of ascertaining when a bevel of the needle rests in the epidural space. Note that the right-handed anesthetist exerts pressure on the barrel of the syringe with his left hand as the right hand *slowly* advances the needle through the interspinous ligament and ligamentum flavum. The back of the right hand rests firmly against the patient's back and the thumb and index finger are used to advance the needle slowly.

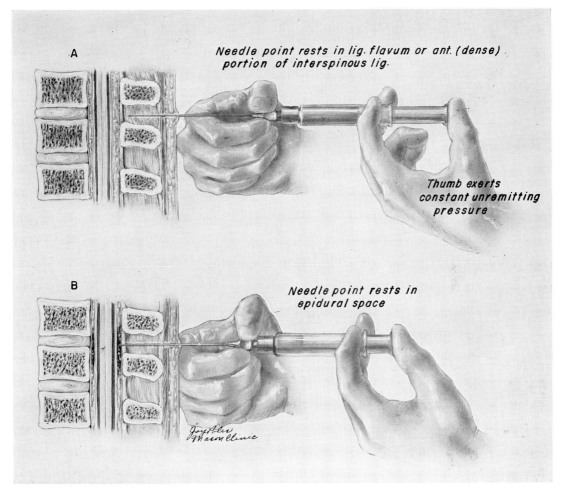

A. Needle point rests in lig. flavum or ant. (dense) portion of interspinous lig.

Thumb exerts constant unremitting pressure

B. Needle point rests in epidural space

Figure 278. Pressure method of ascertaining when the point of the needle rests in the epidural space. A. Needle rests in interspinous ligament. B. Needle rests in epidural space.

of the syringe with the thumb of the left hand. If the solution is easily injected, the needle probably lies in the posterior part of the interspinous ligament (Figure 279, page 418) and it should be slowly advanced a small distance at a time until resistance to pressure on the plunger is met (Figure 278 A, page 417). When the needle lies within the substance of the anterior part of the interspinous ligament or the ligamentum flavum, it is very difficult to force any fluid from the syringe (Figure 278 A, page 417).

The index finger and thumb of the right hand now *very slowly* advance the needle while *constant, unremitting pressure*

is kept on the plunger of the syringe with the left hand (Figure 277, page 416 and Figure 278 A, page 417).

The moment the bevel of the needle enters the epidural space a sudden release of the plunger occurs and the contents of the syringe will be rapidly discharged *if constant, unremitting pressure on the plunger has been exerted* (Figure 278 B, page 417).

The fluid which is under pressure in the needle automatically pushes the dura away from its bevel, and this makes inadvertent spinal taps less likely (Figure 282, page 420). The forward advance-

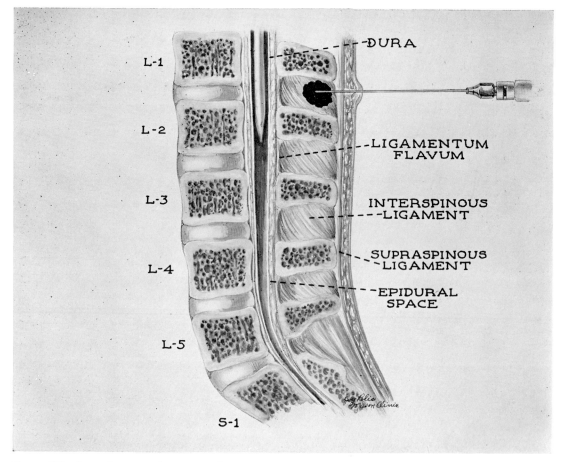

Figure 279. Sagittal section showing needle point resting in posterior portion of interspinous ligament and easy injection of solution.

ment of the needle is immediately stopped, and pressure on the plunger of the syringe suspended. If this advancement has been *very slow* and cautious, the *bevel* of the needle will lie in the epidural space, and ½ to 1½ cc. of the normal saline will remain in the syringe.

9. Careful aspiration tests are made in at least four planes by rotating the needle 90 degrees each time. If no blood or spinal fluid is aspirated, then the anesthetist may continue with the procedure. If blood is obtained, the needle may be inserted one interspace above or below the one in which blood has been obtained. Then should blood still appear, the needle may be advanced into the subarach-

noid space and a single dose or continuous spinal block administered or the regional technique may be abandoned for general anesthesia.

If spinal fluid is obtained, the anesthetist should use spinal block, adjust or reinsert the needle, or he may discard the regional method for general anesthesia. If the needle is placed in the epidural space either by readjustment at the same interspace or by replacement of the needle at another interspace, it has been cautioned that a high or total spinal anesthesia may occur from leakage of the local anesthetic solution from the epidural space into the subarachnoid space through the hole in the dura. This has not been observed by us (see Remarks, page 424).

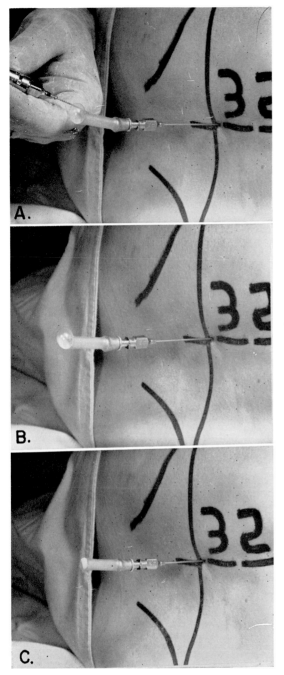

Figure 280. Macintosh balloon method of ascertaining when the bevel of the needle rests in the epidural space. A. Needle rests in ligamentum flavum or anterior portion of the interspinous ligament. With a syringe and needle, air is placed into this apparatus through the thick rubber sleeve just behind metal needle adapter—not into the thin balloon at the end. B. Syringe and needle removed. C. Needle rests in epidural space—balloon has collapsed.

During the aspiration test, the back of the hand not containing the syringe should always rest against the patient's back and the hub of the needle should be held securely between the thumb and index finger of this hand so that the needle will not be moved (Figure 277, page 416).

10. When neither blood nor spinal fluid is obtained, the remaining ½ to 1 cc. of saline in the 3 cc. syringe is discarded and the *rebound test* performed. With this test, 1 to 1.5 cc. of air is aspirated into the 3 cc. syringe. The syringe is connected to the needle and the air rapidly injected. At the end of the downward motion of the plunger of the syringe, quickly release the pressure on the plunger. If the needle is in the epidural space, the syringe will only refill 0.1 cc. to 0.2 cc., or there will be no refill. If the needle is incorrectly placed in a ligament, there will be a refill of from 0.5 cc. to 1.0 cc.

11. Now, 2 cc. of the local anesthetic solution is drawn into the syringe, and it is injected into the epidural space as a test dose.

12. The syringe is disconnected, the stylet is not replaced in the spinal needle, and five minutes time *by the clock* allowed to elapse. *Do not let the patient or the needle be moved.* The needle should be rotated 90 degrees at minute intervals and should be observed constantly for signs of spinal fluid or blood.

Following the placement of the needle in the epidural space and injection of the test dose, it is not uncommon for a few drops of fluid to reflux from the hub of the needle. The question then immediately arises whether the dura has been punctured. This can be determined by the following tests. First, try to aspirate with a syringe containing the local anesthetic agent. If the fluid obtained is of any significant quantity or is of a different viscosity and tends to float into the local anesthetic solution, one should suspect that the dura has been entered. Second, the patient should be asked to take two to three deep breaths. If the drop at the hub of the needle varies with respiration, the bevel probably rests in the epidural space. Third, the drops of the

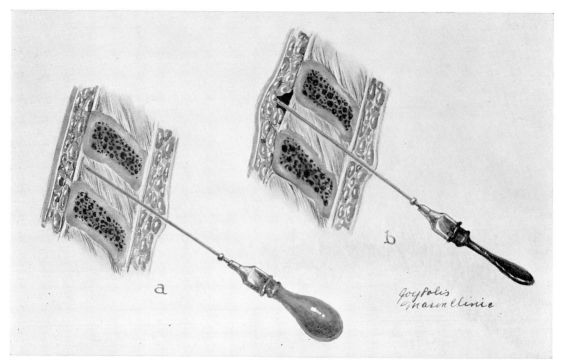

Figure 281. Sagittal section demonstrating Macintosh balloon method of ascertaining when the bevel of the needle rests in the epidural space. A. Needle rests in ligamentum flavum or anterior portion of the interspinous ligament. Air is placed in balloon. B. Needle rests in epidural space—balloon has collapsed.

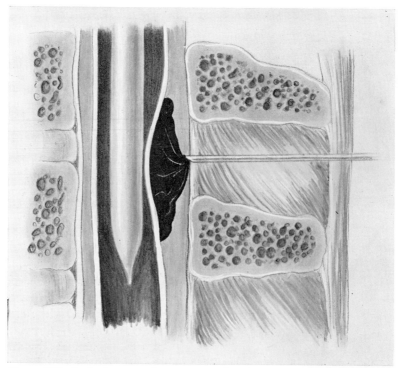

Figure 282. Sagittal section demonstrating that the needle's point rests in epidural space and fluid in syringe is released in a "jet-like" stream pushing contents of epidural space and dura away from the point of the needle.

fluid are allowed to fall on the arm of the physician performing the block. If they are warm, the needle probably rests inside the dura. Lastly, if a 19-gauge or larger gauge needle is used as advocated, the drops of fluid will usually be rapid if the needle rests inside the dura. On the other hand, if the bevel rests in the epidural space, there will be only a few drops of fluid and these will run out relatively slowly.

Carefully monitor the patient's blood pressure, pulse, and sensorium during this period for evidence of a systemic toxic reaction. If one occurs, adjust the needle, remove and reinsert it, advance it, and use spinal anesthesia or abandon the regional technique and administer general anesthesia.

13. If the five minutes pass uneventfully, the lower extremities, abdomen, and chest should be tested for signs of analgesia. When, following a 2 cc. test dose of the local anesthetic solution the area of analgesia is extensive, the dura in all probability has been punctured and further attempts at establishing the epidural block should be discontinued. If the existing spinal block needs to be supplemented, use general anesthesia.

If, as usual, there is no area of analgesia or only a small area of anesthesia or hypesthesia over the distribution of the nerve of the interspace used for the epidural puncture, and if the patient's blood pressure, pulse, and sensorium remain unchanged, it is safe to assume that neither the dura nor a blood vessel has been invaded.

14. Now, the needle is again gripped and steadied with the free hand and after aspiration tests have been performed, another 10 cc. to 20 cc. of the local anesthetic solution is injected—20 cc. is our maximum dose (see page 424 and page 425). The rate of injection, usually ½ to 1 cc. per second, will be regulated by the gauge of the needle and the ability of the epidural space to accommodate the solution. For approximate dosages and site of epidural puncture for a specific surgical procedure see Table IX, page 422. The test dose is disregarded when calculating this dose.

15. At the end of the injection of the local anesthetic solution aspirate for blood or spinal fluid. This serves as a check to assure the anesthetist that the needle was not moved from the epidural space into the subarachnoid space during the injection of the 10 to 20 cc. dosage. Usually, when this aspiration test is performed, 1 to 2 cc. of the local anesthetic agent is withdrawn into the syringe before the plunger stops and no more clear fluid can be aspirated. The 1 to 2 cc. of the local anesthetic solution should be reinjected and the needle withdrawn from the epidural space. This fact is called to the anesthetist's attention so that when he aspirates clear fluid he will not become alarmed and think that he has inadvertently deposited the 10 cc. to 20 cc. dose in the subarachnoid space. After the needle is withdrawn, the patient is placed in the supine position or optimal position to spread the local anesthetic solution (see Table IX, page 422).

If, on the other hand, the plunger does not stop and clear fluid continues to flow into the syringe, the anesthetist may have inadvertently moved the needle and injected 10 cc. to 20 cc. of the local anesthetic solution in the subarachnoid space. When this occurs, he should *slowly* withdraw 20 to 50 cc. of the spinal fluid, withdraw the needle, turn the patient to the supine position, and be prepared to treat a high or total spinal anesthetic. In most instances, if 50 cc. of spinal fluid can be withdrawn *slowly* and *immediately*, a high spinal will not result. Withdrawal of larger amounts of spinal fluid, rapidly, and lavage of the subarachnoid space may not be indicated (see page 353).

DISTRIBUTION OF ANALGESIA

This is not always predictable and varies with the volume of the local anesthetic solution as well as the vertebra at which it is injected. In general it can be assumed that the solution injected spreads equally in a caudad and cephalad direction from the point of the needle, provided the anesthetic solution is injected *slowly*. Likewise it is satisfactory in most instances to assume that 1 cc. of the local

TABLE IX

SITE OF EPIDURAL TAP AND APPROXIMATE DOSAGE
FOR SINGLE-DOSE EPIDURAL BLOCK†

Operation	Interspace for Epidural Tap	Dosage	Position of Operating Table After Injection
Thorax*	T_{12}	16 to 20 cc.	Trendelenburg—10 degrees
Upper abdomen*			
Cholecystectomy	L_2	17 to 20 cc.	Trendelenburg—10 degrees
Gastric resection	L_2	17 to 20 cc.	Trendelenburg—10 degrees
Lower abdomen*			
Appendectomy	L_2 or L_3	16 to 20 cc.	Level
Cesarean section	L_2 or L_3	14 to 18 cc.	Level
Colon resection	L_2	16 to 20 cc.	Level
Hernia (inguinal or umbilical)	L_2 or L_3	14 to 18 cc.	Level
Hysterectomy	L_2 or L_3	16 to 20 cc.	Trendelenburg—10 degrees
Retropubic prostatectomy	L_3 or L_4	16 to 20 cc.	Level
Lower extremities	L_3 or L_4	14 to 18 cc.	Fowler's—10 degrees
Perineum			
Hemorrhoidectomy	L_3 or L_4	12 to 16 cc.	Fowler's—10 degrees
Transurethral prostatectomy	L_3 or L_4	14 to 18 cc.	Level
Vaginal delivery	L_3 or L_4	12 to 16 cc.	Level
Vaginal hysterectomy	L_3 or L_4	16 to 20 cc.	Level
Back and flank			
Nephrectomy	L_2	16 to 20 cc.	Kidney position and Trendelenburg—10 degrees
Pilonidal cystectomy	L_3 or L_4	12 to 16 cc.	Fowler's—10 degrees

† The figures in this table are an approximate "starting point"—they are "a place for the beginner to hang his hat." They must be varied somewhat according to the size, age, weight, and physical status of the patient. The physician who is skilled in performing epidural block may use other dosages, etc., which he has developed by trial and error.

* Abolition of intrapleural and intra-abdominal traction reflexes and noxious stimuli from the diaphragm require blocking of the vagus nerves and phrenic nerves, respectively. No attempt to block such reflexes with an epidural block should be made—the phrenic nerves can be blocked, but the vagus cannot, for the epidural space stops at the foramen magnum. Heavy premedication, light general anesthesia, or both should be used when necessary.

anesthetic solution will anesthetize one somatic dermatome. Therefore if the epidural puncture is performed at the second lumbar interspace and 15 cc. of the local anesthetic solution injected, an area of anesthesia should be established from the seventh or eighth thoracic dermatome to the third or fourth sacral dermatome. Because the area of analgesia varies in this manner and produces a segmental type of anesthesia, most anesthetists skilled in the use of epidural block vary the interspace at which the needle is inserted. In this manner they are able to use less anesthetic solution and produce more constant results. It should be emphasized that it is unwise for the beginner in this technique to change the site of placement of the needle more than one to three interspaces on either side of the second lumbar interspace until he masters the technique. By anatomical dissections it can be demonstrated in the average cadaver that the epidural space, *i.e.*, the distance from the dura to the ligamentum flavum, is greater in the region of the second lumbar vertebra than in any other region used for tap of this space.

COMPLICATIONS

The complications of this block are essentially the same as following spinal block (pages 353 to 361) and include the following.

Hypotension: Hypotension during epidural analgesia can be as sudden and as severe as during spinal block and should be treated in the same way as during spinal block (see page 353).

Nausea and Vomiting: See page 355.

Respiratory Arrest: See page 355.

Systemic Toxic Reactions to Local Anesthetic and Vasoconstrictor Drugs: See page 19 and 40, respectively.

High or Total Spinal Block: See page 353.

Cardiac Failure: See page 356.

Urinary Retention: See page 361.

Headache: This may occur if the dura is inadvertently punctured (see page 356).

Palsies and Paralysis: See page 360.

Local Infections: Extremely rare.

Signs and Symptoms.—These include fever, pain, and, if superficial, the local signs of infection are present.

Etiology.—Failure to adhere to the rules of asepsis.

Treatment.—Chemotherapy, *i.e.*, penicillin, sulfa drugs, etc.; heat; and surgical drainage.

Meningitis or Meningismus: See page 360.

REMARKS

In addition to the remarks below, many of the remarks made for Single-Dose Spinal (Subarachnoid) Anesthesia, pages 361 to 369, apply to this block and should be reviewed before this block is undertaken.

Also, when epidural block is used for obstetrical deliveries, it is advised that the remarks under Continuous (Intermittent) Caudal Block, pages 465 to 472, be read, because they too are applicable to this block.

Site of Action of the Agent Is at the Junction of the Dura and the Epineurium: Relatively strong concentrations and large volumes of local anesthetic drugs must be used in epidural analgesia in comparison to spinal analgesia because the drug site of action is usually considered to be at the point where the spinal nerve leaves the intervertebral foramen. Therefore the solution must be strong enough to penetrate the coverings of the nerves at this point, *i.e.*, junction of the dura and the epineurium.

Size of Epidural Space, Its Contents, and Gravity Regulate Spread of Solution In the Epidural Space: Diffusion of the local anesthetic solution in the epidural space depends on the size of the epidural space, the amount of loose areolar tissue in the epidural space, the capillary action between the two walls of the epidural space, and the anomalous septal divisions. These vary with each patient and may to some extent explain the difficulty in obtaining satisfactory epidural blocks at all times.

Since the epidural space is a compartment, gravity may exert some influence on the spread of the local anesthetic solution. In general the solution tends to gravitate to the dependent portion of the epidural space. When epidural block is used for rectal surgery or lower extremity surgery, the sitting position should be used for the tap to be certain of complete analgesia.

Do Not Attempt to Block Vagus Nerves or Phrenic Nerves When Performing an Epidural Block: Abolition of intrapleural and intraabdominal traction reflexes and noxious stimuli from the diaphragm require blocking of the vagus nerves and phrenic nerves, respectively. No attempt to block such reflexes with an epidural block should be made—the phrenic nerves can be blocked, but the vagus cannot, for the epidural space stops at the foramen magnum. Heavy premedication, light general anesthesia, or both should be used when necessary.

Position of Anesthetist When Performing Block: While placing the needle, the anesthetist should sit on a stool which is adjusted to a comfortable height. After the needle is correctly located in the anterior portion of the interspinous ligament or ligamentum flavum, the anesthetist stands.

Monitor Patient Carefully: A patient under epidural block should never be left unattended, and constant contact by conversation with the patient should be maintained for the first 20 minutes following the injection of the local anesthetic agent. Many of the common complications of this regional procedure occur in these first 20 minutes and complaints of the patient as well as changes in his sensorium are valuable aids in detecting some of the earliest signs of complications.

As Skill of Anesthetist Improves, Interspace May Be Varied: As the physician becomes skilled at epidural puncture and feels perfectly safe in performing it at various levels of the vertebral column, more accurate placement of the anesthetic solution at the dermatomes to be anesthetized usually permits smaller doses than those listed of the local anesthetic solution to be injected with satisfactory results.

Epidural Block Used in Conjunction with Anticoagulant Therapy May Not Be Compatible: If epidural block is used during anticoagulant therapy and a blood vessel is punctured, bleeding into the epidural space may result in neurological complications. And the possibility of profuse hemorrhage into the soft tissues must not be overlooked.

The Advantages of Epidural Block Over Spinal Block: First, duration of single dose injections may be slightly longer; however, with the use of vasoconstrictor drugs subarachnoidally, this is not always true. Second, headaches are very infrequent but backaches still occur occasionally. Lastly, the epidural space ends at the foramen magnum; therefore, the drug cannot reach the brain.

The Disadvantages of Epidural Block when Compared to Spinal Block: First, anesthesia and muscular relaxation are not as predictable. The consistency with which spinal block produces satisfactory analgesia makes it the method of choice for the physician who is not a specialist in anesthesia. Second, massive quantities of the local anesthetic drug must be injected for epidural analgesia. Therefore, the possibility of a massive spinal is ever present. Third, placement of the needle is a tedious procedure, and even if no spinal fluid is obtained on aspiration, spinal anesthesia may occur. Lastly, it has been cautioned that once the dura is tapped, a spinal or general anesthetic should be given because a subsequent epidural injection may result in a high or total spinal anesthesia. This is a reasonable precaution. But, in approximately 250 cases done by us, the dura has been tapped. The needle has been moved to the next interspace and an epidural block established. In none of these cases has a high or total spinal occurred, perhaps because 20 cc. of solution, which is the maximum dose used by us, injected slowly will not exert enough pressure to overcome the pressure within the subarachnoid space and therefore does not enter the spinal fluid.

Is Epidural Block Safer Than Spinal Block?
While the public has been made aware of the problems of spinal block, they are less familiar with the complications of epidural block. Therefore, often patients are willing to accept an epidural block when they refuse to have spinal anesthesia. With epidural block, the minor complications of spinal block, *e.g.*, headache, usually are avoided. However, the incidence of major complications, such as, total spinal block, hypotension, systemic toxic reactions and neurologic complications, is as great or greater with epidural block.

This should be expected because: (1) larger volumes and higher concentrations of the local anesthetic solution must be used; (2) often, the site of the epidural tap is made at or above the second lumbar interspace—the site where the spinal cord usually ends; (3) an inadvertent subarachnoid placement of the needle thought to be in the epidural space may go unrecognized; (4) often, a concentration of epinephrine (Adrenalin) greater than 1:200,000 is employed in the local anesthetic solution injected into the epidural space; (5) with a continuous technique, total subarachnoid block may result after a *reinforcing* dose (see page 467); and (6) the experience of most physicians is not as great with epidural block as with spinal block.

Avoid Solutions Containing Methylparaben and Metabisulfite: These drugs are often added to commercially prepared local anesthetic solutions to prevent oxidation and as a preservative. Solutions containing them are not recommended for epidural block.

Methylparaben.—Methylparaben is a preservative and fungistatic agent.

Metabisulfite.—Metabisulfite is an antioxidizing agent.

More than 20 cc. of Local Anesthetic Solution Need Not be Injected to Effect Satisfactory Epidural Block: For each dermatome to be anesthetized from the point of insertion of the needle in the epidural space, 1.0 cc. of

the local anesthetic solution should be injected. Consistently, 20 cc. of the local anesthetic solution injected into the epidural space spreads a minimum of 16 to 18 dermatomes—20 cc. injected at the first or second lumbar interspace will produce analgesia of at least the fourth thoracic through the second sacral dermatomes. Therefore, to produce satisfactory epidural block, more than 20 cc. need not be used, provided: (1) the epidural space is tapped at the correct vertebral interspace; (2) the entire dosage of the local anesthetic solution is deposited in the epidural space; (3) gravity is allowed to exert its effect, that is, solutions gravitate to the dependent part of the space; (4) the local anesthetic solution is injected at the rate of not less than 1.0 cc. per second; and (5) the interval of time taken in refilling the 10 cc. syringe after the first syringeful has been injected is kept to a minimum—spread of solution within the epidural space is improved by the pressure created by the injection of the local anesthetic solution.

Larger volumes (30 to 40 cc.) of 1.5 to 2.0 percent solutions of the local anesthetic drugs should not be used—such an amount may represent a toxic dose of either lidocaine or mepivacaine. While volumes between 20 cc. and 30 cc. do not necessarily represent toxic doses of these drugs, such volumes should not be employed. One of the rules of regional block, *i.e.*, use the least amount of the local anesthetic drug necessary to produce satisfactory block, still is valid.

At Present, Chloroprocaine (Nesacaine) Is Not Available for Epidural Block: Chloroprocaine has a rapid onset, 8 to 15 minutes, and it seems to have the lowest systemic toxicity of any local anesthetic agent used at the present time. The author and his associates have used it in over 500 epidural blocks for surgical procedures and found it to be a satisfactory agent. Because of packaging difficulties, chloroprocaine is not at the present time available for epidural block (see page 15). However, it is included under Drugs in this chapter because the pharmaceutical house which manufactures the drug indicates that it again may become available.

Do Not Exceed a 1:200,000 Concentration of Epinephrine in the Epidural Space: A stronger concentration, *i.e.,* 1:100,000 will not prolong the duration of anesthesia significantly and it may predispose to complications, *e.g.,* hypertension.

Do Not Use Phenylephrine in the Epidural Space—It May Cause Severe Hypertension: While 3 mg. to 5 mg. of phenylephrine injected into the subarachnoid space will not elevate the blood pressure (see page 484), such dosages will result in a severe hypertension if they are deposited in the epidural space.

Recover Broken Needle(s): All needles should be tested before use. If a needle breaks, every effort to remove it, including surgery, should be made. Unremoved needles have a tendency to migrate and may cause permanent injuries as well as medicolegal complications.

When a spinal needle breaks, there is little doubt in the anesthetist's mind of what has happened. A distinct click is felt. This usually happens when the needle is being inserted and the stylet is still in the needle. If the anesthetist suspects that the needle has broken, he should not remove the stylet. If the needle breaks after the stylet is removed, the portion containing the hub of the needle should not be removed. They are valuable guides to locating the broken end of the needle. When the anesthetist suspects that the needle has been broken, he should release his hold on it and have an x-ray taken immediately.

Repeat Block when Analgesia is Inadequate: If the desired results from the first block attempt are unsatisfactory, do not hesitate to reblock the patient if time permits. Most patients will think nothing about being reblocked if the second attempt is prefaced by a statement such as: "Well, I guess we will have to inject a little more medicine if we are going to freeze this area."

However, do not exceed the maximum safe dosage of the local anesthetic solution for both blocks. If to reblock the patient the maximum safe dose of the local anesthetic solution must be exceeded, 45 minutes should elapse between blocks.

CHAPTER 47

Continuous (Intermittent) Epidural (Peridural) Block

Before using the continuous technique for epidural block the single-dose method should be mastered.

DEFINITION

Same as single-dose epidural block. See page 407.

INDICATIONS

Whenever epidural block is indicated and single-dose epidural block will not produce a sufficient duration of analgesia time, this method may be used.

Surgical: Same as single-dose epidural block. See page 407.

Diagnostic: Same as single-dose epidural block. See page 407.

Therapeutic: Same as single-dose epidural block. See page 407. In addition to these, continuous epidural block is frequently employed to relieve the pain of all stages of labor as well as postoperative pain.

ANATOMY

Same as for single-dose epidural block. See page 407.

PREMEDICATION

Same as for single-dose epidural block. See page 407.

DRUGS

Tetracaine (Pontocaine) or procaine (Novocain) is seldom used for continuous epidural block. The rapid onset and constant results of lidocaine (Xylocaine), mepivacaine (Carbocaine), and chloroprocaine (Nesacaine) make them the agents of choice for this block. Furthermore, tetracaine is not added to a solution of these agents since the continuous technique obviates the need to employ a solution with a prolonged duration. However, the addition of epinephrine (Adrenalin) is advised—not to prolong the duration of anesthesia, but to slow the absorption of the agent.

Solutions containing methylparaben and metabisulfite should not be used (see page 425).

Lidocaine (Xylocaine) or Mepivacaine (Carbocaine)

Dosage.—5 cc. to 20 cc. of 1.0 to 1.5 per-cent solution with or without 0.1 cc. of epinephrine (Adrenalin) 1:1000 in 20 cc. of the local anesthetic solution.*

Onset.—Operating analgesia is established in 10 to 20 minutes.

Duration.—Operating analgesia lasts 1¼ to 2 hours, with stronger concentrations containing epinephrine giving the upper limits.

Chloroprocaine (Nesacaine): See Remarks, page 425.

Dosage.—5 to 20 cc. of a 2.0 percent solution with or without 0.1 cc. of epinephrine (Adrenalin) 1:1000 in 20 cc. of the local anesthetic solution.*

Onset.—Operating analgesia is established in 10 to 20 minutes.

---

*Optimal concentration of epinephrine is 1:200,000, that is, 0.1 cc. of epinephrine 1:1000 in 20 cc. of the local anesthetic solution (see page 438).

Duration.—Operating analgesia lasts ¾ to 1¼ hours, with solutions containing epinephrine giving the upper limits.

MATERIALS

Regional tray (see page 51) or:

1. One ¾-inch (2 cm.), 25-gauge Huber point security Lok-needle.

2. One 1½-inch (3.8 cm.), 22-gauge security Lok-needle.

3. One tuberculin Lok-syringe for measuring epinephrine.

4. One 3 cc. Lok-syringe.

5. One 5 cc. Lok-syringe.

6. One 10 cc. Lok-syringe.

7. One prep cup.

8. One graduated measuring cup, preferably stainless steel, for mixing solution.

9. One Allis forceps.

10. One sponge forceps.

11. One Pitkin or thin-walled needle guide.*

12. Four towels.

13. Four 4 x 4 sponges.

14. One sterilizer control.

To the above basic equipment must be added:

1. One 3-inch (7.5 cm.), 18-gauge thin-walled spinal needle with a Tuohy (directional) bevel (Figure 252, page 389).*

2. One vinyl plastic tubing (Figure 253, page 390 and Figure 263, page 401).* The tubing is marked with a felt marking pen or ball point pen 5¾ inches (14.5 cm.) from the end to be placed in the epidural space. The tubing with wire stylet in it (item 3) is placed in a plastic bag, wrapped with a sterilizer control (Figure 263, page 401), and heat sterilized.

3. One wire stylet for the vinyl tubing (Figure 253, page 390).*

4. One ¾-inch (2 cm.), 23-gauge Lok-needle, preferably with a short bevel, or a Tuohy-Borst female Lok to plastic tubing adapter (Figure 253, page 390, Figure 264, page 402 and Figure 265, page 402).* Either the needle or the adapter is employed so that the syringe containing the local anesthetic solution may be attached to the plastic tubing.

5. One plug for female outlet (Figure 253, page 390 and Figure 264, page 402).*

TECHNIQUE

Landmarks: Same as for single-dose epidural block. See page 411. When this technique is used, the epidural puncture should be made at the first through the fourth lumbar interspace because the anteroposterior diameter of the epidural space is usually considered to be greatest at this point, *i.e.*, approximately ¼-inch (0.6 cm.). Since the bevel of the Tuohy needle is ⅛-inch (0.3 cm.) in length, it must be placed where the epidural space is the largest (see Figure 256, page 393).

Position: Same as for single-dose epidural block—the lateral decubitus (side) position is the most frequently employed (Figure 271 A, page 412). See page 411.

Precautions: Same as for single-dose epidural block. See page 412.

---

*These items may be obtained from Becton, Dickinson and Company, Rutherford, New Jersey. They have the following order numbers: Pitkin needle guide, PNG; thin-walled needle guide, 01-0027; 18-gauge 3-inch (7.5 cm.) Tuohy needle, T466LNRH; vinyl plastic tubing, VX020 and radiopaque, RVX020; wire stylet, 01-0041; Tuohy-Borst adapter, 610A; and plug for female outlet, 417A.

Two types of radiopaque tubing are available—the RVX020 which does not permit observation of the lumen and the CRVX020, which does permit observation of the lumen. The CRVX020 allows detection of blood or spinal fluid more easily when the aspiration tests are performed. It also permits observation of the wire stylet. For illustrations, the RVX020 was employed because photographs of it are better.

Procedure

1. The sterilizer control is checked to be sure the equipment is sterile.

2. The anesthetist aseptically prepares the skin, and places a sterile towel over the up side and under the down side.

3. A skin wheal is raised over the selected interspace with the ¾-inch (2 cm.), 25-gauge Huber point security Lok-needle, using 0.2 cc. to 0.3 cc. of the local anesthetic solution (Figure 271B, page 412).

4. 0.8 cc. to 1.5 cc. of the local anesthetic solution is infiltrated into the interspinous ligament.

5. The Pitkin or thin-walled needle guide is placed through the skin wheal to make a hole in the skin which will accommodate the 18-gauge spinal needle (Figure 271C, page 412). The needle guide is removed. Usually, this prevents the 18-gauge Tuohy needle carrying with it a skin plug and skin bacteria into the epidural space.

6. The 18-gauge Tuohy needle is held by the anesthetist so that the thumb exerts pressure on the stylet's top and the shaft is supported between the index and middle fingers (Figure 271D, page 412). This prevents displacement of the stylet and allows the anesthetist to steady his hand by resting the ring and little fingers on the patient's back (Figure 271D, page 412).

7. The relationship of the opening in the bevel of the Tuohy spinal needle to the markings on the hub is noted. The projection in the top of the stylet which fits into the notch in the hub of the needle is on the same side as the opening in the bevel of the Tuohy needle (Figure 252, page 389).

The Tuohy needle is then inserted through the hole in the skin wheal with the opening in the bevel pointing cephalad and carefully and slowly advanced 1 inch (2.5 cm.) to 1¼ inches (3.2 cm.) until its point lies in the substance of the interspinous ligament (Figure 271D, page 412). If the needle is not inserted through the skin and the ligament with its bevel in this direction, the needle will tend to deviate to one side or the other.

The index and middle (long) fingers of the free hand should straddle the interspace into which the needle is to be placed. Great care should be taken that the needle lies in the same plane as the spinous processes and perpendicular to the transverse processes. If it points upward or downward, or if the patient's back is not at a 90-degree angle in the vertical plane with the table, the spinal needle may not travel a true course (Figure 233, page 349).

8. Either the *negative pressure* or *loss of resistance method* is used to ascertain when the epidural space has been entered by the needle (see step 8, page 413). We prefer the "loss of resistance" method.

9. If the needle was advanced slowly through the ligamentum flavum, the *sign* that the epidural space has been tapped probably occurred when only ¹⁄₁₆ (0.15 cm.) of the bevel entered the epidural space. The bevel of the Tuohy needle is ⅛-inch (0.3 cm.) in length (Figure 256, page 393) and the plastic tubing will not pass through the bevel unless its entire opening is in the epidural space. Therefore, reinsert the stylet in the needle and slowly and carefully advance the needle ¹⁄₁₆-inch (0.15 cm.) to ⅛-inch (0.3 cm.) further into the epidural space.

10. Careful aspiration tests are made in at least four planes by rotating the needle 90 degrees each time. If no blood or spinal fluid is aspirated, then the anesthetist may continue with the procedure. If blood is obtained, the needle may be inserted one interspace above or below the one in which blood has been obtained. Then should blood still appear, the needle may be advanced into the subarachnoid space and a single dose or continuous spinal block administered or the regional technique may be abandoned for general anesthesia.

If spinal fluid is obtained, the anesthetist should use spinal block, adjust or reinsert the needle, or he may discard the regional method for general anesthesia. If the needle is placed in the epidural space either by readjustment at the same interspace or by replacement of the needle at another interspace, it has been cautioned that a high or total spinal anesthesia may occur from leakage of the local anesthetic solution from the epidural space into the subarachnoid space through the hole in the dura. This has not been observed by us (see Remarks, page 424).

During the aspiration test, the back of the hand not containing the syringe should always rest against the patient's back and the hub of the needle should be held securely between the thumb and index finger of this hand so that the needle will not be moved (Figure 277, page 416).

11. When neither blood nor spinal fluid is obtained, the remaining ½ to 1 cc. of saline in the 3 cc. syringe is discarded and the rebound test performed. With this test, 1 to 1.5 cc. of air is aspirated into the 3 cc. syringe. The syringe is connected to the spinal needle and the air rapidly injected. At the end of the downward motion of the plunger of the syringe, quickly release the pressure on the plunger. If the needle is in the epidural space, the syringe will only refill 0.1 cc. to 0.2 cc., or there will be no refill. If the needle is incorrectly placed in a ligament, there will be a refill of from 0.5 cc. to 1.0 cc.

12. When it has been determined that the bevel of the needle rests in the epidural space, the needle is checked to be sure the opening in its bevel points cephalad (Figure 252, page 389).

13. The wire stylet in the plastic tubing is withdrawn ½-inch (1.3 cm.) from the end to be inserted into the Tuohy spinal needle. If the anesthetist is right-handed, the thumb and index finger of the left hand grasp the hub of the Tuohy needle while the remaining fingers hold the plastic tubing. The back of the left hand rests against the patient's back (Figure 283A, page 431). The right hand feeds the plastic tubing through the needle (Figure 283A, page 431). The plastic tubing will stop when its end hits the curve of the point of the needle. Now, the plastic tubing is pushed ½-inch

(1.3 cm.) beyond the bevel of the needle. To push the tubing beyond the bevel may require *moderate* pressure and *therefore the needle must be held securely* (Figure 283 A, page 431).

14. Once the first ½-inch (1.3 cm.) of the plastic tubing passes beyond the point of the Tuohy needle it is no longer necessary to hold the hub of the needle with the left hand. The index finger and thumb of the left hand release their hold on the hub of the needle (Figure 283B, page 431). The tubing is carefully removed from the middle, ring, and little fingers. The tubing is straightened and the stylet is withdrawn 2 inches (5 cm.). Now the tubing is advanced this distance through the needle until the mark on the plastic tubing is at the hub of the needle (Figure 283 B and C, page 431). If the bevel of the needle rests in the epidural space, the tubing should advance easily with *light* and *delicate* pressure—no resistance should be encountered and there should be no need to hold the needle. If the tubing is difficult to thread, the bevel of the needle probably does not lie in the epidural space.

If the stylet is not withdrawn prior to the insertion of the tubing beyond the point of the Tuohy needle, the physician probably will not be able to remove the stylet from the tubing, although he may be able to withdraw the 18-gauge needle over the tubing and the stylet. Even in a situation where the Tuohy needle can be removed, the stylet usually cannot be dislodged from the tubing. Thus, the procedure to this point may have to be repeated. This difficulty occurs because the 18-gauge needle employed has a curved point and the tubing and stylet are bent at an acute angle where they enter the epidural space.

Once the plastic tubing has passed the point of the needle, do not try to withdraw it, as the needle will cut it off or shred it. If a readjustment is necessary, the needle and the plastic tubing must be removed as one, and the procedure to this point repeated.

15. The Tuohy needle is now withdrawn from the patient's back over the plastic tubing

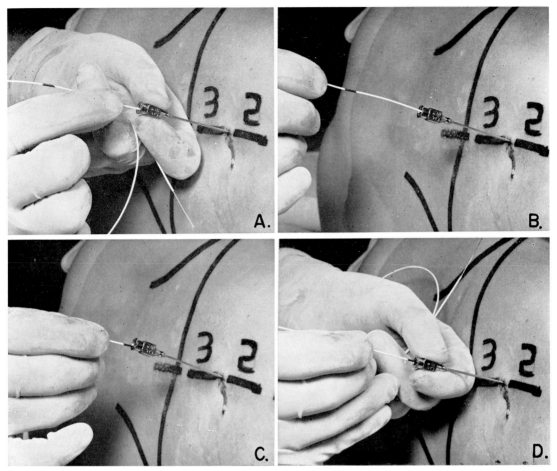

Figure 283. Technique of continuous epidural block. A. Method of holding the needle for the initial ½-inch (1.3 cm.) insertion of the tubing into the epidural space by the right-handed anesthetist. The back of the left hand rests firmly against the patient's back, holding the hub of the needle securely with the thumb and index finger and the tubing with the middle, ring, and little fingers. The thumb and index finger of the right hand feed the tubing into the needle. B. After the plastic tubing has passed the point of the needle, it is no longer necessary for the left hand to steady the needle. The thumb and index finger, with light pressure, thread the tubing into the epidural space. C. Mark on the plastic tubing at the hub of the needle. D. Thumb and index finger of the left hand hold the hub of the needle and thumb and index finger of the right hand grip plastic tubing and stylet 1 inch (2.5 cm.) distal to the needle hub.

and stylet. This is a critical maneuver. Again, the thumb and index finger of the left hand hold the hub of the needle (Figure 283 D, page 431). The plastic tubing with stylet in it is grasped firmly 1 inch (2.5 cm.) distal to the hub of the needle by the thumb and index finger of the right hand (Figure 283 D, page 431). Then the thumb and index finger of the left hand pull the needle out of the patient until the hub touches the thumb and index finger of the right hand—*do not move the right hand* (Figure 284 A, page 432). This maneuver

is repeated two or three times until the point of the needle emerges from the skin. If this maneuver is executed carefully, the plastic tubing will not be dislodged from its position in the epidural space.

16. As soon as the point of the needle emerges from the skin, the plastic tubing is grasped by the thumb and index finger of the left hand at its point of entrance into the skin (Figure 284 B, page 432). The needle is slipped to the end of the plastic tubing (Fig-

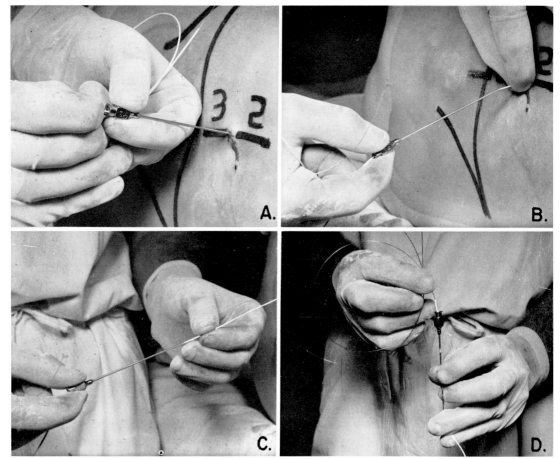

Figure 284. Technique of continuous epidural block (con't.). Thumb and index finger of the left hand pull needle out of the patient until the hub of the needle touches the thumb and index finger of the right hand. B. Tubing grasped at the point of its entrance into the skin. C. Needle being removed from tubing. D. Needle at end of tubing. Thumb and index finger of the left hand hold needle while little and ring fingers hold the tubing. The stylet is being withdrawn.

ure 284 C and D, page 432). The stylet is withdrawn (Figure 284 D, page 432), and the needle removed (Figure 285 A, page 433). The distance of the mark on the plastic tubing from the skin should be checked—by doing this it can be determined whether or not the plastic tubing was dislodged from the epidural space when the Tuohy needle was withdrawn (Figure 285 B, page 433).

17. The Tuohy-Borst adapter or the 23-gauge short beveled ¾-inch (2 cm.) Lok-needle is affixed to the plastic tubing (Figure 285 B, page 433, and Figure 259 B, page 396). We prefer the 23-gauge needle.

18. *Even if all tests indicate that the Tuohy*

needle was correctly placed in the epidural space, and even if there was no difficulty in threading the plastic tubing through the needle, the following tests (steps 19, 20, 21, and 22) must be performed because it is possible for the plastic tubing to puncture and rest either inside the dura or in the lumen of a blood vessel.

19. Attempt to aspirate blood or spinal fluid through the plastic tubing. If spinal fluid is obtained, use continuous spinal anesthesia or abandon the block for general anesthesia. If blood is obtained, either withdraw the tubing and reinsert it or abandon the technique and use a continuous spinal block or general anesthesia.

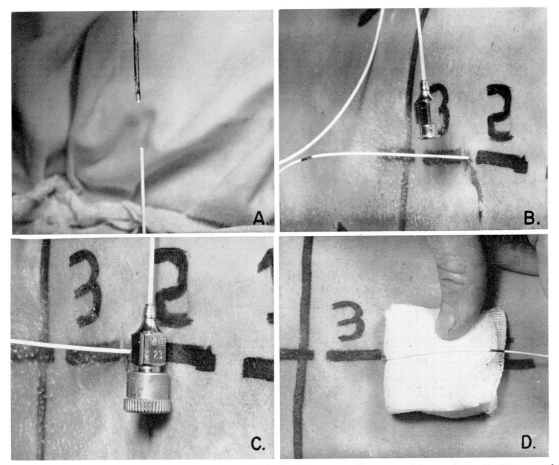

Figure 285. Technique of continuous epidural block (con't.) A. Needle removed from tubing. B. Distance of mark on tubing from skin examined and 23-gauge needle inserted into tubing. C. 23-gauge needle capped with plug. D. Sponge placed under tubing prior to taping it to patient's back.

20. If no blood or spinal fluid is obtained, 2 cc. of the local anesthetic solution is injected at the rate of 1 cc. per 6 to 8 seconds. The syringe is detached and the Tuohy-Borst adapter or 23-gauge needle is capped with the plug for the female outlet (Figure 285 C, page 433).

21. Five minutes by the clock are allowed to pass. Carefully monitor the patient's blood pressure, pulse, and sensorium during this period for evidence of a systemic toxic reaction. If one occurs, remove the plastic tubing and reinsert it, use spinal anesthesia, or abandon the regional technique and administer general anesthesia

22. If the five minutes pass uneventfully, the lower extremities, abdomen, and chest should be tested for signs of analgesia. When, following a 2 cc. test dose of the local anesthetic solution, the area of analgesia is extensive, the dura has in all probability been punctured and further attempts at establishing the epidural block should be discontinued. If the existing spinal anesthesia needs to be supplemented, use the continuous spinal block technique or general anesthesia.

If, as usual, there is no area of analgesia or only a small area of anesthesia or hypesthesia over the distribution of the nerve of the interspace used for the epidural puncture, and if the patient's blood pressure, pulse, and sensorium remain unchanged, it is safe to assume that neither the dura nor a blood vessel has been invaded.

23. When it has been determined that the plastic tubing lies in the epidural space, a piece of gauze is taped under the plastic tubing as it emerges from the skin (Figure 285 D, page 433) and the plastic tubing taped to the back either to the right or left of the spinous processes (Figure 261 A, page 397).

24. The patient is instructed to turn on his back. He may do this himself, providing the anesthetist prevents pull on the tubing by placing his hand over the entrance of the plastic tubing through the skin (Figure 261 B, page 397).

25. The knee restraint straps, shoulder braces, and wrist cuffs are snugly adjusted so that the patient will not move (Figure 261 C, page 397).

26. The table is placed in the optimal position (Table X, page 435).

27. Now the plug is removed from the Tuohy-Borst adapter or 23-gauge needle and an additional 5 cc. to 16 cc. of the local anesthetic solution is added for the initial dose at the rate of 1 cc. per 6 to 10 seconds (see Table X, page 435). The 2 cc. test dose is disregarded when calculating the dose needed to produce anesthesia.

28. The syringe is removed from the adapter or needle and again the opening capped with the plug.

29. A check of the areas of analgesia is made at frequent intervals with an Allis forceps to ascertain the area and height of analgesia.

30. With the continuous epidural block, reinforcing doses of 5 cc. to 16 cc. of the local anesthetic solution are usually adequate. The reinforcing dose should be approximately the same number of cc. as the initial dose—sufficient volume to fill the epidural space and anesthetize the required dermatomes must be used. *It is best to add the reinforcing dose before the patient feels severe pain; otherwise, it may be difficult to re-establish adequate anesthesia.*

Before injecting a reinforcing dose, aspirate for blood or spinal fluid. If either is obtained and the procedure is being used for surgery, discontinue the epidural block and administer general anesthesia. If either is obtained when epidural block is being administered for pain relief during the first stage of labor, discontinue the epidural block and administer either a spinal block or general anesthesia for delivery of the fetus.

31. When the operation is completed, either the tubing may be slowly withdrawn from the patient or it may be left in the epidural space for one to two days postoperatively to provide pain relief, sympathetic block of the lower extremities, or both. Tubing which is left in the epidural space does not cause serious complications, provided antiseptic precautions are taken. If signs of meningeal irritation, *i.e.*, stiff neck or headache, develop, the tubing is removed immediately and the signs of meningeal irritation disappear in 6 to 8 hours. We have left the tubing in the epidural space for 9 days without complications.

When the tubing is withdrawn, it should be examined to be sure it is the same length as it was when it was introduced into the epidural space.

DISTRIBUTION OF ANALGESIA

Same as single-dose epidural. See page 421.

COMPLICATIONS

Same as single-dose epidural block (page 423). Also, total spinal block following reinforcing doses may occur (page 467).

REMARKS

In addition to the remarks below, many of the remarks made for Single-Dose Spinal (Subarachnoid) Anesthesia (page 361) and Single-Dose Epidural (Peridural) Block (page 423), apply to this block and should be reviewed. *Also, when continuous epidural block is used for obstetrical deliveries, it is advised that the remarks under Continuous (Intermittent) Caudal Block (pages 465 to 472) be read, because they are applicable to this block.*

Can the Position of the Plastic Tubing in the Epidural Space Be Predicted Precisely

TABLE X

SITE OF TAP, LOCATION OF TIP OF PLASTIC TUBING AND DOSAGE FOR CONTINUOUS EPIDURAL BLOCK†

Procedure	Interspace Used for Epidural Tap	Approximate Vertebra at Which Tip of Plastic Tubing Lies	Dosage in Cubic Centimeters	Position of Operating Room Table
Chest*	T_{12}	T_{11}	8 to 12 cc.	Trendelenburg—10 degrees
Upper abdomen*				
Cholecystectomy	L_2	L_1	12 to 16 cc.	Trendelenburg—10 degrees
Gastric resection	L_1 or L_2	L_1	12 to 16 cc.	Trendelenburg—10 degrees
Incisional pain relief**	L_2	L_1	7 to 10 cc.	Level
Lower abdomen*				
Colon resection	L_2	L_1	12 to 16 cc.	Trendelenburg—10 degrees
Repair of aneurysm of aorta	L_2	L_1	12 to 16 cc.	Level
Retropubic prostatectomy	L_3	L_2	8 to 12 cc.	Level
Herniorrhaphy	L_3	L_2	8 to 12 cc.	Level
Incisional pain relief**	L_2 or L_3	L_1 or L_2	5 to 7 cc.	Level
Pancreatic pain relief**	L_2	L_1	7 to 10 cc.	Level
Hysterectomy	L_3	L_2	10 to 14 cc.	Level
Lower extremities				
Anesthesia	L_4	L_3	10 to 14 cc.	Fowler's—10 degrees
Sympathetic Block**	L_2	L_1	5 to 7 cc.	Level
Perineum				
Transurethral prostatectomy	L_4	L_3	8 to 12 cc.	Level
Vaginal hysterectomy	L_4	L_3	8 to 12 cc.	Level
Back and flank				
Nephrectomy	L_2	L_1	10 to 14 cc.	Kidney position and Trendelenburg—10 degrees
Anuria**	L_2	L_1	7 to 10 cc.	Level
Vaginal delivery				
Pain relief, first stage of labor	L_3	L_2	5 to 7 cc.	Level
Pain relief, second and third stages of labor	L_3	L_2	10 to 12 cc.	Level

†The figures in this table are an approximate "starting point"—they are "a place for the beginner to hang his hat." They must be varied somewhat according to the size, age, weight, and physical status of the patient. The physician who is skilled in performing continuous epidural block may use other dosages, etc., which he has developed by trial and error.

The entries in this table are based on: (1) using a plastic tubing which has been marked 5¾ (14.5 cm.) from the end to be inserted; (2) using a 3-inch (7.5 cm.), 18-gauge, thin-walled Tuohy needle to place the tubing in the epidural space; and (3) threading the tubing through the 18-gauge needle into the epidural space until the mark is at the hub of the needle.

*Abolition of intrapleural and intra-abdominal traction reflexes and noxious stimuli from the diaphragm require blocking of the vagus nerves and phrenic nerves, respectively. No attempt to block such reflexes with an epidural block should be made—the phrenic nerves can be blocked, but the vagus cannot, for the epidural space stops at the foramen magnum. Heavy premedication, light general anesthesia, or both should be used when necessary.

**The weakest concentration (0.5 to 1.0 percent) of mepivacaine or lidocaine that will effect pain relief should be used *initially*. It is not unusual for patients to become refractory to these drugs and, after 18 to 24 hours, have no pain relief. When this occurs, stronger concentrations of the drug must be used or another local anesthetic agent employed, *e.g.*, lidocaine may be substituted for mepivacaine, or vice versa.

and Consistently Using the Technique Advocated? The answer is "Yes," provided the plastic tubing is inserted for only 2 inches (5 cm.). If it is inserted for a greater distance, then its position can be determined with certainty only if the tubing is radiopaque and roentgenograms are taken.

With the technique described herein, the tubing will rest approximately at the same interspace or one vertebra above the interspace through which the needle was inserted (Figure 286, page 436). When the tubing is inserted for more than 2 inches (5 cm.) beyond the bevel of the needle it may curl back (Figure 287, page 436). For this reason, the tubing

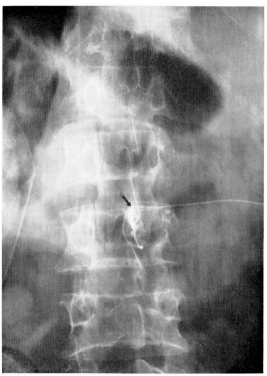

Figure 287. X-ray of plastic tubing in epidural space. Tubing was inserted at the interspace between the second and third lumbar vertebrae with the opening in the Tuohy needle pointed cephalad. The tubing was inserted for 4 inches (10 cm.) It curled back on itself and all 4 inches (10 cm.) rest at the second lumbar interspace (arrow). This patient had a nephrectomy. He is 5 feet, 8 inches tall; weighs 144 pounds; and is 60 years old. The initial dose was 12 cc. of lidocaine (Xylocaine) 1.5 percent. The table was in 10-degree Trendelenburg. Anesthesia level was to the fourth thoracic dermatome.

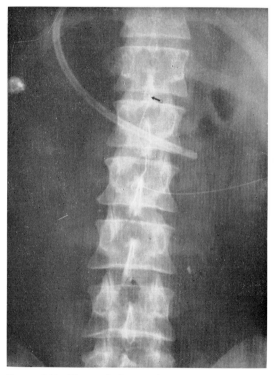

Figure 286. X-ray of plastic tubing in epidural space. Tubing was inserted at the interspace between the first and second lumbar vertebrae with the opening in the point of the Tuohy needle pointing cephalad. The tubing was inserted for 2 inches (5 cm.). It went cephalad and the tip lies at the interspace between the twelfth thoracic and first lumbar vertebrae. This patient had a gastrostomy with removal of a polyp and a bilateral herniorrhaphy. He is 6 feet, 4½ inches tall; weighs 203 pounds; and is 44 years old. The initial dose was 15 cc. of lidocaine (Xylocaine) 1.5 percent. The table was in 10-degree Trendelenburg. Anesthesia level was to the third thoracic dermatome.

seldom is inserted more than 2 inches (5 cm.) in the epidural space. When the tubing is inserted for only 2 inches (5 cm.), the tip's approximate position is known and the dosage can be determined more accurately.

Effecting Continuous Segmental Epidural Block With Small Volumes of Solution Requires Skill, Patience, and Practice: The needle must be placed at the optimal lumbar vertebra through whose intervertebral foramina the spinal nerves to be blocked pass (Figure 319, page 487). The anesthetist cannot rely on inserting an 18-gauge Tuohy needle at one level with the idea of threading plastic tubing through it to a higher or lower level (Figure 287, page 436).

The *paramedian* approach using an 18-gauge thin-walled needle with short, blunt point, *i.e.*, Crawford point, is often employed by the anesthetist skilled in epidural block to thread plastic tubing cephalad in the epidural space.* Principally, this needle and this approach are used for thoracic epidural block where the slope of the spines of the vertebrae makes the midline approach difficult. The placement of this needle requires practice and patience and to thread the tubing cephalad through it requires that the stylet remain in the tubing after the tubing has passed beyond the bevel.

This approach should not be employed until epidural block in the lumbar region using the midline approach is mastered (see page 411). In most instances, we prefer to use the Tuohy needle, place it in the lumbar area at or below the second interspace, thread the tubing 2 inches (5 cm.) into the epidural space and rely on the volume of the local anesthetic solution to produce satisfactory anesthesia.

Position of Anesthetist When Performing Block: While placing the needle, the anesthetist should sit on a stool which is adjusted to a comfortable height. After the needle is correctly located in the anterior portion of the interspinous ligament or the ligamentum flavum, the anesthetist stands.

Difficulties May Be Encountered When Plastic Tubing Is Inserted More Than 2 Inches (5 cm.) into Epidural Space: If the plastic tubing is inserted more than 2 inches (5 cm.) into the epidural space, the following may occur: (1) it may kink; (2) turn 180 degrees and go in the opposite direction to that in which it was inserted; (3) pass out an intervertebral foramen; (4) wrap around a nerve and be difficult to remove; or (5) a combination of these.

---

*Crawford point needle may be obtained from Becton, Dickinson and Company, Rutherford, New Jersey, order numbers TK 461 LNR (large spool hub) or TK 426 LNR (regular hub).

Tachyphylaxis to the Local Anesthetic Drug Occurs: When continuous epidural is used for pain relief for 36 hours or more, tachyphylaxis to the local anesthetic drug may occur. Therefore, the weakest concentration (0.5 to 1.0 percent) of mepivacaine or lidocaine that will effect pain relief or block of the sympathetic nervous system should be used initially. It is not unusual for patients to become refractory to the drug being used and after 24 to 36 hours have no relief from the concentration of the drug being employed. When this occurs, stronger concentrations of the drug must be used or another local anesthetic solution employed, *e.g.*, lidocaine may be substituted for mepivacaine or vice versa.

Pass Plastic Tubing Slowly Into Epidural Space: If the tubing meets resistance or stimulates a nerve, do not force the tubing past the obstruction—the obstruction may be the dura or a blood vessel. Leave the catheter where it is and inject the local anesthetic solution.

Mark Plastic Tubing 5¾ Inches (14.5 cm.) from End to be Placed in Epidural Space: When the plastic tubing is used, the distance it is to be inserted should be marked with a felt marking pen or ball point pen prior to sterilization. Marking of the tubing serves two purposes: (1) it permits placement of the tubing the correct distance into the caudal canal, and (2) it allows the physician to recognize whether the tubing was dislodged from the epidural space when the 18-gauge needle and wire stylet are withdrawn.

Use Wire Stylet in Plastic Tubing: The stylet remains in the plastic tubing while threading it through the 18-gauge needle to facilitate its introduction into the epidural space. The plastic tubing for continuous epidural blocks does not come with a stylet and the manufacturer states that none is necessary for its insertion. However, it has been found through unfortunate experiences that this is not true, particularly when the tubing has been sterilized in the autoclave. A stylet may be purchased (see footnote, page 428), gotten from the urology department—a suitable one comes in a number 5 ureteral catheter, or made from 28- to 26-gauge stainless steel surgical wire available in the supply room of most operating suites.

Should Regular or Radiopaque Plastic Tubing be Used? The principal disadvantage of the non-radiopaque tubing is that its location cannot be determined if the block is inadequate or if the tubing breaks. The principal disadvantage of the radiopaque tubing is the ability to locate it if it does break.

Vinyl plastic tubing is inert and when left in the body, seldom, if ever, causes any difficulty. But if it can be located in the subarachnoid, epidural, or caudal space, the question arises: Should it be removed? To remove it may subject the patient to an unnecessary, hazardous operation. To not remove it may provoke a medicolegal situation—the ramifications of which are too numerous to list.

Therefore, the type of tubing a physician selects is one of personal choice. Regardless of which type is selected, a broken piece of tubing in a patient presents a difficult problem. Whether an attempt to retrieve the tubing is made depends on the circumstances and should involve consultation with other specialists and the anesthetist's insurance company. Nonetheless, the patient must be informed of such a mishap and should participate in the decision as to whether the tubing should be removed.

Sterilization of Tuohy Needle, Plastic Tubing, Tuohy-Borst Adapter, One-way Stopcock, and Plug for Stopcock: See page 400.

Do Not Exceed a 1:200,000 Concentration of Epinephrine in the Epidural Space: A stronger concentration, *i.e.*, 1:100,000 will not prolong the duration of anesthesia significantly and it may predispose to complications, *e.g.*, hypertension.

Do Not Use Phenylephrine in the Epidural Space—It May Cause Severe Hypertension: While 3 mg. to 5 mg. of phenylephrine injected into the subarachnoid space will not elevate the blood pressure (see page 484), such dosages will result in a severe hypertension if they are deposited in the epidural space.

Recover Broken Needle(s): See page 426.

CHAPTER 48

Single-Dose Caudal Block

DEFINITION

E PIDURAL ANALGESIA is analgesia produced by placing the local anesthetic solution in the space between the dura and the ligaments and periosteum lining the vertebral canal (Figure 268, page 408 and Figure 269, page 408). Caudal block as referred to in this chapter means analgesia of the lower thoracic nerves (T9, 10, 11, and 12), the lumbar nerves, the sacral nerves, and the coccygeal plexus by placement of the local anesthetic solution in the epidural space via the sacral hiatus and caudal canal. It is a relatively simple procedure and may be mastered easily by careful attention to details.

INDICATIONS

Surgical: Operations or manipulations involving the anus, rectum, sigmoid colon, prostate gland, urethra, uterus, bladder, penis, vulva, vagina, cervix, and clitoris.

Often it is used for vaginal deliveries.

It is not indicated for intra-abdominal procedures. To anesthetize the abdomen and peritoneum, a T4 level is needed and this requires too large a dose—approximately 60 cc. to 80 cc. (see Remarks, page 449). Spinal or epidural block is the regional procedure most used for intra-abdominal surgery.

Diagnostic: Differentiation of vasospastic diseases from organic diseases of the lower extremities.

Therapeutic: Relief of vasospastic diseases of the extremities caused by embolic diseases, traumatic injuries, frostbite, thrombophlebitis, drug therapy (example: ergotrate poisoning), etc.

Relief of acute sciatica in the absence of a ruptured or protruding nucleus pulposus. The pain associated with this type of sciatica is often dramatically improved (see Remarks, page 450).

Increase of circulation of the lower extremities following operations on them where evidence of decreased circulation has been shown, *i.e.*, there is no healing or healing is slow.

ANATOMY

The sacrum is a large triangular bone formed by the fusion of five bones. It is inserted like a wedge between the two iliac bones (Figure 288, page 440). The dorsal surface is convex and in the midline is a crest, the median sacral crest (Figure 288, page 440). On either side of the middle sacral crest and separated from it by the sacral groove are linear series of tubercles produced by the fusion of the articular processes of the five sacral bones. These are called the sacral articular crests. The superior articular processes of the first sacral vertebra articulate with the inferior articulating processes of the fifth lumbar vertebra (Figure 288, page 440). The inferior articular processes of the fifth sacral vertebra are prolonged downward and are known as the sacral cornu (Figure 288, page 440). These lie on either side of the small triangular opening, the sacral hiatus at the apex of the sacrum. The sacral hiatus is the means of access to the caudal canal (Figure 288, page 440). Lateral to the articular crests and almost parallel to the midline are the four posterior sacral foramina which are approximately 1 cm. in diameter (Figure 288, page 440). These sacral foramina are the means of access to the sacral nerves, and the posterior primary division of the sacral nerves passes through them. The

439

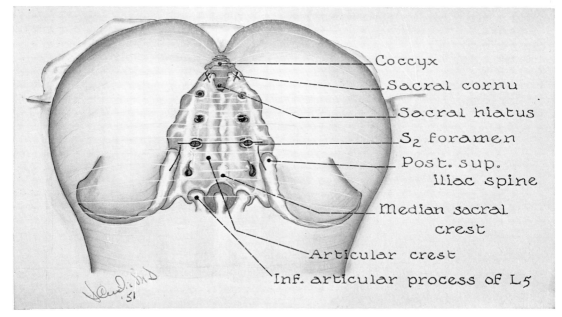

Figure 288. Topographical landmarks and anatomical considerations involved in a caudal block.

pelvic or anterior surface of the sacrum is of no consequence in this block and will not be described. The plexuses involved in this block are the lumbar plexus formed by the first, second, third, and fourth lumbar nerves together with a branch from the twelfth thoracic nerve; the sacral plexus formed by the fourth and fifth lumbar nerves together with the first, second, and third sacral nerves; and the coccygeal plexus formed by the fourth and fifth sacral nerves and the coccygeal nerve. The dural sac usually ends at the level of the second sacral foramina but on occasion may reach to the third or fourth sacral foramina (Figure 223, page 343). However, the filum terminale externum, closely invested by a sheath of dura, continues downward to be fused with the back of the coccyx.

The lumbar and sacral plexuses are together referred to as the lumbosacral plexus. It is to be noted that they each receive a portion of the fourth lumbar nerve (hence its name, nervus furcalis).

PREMEDICATION

Paresthesias are not sought. Therefore, heavy medication is advised except in obstet-rical cases, where light medication is chosen in order to avoid narcotizing the fetus.

Heavy Premedication: The average patient (age 20 to 50, weight 150 pounds or over, approximate height 5 feet, 5 inches or over, good physical status), receives:

1. 200 mg. (3 gr.) of pentobarbital (Nembutal) by mouth at hour of sleep the night before surgery.

2. 100 mg. (1½ gr.) to 200 mg. (3 gr.) of pentobarbital with one ounce of water by mouth 1½ to 2 hours before estimated *block* time.

3. 15 mg. (¼ gr.) of morphine and 0.6 mg. (1/100 gr.) of scopolamine intramuscularly ¾ to 1 hour before estimated *block* time.

Reduction of Premedication: It is seldom necessary to increase this premedication irrespective of the over-all size of the patient until the patient arrives in either the anesthesia or operating room. However, it is very common to reduce this medication under various circumstances; for example, in the case of the geriatric patient, the obstetrical patient, the adolescent patient or child, the debilitated or cachectic patient, and for those whose surgery is complicated by other disease, *e.g.*, myxedema, diabetes, heart disease, etc. In the patient over 60 years of age, barbiturates and especially scopolamine often cause disorientation. Therefore, in such a patient atropine is usually substituted for scopolamine and the dosages of the barbiturate omitted or greatly reduced, *i.e.*, to 50 mg. (¾ gr.) or less. *Always err on the light side.*

Inadequate Premedication: If the medication is inadequate, either for the block or for the surgical procedure, intravenous pentobarbital 50 mg. (¾ gr.) to 100 mg. (1½ gr.) or intravenous morphine 8 mg. (⅛ gr.) to 15 mg. (¼ gr.) may be given slowly. Judicious use of added sedation is extremely important. Often small supplementary doses of morphine or pentobarbital will make a block successful when a patient interprets touch and motion as pain.

Premedication of the Patient in Labor: All barbiturates, narcotics, belladonna derivatives, tranquilizers, and combinations of these drugs will pass the placenta and equilibrate in the fetus in the same period of time as they do in the mother. Therefore, little or no premedication is advised—the caudal block will relieve the pain.

If premedication is to be given to allay the parturient's fears and apprehensions *only,* a reasonable dosage of drugs which will not significantly depress the fetus should be used, *e.g.*, meperidine (Demerol) 50 mg. and promethazine (Phenergan) 25 mg.

DRUGS

Solutions containing methylparaben and metabisulfite should not be used (see page 451).

Lidocaine (Xylocaine) or Mepivacaine (Carbocaine): The rapid onset and constant results with either of these two drugs make them the drugs of choice for this procedure.

Dosage.—20 cc. to 40 cc. of 1.0 to 1.5 percent solution with or without 0.1 cc. of epinephrine (Adrenalin) 1:1000 in each 20 cc. of solution, depending on the size of the patient, *i.e.*, 5

feet, 6 inches or under, 20 cc. to 25 cc.; and over 5 feet, 6 inches, 25 cc. to 40 cc.* *Do not exceed 500 mg. (0.5 gm.) of lidocaine or mepivacaine.* We do not add epinephrine to a mepivacaine solution, but do add it when lidocaine is employed (see page 18).

Onset.—Operating analgesia is established in 10 to 20 minutes.

Duration.—Operating analgesia lasts 1¼ to 2 hours, with stronger concentrations and solutions containing epinephrine giving the upper limits.

Addition of Tetracaine (Pontocaine).—1 to 2 mg. of tetracaine may be added to each 1 cc. of lidocaine or mepivacaine to prolong its duration (see Chapter 2, page 15). When this is done, epinephrine is added to the solution.

Piperocaine (Metycaine)

Dosage.—20 cc. to 40 cc. of a 1.5 percent solution with or without 0.1 cc. of epinephrine (Adrenalin) 1:1000 in each 20 cc. of solution, depending on the size of the patient, *i.e.*, 5 feet, 6 inches or under, 20 cc. to 25 cc.; and over 5 feet, 6 inches, 25 cc. to 40 cc.*

Onset.—Operating analgesia is established in 15 to 30 minutes, with an average of 20 minutes.

Duration.—Operating analgesia lasts ¾ to 1¼ hours, with epinephrine solutions giving the upper limits.

Procaine (Novocain)

Dosage.—20 cc. to 40 cc. of 1.0 to 2.0 percent solution with or without 0.1 cc. of epinephrine (Adrenalin) 1:1000 in each 20 cc. of solution, depending on the size of the patient, *i.e.*, 5 feet, 6 inches or under, 20 cc. to 25 cc.; and over 5 feet, 6 inches, 25 cc. to 40 cc.*

Onset.—Operating analgesia is established in 15 to 30 minutes, with an average of 20 minutes.

---

*Optimal concentration of epinephrine is 1:200,000, that is, 0.1 cc. of epinephrine 1:1000 in 20 cc. of the local anesthetic solution (see page 451).

Duration.—Operating analgesia lasts ¾ to 1¼ hours, with stronger concentrations and solutions containing epinephrine giving the upper limits.

Tetracaine (Pontocaine)

Dosage.—20 cc. to 40 cc. of 0.15 to 0.25 percent solution with or without 0.1 cc. of epinephrine (Adrenalin) 1:1000 in each 20 cc. of solution, depending on the size of the patient, *i.e.,* 5 feet, 6 inches or over, 20 cc. to 25 cc.; and over 5 feet, 6 inches, 25 cc. to 40 cc.*

Onset.—Operating analgesia is established in 15 to 30 minutes, with an average of 25 minutes.

Duration.—Operating analgesia lasts 1¾ hours to 4½ hours, with stronger concentrations and solutions containing epinephrine giving the upper limits.

Chloroprocaine (Nesacaine): See page 451.

Dosage.—20 cc. to 40 cc. of a 2.0 percent solution with or without 0.1 cc. of epinephrine (Adrenalin) 1:1000 in each 20 cc. of solution, depending on the size of the patient, *i.e.,* 5 feet, 6 inches or under, 20 cc. to 25 cc.; and over 5 feet, 6 inches, 25 cc. to 40 cc.*

Onset.—Operating analgesia is established in 5 to 15 minutes, with an average of 8 to 10 minutes.

Duration.—Operating analgesia lasts ¾ to 1¼ hours, with solutions containing epinephrine giving the upper limits.

MATERIALS

Regional tray (see page 51) or:

1. One ¾-inch (2 cm.), 25-gauge Huber point security Lok-needle.

2. One 1½-inch (3.8 cm.), 22-gauge security Lok-needle, preferably with short bevel.

3. One 3-inch (7.5 cm.), 19-gauge spinal Lok-needle, preferably with short bevel.

4. One tuberculin Lok-syringe for measuring epinephrine.

5. One 10 cc. Lok-syringe, preferably with finger rings.

6. One Pitkin or a thin-walled needle guide.*

7. One graduated measuring cup, preferably stainless steel, for mixing solution.

8. One prep cup, preferably stainless steel.

9. Four sterile towels.

10. Six sterile sponges.

11. One sterilizer control.

TECHNIQUE

Position and Landmarks

1. The patient lies on a cart in the prone position with a large pillow under the iliac bones so that the sacrum is elevated and tilted approximately at a 35-degree angle to the table (Figure 289, page 442). On the operating

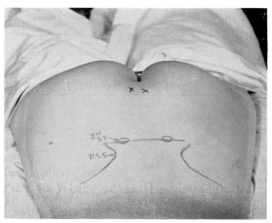

Figure 289. Landmarks for a caudal anesthesia. Patient lies in the prone position with a pillow under the iliac bones. X's, sacral cornu. S.F., sacral foramina. P.S.S., posterior superior spine of the iliac bone.

---

*Optimal concentration of epinephrine is 1:200,000, that is, 0.1 cc. of epinephrine 1:1000 in 20 cc. of the local anesthetic solution (see page 451).

*These items may be obtained from Becton, Dickinson and Company. Order number for Pitkin needle guide is PNG and for thin-walled needle guide is 01-0027.

table the position may be simulated by raising the kidney bar and flexing the table (Figure 290, page 443). If the caudal is being performed for an obstetrical delivery, the knee-chest position of the patient is the one of choice for the beginner as landmarks are not distorted by it (Figure 299, page 455).

2. When the prone position is employed, the patient is instructed to abduct his legs and turn his toes in and his heels out. This maneuver relaxes the gluteal muscles and makes it difficult for the patient to tense them (Figure 290 A and B, page 443).

3. The sacral cornu are palpated and marked with X's (Figure 289, page 442). The fingers of one hand are used to palpate while the other hand is used to exert pressure (Figure 10, page 58). If the sacral cornu cannot be palpated, the tip of the coccyx should be located and the sacral hiatus is usually found 2 inches (5 cm.) to 2½ inches (6.3 cm.) from its tip.

4. The posterior superior spines of the iliac bones are palpated and 0's are marked on the skin ½ inch (1.3 cm.) caudad and ½ inch (1.3 cm.) medial to these spines (Figure 289, page 442). The 0's should overlie the second sacral foramina. A line is usually drawn between these two 0's (Figure 289, page 442).

Precautions

Do Not Burn Perineum with Antiseptic Solution.—A sponge must be placed between the gluteal folds to prevent the antiseptic solution from running over the perineum and burning the patient.

3-inch (7.5 cm.), 19-Gauge Spinal Needle is Preferred to 1½-inch (3.8) 21- or 22-Gauge Needle.—A 3-inch (7.5 cm.), 19-gauge needle is preferable to a short, narrow-gauge needle. Since the caudal canal is narrowest at the sacral hiatus and this area is highly vascular, a longer needle can be placed beyond this area and thus minimize the chance of an intravas-

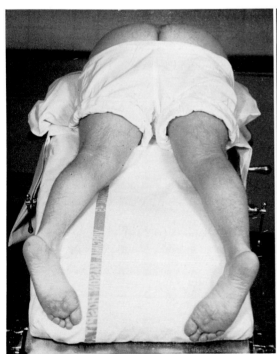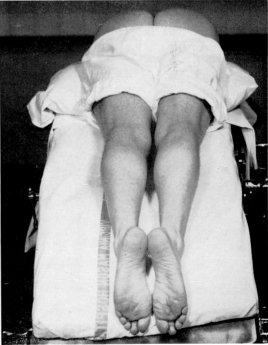

Figure 290. A. and B. A. *(Left)* Relaxation of the gluteal muscles and intergluteal fold by having the patient put his legs apart with toes in and heels out for a caudal block. In this position it is very difficult to tense the gluteal muscles. B. *(Right)* Tensing of the gluteal muscles and narrowing of the intergluteal fold when patient tenses muscles with the feet together.

cular injection. The greater gauge needle is used because it is easier to aspirate blood through it if its point rests in a blood vessel.

Point of 3-inch (7.5 cm.), 19-Gauge Spinal Needle Should Not Extend To or Above Second Sacral Foramina.—The point of the needle should never extend in the caudal canal above the second sacral foramina since the dural sac usually ends at or above this spot.

Carefully Identify Landmarks.—The tip of the coccyx must not be mistaken for the sacrococcygeal joint or the needle when inserted may enter the pelvic viscera, probably the rectum.

Aspirate for Blood or Spinal Fluid.—Careful aspiration for blood and spinal fluid should always be made.

Procedure

1. The sterilizer control is checked to be sure the equipment has been sterilized.

2. The area is aseptically prepared and draped.

3. If the anesthetist is right-handed, he stands at the patient's left side and vice versa (Figure 291, page 444).

4. An intradermal skin wheal is raised between the two X's marking the position of the

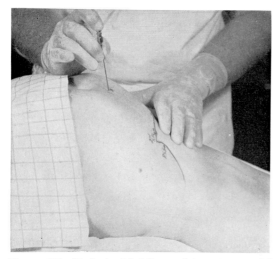

Figure 291. Method of holding and inserting caudal needle.

sacral cornu with the ¾-inch (2 cm.), 25-gauge Huber point security Lok-needle. This wheal should overlie the sacral hiatus.

5. With a 1½-inch (3.8 cm.), 22-gauge security Lok-needle, the subcutaneous tissue over and around the sacral hiatus is infiltrated. The periosteum around the sacral hiatus is particularly sensitive and should also be carefully injected. While infiltrating, an attempt to locate the sacrococcygeal ligament and the sacral hiatus should be attempted, since their location will give the anesthetist an idea of the inclination of the caudal canal.

6. A hole in the skin wheal is made with the needle guide and the guide withdrawn. Usually, this prevents the 19-gauge needle carrying with it a skin plug and skin bacteria into the caudal space.

7. The 3-inch (7.5 cm.), 19-gauge standard spinal needle with stylet in place is grasped so that the shaft is held by the thumb and middle fingers and the index finger rests on the head of the stylet (Figure 291, page 444). The index finger prevents the displacement of the stylet. The relationship of the markings on the hub of the needle to the bevel of the needle are noted and the needle with the bevel up is advanced at a 70- to 80-degree angle through the skin wheal until the point contacts the sacrum (Figure 292B, needle 1, page 445).

8. The needle is now slightly withdrawn and the anesthetist slowly reduces the angle of the needle, feeling his way each time until the needle point encounters the sacrococcygeal membrane (Figure 292B, needle 2, page 445). This may be at a depth of ¼ inch (0.6 cm.) to 1½ inches (3.8 cm.) from the skin, depending on the build of the patient.

9. The bevel of the needle is turned downward to facilitate the passage of the needle into and through the sacral canal (Figure 292B, needle 2, page 445).

10. The hub of the needle is now swung downward to an angle of 20 degrees to the surface of the skin for a male, but only to an angle of 35 degrees to 40 degrees to the surface of the skin for a female (Figure 293, page

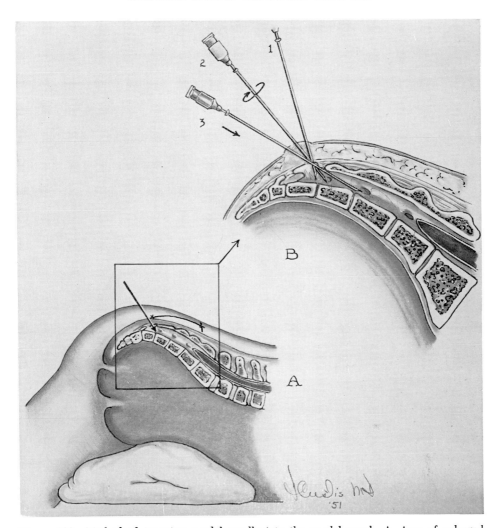

Figure 292. Method of inserting caudal needle into the caudal canal. A. Area of enlarged section. B. 1. Needle point with the bevel up has pierced the ligament covering the opening of the caudal canal. 2. Needle lowered to an approximate 50-degree angle with the skin and advanced into the caudal canal. The bevel is now rotated so that it points downward. This facilitates its passage over the periosteum of the sacral canal. 3. Needle is now lowered to an approximate 30-degree to 45-degree angle in the female and a 10-degree to 20-degree angle in the male and advanced into the caudal canal.

446 and Figure 292B, needle 3, page 445). The tilt of the female sacrum is normally greater than that of the male (Figure 293, page 446).

11. The needle is advanced through the sacrococcygeal ligament and into the caudal canal for approximately 1½ inches (3.8 cm.) (Figure 294, page 446). If the needle should contact bone, gentle pressure downward on the shaft of the needle with the index finger

of the free hand may depress the needle to aid its passage in the canal (Figure 295, page 447).

12. The stylet is withdrawn and the distance of the needle in the canal checked. This is easily done by placing the stylet on the skin overlying the sacrum (Figure 296, page 448). The needle point should not extend to the line drawn between the second sacral foramen.

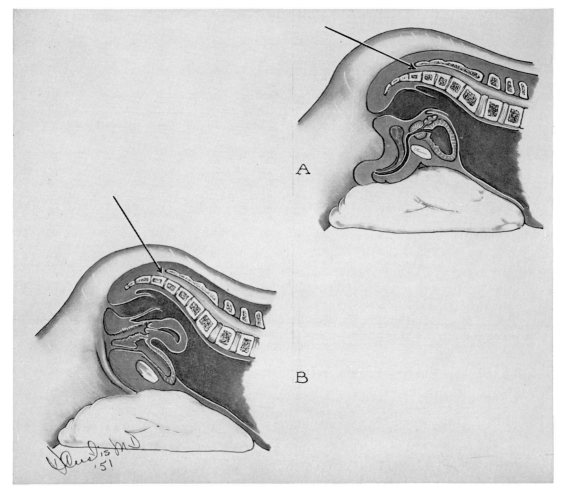

Figure 293. Variations in the tilts of the human pelvis depending on whether the patient is a male or female. A. Male. B. Female.

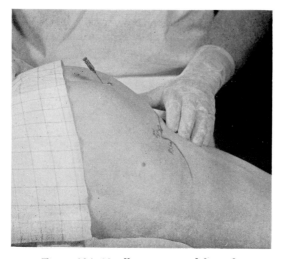

Figure 294. Needle rests in caudal canal.

13. The syringe is attached and an attempt to aspirate blood or spinal fluid is made. The needle is then rotated 180 degrees and aspiration repeated. If spinal fluid is aspirated, another regional procedure such as spinal block is instituted. If blood is aspirated, the needle should be advanced ¼ inch (0.6 cm.), the stylet reinserted to clear the blood from the lumen of the needle before it coagulates, and the needle allowed to remain untouched for 2 to 3 minutes by the clock. This maneuver allows the needle point to be disengaged from the lumen of a vessel and allows time for the vessels that have been damaged by trauma during the introduction of the needle to stop oozing. After the 2- to 3-minute interval, the

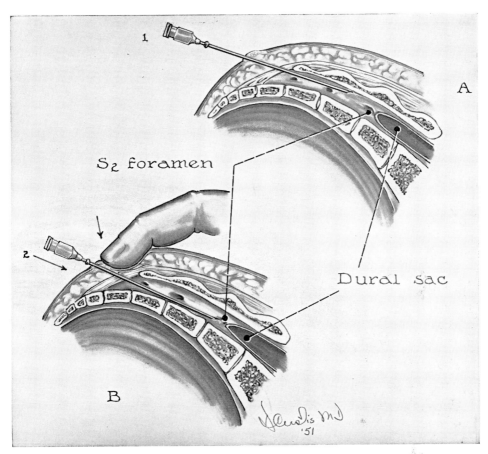

Figure 295. Use of the index finger to depress the shaft of the needle to facilitate its passage into the caudal canal. A. Needle point rests against posterior bone plate of the sacrum. B. Index finger exerting pressure on the shaft of the needle so that it may be advanced in the caudal canal.

stylet is withdrawn and aspiration in two planes repeated. If blood is still aspirated the block should be stopped and a spinal block, epidural block, or general anesthesia used.

14. If no blood or spinal fluid is obtained, 5 cc. of air is injected rapidly while the anesthetist observes the area over the sacrum. When the needle is posterior to the sacrum, air causes the tissues over the sacrum to swell, and crepitation, which shows the air in the tissue, may be palpated. Should this occur, withdraw the needle and make another attempt to place it in the caudal canal. If, as usual, the needle lies in the caudal canal, the patient may experience a "funny sensation in the legs." Prior to injecting air, the patient should be warned that this may occur.

15. When the air test indicates the needle lies in the caudal canal, 3 to 5 cc. of the local anesthetic solution is injected rapidly as a test dose. During injection, the tissue over the sacrum should be observed for swelling. At the end of the downward motion of the plunger of the syringe, quickly release the pressure on the plunger. If the needle is posterior to the sacrum, there will be a refill of from 0.5 cc. to 1.0 cc. If it lies inside the canal, there will be a refill of 0.1 cc. to 0.2 cc., or there will be no refill. If the needle lies posterior to the sacrum, withdraw it and make another attempt to place it in the caudal canal.

16. Now, the syringe is detached from the needle and the stylet replaced. Five minutes are allowed to elapse *by the clock*. Carefully

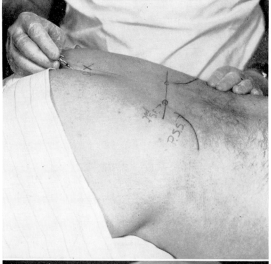

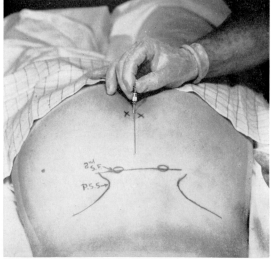

Figure 296. Method of checking height of the needle in the caudal canal. A. *(Top)* Lateral view. B. *(Bottom)* Posterior view.

monitor the patient's blood pressure, pulse, and sensorium during this period for evidence of a systemic toxic reaction. If one occurs, adjust the needle, remove and reinsert it, use another regional technique, or abandon the regional technique and administer general anesthesia.

If the five minutes pass uneventfully, the lower extremities, abdomen, and chest should be tested for signs of anesthesia. When following a 3 cc. to 5 cc. test dose of the local anesthetic solution the area of analgesia is extensive, the dura has in all probability been

punctured and further attempts at establishing the caudal block should be discontinued. If the existing spinal anesthesia needs to be supplemented, use general anesthesia.

If, as usual, there is no area of analgesia or only a small area of anesthesia or hypesthesia limited to the immediate perianal region or the tissue over the coccyx, and if the patient's blood pressure, pulse, and sensorium remain unchanged, it is safe to assume that neither the dura nor a blood vessel has been invaded.

17. Now, an additional 15 cc. to 30 cc. of the anesthetic solution should be added.

18. As the needle is withdrawn, 5 cc. of the anesthetic solution is injected.

EXTENT OF ANALGESIA

Analgesia exists from approximately the tenth thoracic dermatome to the tips of the toes (Figure 242, page 354). However, operating analgesia of the thighs and legs, particularly on the anterior surface, is often incomplete. This is probably due to the fact that enough anesthetic solution to anesthetize these nerves completely does not penetrate the nerve coverings.

COMPLICATIONS

Hypotension: See page 353. Hypotension during caudal analgesia should be treated in the same way as during spinal block (see page 354).

Nausea and Vomiting: See page 355.

Respiratory Arrest: See page 355.

Systemic Toxic Reactions to Local Anesthetic and Vasoconstrictor Drugs. See pages 19 and 40, respectively.

High or Total Spinal Block: This is not considered individually, since its signs and symptoms are hypotension, nausea and vomiting, respiratory arrest, and, if these go untreated, cardiac arrest. See pages 353 to 356.

Cardiac Failure: See page 356.

Urinary Retention: Frequently, this complication occurs following caudal anesthesia.

However, its incidence is not much greater than that after general anesthesia. Treatment consists of one or two catheterizations, following which the patient usually voids voluntarily. Voluntary urination may be encouraged by hot packs to the perineum, standing or sitting the patient in the upright position, and suggesting another catheterization in the patient's presence. If the bladder was traumatized at operation, it should be placed at rest for 24 to 48 hours by catheter drainage (see page 361).

Headache: This may occur if the dura is inadvertently punctured (see page 356).

Palsies and Paralysis: See page 360.

Placement of Needle Anterior to Sacrum: On the very rare occasion, the caudal needle may be inserted anterior to the sacrum or into the rectum. When this occurs, no anesthesia will result. Usually, no sequelae, e.g., infection or fistula, result.

Local Infections: Extremely rare.

Signs and Symptoms.—These include fever, pain over the sacrum, and, if superficial, the local signs of infection are present.

Etiology.—Failure to adhere to the rules of asepsis.

Treatment.—Chemotherapy, i.e., penicillin, sulfa drugs, etc.; heat over the sacrum; and surgical drainage.

Meningitis or Meningismus: See page 360.

REMARKS

In addition to the remarks below, many of the remarks under Single-Dose Spinal (Subarachnoid) Anesthesia, page 361, are applicable to this block and they should be read. *Also, when caudal block is used for obstetrical deliveries, it is advised that the remarks under Continuous (Intermittent) Caudal Block, pages 465 to 472 be read, because they are applicable to this block.*

Do Not Attempt to Produce Anesthesia Above Tenth Thoracic Dermatome with Cau- dal Block: Injection of local anesthetic solutions in the caudal canal should be limited to 30 cc. to 40 cc. This will produce analgesia to approximately the tenth or, occasionally, the ninth thoracic somatic dermatome. High caudal anesthesia, i.e., analgesia above the tenth thoracic dermatome, produced by injecting a large volume (50 to 80 cc.) of anesthetic solution into the caudal canal, may be quite dangerous because this volume of solution usually represents a toxic dose of the local anesthetic agent. If a regional block of the abdominal cavity or other area innervated by nerves above the tenth thoracic somatic nerve is sought, spinal or epidural block should be chosen rather than high caudal block, as it is more controllable and the results are more predictable.

Height of Caudal Block Depends on Size of Epidural Space, Gravity, etc.: The height as well as the adequacy of analgesia obtained by a caudal injection depend on: (1) the size of the epidural space; (2) the amount of areolar tissue in the epidural space; (3) the various septa of the epidural space; (4) the permeability of the neural and dural sheath to the drug; (5) the capillary action exerted on fluids by the space between the dural wall and the ligaments and periosteum lining the vertebral canal; and (6) since the epidural space is a compartment, gravity may exert some influence on the spread of the local anesthetic solution—in general, the solution tends to gravitate to the dependent portion of the epidural space.

Contraindications to Caudal Block: Most of the contraindications to spinal block apply to caudal block (see Chapter 43, page 363). To these may be added a pilonidal cyst and malformations of the sacrum. Approximately 20 to 25 percent of patients have deformities of the sacrum but in only 5 percent or less do these deformities prevent insertion of the needle into the caudal canal.

Is Caudal Block Safer Than Spinal Block? While the public has been made aware of the problems of spinal block, they are less familiar with the complications of caudal block. Therefore, often patients are willing to accept this block when they refuse to have spinal anesthesia. With caudal block, the minor complications of spinal block, e.g., headache, usually are avoided. However, the incidence of major complications, such as, total spinal block, hypotension, systemic toxic reactions, and neurologic complications, is as great or greater with caudal block.

This should be expected because: (1) large volumes and higher concentrations of the local anesthetic solution must be used; (2) an inadvertent subarachnoid placement of the needle thought to be in the caudal canal may go unrecognized; (3) often, a concentration of epinephrine (Adrenalin) greater than 1:200,-000 is employed in the local anesthetic solution; (4) with a continuous technique, total subarachnoid block may result after a *reinforcing* dose (page 467); and (5) the experience of most physicians is not as great with caudal block as with spinal block.

Single-Dose Caudal Block Is Preferred to Single-Dose Spinal Block for: (1) Operations on the Rectum, Vulva, and Coccyx; and (2) Vaginal Delivery: The author prefers caudal block for these procedures because the relaxation is excellent and postspinal headache is eliminated unless the dura is punctured inadvertently. Furthermore, for hemorrhoidectomy, fistulectomy, and polypectomy, the jackknife position (Buie) may be used without a high level of anesthesia ensuing.

Atypical Sciatica May Be Relieved by Pressure Caudal: Not infrequently a "pressure" caudal with or without a back manipulation is done to relieve atypical sciatica or back pain. This entails the rapid injection of 50 to 90 cc. of a saline solution into the caudal canal. The solution must be injected rapidly so that it will not escape through the foramina and thus fail to elevate the pressure in the epidural space.

To perform a pressure caudal and back manipulation it has been our custom to: (1) place the needle in the caudal canal; (2) inject 30 cc. of 1.0 percent lidocaine or mepivacaine solution; (3) wait 15 to 20 minutes for the anesthetic effects of either agent to be-

come well established; (4) then inject 50 to 90 cc. of normal saline rapidly until the patient complains of either an aching between the scapula or a headache; and (5) have the referring physicians, e.g., the orthopedist, vigorously manipulate the back and legs.

On a number of occasions after 40 to 50 cc. of the saline had been injected rapidly and before the complaint of headache, the patient had a convulsion which lasted 10 to 20 seconds. Presumably this is due: (1) to motion of the cord caused by the rapid injection of the saline or (2) to the increase in the spinal fluid pressure which results from filling the epidural space, which then forces the cerebrospinal fluid from the dural sac into the cranial cavity increasing intracranial pressure. To date, we have seen no untoward effects from either the injection, the convulsion, or the manipulation.

These patients are never given heavy sedation or general anesthesia prior to such an injection, and whenever the patient complains of pain between the scapula, headache, or has a convulsion, the injection is suspended; but the manipulation is performed. It is the author's opinion that giving heavy sedation or general anesthesia may create a dangerous situation because the signs that the epidural space has been almost filled with saline, i.e., complaint of headache, pain between the shoulders, or convulsion, are not available. Thus, a dosage of the saline in excess of that which is needed to fill and exert pressure in the epidural space may be administered. When pressure caudals are performed under general anesthesia and manipulation of the legs and back done, retinal hemorrhage has resulted.

Pain, Cramping, or Feeling of Fullness in Thighs or Calves Indicates Needle Is Correctly Placed: Pain, cramping, or the feeling of fullness in the legs during injection of the local anesthetic solution in the caudal canal is of no significance other than the fact that it indicates the needle is correctly placed in the caudal canal.

Caudal Block May Be Used to Block Lumbar and Pelvic Sympathetic Nerves: When acute vascular emergencies of the lower extremities arise (see page 211), and proficiency at lumbar sympathetic block has not been acquired, caudal block should be considered as it may save all or part of the extremity. If prolonged analgesia is needed, continuous caudal block should be considered.

Monitor Patient Carefully: A patient under caudal block must never be left unattended and constant contact by conversation with the patient should be maintained for the first twenty minutes following the injection of the local anesthetic agent. Many of the common complications following this regional procedure occur in these first twenty minutes and complaints of the patient as well as changes in his blood pressure and pulse are valuable aids in detecting some of the earliest signs of complications.

Avoid Solutions Containing Methylparaben and Metabisulfite: These drugs are often added to commercially prepared local anesthetic solutions to prevent oxidation and as a preservative. Solutions containing them are not recommended for caudal blocks.

Methylparaben.—Methylparaben is a preservative and fungistatic agent.

Metabisulfite.—Metabisulfite is an antioxidizing agent.

Chloroprocaine (Nesacaine): Chloroprocaine has a rapid onset, 8 to 15 minutes, and it seems to have the lowest systemic toxicity of any local anesthetic agent used at the present time. The author and his associates have used it in over 2,500 continuous caudal blocks for obstetrical delivery and found it to be a satisfactory agent. Because of packaging difficulties, chloroprocaine is not at the present time available for epidural block (see page 15). However, it is included under Drugs in this chapter because the pharmaceutical house which manufactures the drug indicates that it again may become available.

Do Not Exceed a 1:200,000 Concentration of Epinephrine in the Caudal Canal: A stronger concentration, *i.e.,* 1:100,000 will not prolong the duration of anesthesia significantly and it may predispose to complications, *e.g.,* hypertension.

Do Not Use Phenylephrine in the Caudal Canal—It May Cause Severe Hypertension: Phenylephrine, 3 mg. to 5 mg., injected into the caudal canal will result in a severe hypertension.

Recover Broken Needle(s): All needles should be tested before use. If a needle breaks, every effort to remove it, including surgery, should be made. Unremoved needles have a tendency to migrate and may cause permanent injuries as well as medicolegal complications.

When a spinal needle which is being placed in the caudal canal breaks, there is little doubt in the anesthetist's mind as to what has happened. A distinct click is felt. This usually happens when the needle is being inserted and the stylet is still in the needle. If the anesthetist suspects that the needle has broken, he should not remove the stylet. If the needle breaks after the stylet is removed, the portion containing the hub of the needle should not be removed. They are valuable guides to locating the broken end of the needle. When the anesthetist suspects that the needle has been broken, he should release his hold on it and have an x-ray taken immediately.

Repeat Block When Analgesia Is Inadequate: If the results from the first block attempt are unsatisfactory, do not hesitate to reblock the patient if time permits. Most patients will think nothing about being reblocked if the second attempt is prefaced by a statement such as: "Well, I guess we will have to inject a little more medicine if we are going to freeze this area."

However, do not exceed the maximum safe dosage of the local anesthetic solution for both blocks. If to reblock the patient the maximum safe dose of the local anesthetic solution must be exceeded, 45 minutes should elapse between blocks.

CHAPTER 49

Continuous (Intermittent) Caudal Block

INDICATIONS

INDICATIONS for this block are the same as for single-dose caudal block (see page 439), and this procedure is instituted where prolonged analgesia is required. Continuous caudal analgesia is used most frequently by us for vaginal deliveries. Therefore, in this chapter, the pregnant female is used to illustrate this block procedure. Nevertheless, the fundamental principles involved in the technique of placing the malleable needle or plastic tubing are largely applicable to other operations and therapeutic and diagnostic blocks in which this method is indicated.

ANATOMY

Same as in single-dose caudal block (see page 439).

PREMEDICATION

Same as for single-dose caudal block (see page 440).

DRUGS

The drugs used for this block are the same as those used for single-dose caudal block (see page 441). Solutions containing methylparaben and metabisulfite should not be used (see page 469). Tetracaine (Pontocaine) or procaine (Novocain) is seldom used for continuous caudal block. The rapid onset and constant results of lidocaine (Xylocaine), mepivacaine (Carbocaine), and chloroprocaine (Nesacaine) make them the agents of choice for this block. Tetracaine is seldom added to solutions of these three agents since the continuous technique obviates the need to employ a solution with a prolonged duration. However, epinephrine (Adrenalin) may be added—not to prolong the duration of anesthesia, but to slow the absorption of the agent.

Onset and duration are the same with continuous caudal block as with single-dose caudal block, depending on the agent employed (see page 441). *However, the dosage depends on whether the malleable needle technique or the plastic tubing technique is employed.*

Malleable Needle Technique: The malleable needle is placed approximately 1½ inches (3.8 cm.) to 2 inches (5 cm.) into the caudal canal and lies below the level of the second sacral foramina. The initial dose of local anesthetic solution injected depends on the size of the patient, *i.e.,* 5 feet, 6 inches or under, 20 cc. to 25 cc.; and over 5 feet, 6 inches, 25 cc. to 35 cc. Each reinforcing dose is approximately the same or slightly less than the initial dose, *i.e.,* if the initial dose was 30 cc., each reinforcing dose would be 25 cc. to 30 cc. Reinforcing doses should not be given until ¾ to 1 hour has elapsed unless the previous dose and the dose to be given do not exceed the toxic dose of local anesthetic agent. With the exception of mepivacaine, the other local anesthetic agents do not seem to have a cumulative effect (see page 23).

Reinforcing doses must be given immediately when the patient first starts to feel pain. If administration is delayed until pain is severe, it may be difficult to re-establish the block.

Plastic Tubing Technique: The plastic tubing is placed approximately 5 inches (12.5 cm.) to 6 inches (15 cm.) into the caudal canal and lies at the level of approximately the fifth lumbar vertebra (Figure 310, page 470). Therefore, less anesthetic solution can be employed. The initial dose of the local anesthetic solution with this technique is 12 to 20 cc. depending of the height of the patient, *i.e.*, 5 feet, 6 inches or under, 12 cc. to 15 cc.; and over 5 feet, 6 inches, 15 cc. to 20 cc. These dosages are "rule of thumb" dosages and may be varied slightly.

The volume of the reinforcing dose is the same as the initial dose. As soon as the patient feels pain, it should be given. If administration is delayed until the pain is severe, it may be difficult to re-establish the block.

MATERIALS

Same as for single-dose caudal block (see Chapter 48, page 442). To this equipment should be added the following items, depending on whether the malleable needle or the plastic tubing technique is to be used.

Malleable Needle Method

1. One 2-inch (5 cm.), 19-gauge malleable hubless security bead needle with stylet (Figure 297, page 453).*

2. One 2½-inch (6.3 cm.), 19-gauge malleable hubless security bead caudal needle with stylet (Figure 297, page 453).*

3. One 3-inch (7.5 cm.), 19-gauge malleable hubless security bead caudal needle with stylet (Figure 297, page 453).*

4. One 6-inch (15 cm.) piece of hard-walled rubber tubing with a diameter of 3 mm. (Figure 298, page 454). **

Malleable Needle Method.—These items may be obtained from Becton, Dickinson and Company, Rutherford, N. J. The order numbers are: 2-inch (5 cm.), 2½-inch (6.3 cm.), and 3-inch (7.5 cm.) malleable hubless continuous caudal needles with security bead, F460R; female Lok to hose end adapter, L/609; and plug for female Lok outlet, 417A.

**This item may be obtained from the Davol Rubber Company, Providence, R. I. The order number is 2841 and the measurements of the tubing are 1/16-inch by 7/128-inch (13 F.S., O. diameter).

5. A female Lok to hose end adapter—one end fits the Lok-syringe, the other, the hard-walled rubber tubing (Figure 298, page 454).*

6. One plug for the female Lok outlet adapter in 5 above so that when the syringe is detached the hub of the needle may be kept sterile (Figure 298, page 454).*

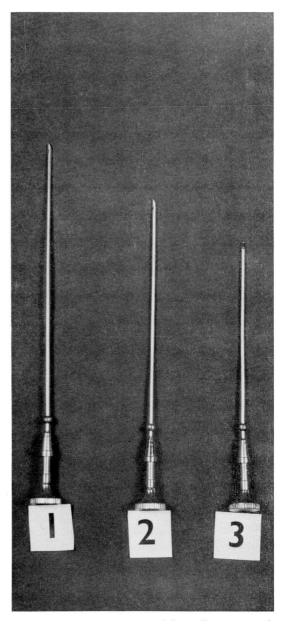

Figure 297. Continuous caudal needles. 1. 3-inch (7.5 cm.). 2. 2½-inch (6.3 cm.). 3. 2-inch (5 cm.).

Plastic Tubing Method

1. One 3-inch (7.5 cm.), 18-gauge thin-

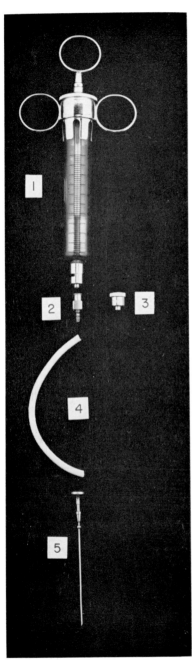

Figure 298. Continuous caudal equipment. 1. 10 cc. Lok-syringe with finger rings. 2. Female Lok-adapter. 3. Plug for female Lok-adapter. 4. 6-inch (15 cm.) rubber tubing with a $\frac{1}{16}$-inch (3 mm.) lumen. 5. 2½-inch (6.3 cm.) continuous caudal needle with stylet.

walled spinal needle with a *regular bevel* and a stylet.†

2. One plastic tubing (Figure 253, page 390 and Figure 263, page 401).† The plastic tubing is marked prior to sterilization 7¾ inches (19.5 cm.) from the end to be inserted into the caudal canal with a felt marking pen or a ball point pen—3 inches (7.5 cm.) for the length of the shaft of the needle; ¾-inch (2.0 cm.) for the length of the hub of the needle; and 4 inches (10 cm.) for beyond the point of the needle. The tubing with wire stylet in it (item 3) is placed in a plastic bag, wrapped with a sterilizer control (Figure 263, page 401), and heat sterilized.

3. One wire stylet (Figure 253, page 390).† If a wire stylet is not used in the plastic tubing, it may be difficult to thread the plastic tubing cephalad in the caudal canal, and it will be hard to slide the needle off the tubing without dislodging the tubing.

4. One Tuohy-Borst female Lok to plastic tubing adapter or one ¾-inch (2 cm.), 23-gauge Lok-needle, preferably with a short bevel (Figure 253, page 390 and Figure 265, page 402).†

5. One plug for female Lok outlet in 4 so that when syringe is detached the female outlet of the needle or adapter may be kept sterile (Figure 253, page 390 and Figure 264, page 402).†

†*Plastic Tubing Method.*—These items may be obtained from Becton, Dickinson and Company, Rutherford, N. J. The order numbers are: 3-inch (7.5 cm.), 18-gauge thin-walled needle, T462LNR; plastic tubing, regular VX020 and radiopaque RVX020 or CRVX020; wire stylet, 01-0041; Tuohy-Borst female Lok to plastic tubing adapter, 610A; and plug for female Lok outlet, 417A.

Two types of radiopaque tubing are available— the RVX020 which does not permit observation of the lumen and the CRVX020, which does permit observation of the lumen. The CRVX020 allows detection of blood or spinal fluid more easily when the aspiration tests are performed. It also permits observation of the wire stylet. For illustrations, the RVX020 was employed because photographs of it are **better.**

TECHNIQUE

Position and Landmarks: Same as in single-dose caudal block (see page 442). For obstetrical cases, the knee-chest position is the position of choice while mastering this technique (Figure 299, page 455). After the tech-

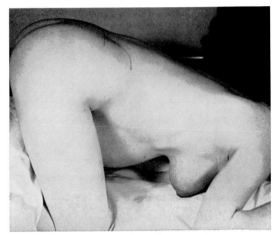

Figure 299. Knee-chest position.

nique is mastered, a modified Sims' (side) position may be employed (Figure 303, *Top*, page 457).

Precautions: Same as for single-dose caudal block. See page 443.

Procedure: This depends on the method to be employed. Regardless of the method, the sterilizer control should be carefully checked to see that the equipment is sterile.

Malleable Needle Method

1. The area is aseptically prepared and draped.

2. If the anesthetist is right-handed, he stands at the patient's left side (Figure 300, page 455).

3. An intradermal skin wheal is raised between the two X's marking the position of the sacral cornu with the ¾-inch (2 cm.), 25-gauge Huber point security Lok-needle. This wheal should overlie the sacral hiatus.

4. With a 1½-inch (3.8 cm.), 22-gauge security Lok-needle the subcutaneous tissue over

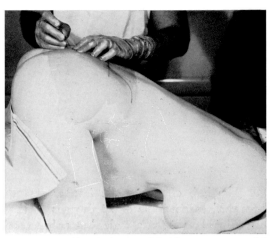

Figure 300. 2½-inch (6.3 cm.) hubless security caudal needle being inserted at an 80-degree angle to the skin until the sacrum is contacted.

and around the sacral hiatus is infiltrated. The periosteum around the sacral hiatus is particularly sensitive and should also be carefully injected. While infiltrating, an attempt to locate the sacrococcygeal ligament and the sacral hiatus should be attempted to give the anesthetist an idea of the inclination of the caudal canal.

5. A hole is made in the skin wheal with the Pitkin or thin-walled needle guide and the guide withdrawn. Usually, this prevents the 19-gauge needle carrying with it a skin plug and skin bacteria into the caudal space.

6. Depending on the size of the patient and the fat pad over the sacrum, either the 2-inch (5 cm.), the 2½-inch (6.3 cm.), or the 3-inch (7.5 cm.), 19-gauge malleable hubless security bead caudal needle with stylet in place is grasped so that the shaft is held by the thumb and middle finger and the index finger rests on the head of the stylet (Figure 300, page 455). The index finger prevents the displacement of the stylet. The relationship of the notch at the hubless end of the needle to the point's bevel is noted and the needle with the bevel up is advanced at a 70- to 80-degree angle to the skin through the skin wheal until the point contacts the sacrum (Figure 292 B, needle 1, page 445).

7. The needle is now withdrawn slightly and the anesthetist slowly reduces the angle

of the needle, feeling his way each time until the needle point encounters the sacrococcygeal ligament (Figure 292B, needle 2, page 445). This may be at a depth of ¼ inch (0.6 cm.) to 1½ inches (3.8 cm.) from the skin depending on the build of the patient.

8. The bevel of the needle is turned downward to facilitate the passage of the needle into and through the sacral canal (Figure 292B, needle 2, page 445).

9. The hub of the needle is now swung downward to an angle of 20 degrees to the surface of the skin in a male, but only to an angle of 35 degrees to 40 degrees to the surface of the skin in a female (Figure 292B, needle 3, page 445 and Figure 293, page 446). The tilt of the female sacrum is normally greater than that of a male.

10. The needle is advanced through the sacrococcygeal ligament and into the caudal canal for approximately 1½ inches (3.8 cm.) (Figure 301, page 456 and Figure 302A, page 456).

11. The stylet is withdrawn and the distance of the needle in the canal checked. This is easily done by placing the stylet on the skin overlying the sacrum (Figure 302B, page 456). The needle point should not extend to a line drawn between the second sacral foramina.

12. The end of the 6-inch (15 cm.) hard wall rubber tubing opposite the female Lok-

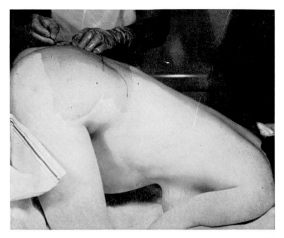

Figure 301. 2½-inch (6.3 cm.), hubless security caudal needle has been lowered to a 45-degree angle with the skin. The needle has slipped into the caudal canal and is slowly being advanced up the caudal canal.

adapter is attached to the hubless needle (Figure 303, page 457).

13. The syringe is attached to the end of the rubber tubing with a female Lok-adapter and an attempt to aspirate blood or spinal fluid is made. The needle is then rotated 180 degrees and aspiration repeated. If spinal fluid is aspirated, another regional procedure such as spinal block is considered. If blood is aspirated, the needle should be advanced ¼ inch (0.6 cm.), the stylet reinserted to clear the blood from the lumen of the needle before it coagulates, and the needle allowed to remain untouched for 2 or 3 minutes by the

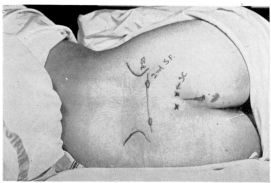
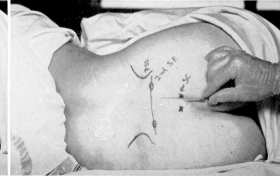

Figure 302. A. (Left) Patient turned in lateral position. B. (Right) Note measurement of distance needle lies in the caudal canal. PSS, posterior superior spine of the iliac bone. SF, sacral foramen. SC, sacral cornu. Note the patient at these steps in the procedure is still in the knee-chest position. However, to clearly illustrate important points the patient was turned into the modified Sims' (side) position.

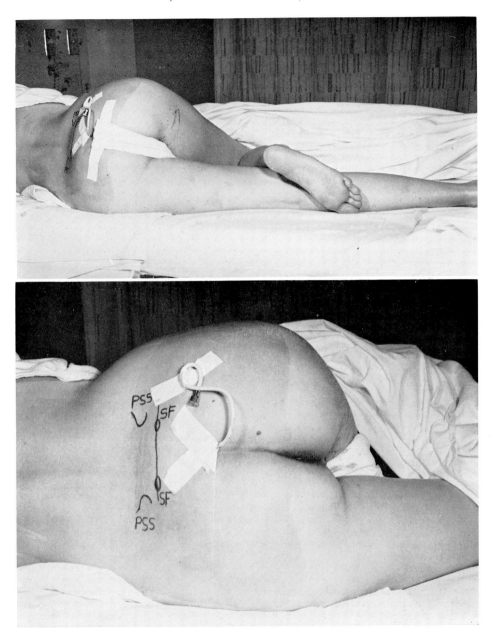

Figure 303. Patient in modified Sims' position with needle taped in place. A pillow (not shown in figure) is placed at back of the patient to remind her not to turn into the supine position. PSS, posterior superior spines of the iliac bone. SF, second sacral foramina. *(Top)* Full view showing patient's position when needle was inserted. *(Bottom)* Closeup of needle taped in place.

clock. This maneuver allows the needle point to be disengaged from the lumen of a vessel and allows time for the vessels that have been damaged by trauma during the introduction of the needle to stop oozing. After the 2- or 3-minute interval, the stylet is withdrawn and aspiration in two planes repeated. If blood is still aspirated, the caudal block should be discontinued and spinal block, epidural block, or general anesthesia employed.

14. If no blood or spinal fluid is obtained, 5 cc. of air is injected rapidly while the anesthetist observes the area over the sacrum.

When the needle is posterior to the sacrum, air causes the tissues over the sacrum to swell, and crepitation, which shows the air in the tissue, may be palpated. Should this occur, withdraw the needle and make another attempt to place it in the caudal canal. If, as usual, the needle lies in the caudal canal, the patient may experience a "funny sensation in the legs." Prior to injecting air, the patient should be warned that this may occur.

15. When the air test indicates the needle lies in the caudal canal, 3 to 5 cc. of the local anesthetic solution is injected rapidly as a test dose. During injection, the tissue over the sacrum should be observed for swelling. At the end of the downward motion of the plunger of the syringe, quickly release the pressure on the plunger. If the needle is posterior to the sacrum, there will be a refill of from 0.5 cc. to 1.0 cc. If it lies inside the canal, there will be a refill of 0.1 cc. to 0.2 cc., or there will be no refill. If the needle lies posterior to the sacrum, withdraw it and make another attempt to place it in the caudal canal.

16. The syringe is detached from the rubber tubing and the plug is placed in the opening of the female Lok-adapter (Figure 303, page 457). If the needle was placed with the patient in the knee-chest position, she is placed in the modified Sims' (side) position. Five minutes are allowed to elapse *by the clock*. Carefully monitor the patient's blood pressure, pulse, and sensorium during this period for evidence of a systemic toxic reaction. If one occurs, adjust the needle, remove and reinsert it, use another regional technique, or abandon the regional technique and administer general anesthesia.

If the five minutes pass uneventfully, the lower extremities, abdomen, and chest should be tested for signs of analgesia. When, following a 3 cc. to 5 cc. test dose of the local anesthetic solution the area of analgesia is extensive, the dura has in all probability been punctured and further attempts at establishing the continuous caudal block should be discontinued. If the existing spinal anesthesia needs to be supplemented, use general anesthesia.

If, as usual, analgesia is absent or limited to the immediate perianal region or the tissue over the coccyx and if the patient's blood pressure, pulse, and sensorium remain unchanged, it is safe to assume that neither the dura nor a blood vessel has been invaded. Then, an additional 20 cc. to 35 cc. of the anesthetic solution is added, depending on the size of the patient. The test dose is disregarded when calculating this initial dose.

17. The caudal needle is taped in place (Figure 303, page 457).

18. Reinforcing doses should be approximately the same or slightly less than the initial dose, *i.e.*, if 30 cc. was given initially, the second dose would be 25 cc. to 30 cc. It is best to give the subsequent doses when the patient first notices discomfort. Once severe pain has been felt, it is often difficult to re-establish adequate analgesia.

19. When the parturient with a malleable caudal needle in place is ready to be delivered, a reinforcing dose should be given, the malleable caudal needle withdrawn, and she is turned supine. When the parturient is turned to the supine position, she must be observed for the supine hypotensive syndrome.

Plastic Tubing Method

1. The area is aseptically prepared and draped.

2. If the anesthetist is right-handed, he stands at the patient's left side (Figure 300, page 455).

3. An intradermal skin wheal is raised between the two X's marking the position of the sacral cornu with the ¾-inch (2 cm.), 25-gauge Huber point security Lok-needle. This wheal should overlie the sacral hiatus.

4. With a 1½-inch (3.8 cm.), 22-gauge security Lok-needle the subcutaneous tissue over and around the sacral hiatus is infiltrated. The periosteum around the sacral hiatus is particularly sensitive and should also be carefully injected. While infiltrating, an attempt to locate the sacrococcygeal ligament and the sacral

hiatus should be attempted to give the anesthetist an idea of the inclination of the caudal canal.

5. A hole is made in the skin wheal with the Pitkin or thin-walled needle guide and the guide withdrawn. Usually, this prevents the 18-gauge needle carrying with it a skin plug and skin bacteria into the caudal space.

6. The 3-inch (7.5 cm.), 18-gauge thin-walled spinal needle with a regular point and a stylet in place is grasped so that the shaft is held by the thumb and middle finger with the index finger resting on the head of the stylet (Figure 300, page 455). The index finger prevents the displacement of the stylet. The relationship of the markings on the hub of the needle to the bevel are noted and the needle with the bevel up is advanced at a 70- to 80-degree angle to the skin through the skin wheal until the point contacts the sacrum (Figure 292B, needle 1, page 445).

7. The needle is now withdrawn slightly and the anesthetist slowly reduces the angle of the needle, feeling his way each time until the needle point encounters the sacrococcygeal ligament (Figure 292B, needle 2, page 445). This may be at a depth of ¼ inch (0.6 cm.) to 1½ inches (3.8 cm.) from the skin, depending on the build of the patient.

8. The bevel of the needle is turned downward to facilitate the passage of the needle into and through the sacral canal (Figure 292B, needle 2, page 445).

9. The hub of the needle is now swung downward to an angle of 20 degrees to the surface of the skin in a male, but only to an angle of 35 degrees to 40 degrees to the surface of the skin in a female (Figure 292, needle 3, page 445 and Figure 293, page 446). The tilt of the female sacrum is normally greater than that of a male.

10. The needle is advanced through the sacrococcygeal ligament and into the caudal canal for approximately 1½ inches (3.8 cm.) (Figure 304, page 459).

11. The stylet is withdrawn and the distance of the needle in the canal checked. This is easily done by placing the stylet on the skin overlying the sacrum (Figure 305, page 460). The needle point should not extend to the line drawn between the second sacral foramina.

12. The syringe is attached and an attempt to aspirate blood or spinal fluid is made. The needle is then rotated 180 degrees and aspiration repeated. If spinal fluid is aspirated, another regional procedure such as spinal block is performed. If blood is aspirated, the needle should be advanced ¼ inch (0.6 cm.), the stylet reinserted to clear the blood from the lumen of the needle before it coagulates, and the needle allowed to remain untouched for 2 to 3 minutes by the clock. This maneuver allows the needle point to be disengaged from

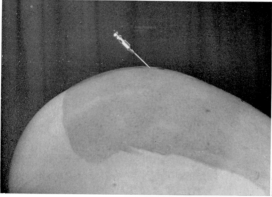 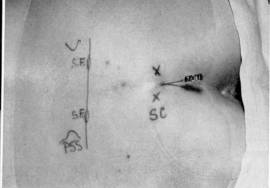

Figure 304. Needle rests in caudal canal. *(Left)* Lateral view. *(Right)* Posterior view. PSS, posterior superior spine of iliac bone. S.F., second sacral foramina. SC, sacral cornu.

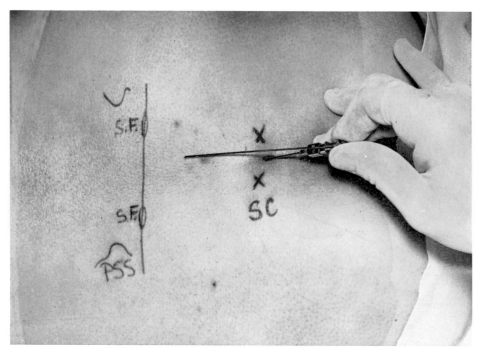

Figure 305. Method of checking the height of the needle in the caudal canal. PSS, posterior superior spine of the iliac bone. S. F., second sacral foramina. SC, sacral cornu.

the lumen of a vessel and allows time for the vessels that have been damaged by trauma during the introduction of the needle to stop oozing. After the 2 to 3 minute interval, the stylet is withdrawn and aspiration in two planes repeated. If blood is still aspirated, the block should be stopped and a spinal block, epidural block, or general anesthesia used.

13. If no blood or spinal fluid is obtained, 5 cc. of air is injected rapidly while the anesthetist observes the area over the sacrum. When the needle is posterior to the sacrum, air causes the tissues over the sacrum to swell, and crepitation, which shows the air in the tissue, may be palpated. Should this occur, withdraw the needle and make another attempt to place it in the caudal canal. If, as usual, the needle lies in the caudal canal, the patient may experience a "funny sensation in the legs." Prior to injecting air, the patient should be warned that this may occur.

14. When these tests indicate that the needle lies in the caudal canal, the plastic tubing with stylet ½ inch (1.3 cm.) from the end to be

inserted is fed into the 18-gauge needle (Figure 306 A, page 461) and advanced until the mark on the tubing is even with the hub of the needle (Figure 306B, page 461). The plastic tubing now lies approximately 5 inches (12.5 cm.) to 6 inches (15 cm.) inside the caudal canal at about the level of the fifth lumbar vertebra (Figure 310, page 470). *Once the plastic tubing has passed the point of the introducing needle, it should not be withdrawn, as the needle edge may cut or shred it off.*

When the plastic tubing is inserted into the needle, the hub need not be held securely (Figure 306A, page 461). Usually, the tubing passes easily through the straight bevel, meets little or no resistance in the caudal canal, and can be inserted to the mark with light and delicate pressure. If the plastic tubing meets resistance, do not force it by the obstruction. Leave the tubing at the point of obstruction and continue the technique—the obstruction may be the dura, a nerve, or a blood vessel.

15. The Tuohy needle is now withdrawn

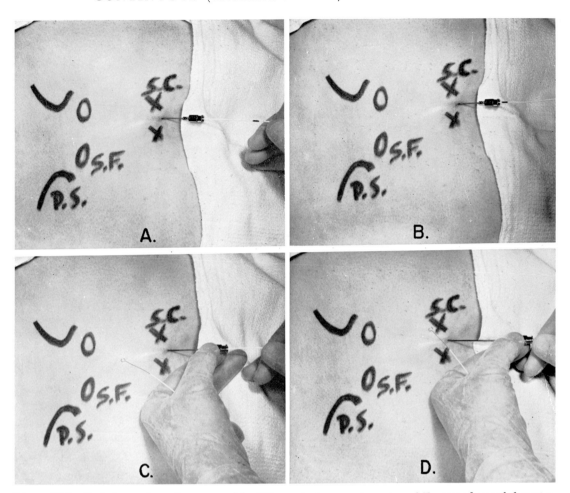

Figure 306. Technique of continuous caudal. P.S., posterior superior spine. S.F., second sacral foramina. S.C., sacral cornu. A. Tubing being threaded through needle into caudal canal with light and gentle pressure. B. Mark on tubing—7¾ inches (19.5 cm.) from end of tubing—at hub of needle. C. Left hand rests against buttocks of patient and thumb and index finger grip hub of needle. Thumb and index finger of the right hand fix the tubing in place 1 inch distal to the hub of the needle. D. Thumb and index finger of the left hand pull needle from patient until the hub touches the thumb and index finger of the right hand—do not move right hand.

from the patient's back over the plastic tubing and stylet. This is a critical maneuver. The thumb and index finger of the left hand hold the hub of the needle (Figure 306C, page 461). The plastic tubing with stylet in it is grasped firmly 1 inch (2.5 cm.) distal to the hub of the needle by the thumb and index finger of the right hand (Figure 306C, page 461). Then, the thumb and index finger of the left hand pull the needle out of the patient until the hub touches the thumb and index finger of the right hand—*do not move the right hand* (Figure 306D, page 461). This maneuver is repeated two or three times until the point of

the needle emerges from the skin. If this maneuver is executed carefully, the plastic tubing will not be dislodged from its position in the caudal canal.

16. As soon as the point of the needle emerges from the skin, the plastic tubing is grasped by the thumb and index finger of the left hand at its point of entrance into the skin (Figure 307A, page 462). The needle is slipped to the end of the plastic tubing (Figure 307B, page 462). The stylet is withdrawn (Figure 307C and D, page 462), and the needle removed (Figure 308A, page 463). The

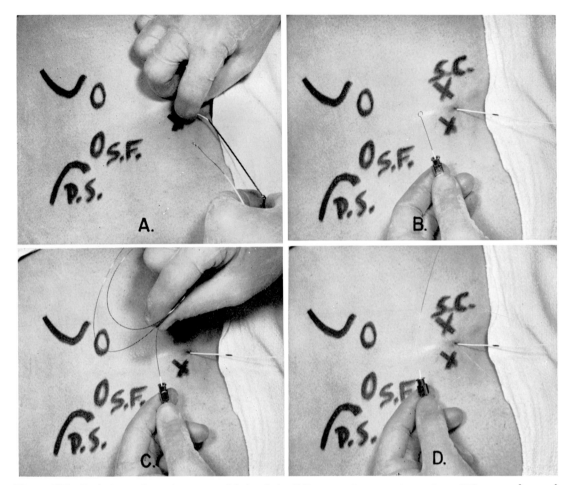

Figure 307. Technique of continuous caudal (con't.). P.S., posterior superior spine. S.F., second sacral foramina. S.C., sacral cornu. A. Thumb and index finger of the right hand grip tubing at its entrance into the skin. B. Needle at end of tubing. C. Wire stylet being removed from tubing. D. Wire stylet out of tubing.

distance of the mark on the plastic tubing from the skin should be checked—by doing this it can be determined whether or not the plastic tubing was dislodged from the epidural space when the 18-gauge, thin-walled needle was withdrawn (Figure 308B, page 463).

17. The Tuohy-Borst female Lok to plastic tubing adapter (Figure 259B, page 396) or ¾-inch (2 cm.), 23-gauge needle is affixed to the plastic tubing (Figure 308C, page 463). We prefer the 23-gauge needle.

18. The plug is placed on the adapter or 23-gauge needle (Figure 308D, page 463).

19. The plugged end is placed on the patient's back (Figure 309A, page 464). A ster-

ile sponge is taped under the plastic tubing at its entrance into the skin to avoid a right-angle or greater bend (Figure 309A and B, page 464). The tubing is taped to the patient's up side (Figure 309C, page 464).

20. If the plastic tubing was placed with the patient in the knee-chest position, she is placed in the modified Sims' (side) position. *Now it is mandatory to repeat aspiration tests for blood and spinal fluid and inject a test dose of 3 cc. to 5 cc. of the local anesthetic solution*—when the plastic tubing is placed, it may puncture a blood vessel or the dura. If blood is obtained, either the tubing must be reinserted or the technique abandoned for another regional block or general anesthesia. If spi-

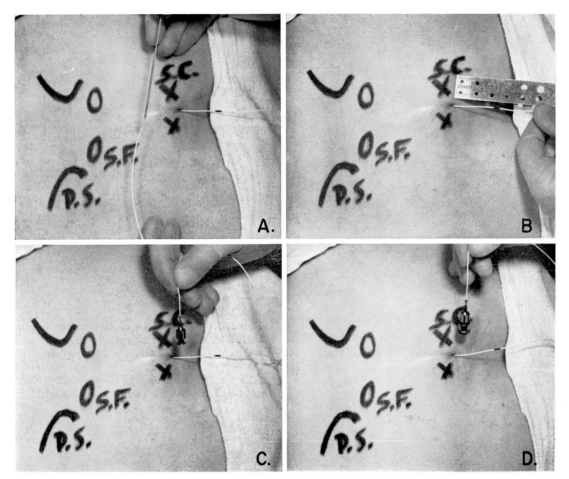

Figure 308. Technique of continuous caudal (con't.). P.S., posterior superior spine. S.F., second sacral foramina. S.C., sacral cornu. A. Needle withdrawn from the tubing. B. Distance of mark from skin examined. C. 23-gauge needle inserted into the tubing. D. 23-gauge needle capped with plug.

nal fluid is obtained, spinal anesthesia may be administered or the technique abandoned for another regional block or general anesthesia. If neither is obtained, then 3 cc. to 5 cc. of the local anesthetic solution is injected at the rate of approximately 1 cc. per 6 to 10 seconds (Figure 309C, page 464).

21. Five minutes are allowed to elapse *by the clock.* Carefully monitor the patient's blood pressure, pulse, and sensorium during this period for evidence of a systemic toxic reaction. If one occurs, remove the plastic tubing and reinsert it, use another regional procedure, or abandon the regional technique and administer general anesthesia.

If the five minutes pass uneventfully, the lower extremities, abdomen, and chest should be tested for signs of analgesia. When, following a 3 cc. to 5 cc. test dose of the local anesthetic solution the area of analgesia is extensive, the dura has in all probability been punctured and further attempts at establishing the continuous caudal block should be discontinued. If the existing spinal block needs to be supplemented, use general anesthesia.

If, as usual, analgesia is absent or limited to the immediate perianal region or the tissue over the coccyx and if the patient's blood pressure, pulse, and sensorium remain unchanged, it is safe to assume that neither the dura nor a blood vessel has been invaded. Then, an additional 12 to 20 cc. of the anes-

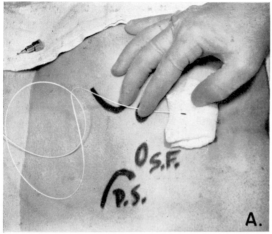

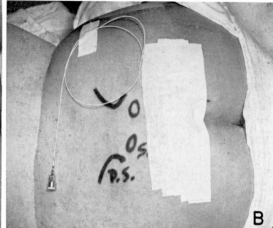

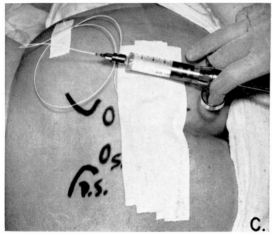

Figure 309. Technique of continuous caudal (con't.). P.S., posterior superior spine. S.F., second sacral foramen. A. Capped needle placed on the patient's back and sponge placed under the tubing at its entrance into the skin. B. Tubing taped in place. C. Test dose administered.

thetic solution is added, depending on the size of the patient (see page 452)—the test dose is not considered as part of this initial dose.

22. Reinforcing doses should be approximately the same as or slightly less than the initial dose, i.e., if 15 cc. was given initially, the second dose would be 12 cc. to 15 cc. It is best to give the reinforcing doses when the patient first becomes uncomfortable. Once severe pain has been felt, it is often difficult to reestablish adequate analgesia.

Before injecting a reinforcing dose, aspirate for blood or spinal fluid. If either is obtained and the procedure is being used for surgery, discontinue the continuous caudal block and administer general anesthesia. If either is obtained when continuous caudal block is being administered for pain relief during the first

stage of labor, discontinue the caudal block and administer either a spinal block, epidural block, or general anesthesia for delivery of the fetus (see page 467).

23. When the parturient with plastic tubing in place is ready to be delivered, she is turned to the supine position—the tubing remaining in place. Reinforcing doses are given when necessary, and the tubing is removed when the delivery is completed. When the parturient is turned to the supine position, she must be observed for the supine hypotensive syndrome.

EXTENT OF ANALGESIA

Same as after single-dose caudal block. See page 448.

COMPLICATIONS

Same as those which may occur after single-dose caudal block (page 448) and the following.

Placement of the Needle Anterior to the Sacrum: On the very rare occasion, the caudal needle may be inserted anterior to the sacrum, into the rectum, into the head of the fetus, or all three. Therefore, *immediately* after placing the caudal needle or plastic tubing, a routine rectal examination should be made prior to the injection of a large quantity of the local anesthetic solution. Removal of the needle or plastic tubing at this time may prevent a serious complication, *e.g.*, infection or death of the infant.

Total Spinal Block Following Reinforcing Doses: See page 467.

Air Embolism: With the patient in the knee-chest position, this complication may occur when the stylet is withdrawn from the spinal needle if the needle's point inadvertently lies in a blood vessel.

Signs and Symptoms.—These include pain in the chest, coughing, cyanosis, and cardiac arrest.

Treatment.—Place patient on the left side, administer oxygen, maintain blood pressure, and if cardiac arrest occurs, institute closed cardiac massage. We have seen only one such case in over 15,000 continuous caudal blocks, and she responded to positioning and administering of oxygen by bag and mask.

REMARKS

Continuous caudal analgesia is usually limited in its use to vaginal obstetrical deliveries and an occasional therapeutic problem, because prolonged single-dose spinal block, continuous spinal block, single-dose epidural block, or continuous epidural block presents less technical difficulties and produces more predictable results for intra-abdominal and lower extremity surgery. The remarks found under Single-Dose Caudal Block (page 449) and many of those under Single-Dose Spinal (Subarachnoid) Block (page 361) are applicable also to continuous caudal block and should be reviewed before this block procedure is performed. Therefore, the following statements are confined principally to continuous caudal analgesia in the obstetrical case.

Conditions for which Continuous Caudal Block Is Particularly Suitable: Continuous caudal is indicated for: (1) premature labor; (2) eclampsia—caudal block may lower blood pressure, but whether it improves kidney function is debatable; (3) diseases of the mother in which a long labor is contraindicated, *i.e.*, heart disease, tuberculosis, pneumonia, etc.; and (4) tense patients with severe labor pains who are cooperative but cannot relax, and whose cervix will not dilate more than 6 to 7 cm.

Conditions in which Continuous Caudal Block Is Inadvisable: Continuous caudal is inadvisable when: (1) the sacrum is markedly deformed; (2) there is disproportion between the birth canal and the fetus; (3) version and extraction or similar operative obstetrics are indicated; (4) pilonidal cysts and infections over the sacral hiatus are present; (5) the patient has septicemia; (6) bleeding from placenta praevia, etc., is profuse and there is moderate to severe hypovolemia; and (7) the highly emotional patients who are uncooperative.

Do Not Start Block Until Patient Is in Active Labor and at Least 5 to 6 cm. Dilated: Continuous caudal anesthesia should never be started unless the obstetrician is positive the patient is in active labor. A parturient who is delivering her first child should be at least 6 to 7 cm. dilated and the parturient who has delivered one or more children, 5 to 6 cm. Otherwise, labor may be slowed and the caudal anesthesia may have to run for 10 to 12 hours before the patient delivers, or it may have to be discontinued.

If Block Slows Labor, the Uterus Will Respond to Oxytocic Drugs: Caudal block may slow labor, but the exact underlying etiology is not clearly established. While regional block can abolish the pain of labor, it does not interfere with the contractility of the uterus. Uterine contractility during labor is considered to be autonomous and not affected by the regional block technique itself. Regardless of the regional block procedure employed, the uterus will respond to oxytocic drugs.

Caudal Block Abolishes Only Pain Impulse from the Uterus: Caudal analgesia blocks *only* the sensory pathways from the uterus—motor impulses are not interrupted. Contractions still occur and if manipulations inside the uterus, such as version and extraction, are to be accomplished, caudal analgesia may not effect adequate relaxation of the uterus. For version and extractions general anesthesia should be considered.

Obstetrician May Need to Use Forceps: When a continuous caudal block is administered to alleviate pains during labor, the obstetrician should be competent to use midforceps. The percentage of posteriors seems to be increased by caudal analgesia and often a midforceps with or without rotation of the baby's head may be necessary to terminate the labor.

The incidence of forceps deliveries with caudal block is increased because the involuntary urge to bear down, which is necessary during the second stage of labor, is absent—Fergusson's reflex is blocked by this block. However, when the analgesic level is not above the tenth thoracic dermatome with this block and when the parturient is cooperative, she can bear down and often she can deliver the fetus. She should be coached to do so during her contractions by either the anesthetist or the obstetrician, and moderate pressure should be exerted on the fundus of the uterus to prevent the uterus being pushed anteriorly as the diaphragm moves caudad.

When Head of Fetus Is On Perineum Avoid Caudal Block: Caudal analgesia of any type is usually best avoided at the terminal stage of labor because: (1) time to correct any technical difficulties, *e.g.*, misplaced needle, and time to establish analgesia may be inadequate; (2) when the head is on the perineum, even the patient who is normally cooperative may become uncooperative because of the almost constant labor pains; and (3) distortion of landmarks caused by the straightening of the coccyx, as well as the patient straining with each pain, may make insertion of the needle in the caudal canal extremely difficult. *If regional anesthesia is to be used under these circumstances, spinal analgesia is preferable* (page 384).

Pain, Cramping, or Feeling of Fullness in Thighs or Calves Indicate Needle Is Correctly Placed: Pain or cramping in the legs during injection of the local anesthetic solution in the caudal canal is of no significance other than the fact that it indicates the needle is correctly placed in the caudal canal.

Oxytocics Intensify Contractions: Pitocin or like substances, *i.e.*, synthetic oxytocin (Syntocinon) intensify uterine contractions. Therefore, if a patient is to receive pitocin it is often necessary to increase the initial and reinforcing doses of the local anesthetic solution by 5 to 10 cc.

Vasoconstrictor Drugs, Oxytocic Drugs, or a Combination of These May Cause Severe Hypertension: If continuous caudal block is employed for obstetrical delivery, a vasoconstrictor drug to prevent or correct hypotension should be given with care. A severe, persistent, dangerous hypertension and even rupture of a cerebral blood vessel which may cause brain damage and hemiplegia can result from the combined effect of a vasoconstrictor and an oxytocic drug which have been administered to a patient within three to six hours of one another (see page 41).

Long-acting vasoconstrictor drugs, *e.g.*, methoxamine (Vasoxyl), must not be used either to prevent or correct a hypotension in the obstetrical patient or any other patient who may receive an oxytocic drug (see pages 41, 42, 372, 387).

This does not preclude the addition of 0.1 cc. of epinephrine 1:1000 to each 20 cc. of solution to be injected into the caudal canal. This small amount of epinephrine has not, in our experience with over 25,000 caudal and epidural blocks, caused this complication, *i.e.,* persistent hypertension (see page 41).

Monitor Patient: Constant supervision by a physician is of prime importance. The initial injection as well as reinforcing injections should be done under his supervision. Therefore, a busy obstetrician usually prefers a terminal caudal or spinal block unless there is medical anesthesia available at the hospital.

The blood pressure and pulse of the parturient and the heart rate of the fetus should be checked frequently and persistent hypotension should be treated immediately with vasoconstrictor drugs.

Total Spinal Block Following Reinforcing Doses: One of the most unexpected complications of continuous caudal block or continuous epidural block is a high or total subarachnoid block occurring after reinforcing doses are given. Three of these complications have been observed by us—continuous caudal block was being administered and 2½-inch (6.3 cm.) hubless malleable needles were being used. In each instance, the initial dose of 20 cc. or more of the local anesthetic solution had been administered with satisfactory anesthetic levels of the tenth thoracic dermatome or below with no indication of the local anesthetic solution mixing with the spinal fluid. In one patient on the second refill dose, and in two patients on the third refill dose, total spinal block developed.

In none of the three cases could the drugs be incriminated. While it is possible that the malleable needle could have perforated the dura as a result of the patient's movements, this complication has also occurred when plastic tubing is inserted into the caudal canal or epidural space. Also, permeability of the dura could be altered by repeated injections of the local anesthetic drug, although this seems unlikely.

Pulsations of the dura may be the cause of this complication. The dura does not pulsate as long as the aerodynamics of epidural space are normal. However, when they are altered by the introduction of air from insertion of the needle, plastic tubing, or both, the dura will pulsate. It is, therefore, possible that such pulsations against the needle or tubing could result in the dura being eroded and the needle or tubing then entering the subarachnoid space.

When Total Spinal Block Occurs, Should Spinal Fluid be Withdrawn and Should the Subarachnoid Space by Lavaged? In most instances, when a total spinal block occurs, the anesthetist is too busy resuscitating the patient to withdraw spinal fluid and lavage the subarachnoid space—the correction of hypotension, respiratory arrest, and cardiac arrest must come first. By the time the patient's vital signs are stable, withdrawal of spinal fluid and lavage may not be indicated.

Withdrawal of Spinal Fluid.—A total of 50 to 60 cc. of spinal fluid may be withdrawn, provided: (1) it can be done slowly without herniating the medulla; and (2) immediately—most local anesthetic drugs "fix" in 15 to 30 minutes.

Lavage of Subarachnoid Space.—Lavage with normal saline or distilled water is not indicated, since both are unphysiologic solutions and could cause irreparable damage to the cord. If lavage is to be done, a physiologic solution, *e.g.,* Ringer's, must be used.

Neurologic Sequelae Should Not Automatically Be Attributed to the Regional Block Procedure: In obstetrics the femoral nerves, the sciatic nerves, and the lateral femoral cutaneous nerves are particularly vulnerable. The femoral nerves can be damaged from pressure of retractors during cesarean section. The sciatic nerves can be traumatized by the head of the fetus—it is not uncommon to see one of the legs of the parturient twitch as the head of the fetus is rotated by forceps. And, the lateral femoral cutaneous nerve can be traumatized from pressure if the stirrups are opened widely and tilted too far cephalad —six such cases have been observed in our institution.

When neurological sequelae result, treatment includes consultation with a neurologist or neurosurgeon, establishing the level and on-set of nerve damage by electromyography, drug therapy, *e.g.*, thiamine chloride and nico-tinic acid, physiotherapy, and rehabilitation. Such treatment is usually directed by a neurol-ogist or neurosurgeon.

Hypotension in the Pregnant Patient Must Be Corrected Immediately: Fetal oxygenation depends on adequate perfusion of the uterus, and maternal blood pressure must be main-tained at a reasonable level or fetal oxygena-tion will be compromised. There is no magic level of systolic pressure in the pregnant pa-tient at which treatment of hypotension with a vasoconstrictor drug must be instituted. Whenever, following a regional block, the sys-tolic pressure falls to thirty percent of its pre-operative level or below 100 mm. of mer-cury, the anesthetist should be prepared to use vasoconstrictor drugs to elevate the pres-sure. If blood pressure falls to 80 to 85 mm. of mercury, treatment with a short-acting vaso-constrictor drug, *e.g.*, 25 mg. of ephedrine sulfate intravenously, is indicated. If this dos-age does not correct the hypotension, it may be repeated once. Then, if the blood pres-sure does not stabilize, an intravenous drip of phenylephrine (Neo-Synephrine) is indicated (see page 36).

While the rapid administration of 500 cc. to 700 cc. of fluid is advocated in certain instances, *e.g.*, cesarean section, to raise the blood pressure following a regional block pro-cedure, its use during a continuous caudal block which may last for 2 to 3 hours prior to the delivery of an infant is debatable (see page 372).

During Continuous Caudal Block, the Pa-tient Remains in a Modified Sims' Position: With the malleable caudal needle or plastic tubing in place, the patient should remain in the modified Sims' (side) position to avoid: (1) breaking of the malleable needle, (2) dis-lodging of the needle or tubing, and (3) the supine hypotensive syndrome. Since the cau-dal space is a compartment, gravity may exert some influence on the spread of the local anes-thetic solution. In general, the solution tends to gravitate to the dependent portion of the epidural space. Therefore, it is not uncom-mon for these patients to get more analgesia on the "down" side. If the patient complains of pain, check to see if the pain is limited to the "up" side. If this is the case, the patient should be turned to the other side before the next reinforcing dose is adminis-tered. When turning a patient with a mal-leable needle or plastic tubing in place, always have her reassume the knee-chest position, and then the side position. Do not allow her to roll over on her back, as this may break the needle or dislodge either the needle or the tubing.

When the parturient is turned to the supine position, she must be observed for the supine hypotensive syndrome.

Catheterize Patient: During a prolonged labor conducted under continuous caudal analgesia, the patient's bladder should be frequently checked and catheterized if dis-tended. A distended bladder may cause pain in the presence of a satisfactory caudal anes-thesia, as well as slow the labor.

Do Not Mistake Psychogenic Reaction for High Caudal or Spinal Block: Obstetrical pa-tients are often under great strain and may make various complaints that are purely psy-chogenic. These include inability to breathe, feeling of faintness, crying, nausea, the inter-pretation of touch as pain, hysteria, and a host of others. Reassurance that everything is as it should be is often the only treatment neces-sary. Should symptomatic treatment be indi-cated, it consists of the administration of oxy-gen and, if necessary, meperidine (Demerol) 50 mg. and promethazine (Phenergan) 25 mg. intravenously. Do not exceed this amount or depression of the baby may occur. These cases are called to the anesthetist's attention so that before he automatically treats any symptoms, he checks the blood pressure, pulse, respirations, and the anesthetic level to ascer-tain the cause of the complaint. Many of these psychogenic responses simulate the com-plications of high caudal or spinal block.

Cumulative Reaction to Mepivacaine (Car-

bocaine): Of all the commonly employed local anesthetic agents, only mepivacaine has shown evidence of cumulating in the body (see page 23). Therefore, its dosage is limited in continuous caudal block to a total of 100 cc. of a 1.0 percent solution. Since using this criterion for dosage, no cumulative-type reactions have been observed. Furthermore, the use of the 1.0 percent solution in over 1,500 patients indicates that this concentration is probably optimal for this block.

Spinal or Epidural Block—Not Caudal Block —Is Indicated for Cesarean Section: For cesarean section, we prefer spinal or epidural block. The amount of the local anesthetic agent which must be injected through the caudal canal, *i.e.*, 50 cc. to 60 cc., to effect adequate anesthesia for cesarean section represents a near toxic or toxic dose of the commonly used local anesthetic drugs.

Avoid Solutions Containing Methylparaben and Metabisulfite: These drugs are often added to commercially prepared local anesthetic solutions to prevent oxidation and as a preservative. Solutions containing them are not recommended for caudal block.

Methylparaben.—Methylparaben is a preservative and fungistatic agent.

Metabisulfite.—Metabisulfite is an antioxidizing agent.

Can the Position of the Plastic Tubing in the Caudal Canal Be Predicted Precisely and Consistently Using the Technique Advocated? The answer is Yes, provided: (1) the wire stylet remains in the tubing when it is advanced up the caudal canal; (2) the tubing is threaded with light and delicate pressure into the caudal canal; (3) it is inserted no more than 6 inches (15 cm.); and (4) a needle with a straight bevel is used for inserting the plastic tubing.

When this technique is used, the tip of the tubing consistently is located at approximately the fifth lumbar vertebra (Figure 310, page 470).

Thread Tubing into Caudal Canal with Light and Delicate Pressure: If the tubing meets resistance or elicits severe or persistent paresthesias, do not force the tubing past the obstruction or the paresthesia. Leave it where it is and inject the local anesthetic solution. If the tubing is forced past the obstruction or paresthesia, it may: (1) enter the dura or a blood vessel; (2) pass out a sacral foramen; (3) damage a nerve; or (4) a combination of these.

Mark Plastic Tubing 7¾ Inches (19.5 cm.) from End To Be Placed in Caudal Canal: When the plastic tubing is used, the distance it is to be inserted should be marked with a felt marking pen or ball point pen prior to sterilization. Marking of the tubing serves two purposes: (1) it permits placement of the tubing the correct distance into the caudal canal, and (2) it allows the physician to recognize whether the tubing was dislodged from the caudal canal when the 18-gauge needle and wire stylet are withdrawn.

Use Wire Stylet in Plastic Tubing: The stylet remains in the plastic tubing while placing it to prevent its kinking in the caudal canal and to facilitate its introduction through the 18-gauge needle. The plastic tubing for continuous caudal blocks does not come with a stylet and the manufacturer states that none is necessary for its insertion. However, it has been found through unfortunate experiences that this is not true, particularly when the tubing has been sterilized in the autoclave. A stylet may be purchased (footnote, page 454), obtained from the urology department—a suitable one comes in a number 5 ureteral catheter, or made from 28- to 26-gauge stainless steel surgical wire available in the supply room of most operating suites.

Should Regular or Radiopaque Plastic Tubing be Used: The principal disadvantage of the non-radiopaque tubing is that its location cannot be determined if the block is inadequate or if the tubing breaks. The principal disadvantage of the radiopaque tubing is the ability to locate it if it does break.

Vinyl plastic tubing is inert and when left in the body, seldom, if ever, causes any difficulty. But if it can be located in the subarachnoid,

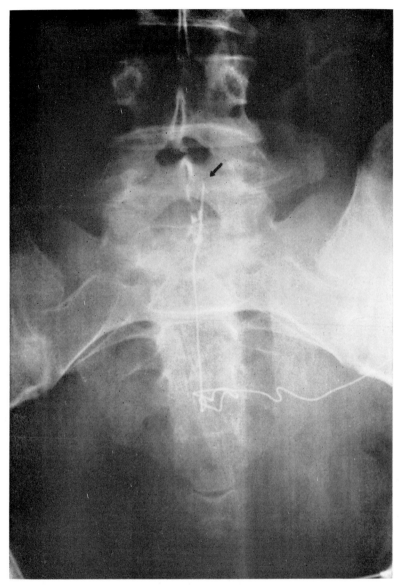

Figure 310. X-ray of plastic tubing in sacral canal. Tubing inserted through 3-inch (7.5 cm.), 18-gauge thin-walled needle with *regular* bevel. The needle was inserted for 1½ inches (3.8 cm.) into canal. The marked distance from the tip of catheter was 7¾ inches (19.5 cm.). Tip of catheter (arrow) lies at the interspace between the fourth and fifth lumbar vertebrae. This patient was in labor. She was 5 feet, 8 inches tall, weighed 150 pounds, and was 26 years old. The initial dose was 17 cc. of mepivacaine (Carbocaine) with the patient in the modified Sims' (side) position. Anesthesia level to the tenth thoracic dermatome resulted.

epidural, or caudal space, the question arises: Should it be removed? To remove it may subject the patient to an unnecessary, hazardous operation. To not remove it may provoke a medicolegal situation—the ramifications of which are too numerous to list.

Therefore, the type of tubing a physician selects is one of personal choice. Regardless of which type is selected, a broken piece of tubing in a patient presents a difficult problem. Whether an attempt to retrieve the tubing is made depends on the circumstances and should involve consultation with other specialists and the anesthetist's insurance company. Nonetheless, the patient must be informed of such a mishap and should participate in the decision as to whether the tubing should be removed.

Sterilization of Tuohy Needle, Plastic Tubing, Tuohy-Borst Adapter, One-way Stopcock, and Plug for Stopcock: See page 400.

Plastic Tubing Is Not Inserted Into the Caudal Canal for More Than 6 Inches (15 cm.) Nor Is It Inserted Without a Wire Stylet: If it is inserted for more than 6 inches (15 cm.) and if a wire stylet is not used, the following may occur: (1) it may kink; (2) turn 180 degrees and go in the opposite direction to that in which it was inserted; (3) pass out a sacral or intervertebral foramen; (4) wrap

around a nerve and be difficult to remove; or (5) a combiantion of these.

At Present, Chloroprocaine (Nesacaine) is Not Available for Epidural Block: Chloroprocaine has a rapid onset, 8 to 15 minutes, and it seems to have the lowest systemic toxicity of any local anesthetic agent used at the present time. The author and his associates have used it in over 2,500 continuous caudal blocks for obstetrical delivery and found it to be a satisfactory agent. Because of packaging difficulties, chloroprocaine is not at the present time available for epidural block (see page 15). However, it is included under Drugs in this chapter because the pharmaceutical house which manufactures the drug indicates that it again may become available.

Recover Broken Needle(s): All needles should be tested before use. If a needle breaks, every effort to remove it, including surgery, should be made (Figure 311, page

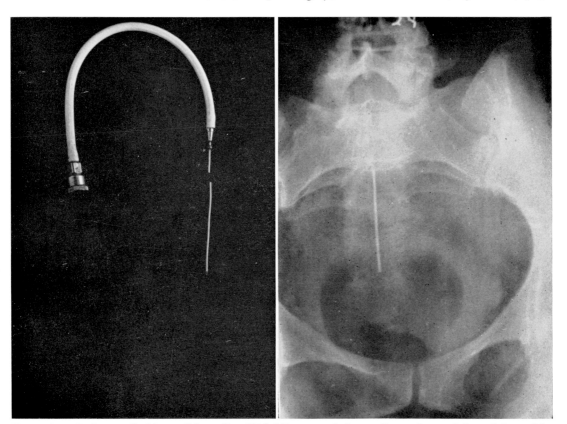

Figure 311. Broken malleable caudal needle. *(Right)* Position of the needle in the caudal canal located by x-ray. *(Left)* Broken part of needle recovered by surgery.

471). Unremoved needles have a tendency to migrate and may cause permanent injuries as well as medicolegal complications.

When a spinal or caudal needle breaks, there is little doubt in the anesthetist's mind of what has happened. A distinct click is felt. This usually happens when the needle is being inserted and the stylet is still in the needle. If the anesthetist suspects that the needle has broken, he should not remove the stylet. If the needle breaks after the stylet is removed, the portion containing the hub of the needle should not be removed. They are valuable guides to locating the broken end of the needle. When the anesthetist suspects that the needle has been broken, he should release his hold on it and have an x-ray taken immediately.

Repeat Block when Analgesia is Inadequate: Adequate time should always be allowed for the local anesthetic agent to exert its maximum effect before giving additional amounts of the solution. This usually is 15 to 30 minutes. Then, if the desired results from the first block attempt are unsatisfactory, do not hesitate to reblock the patient if time permits. Most patients will think nothing about being reblocked if the second attempt is prefaced by a statement such as: "Well, I guess we will have to inject a little more medicine if we are going to freeze this area."

However, do not exceed the maximum safe dosage of the local anesthetic solution for both blocks. If to reblock the patient the maximum safe dose of the local anesthetic solution must be exceeded, 45 minutes should elapse between blocks.

CHAPTER 50

Transsacral Block

INDICATIONS

Surgical: Operations on the anus, rectum, coccyx, and lower sacrum, *i.e.*, hemorrhoidectomy, coccygectomy, and pilonidal cystectomy, may be performed under this block alone. Many anesthetists, except in obstetrical deliveries, combine transsacral block and caudal block, in the belief that the onset of analgesia is more rapid and that more profound and prolonged analgesia results.

Diagnostic: Localization of pain problems of the lower extremities.

Therapeutic: Relief of sciatic pain, particularly that which is often associated with carcinoma of the prostate.

In paraplegia due to spinal cord injuries where the patient cannot void, but catheterization and cystometric readings show the bladder to have good tone, often a block of either the second or third sacral nerves, usually the third, bilaterally will release the sphincter spasm and the patient will be able to void. The exact cause of this is undetermined. If a block of the individual pairs of sacral nerves bilaterally does not produce results, then block of the second and third sacral nerves bilaterally at the same time will usually do so.

ANATOMY

The sacrum is a large, triangular bone formed by the fusion of five bones. It is inserted like a wedge between the two iliac bones (Figure 314, page 477). The dorsal surface is convex and in the midline is a crest, the median sacral crest. On either side of the median sacral crest, separated from it by the sacral groove are linear series of tubercles

produced by the fusion of the articular processes of the five sacral bones. These are called the sacral articular crests. The superior articular processes of the first sacral vertebra articulate with the inferior articulating process of the fifth lumbar vertebra (Figure 288, page 440). The inferior articular processes of the fifth sacral vertebra are prolonged downward and are known as the sacral cornu (Figure 314, page 477). Lateral to the articular crests and almost parallel to the midline are the four posterior sacral foramina, which are approximately 1 cm. in diameter (Figure 312, page 474). These sacral foramina are the means of access to the sacral nerves, and the posterior primary divisions of the sacral nerves pass through them. The foramina lie approximately ⅝ inch (1.5 cm.) to ¾ inch (2 cm.) apart, depending on the build of the patient.

PREMEDICATION

Paresthesias are not sought, so heavy medication is advised for surgical patients.

Heavy Premedication: The average patient (age 20 to 50, weight 150 pounds or over, height 5 feet, 5 inches or over, and good physical status) receives:

1. 200 mg. (3 gr.) of pentobarbital (Nembutal) by mouth at hour of sleep the night before surgery.

2. 100 mg. (1½ gr.) to 200 mg. (3 gr.) of pentobarbital with one ounce of water by mouth 1½ to 2 hours before estimated *block* time.

3. 15 mg. (¼ gr.) of morphine and 0.6 mg. (1/100 gr.) of scopolamine intramuscularly ¾ to 1 hour before estimated *block* time.

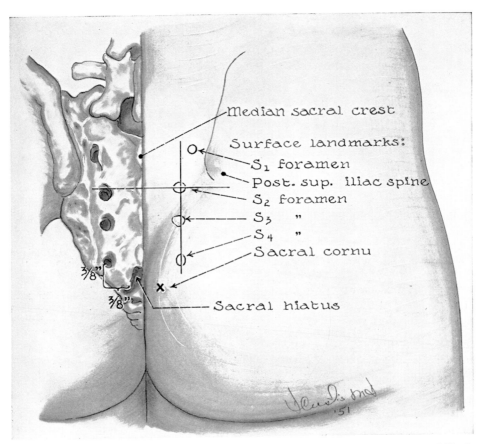

Figure 312. Topographic and deep anatomical considerations involved in a transsacral block.

Reduction of Premedication: It is never necessary to increase this premedication irrespective of the over-all size of the patient until the patient arrives in either the anesthesia or operating room. However, it is very common to reduce this medication under various circumstances; for example, in the case of the geriatric patient, the adolescent patient or child, the debilitated or cachectic patient, and patients whose surgery is complicated by other disease, e.g., myxedema, diabetes, heart disease, etc. In the patient over 60 years of age, barbiturates and especially scopolamine often cause disorientation. Therefore, in these patients atropine is usually substituted for scopolamine and the dosages of the barbiturate omitted or greatly reduced, i.e., to 50 mg. (¾ gr.) or less. *Always err on the light side.*

Inadequate Premedication: If the medication is inadequate, either for the block or

for the surgical procedure, pentobarbital 50 mg. (¾ gr.) to 100 mg. (1½ gr.) or morphine 8 mg. (⅛ gr.) to 15 mg. (¼ gr.) may be slowly given intravenously. Judicious use of added sedation is extremely important. Often small supplementary doses of morphine or pentobarbital will make a block successful when a patient interprets touch and motion as pain.

DRUGS

Tetracaine (Pontocaine) or procaine (Novocain) alone is seldom used for transsacral block or a combination of a transsacral block with a caudal block. The rapid onset and constant results of lidocaine (Xylocaine), mepivacaine (Carbocaine), and chloroprocaine (Nesacaine) make them the agents of choice for this block.

When caudal block and transsacral block are combined, the volumes of local anesthetic solutions listed below must not be exceeded for both procedures; otherwise, toxic reactions will occur with greater frequency.

Lidocaine (Xylocaine) or Mepivacaine (Carbocaine)

Dosage.—20 cc. to 50 cc. of a 1.0 percent solution or 50 cc. to 100 cc. of a 0.5 percent solution with or without 0.25 cc. of epinephrine (Adrenalin) 1:1000 in 50 cc. of solution.*

Onset.—Operating analgesia is established in 10 to 20 minutes.

Duration.—Operating analgesia lasts 1¼ to 2 hours, with the stronger concentrations and solutions containing epinephrine giving the upper limits.

Lidocaine (Xylocaine) or Mepivacaine (Carbocaine) with Tetracaine (Pontocaine): Tetracaine may be incorporated in a lidocaine or mepivacaine solution to prolong the duration of action of these two solutions. Either of these mixtures is the author's choice for executing a transsacral block or a combination of a transsacral block with a caudal block.

Dosage.—No more than 60 cc. is employed —10 cc. for local infiltration, 20 cc. in the caudal canal, 7 cc. in each of the second sacral foramina, 5 cc. in each of the third foramina, and 3 cc. in each of the fourth foramina.

60.00 cc. of a 0.8 percent solution of lidocaine or mepivacaine.

60.00 mg. of tetracaine crystals.

0.25 cc. of epinephrine (Adrenalin) 1:1000.*
_____
60.25 cc.

Onset.—Operating analgesia is established in 10 to 20 minutes.

Duration.—Operating analgesia lasts 2½ to 3 hours.

Piperocaine (Metycaine)

Dosage.—20 cc. to 50 cc. of a 1.5 percent solution or 50 cc. to 100 cc. of a 1.0 percent

solution with or without 0.25 cc. of epinephrine (Adrenalin) 1:1000 in 50 cc. of solution.*

Onset.—Operating analgesia is established in 10 to 30 minutes, with an average of 15 minutes.

Duration.—1 to 1¼ hours, with stronger concentrations and solutions containing epinephrine giving the upper limits.

Procaine (Novocain)

Dosage.—20 cc. to 50 cc. of a 2.0 percent solution or 50 cc. to 100 cc. of a 1.0 percent solution with or without 0.25 cc. of epinephrine (Adrenalin) 1:1000 in 50 cc. of solution.*

Onset.—Operating analgesia is established in 10 to 30 minutes, with an average of 15 minutes.

Duration.—¾ to 1¼ hours, with stronger concentrations and solutions containing epinephrine giving the upper limits.

Tetracaine (Pontocaine)

Dosage.—20 cc. to 100 cc. of a 0.15 percent solution with or without 0.25 cc. of epinephrine (Adrenalin) 1:1000 in 50 cc. of solution.*

Onset.—Operating analgesia is established in 15 to 30 minutes, with an average of 20 minutes.

Duration.—2½ to 5 hours, with solutions containing epinephrine giving the upper limits.

Chloroprocaine (Nesacaine): See Remarks, page 451.

Dosage.—20 cc. to 50 cc. of a 2.0 percent solution or 50 cc. to 100 cc. of a 1.0 percent solution with or without 0.25 cc. of epinephrine (Adrenalin) 1:1000 in 50 cc. of solution.*
_____

*Optimal concentration of epinephrine is 1:200,000, that is, 0.1 cc. of epinephrine 1:1000 in 20 cc. of the local anesthetic solution. Do not exceed 0.25 cc. of epinephrine 1:1000 even if amount of local anesthetic solution exceeds 50 cc. (see page 39).

Onset.—Operating analgesia is established in 5 to 15 minutes, with an average of 8 to 10 minutes.

Duration.—Operating analgesia lasts ¾ to 1¼ hours, with stronger concentrations and solutions containing epinephrine giving the upper limits.

MATERIALS

Complete regional tray (see Chapter 9, page 51) or:

1. One ¾-inch (2 cm.), 25-gauge, Huber point security Lok-needle.

2. Two 1½-inch (3.8 cm.), 22-gauge, security Lok-needles, preferably with short bevel.

3. Two 2½-inch (6.3 cm.), 22-gauge, security Lok-needles, preferably with short bevel.

4. Two 3-inch (7.5 cm.), 22-gauge, security Lok-needles, preferably with short bevels.

5. One tuberculin Lok-syringe for measuring epinephrine.

6. One 10 cc. Lok-syringe, preferably with finger rings.

7. One graduated measuring cup, preferably stainless steel, for mixing solution.

8. One prep cup, preferably stainless steel.

9. Four sterile towels.

10. Six sterile sponges.

11. One sterilizer control.

TECHNIQUE

Position and Landmarks

1. The patient lies in the prone position with a large pillow under the iliac bones so that the sacrum is elevated and tilted at a 45-degree angle to the table (Figure 313, page 476 and Figure 314, page 477).

2. The patient is instructed to abduct his legs and turn his toes in and his heels out (Figure 290A, page 443). The maneuver relaxes the gluteal muscles and makes it diffi-

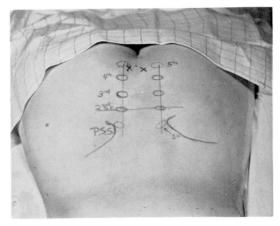

Figure 313. Landmarks for a transsacral block. Patient is in the prone position with iliac bones resting on a pillow. X's, sacral cornua. S.F., sacral foramen. P.S.S., posterior superior spine of the iliac bone.

cult for the patient to tense them (Figure 290B, page 443).

3. The sacral cornua are palpated and marked with X's (Figure 313, page 476 and Figure 314, page 477).

4. The posterior superior iliac spines are located and O's are marked on the skin ½ inch (1.3 cm.) caudad and ½ inch (1.3 cm.) medial to the spines (Figure 313, page 476 and Figure 314, page 477). The O's should overlie the second sacral foramina.

5. O's are marked on the skin ⅜ inch (1 cm.) lateral and ⅜ inch (1 cm.) cephalad to the X's marking the sacral cornua. These O's mark the fourth sacral foramina (Figure 312, page 474; Figure 313, page 476; and Figure 314, page 477).

6. Lines are drawn between the two O's through their approximate centers. These lines are bisected in order to locate the third sacral foramina (Figure 313, page 476 and Figure 314, page 477). The two lines drawn between the O's should be *parallel* to each other and the median sacral crest (Figure 313, page 476 and Figure 314, page 477). They should be 1 inch (2.5 cm.) to 1¼ inch (3.2 cm.) lateral to the median sacral crest.

7. To locate the other sacral nerves, the lines drawn through the O's are extended

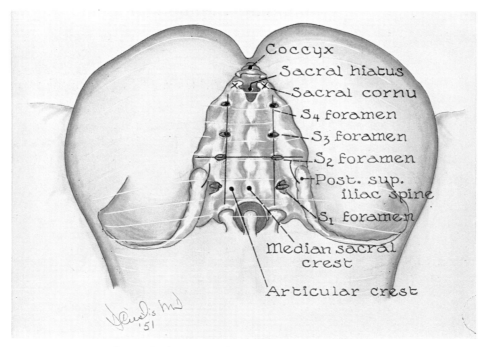

Figure 314. Deep and superficial anatomy of the sacrum with landmarks necessary for a caudal transsacral block marked on the skin.

cephalad and caudad. The first sacral fora-mina lie underneath points on these lines ¾ inch (2 cm.) cephalad and slightly lateral to the O's which mark the second sacral fora-mina (Figure 312, page 474 and Figure 314, page 477). There are no fifth sacral foramina but the fifth sacral nerves lie underneath points on these lines ¾ inch (2 cm.) caudad to the O's which mark the fourth sacral foramina.

Precautions

Aspirate.—Aspirate for blood or spinal fluid.

Do Not Allow Antiseptic Solution to Burn Perineum.—Always place a sponge between the gluteal folds to prevent the antiseptic solution from running over the perineum and burning the patient.

Procedure: When a transsacral block is used for rectal work by itself or in conjunction with a caudal, the second, third, and fourth sacral nerves are usually the only ones injected. Therefore in this chapter the block of these nerves has been used for the illustrations.

However, the technique used to inject them is applicable to the first and fifth sacral nerves.

1. The sterilizer control is checked to be sure the equipment has been sterilized.

2. The area is aseptically prepared and draped.

3. The anesthetist stands at the side of the patient to be blocked.

4. Skin wheals are raised over the second, third, and fourth sacral foramina bilaterally with the ¾-inch (2 cm.), 25-gauge Huber point security Lok-needle.

5. Local infiltration from the skin to and including the periosteum of the sacrum is car-ried out with the 1½-inch (3.8 cm.), security Lok-needle.

6. First, an attempt is made to place a 3-inch (7.5 cm.) needle in the second sacral foramen on one side. Then, on the same side, a 2½-inch (6.3 cm.) needle is placed in the third sacral foramen. And, finally, a 1½-inch (3.8 cm.) needle is placed in the fourth sacral foramen.

The 3-inch (7.5 cm.) security Lok-needle is inserted almost perpendicular in all planes to the skin through the skin wheal over the second sacral foramen and advanced until the posterior surface of the sacrum is contacted. If the sacral foramina are to be found easily, the anesthetist should always keep in mind the anatomical curve and tilt of the sacrum when placing the needles (Figure 315, page 478 and Figure 316, page 478). The depth to which the needle must be inserted at the second sacral foramen to contact bone varies with the build of the patient, e.g., thin patient, ½

inch (1.3 cm.) or less; medium build patient, ½ inch (1.3 cm.) to 1¼ inches (3.2 cm.); and, obese patient, 1¼ inches (3.2 cm.) to 2 inches (5 cm.).

7. If the 3-inch (7.5 cm.) needle does not

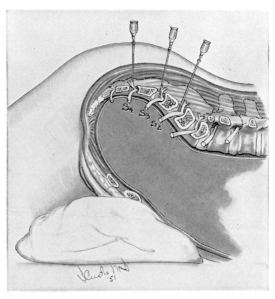

Figure 316. Transsacral needles in the second, third, or fourth sacral foramina. Note the tilt of the needles to conform to the anatomical tilt of the sacrum.

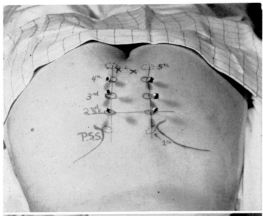

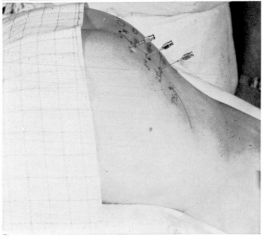

Figure 315. Needles resting in the sacral foramina. A. (Top) Posterior view. B. (Bottom) Lateral view. X's, sacral cornua. S.F., sacral foramen. P.S.S., posterior spine of the iliac bone. 3-inch (7.5 cm.) needles rest in the second sacral foramina. 2½-inch (6.3 cm.) needles rest in the third sacral foramina. 1½-inch (3.8 cm.) needles rest in the fourth sacral foramina.

contact the posterior surface of the sacrum at the estimated depth from the skin when attempting to locate the second sacral foramina, it may have slipped into the foramen or it may not have been inserted deep enough. If by advancing the needle the sacrum is not contacted, then it may have slipped into the foramen and it should be withdrawn and contact with the posterior surface of the sacrum made. It is essential to contact this surface of the sacrum so that the depth which the needle is inserted into the sacral foramen can be measured accurately.

8. Once the posterior surface of the sacrum is contacted, the "hunt and peck" method is used until the foramen is found. Then, the needle is advanced a *measured distance* into the lumen of the foramen. This depth depends on the foramen into which the needle

is being inserted. For the second sacral fora-men, the 3-inch (7.5 cm.) needle is advanced ½ (1.3 cm.) to ¾ inch (2 cm.) deeper than the posterior surface of the sacrum.

9. Now, the 2½-inch (6.3 cm.) needle is placed in the third sacral foramen and the 1½-inch (3.8 cm.) needle is placed in the fourth sacral foramen using the same prin-ciples for placement as described for the plac-ing of the 3-inch (7.5 cm.) needle.

Usually, when attempting to locate the third and fourth sacral foramina, the depth from the skin to the posterior surface of the sacrum is less than the depth at the second sacral fora-men (Figure 316, page 478). Furthermore, the depth to which the needles are placed into these foramina also is less—for the third sacral foramen, the needle is advanced ⅜-inch (1 cm.) to ½-inch (1.3 cm.), and for the fourth sacral foramen, the needle is advanced ¼ inch (0.6 cm.) to ⅜-inch (1 cm.). This depth is regulated by the anatomical taper of the sac-rum—the sacrum is thicker cephalad and thin-ner caudad (Figure 316, page 478).

10. After the needles are correctly placed on one side, needles of similar size are inserted in the second, third, and fourth foramina on the other side. The directions and depths of the needles which are already in place are valuable guides for the correct placement of the second group of needles.

11. When all six needles are located cor-rectly, 3 to 10 cc. of the anesthetic solution is deposited. If paresthesias, which are felt by the patient in the leg, penis, vagina, buttock, or rectum, are encountered at any point when placing a needle, the advancement of the needle is stopped and the injection of the an-esthetic solution is made.

12. As the needles are withdrawn from the foramina and removed from the patient, usu-ally 3 cc. of the anesthetic solution is injected.

EXTENT OF ANALGESIA

Over the distribution of the sacral nerves blocked (Figure 242, page 354).

COMPLICATIONS

Toxic Reactions (intravascular injections, etc.: See Chapter 3, page 19.

Subarachnoid Injection: See page 353.

Local Infections: May occur as after single-dose caudal block. See page 449.

REMARKS

Perform Transsacral Block along with Cau-dal Block: Transsacral block is not an easy procedure to master, but since there is little danger connected with it and since it is of val-ue in certain cases, it should be done along with most caudal blocks whenever time per-mits, so that the anesthetist may learn the technique (Figure 317, page 479). Usually

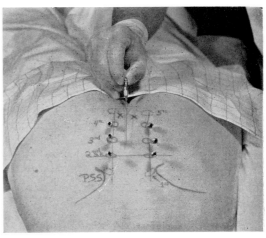

Figure 317. Needles of advocated sizes in place for a combined caudal and transsacral block. X's, sacral cornu. S.F., sacral foramen. P.S.S., posterior superior spine of the iliac bone.

when this block is combined with caudal anal-gesia, attempts are made to block only the second, third, and fourth sacral nerves since these are responsible for sensory innervation of the coccygeal region, sacral region, anus, and rectum.

Sacrum is Deformed in 20 to 25 Percent of Patients: Deformities of the sacrum are quite frequent and it is not unusual to find the sac-ral foramina on one side of the sacrum a greater distance from the median sacral crest than the other side (Figure 315, page 478, and Figure 317, page 479). In spite of the incidence of deformities, transsacral blocks can be administered in 90 to 95 percent of the patients.

Avoid Transsacral Block in Markedly Obese Patients: In such patients, the landmarks are obscure, the incidence of unsatisfactory anesthesia is increased, and complications are more likely.

It is the author's opinion that in such patients other regional block techniques, *e.g.*, spinal or epidural block, are more satisfactory methods of producing block anesthesia.

Block of the First Sacral Nerves and the Fifth Sacral Nerves: If the first sacral nerves or the fifth sacral nerves are to be blocked the technique is comparable (see Procedure, page 477) but the following should be remembered: (1) the depth from the skin to the posterior surface of the sacrum at the first sacral foramina may be slightly deeper than the distance at the second sacral foramina; (2) the distance the needles are inserted after the posterior surface of the sacrum is contacted at the first sacral foramina is approximately the same as the distance they are inserted when blocking the second sacral nerves; (3) the depth from the skin to the posterior portion of the sacrum at the fifth sacral nerves is slightly less than the distance at the fourth sacral foramina; and (4) the distance the needles are inserted after the posterior surface of the sacrum is contacted at the fifth sacral nerves is approximately the same as the distance they are inserted when blocking the fourth sacral nerves.

Recover Broken Needle(s): All needles should be tested before use. If a needle breaks, every effort to remove it, including surgery, should be made. Unremoved needles have a tendency to migrate and may cause permanent injuries as well as medicolegal complications.

Repeat Block when Analgesia is Inadequate: If the desired results from the first block attempt are unsatisfactory, do not hesitate to reblock the patient if time permits. Most patients will think nothing about being reblocked if the second attempt is prefaced by a statement such as: "Well, I guess we will have to inject a little more medicine if we are going to freeze this area."

However, do not exceed the maximum safe dosage of the local anesthetic solution for both blocks. If to reblock the patient the maximum safe dose of the local anesthetic solution must be exceeded, 45 minutes should elapse between blocks.

CHAPTER 51

The Use of Vasoconstrictor Drugs in the Subarachnoid Space to Prolong Spinal Block

INDICATIONS

To PROLONG duration of spinal analgesia. Epinephrine (Adrenalin) and phenylephrine (Neo-Synephrine) definitely prolong the duration of spinal analgesia and can be used in hypobaric, isobaric, and hyperbaric local anesthetic solutions without significantly altering the specific gravity of these solutions. Furthermore, they may be employed with safety and with constant results.

MODE OF ACTION

The exact mode of action of vasoconstrictor drugs on the central nervous system is undetermined. However, most experimental data would indicate that the vasoconstrictor agent constricts the local vascular system of the dura and its contents. The venous system of the dura and its contents is considered to be the direct route of drainage from the subarachnoid space; at least this is so in experimental animals. Therefore, the normal rate of absorption of the anesthetic agent from the spinal fluid may be greatly retarded by the vasoconstriction of the blood vessels.

DRUGS

Small ampules of the vasoconstrictor drugs should be used, i.e., 1 cc. size, rather than large rubber-stoppered bottles. Vasoconstrictor agents other than those listed below have not been given subarachnoidally by us.

Epinephrine (Adrenalin)

Dosage.—0.2 cc. (0.2 mg.) of a 1:1000 solution mixed with the local anesthetic solution to be injected into the subarachnoid space. A 1:1000 epinephrine solution contains 1 mg. of the drug in 1 cc. of solution.

Effect on the Specific Gravity of the Local Anesthetic Solution.—None. The addition of this small amount of solution together with the small fraction of a milligram of epinephrine involved is insignificant. Solutions of epinephrine 1:1000 are hypobaric (lighter than the specific gravity of spinal fluid).

Effect on the Duration of Analgesia.—Duration varies with the patient and height of anesthesia, but 0.2 cc. epinephrine prolongs the duration of analgesia 40 to 50 percent. The prolongation of the duration of analgesia does not seem to be influenced by the amount of epinephrine employed, i.e., it makes no difference whether 0.2 cc. (0.2 mg.) or 0.5 cc. (0.5 mg.) is incorporated in the anesthetic solution.

Phenylephrine (Neo-Synephrine)

Dosage.—0.2 cc. (2 mg.) to 0.5 cc. (5 mg.) of a 1 percent solution. Phenylephrine is packaged in 1 cc. ampules with 10 mg. in a cubic centimeter, i.e., a 1.0 percent solution.

Effect on the Specific Gravity of the Local Anesthetic Solution.—None. A 1 percent (10 mg. per cc.) solution is isobaric, i.e., its specific gravity falls within the normal range of spinal fluid.

Effect on the Duration of Analgesia.—This varies with the patient, the height of analgesia, and the amount of phenylephrine, but the addition of this drug usually prolongs the duration of analgesia from 30 to 100 percent.

The prolongation of the duration of analgesia seems to be influenced by the amount of phenylephrine employed, the larger doses, i.e., 0.4 to 0.5 cc., giving the longer durations. This is particularly true in intra-abdominal and high retroperitoneal surgery where 0.5 cc. (5 mg.) of phenylephrine prolongs the duration of tetracaine (Pontocaine) by 70 to 100 percent (Table XI, page 482).

Ephedrine Sulfate: This vasoconstrictor drug is no longer used by us, but it is included herein so that the reader may understand why.

Dosage.—0.5 cc. to 1.0 cc. of a 5 percent (50 mg. per cc.) solution.

Effect on the Specific Gravity of the Local Anesthetic Solution.—5 percent ephedrine solutions are hyperbaric, *i.e.*, their specific gravity is greater than spinal fluid. The relatively large doses employed contain 25 to 50 mg., which, when added to a hyperbaric anesthetic solution, may make it extremely hyperbaric. Also, when it is added to hypobaric solutions such as light dibucaine (Nupercaine) or light tetracaine, it may change them from a hypobaric to a hyperbaric solution irrespective of the quantity of the local anesthetic solution.

These points are extremely important to the anesthetist because: (1) ephedrine increases the usual rate of gravitation of hyperbaric or isobaric solutions, and (2) ephedrine reverses the direction of gravitation of a hypobaric solution resulting in a high level of analgesia when a low level is expected, or vice versa.

Effect on the Duration of Analgesia.—The effect of ephedrine on the duration of analgesia has been variously reported, but most investigators feel that ephedrine does not significantly increase the duration of analgesia to warrant its use. However, it is significant to note that ephedrine, itself, has analgesic properties when administered subarachnoidally. The early clinical experiments with it did not particularly emphasize that it prolonged analgesia but rather the fact that, when used with smaller amounts of the local anesthetic agent, the same duration of analgesia occurred as with larger amounts of the local anesthetic agent. Perhaps the results in these cases were due to the synergistic effect of the anesthetic properties of ephedrine combined with local anesthetic agents.

REMARKS

Epinephrine and Phenylephrine Prolong Duration of Spinal Block: Many of the questions concerning the subarachnoid use of vasoconstrictor drugs are still unanswered. The clinical results of many investigators on this subject differ. Nevertheless, it can be stated with certainty that epinephrine and phenylephrine do prolong spinal anesthesia to the extent stated.

When a local anesthetic solution is injected into the subarachnoid space, analgesia of the perineum and lower extremities normally lasts longer than intra-abdominal analgesia. For example, see Table XI, page 482.

TABLE XI

APPROXIMATE MINIMUM AND MAXIMUM
DURATION OF TETRACAINE SPINAL
ANALGESIA WITH AND WITHOUT
VASOCONSTRICTOR DRUGS

Drugs	Intra-abdominal Analgesia*	Perineal and Lower Extremity Analgesia*
Tetracaine	1¼ to 1¾ hrs.	2 to 2½ hrs.
Tetracaine with 0.2 cc. (0.2 mg.) epinephrine 1:1000	2 to 2¼ hrs.	3 to 3¾ hrs.
Tetracaine with 0.5 cc. (5 mg.) phenylephrine, 1.0 percent solution	2¼ to 3½ hrs.	5 to 5¾ hrs.

*Figures are based on "operative duration" (see page 484).

Clinical Experience Indicates That Injection of a Vasoconstrictor Drug into the Subarachnoid Space Is Not Contraindicated: Anatomically, the blood supply to the spinal cord comes from three sources: the posterior spinal arteries, the anterior spinal artery, and the spinal rami (Figure 318 A and B, page 483).

The *posterior spinal arteries* arise from the vertebral arteries at the sides of the medulla oblongata. They are reinforced by a succession of small branches which enter the vertebral canal through the intervertebral foramina; by means of these they continue to the lower

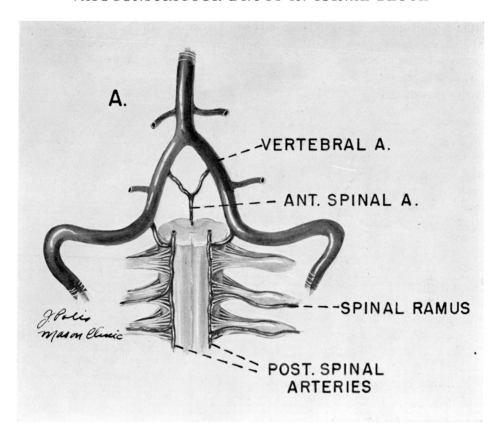

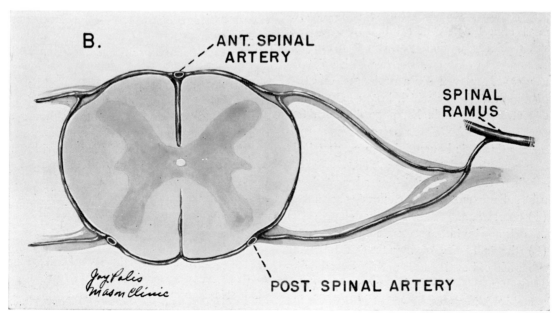

Figure 318. Anatomy of the blood supply of the spinal cord. A. Origin of the anterior and posterior spinal arteries. B. Cross section showing reinforcement of anterior spinal artery and posterior spinal arteries by small branches which enter the vertebral canal through the intervertebral foramina. These branches are derived from the vertebral and ascending cervical branch of the inferior thyroid arteries in the neck; from the intercostal arteries in the thorax; and from the lumbar, iliolumbar, and lateral sacral arteries in the abdomen and pelvis.

part of the medulla spinalis and to the cauda equina (Figure 318 A, page 483).

The *anterior spinal artery* is a small branch, which arises near the termination of the vertebral artery and, descending in front of the medulla oblongata, unites with its fellow of the opposite side at the level of the foramen magnum. The single trunk, thus formed, descends on the front of the medulla spinalis and is reinforced by a succession of small branches which enter the vertebral canal through the intervertebral foramina. The anterior spinal artery extends as far as the lower part of the medulla spinalis and is continued as a slender twig on the filum terminale (Figure 318, page 483).

This blood supply is somewhat meager in comparison with the blood supply of other organs. Furthermore, anomalies do exist. Physicians who object to the use of vasoconstrictor drugs in the subarachnoid space object to the placement of any drug in the subarachnoid space which may compromise this blood supply.

We have used 0.2 cc. (0.2 mg.) of epinephrine 1:1000 in over 7000 spinal blocks and phenylephrine 0.2 cc. (2 mg.) to 0.5 cc. (5 mg.) of a 1.0 percent solution in over 2000 spinal blocks without permanent neurologic sequelae. In only one case in which epinephrine was employed did a prolonged duration of anesthesia occur which lasted longer than expected (see Table XI, page 482). In this one case, anesthesia was present for approximately thirty-six hours and then progressively cleared with no detectable residua.

When the vasoconstrictors advocated are used subarachnoidally, the following are noted: (1) onset of analgesia is slightly delayed; (2) there is no rise in the systemic blood pressure; (3) the incidence of hypotension following subarachnoid analgesia is not decreased or increased; and (4) ischemia of the dura and spinal cord, if caused by vasoconstrictor drugs, does not increase the incidence of neurological complications.

Epinephrine and Phenylephrine May Be Heat Sterilized: See page 38.

Vasoconstrictor Drugs Injected into the Subarachnoid Space Do Not Cause Systemic Toxic Reactions: While the injection of epinephrine or phenylephrine subcutaneously, intramuscularly, intravenously, or into the epidural space may produce a severe hypertension, they do not do so when injected into the subarachnoid space. Probably this is true because the blood supply to the spinal cord is relatively poor and is limited to small blood vessels which are constricted immediately by the vasoconstrictor drug, thereby automatically delaying rapid absorption.

Phenylephrine in the Epidural Space May Cause Severe Hypertension: While 3 mg. to 5 mg. of phenylephrine injected into the subarachnoid space will not elevate the blood pressure (see page 484), such dosages will result in a severe hypertension if they are inadvertently deposited in the epidural space.

Operative Duration and Pain Relief Are Not Synonymous: Usually, the operative duration (time the surgeon may "cut") which a local anesthetic drug permits is less than the duration of pain relief which that drug affords. The addition of a vasoconstrictor drug does not alter this property—it prolongs both operating duration and the duration of pain relief. For example, a tetracaine-phenylephrine spinal block for lower extremity surgery will, from the time anesthesia is established, provide six to eight hours of pain relief but only five to five and three-fourths hours of operating duration. For intra-abdominal surgery, this combination of drugs provides an operative duration of two and one-fourth to three and one-half hours, abdominal pain relief up to five hours, and the patient may not be able to move his legs for six to eight hours (see Table XI, page 482).

Occasionally, with phenylephrine prolonged hypesthesia in the legs and feet, lasting eight to twelve hours, may occur. This prolonged analgesia is more likely to result in the elderly patient and in the patient with an initial high dermatome level of anesthesia. The anesthetist's attention is called to this, since it may cause consternation to anyone using this combination for the first time.

CHAPTER 52

Spinal (Subarachnoid) Block With Absolute Alcohol

THE INJECTION of alcohol into the subarachnoid space is often unsatisfactory and time-consuming, and unless the physician is specifically interested in pain problems, he had best avoid the use of alcohol. Likewise, in most instances the use of alcohol should be limited to larger institutions or specialists whose reputation in this type of work can compensate for poor results. For properties of absolute alcohol, see page 329.

INDICATIONS

Surgical: None.

Diagnostic: None.

Therapeutic: Relief of intractable pain from: (1) postherpetic neuralgia; (2) malignant disease where cordotomy is inadvisable; and (3) metastasis to the spinal column, spinal cord or its nerves.

Relief of muscle spasm of the lower extremities from partial sectioning of the spinal cord. Following traumatic injury to the back, alcohol is injected to effect complete transsection of the cord.

PREMEDICATION

During injection of alcohol into the subarachnoid space, *the patient must maintain the position in which he has been placed.* A change in the optimum position during the injection of the alcohol may result in complications, a poor result, or a combination of the two. The patient must be completely awake and cooperative or else it is best to have him anesthetized. Heavy medication may produce an uncooperative patient and this cannot be tolerated during the execution of a subarachnoid alcohol block. If small amounts of alcohol (0.5 cc. to 0.7 cc.) are to be used, no premedication is needed as the pain passes within a few seconds. On the other hand, if a greater amount of alcohol is to be introduced, the patient should probably be anesthetized, as the pain from the injection is severe and may last longer.

DOSAGE

Ampules are favored in preference to a multiple dose bottle to avoid contamination by spores and dilution by the moisture in the air.

It is best not to exceed 0.5 cc. to 0.7 cc. of alcohol in the ambulatory patient who has a pain problem limited to 1 or 2 dermatomes.

Large quantities, *i.e.,* 1 cc. to 10 cc., of alcohol may be employed subarachnoidally in the following cases: (1) cases that are permanently bedridden; (2) cases in whom there is little concern for rectal and bladder function; and (3) patients in whom the primary concern is the relief of pain regardless of the associated motor dysfunction of the legs, bladder, or rectum. Alcohol in large quantities, *i.e.,* 5 to 10 cc., injected subarachnoidally affects a transsection of the spinal cord.

MATERIALS

Same as for spinal block. See page 343.

TECHNIQUE

Landmarks: The nerve(s) to be blocked is determined and the correct interspace is located by counting cephalad from either the third lumbar interspace or the spinous process of the fourth lumbar vertebra as described under Single-Dose Spinal (Subarachnoid) Anesthesia, page 344.

The rootlets of a spinal nerve do not have their origin at the level of the corresponding vertebra. Therefore, the point of the needle should be placed in the subarachnoid space where the nerve rootlets which form the spinal nerve leave the cord—not at the level of the vertebra through whose foramina the spinal nerve exits. For example, to block the eighth spinal thoracic nerve the needle must be inserted through the sixth thoracic interspace (Figure 319, page 487).

Position: When positioning the patient, it must be remembered that the specific gravity of alcohol is less than that of spinal fluid. Therefore, it is hypobaric when compared with spinal fluid and gravitates upward when injected into it.

Semiprone, Lateral Decubitus (Side) Position.—This is the position of choice for unilateral block of one or two thoracic, lumbar, or sacral somatic nerves when 0.5 cc. to 0.7 cc. is to be injected (Figure 320, page 488).

However, often the patient is placed in the lateral decubitus (side) position for the spinal tap (Figure 321, page 488). When it has been done, the patient is turned slowly into a semiprone position so that his body forms a 45-degree angle with the table (Figure 320, page 488). He is supported in this position by pillows and sandbags. This position is assumed so that a maximum concentration of alcohol will bathe the sensory root of the spinal nerve which emerges from the posterior lateral surface of the spinal cord (Figure 322, page 489).

A sandbag or the raised kidney bar should be placed under the patient at the point to be blocked so that this point is the highest in relation to the rest of the vertebral column (Figure 321, page 488). When the alcohol injection is made in the middle thoracic, the lower thoracic, or the lumbar region the table should be in a 10-degree *Fowler's* position so that the alcohol will rise toward the thoracic rather than the sacral region. This will aid in avoiding motor involvement of the lower ex-

tremities, bladder, and rectum. When alcohol is placed in the upper thoracic region the table should be in a 10-degree *Trendelenburg* position to prevent rise of alcohol into the cervical region. This will aid in avoiding motor involvement of the upper extremities. *In subarachnoid alcohol injections the principal aim is to destroy the sensory component of the spinal nerve without involving the motor component.*

Prone Position.—This position is usually employed when large amounts of alcohol (5 to 10 cc.) are to be injected to transsect the spinal cord. The tap of the subarachnoid space is usually performed with the patient in the prone position and the table level. Then, the kidney bar is raised or a sandbag is placed under the iliac bones and the head of the table lowered about 10 degrees. If the spinal tap cannot be done in the prone position, the tap of the subarachnoid space is done with the patient in the lateral decubitus (side) position. Then he is slowly turned to the prone position, the kidney bar raised, and the table placed in 10-degree Trendelenburg position (Figure 323, page 489).

Precautions

Do Not Exceed the Maximum Advised Dose. —The maximum advised dose of alcohol should not be exceeded in the ambulatory patient who has a pain problem of 1 or 2 dermatomes. Because of the caudad slope of the spinal nerves within the subarachnoid space, a small amount (0.5 cc. to 0.7 cc.) of alcohol injected through a correctly placed needle may bathe more than one spinal nerve. This is particularly true of the lower thoracic, lumbar, and sacral somatic spinal nerves (Figure 319, page 487).

Alcohol is Hypobaric.—Remember alcohol is hypobaric and gravitates upward.

Note Position of Bevel of Spinal Needle.— The relationship of the markings on the hub of the needle to the bevel of the needle should be noted.

Procedure: The subarachnoid space is

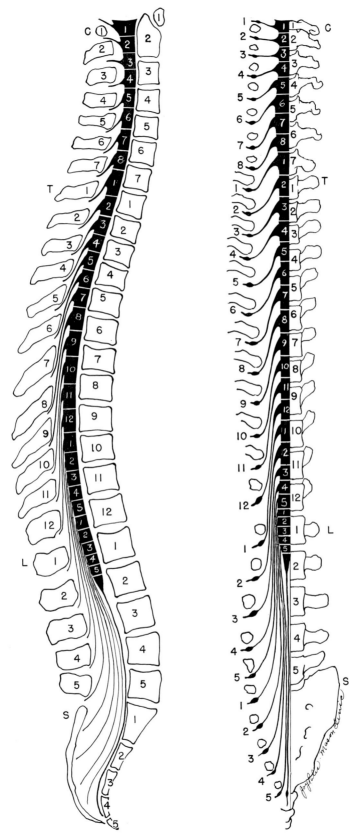

Figure 319. Schematic drawing of relationship of the interspinous spaces and the intervertebral foramina to the spinal nerves and their origin.

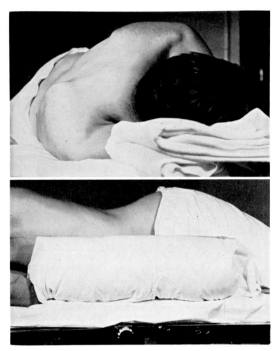

Figure 320. Position of the patient for the subarachnoid alcohol injection. A. *(Top)* Posterior view shows the 45-degree angle of the patient's body in relationship to the table. B. *(Bottom)* Anterior view shows pillow rolled to support the patient at a 45-degree angle.

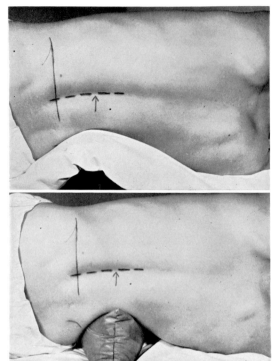

Figure 321. Position for spinal tap. A. *(Top)* Shows use of the kidney bar to elevate the vertebral column. B. *(Bottom)* Shows the use of a sandbag to accomplish the same position as A.

tapped as described in Chapter 43, page 347, at the optimal interspace. The procedure from here on depends on whether 1 or 2 dermatomes are to be blocked or the spinal cord transsected.

Block of 1 or 2 Dermatomes

1. With the patient in the semiprone lateral decubitus position, the bevel of the spinal needle is turned toward the "up" side, *i.e.*, the side to be rendered analgesic.

2. 3 cc. to 5 cc. of spinal fluid is withdrawn and discarded or saved for analysis. This is done to decrease the level of spinal fluid around the nerve or nerves in question so that the alcohol will float to the top of the spinal fluid, as oil does on water, and exert its maximum effect on the nerve tissue.

3. If the patient is awake, he should be instructed to hold very still, and told that if he feels pain, it will disappear rapidly.

4. The calculated amount of absolute alcohol, usually 0.5 cc. to 0.7 cc., is now injected at the rate of 0.1 cc. every thirty seconds.

5. The patient may complain of a warm sensation or pain over the dermatome or dermatomes supplied by the nerve or nerves injected. He should be urged to remain quiet until the injection is completed.

6. The patient is allowed to remain in the semiprone position for 30 to 45 minutes (Figure 320, page 488 and Figure 322, page 489).

Transsection of the Spinal Cord

1. With the patient in the prone position, the bevel of the needle is pointed caudad.

2. The patient is usually lightly anesthetized (lid reflex almost or just absent) with 0.6 percent thiopental (Pentothal) or 0.2 percent methohexital (Brevital).

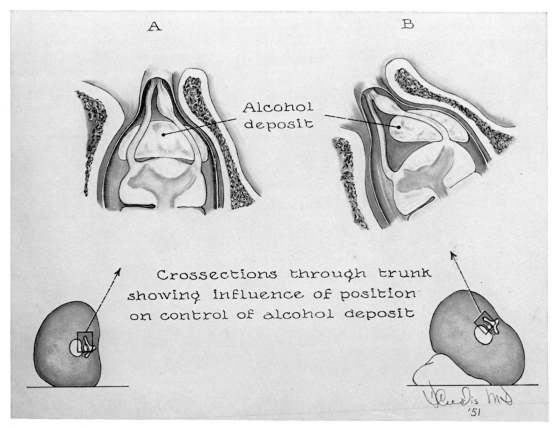

Figure 322. Schematic drawing showing the advantage of placing the patient at a 45-degree angle before the injection of absolute alcohol. A. When the patient's back is perpendicular to the table, the alcohol contacts both the sensory and motor roots of the spinal nerve. B. When the patient's back is at a 45-degree angle to the table, the alcohol contacts only the sensory root of the spinal nerve.

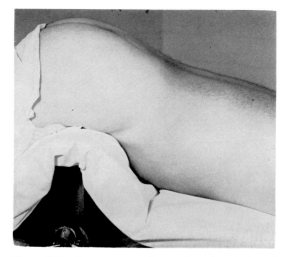

Figure 323. Prone position for a subarachnoid alcohol injection to transsect the spinal cord.

3. 5 cc. of spinal fluid is aspirated into a syringe.

4. The spinal fluid is discarded or saved for analysis.

5. The syringe containing 5 cc. to 10 cc. of alcohol is connected to the spinal needle and injected at the rate of 1.0 cc. per 15 seconds into the subarachnoid space.

6. The patient is allowed to regain consciousness but remains in the prone position for 30 to 45 minutes (Figure 323, page 489).

EXTENT OF ANALGESIA

Analgesia of the dermatome innervated by the nerve injected and usually of the dermatomes on each side of it when 0.5 cc. to 0.7 cc. doses are used. When 1.0 cc. to 1.5 cc. doses are employed, the extent of the area anesthetized is not predictable but both sensory and motor involvement usually result. And, with 5 cc. to 10 cc. doses the spinal cord is transsected.

REMARKS

Allow at Least 24 Hours between Blocks: More than one subarachnoid injection of alcohol should not be attempted on the same day. If the desired results are not obtained at the first injection, the injection should be repeated on a subsequent day. Often it is best to allow six to ten days between injections if circumstances permit since it often takes this long to reach the optimal benefit from an alcohol injection.

Spinal Block Preferable to Peripheral Nerve Block of Thoracic, Lumbar, or Sacral Somatic Nerves: When sensory nerves other than the cranial nerves, the autonomic nerves, and the cervical nerves are to be rendered analgesic with alcohol, the subarachnoid route is the one of choice since peripheral alcohol neuritis, which may be as severe as the original complaint, is avoided.

Block of Thoracic Nerves may be Difficult: In the thoracic region the spinal tap may be technically difficult because of the 45-degree slope of the transverse processes. Also, one should avoid traumatizing or injecting alcohol into the spinal cord *per se.* Alcohol destroys nervous tissue by its dehydrating and sclerosing action and, since the action takes place subarachnoidally, the nervous tissue usually will not regenerate once it has been destroyed.

Surgery may be Preferable to Alcohol Block: Subarachnoid alcohol injections are not always satisfactory and the duration of analgesia may vary. Careful selection of cases for this procedure is essential. Central pain will not be corrected and the drug addict will still complain of pain in hopes of receiving more narcotics. *Where cordotomy, lobotomy, or root section may be performed, this is the procedure of choice, especially in the ambulatory patient whose life expectancy is good.* Even in the specialist's hands motor paralysis from subarachnoid alcohol injections may be a sequelae even if 0.7 cc. of absolute alcohol is not exceeded at any one injection. In most instances when small amounts are used the motor paralysis, usually of the legs, is transient and will clear in 3 to 10 days. Motor paralysis of the bladder or rectum may persist indefinitely. Therefore, the patient and his relatives should understand the risk involved. Depending on the circumstances, witnessed and written permission for the procedure should be obtained if medicolegal suits are to be avoided. Subarachnoid alcohol administrations are in general best employed in terminal cancer cases where motor paralysis is not a major problem.

Postherpetic pain does not respond well to peripheral nerve injections with local anesthetic agents, and alcohol will often cause a neuritis if injected on the peripheral nerves other than the cranial nerves. Therefore, if alcohol is to be employed, it should be given subarachnoidally. In these cases sensory root section is probably the most satisfactory treatment.

Anesthetize Patient When 5 cc. to 10 cc. Doses of Alcohol Are To Be Injected: If transsection of the spinal cord with large quantities of absolute alcohol, i.e., 5 cc. to 10 cc., is to be undertaken, the patient must be well sedated or anesthetized with light inhalation or intravenous anesthesia. Otherwise, the associated pain may cause great discomfort, and a change in the optimal position of the patient as the alcohol is injected may result.

Recover Broken Needle(s): All needles should be tested before use. If a needle breaks, every effort to remove it, including surgery, should be made. Unremoved needles have a tendency to migrate and may cause permanent injuries as well as medicolegal complications.

When a spinal needle breaks, there is little doubt in the anesthetist's mind of what has happened. A distinct click is felt. This usually happens when the needle is being inserted and the stylet is still in the needle. If the anesthetist suspects that the needle has broken, he should not remove the stylet. If the needle breaks after the stylet is removed, the portion containing the hub of the needle should not be removed. They are valuable guides to locating the broken end of the needle. When the anesthetist suspects that the needle has been broken, he should release his hold on it and have an x-ray taken immediately.

Index

493